Applied Laparoscopic Anatomy: Abdomen and Pelvis

This book was written by Dr. Gary Wind in consultation with Drs. Moshe Dudai, Judd Moul (consulting editor, urology) and John Byron (consulting editor, gynecology) in their private capacities. The preceding are solely responsible for its content. No official support or endorsement by the Uniformed Services University of the Health Sciences or the Department of Defense is intended or should be inferred. The opinions or assertions contained herein are the private views of the authors and should not be construed as official or as necessarily reflecting the views of the Uniformed Services University of the Health Sciences or the Department of Defense.

Applied Laparoscopic Anatomy: Abdomen and Pelvis

GARY G. WIND, MD, FACS

Professor of Surgery
Departments of Surgery and Anatomy
Uniformed Services University of the Health Sciences
Staff Surgeon, National Naval Medical Center
Bethesda, Maryland

Consulting Editor
Moshe Dudai, MD, FACS

Assistant Professor of Surgery
Uniformed Services University of the Health Sciences
Command Consultant in Surgery, National Naval Medical Center
Bethesda, Maryland

SANS TACHE

Williams & Wilkins
A WAVERLY COMPANY

BALTIMORE • PHILADELPHIA • LONDON • PARIS • BANGKOK
BUENOS AIRES • HONG KONG • MUNICH • SYDNEY • TOKYO • WROCLAW

Editor: Carroll Cann
Managing Editor: Susan Hunsberger
Production Coordinator: Cindy Park
Book Project Editor: Robert D. Magee
Designer: Ellen B. Zanolle
Illustration Planner: Cindy Park and Donna M. Smith
Cover Designer: Ellen B. Zanolle
Compositor: Donna M. Smith
Printer: Edwards Brothers
Digitized Illustrations: All Systems Color
Binder: Edwards Brothers

Williams & Wilkins
351 West Camden Street
Baltimore, Maryland 21201-2436 USA

Rose Tree Corporate Center
1400 North Providence Road
Building II, Suite 5025
Media, Pennsylvania 19063-2043 USA

Accurate indications, adverse reactions and dosage schedules for drugs are provided in this book, but it is possible that they may change. The reader is urged to review the package information data of the manufacturers of the medications mentioned.

Printed in the United States of America

Wind, Gary G.
Applied laparoscopic anatomy: abdomen and pelvis/Gary Wind; consulting editor, Moshe Dudai.
p. cm.
Includes bibliographical references and index.
ISBN 0-683-09136-0
1. Abdomen—Anatomy. 2. Pelvis—Anatomy. 3. Anatomy, Surgical and topographical. I. Dudai, Moshe. II. Title.
[DNLM: 1. Abdomen—surgery. 2. Abdomen—anatomy & histology. 3. Pelvis—surgery. 4. Pelvis—anatomy & histology. 5. Surgery, Laparoscopic. WI 900 W763a 1997]
QM543.W55 1997
617.5'5—dc20
DNLM/DLC 96-8433
for Library of Congress CIP

The publishers have made every effort to trace the copyright holders for borrowed material. If they have inadvertently overlooked any, they will be pleased to make the necessary arrangements at the first opportunity.

To purchase additional copies of this book, call our customer service department at **(800) 638-0672** or fax orders to **(800) 447-8438**. For other book services, including chapter reprints and large quantity sales, ask for the Special Sales department.

Canadian customers should call **(800) 268-4178**, or fax **(905) 470-6780**. For all other calls originating outside of the United States, please call **(410) 528-4223** or fax us at **(410) 528-8550**.

Visit Williams & Wilkins on the Internet: **http://www.wwilkins.com** or contact our customer service department at **custserv@wwilkins.com**. Williams & Wilkins customer service representatives are available from 8:30 am to 6:00 pm, EST, Monday through Friday, for telephone access.

96 97 98 99
1 2 3 4 5 6 7 8 9 10

Preface

This is a book about abdominal and pelvic anatomy presented from the perspective of the laparoscopic surgeon. In the short time since the domain of operative laparoscopy began to dramatically expand, many excellent books have appeared which document laparoscopic technology, instrumentation, surgical indications and strategy, and operative procedures. What is lacking to date is a reformulation of the way surgeons view anatomy to coincide with the demands of the laparoscopic approach. The material in this book departs from conventional anatomic images and is formulated from scratch for the laparoscopic viewpoint. The anatomy is conceptualized in three dimensions from the start.

This book focuses on areas of current laparoscopic interest as starting points and puts them in the context of the surrounding regional anatomy. The biliary system leads to an exploration of the right upper quadrant, the spleen is the focal point of the left upper quadrant and the stomach is the lead point for the mid upper abdomen. The colon opens up the mid and lower abdomen and exploration of the pelvis centers around the gynecological organs. The urological system is the focus for retroperitoneal anatomy and inguinal anatomy centers around hernia pathology. There is considerable overlap between sections and the same anatomy is presented from different perspectives to try and tie everything together in a unified package.

After presenting embryology, anatomy and variation, each chapter focuses on one or more surgical procedures selected to illustrate the widest range of the anatomy in question. The biliary, inguinal and gastric procedures are widely practiced at the present time and are given proportionate emphasis. Surgery of the spleen, colon, gynecologic and urologic organs is not yet at the same level of acceptance. The focus of the operative examples is on the performance of safe, effective surgery through knowledge of anatomy and variations. Anatomic pitfalls and complications from the insertion of the trochars to exiting the abdomen are emphasized. The surgical playing field is wider in laparoscopy than the tunnel vision of a narrow open surgical wound filled with hands and retractors, and the magnification and clarity of the view are great advantages. The importance of understanding the anatomy as a whole is equally magnified.

The special demands of laparoscopic surgery are addressed in a section outlining the principles of laparoscopic operations. The major role of position is seen in port placement, the disposition of the operating team and the patient and the orientation of the camera. Safe and coordinated use of laparoscopic instruments plays a major role in the successful completion of a case.

Instrumentation is constantly changing and improving. The technology of video equipment, insufflation and cautery devices, and specific surgical ports and instruments is not the domain of this book. I have avoided proprietary names and depict such devices in terms of the principles of operation, e.g., monopolar, bipolar, argon beam, spray modes of cautery. In keeping with the emphasis of the book, conventional cutting modalities are depicted instead of the more complex and potentially dangerous laser technology. New devices such as the ultrasonic scalpel, three-dimensional video, miniaturization and telesurgery will make surgery more efficient and expand our capabilities but will not change the need for a thorough understanding of the anatomy.

The abundance of anatomic references and the plethora of early surgical reports make it difficult to cite specific sources for individual bits of information in either category. I have cited specific sources in the text only for large collected series where incidence percentages are quoted or a particular piece of information is unique. A list of the general anatomic resources I have most relied on is provided at the start of the book and specific anatomic sources are listed at the end of each chapter.

I have chosen laparoscopic surgical approaches that are based on established surgical principles and appear durable at the present time, and have avoided individual idiosyncratic approaches. The references for those procedures I have chosen to list by category for additional reading at the end of each chapter

Proper anatomic names are used throughout the book and common eponyms are provided in parentheses where appropriate to reconcile common usage with the anatomic vocabulary. Both the anatomy and the surgical procedures are described in plain language in the belief that technical jargon does not make a work more scientific, accurate or useful but only slows the reader down.

Gary Wind, MD, FACS

Acknowledgments

The author gratefully acknowledges the help of Dr. John Byron in reviewing the chapter on pelvic anatomy and gynecologic procedures and of Dr. Judd Moul in reviewing the chapter on the urologic system.

John Byron, MD, FACOG, FACS
Assistant Professor of Obstetrics and Gynecology
Course Director, Advanced Gynecologic Laparoscopy
Uniformed Services University of the Health Sciences
Chief of Gynecology
Walter Reed Army Medical Center
Washington, DC

Judd Moul, MD, FACS
Associate Professor of Surgery
Director, Center for Prostate Disease Research
Uniformed Services University of the Health Sciences
Staff Urologist
Walter Reed Army Medical Center
Washington, DC

Acknowledgments

[illegible]

Contents

3

The Inguinal Region

4

The Stomach

5

The Spleen

6

The Colon

7

The Pelvis

8

The Urologic System

Index

Selected Anatomic References

EMBRYOLOGY

England MA. Color Atlas of Life Before Birth, Normal Fetal Development. Chicago: Year Book Medical Publishers, 1983.
O'Rahilly, Muller F. Human Embryology & Teratology, New York: Wiley-Liss, 1992.
Skandalakis JE, Gray SW. Embryology for Surgeons, ed 2, Baltimore: Williams & Wilkins, 1994.

ANATOMY TEXTS

Gray H, Clemente C, (Ed). Anatomy of the Human Body, 30th American ed. Philadelphia: Lea & Febiger, 1985.
Hollinshead WH. Textbook of Anatomy, ed 4. Philadelphia: Harper & Rowe, 1985.
Lockhart RD, Hamilton GF, Fyfe FW. Anatomy of the Human Body, Philadelphia: Lippincott, 1969.
Woodburne RT. Essentials of Human Anatomy, ed 8, New York: Oxford University Press, 1988.

ANATOMY ATLASES

Clemente CD. Anatomy, a Regional Atlas of the Human Body, ed 3, Baltimore: Urban & Schwarzenberg, 1987.
Grant JCB. Grant's Atlas of Anatomy, ed 9, Baltimore: Williams & Wilkins, 1991.
Hinman Jr. F. Atlas of Urosurgical Anatomy, Philadelphia: WB Saunders Co, 1993.
McMinn RMH. A Color Atlas of Human Anatomy, ed 2, Chicago: Yearbook Medical Publishers, 1988.
Pernkopf E. Atlas of Topographic and Applied Human Anatomy, Eng ed 3, Baltimore: Urban & Schwarzenberg, 1990.
Taylor AN, ed. Sobotta Atlas of Human Anatomy, Eng ed 11, Baltimore: Urban & Schwarzenberg, 1991.

CROSS-SECTIONAL ATLASES

Bergman RA, et al. Atlas of human Anatomy in Cross Section, Baltimore: Urban & Schwarzenberg, 1991.
Cahill D. Atlas of Human Cross-sectional Anatomy, Philadelphia: Lea & Febiger, 1984.
Eycleshymer AC. A cross-section Anatomy, New York: D Appleton, 1911.
Koritke J, Sick H. Atlas of Sectional Human Anatomy, ed 2, Baltimore: Urban & Schwarzenberg, 1988.

VARIATION

Bergman RA, et al. Compendium of Human Anatomic Variation, Baltimore: Urban & Schwarzenberg, 1988.

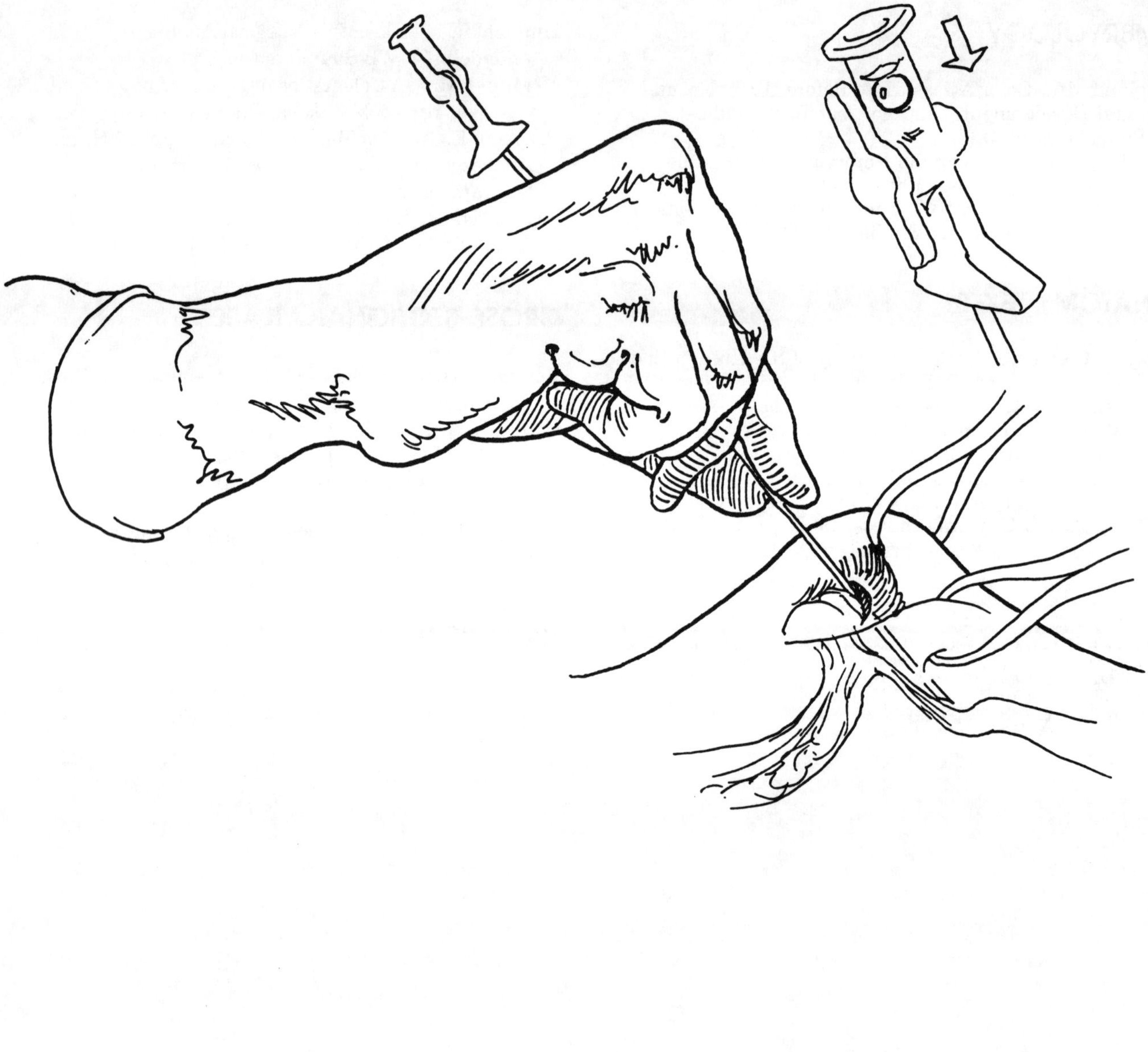

1

Special Operative Considerations

GENERAL ORGANIZATION

Patient Preparation

Laparoscopic surgery requires the same standard rigorous preoperative patient preparation as open intracavitary surgery. Twenty-four-hour prophylactic antibiotic coverage with a first-generation cephalosporin starting with a preoperative dose is routine. In addition, special needs associated with laparoscopy dictate additional measures.

There is increased risk of deep venous thrombosis due to increased levels of CO_2 in the blood and from stasis resulting from positioning (e.g, reverse Trendelenburg) and increased intraabdominal pressure. Intermittent pneumatic compression starting in the preoperative period and continuing through surgery and the first 2 postoperative days helps prevent the occurrence of deep venous thrombosis.

Precautions must also be taken against the increased risk of aspiration. Both the increased intraabdominal pressure and the head down position of the reverse Trendelenburg position predispose to aspiration. Administration of an H_2 blocker to decrease the acid content of the gastric secretions and metoclopromide to promote gastric emptying and increase resting lower esophageal sphincter tone can reduce the risk.

Gastric and intestinal distention increase the risk of perforation both at trochar insertion and during surgical manipulation and cautery. Distention also obscures the field and makes surgery more difficult and dangerous. Gastric tube decompression is mandatory, and mechanical bowel preparation is beneficial. Bladder catheterization is done for lower abdominal procedures and when there is a possibility that the procedure will take a long time.

Operating Room Organization

The configuration of the operating room and the laparoscopic equipment are vital to the success of the operative intervention. The operating room must be large to accommodate the array of technical equipment necessary for laparoscopic surgery. The operating table must have proper cushioning and support to secure the patient without causing injury during position changes. In addition to height adjustment, the table must also be able to tilt head to foot and side to side and to break into a semi-sitting position. The key technology that led to the explosion in laparoscopic surgery, the video equipment, must be optimized. In addition to high-quality camera and monitors, quality 30- and 45-degree operating scopes must be available; there must be two large monitors and a strong cold light source. A second light source is highly desirable for transilluminating bowel mesentery.

The cautery unit should have safeguards against current leakage and should have a spray mode for superficial hemostasis and a finely adjustable bipolar mode. All equipment must be mobile to immediately assume new configurations as circumstances dictate during the procedure.

High volume insufflation and suction/irrigation devices are necessary to maintain visualization. The rate of gas flow is especially critical for procedures using multiple trochars, in which multiple sutures must be passed, cannulas are removed and reinserted, or a supplementary incision must be made. A second insufflator is beneficial in those circumstances.

Positioning

Adherence to certain principles for the positions of the operating personnel and equipment relative to the patient is critical for operating comfortably and safely. The surgeon stands on the side opposite the pathology (except in the case of upper midline operations in which the surgeon stands between the patient's legs). The viewpoint of the camera should be from between the surgeon's hands, and the angle of the camera relative to the surgeon's axis of work must be no wider than 30 degrees (Fig. 1.1). The surgeon's monitor screen similarly should be within 30 degrees of the surgeon's axis of work. Eyes, hands, camera, and monitor should ideally be along a single axis to prevent directional disorientation.

After telemonitoring equipment is attached, the patient's arms should be tucked in at the patient's sides to avoid limiting the surgeon's mobility (e.g., the surgeon stands at the level of the patient's shoulder for repair of a groin hernia and must have access to both sides for bilateral hernias).

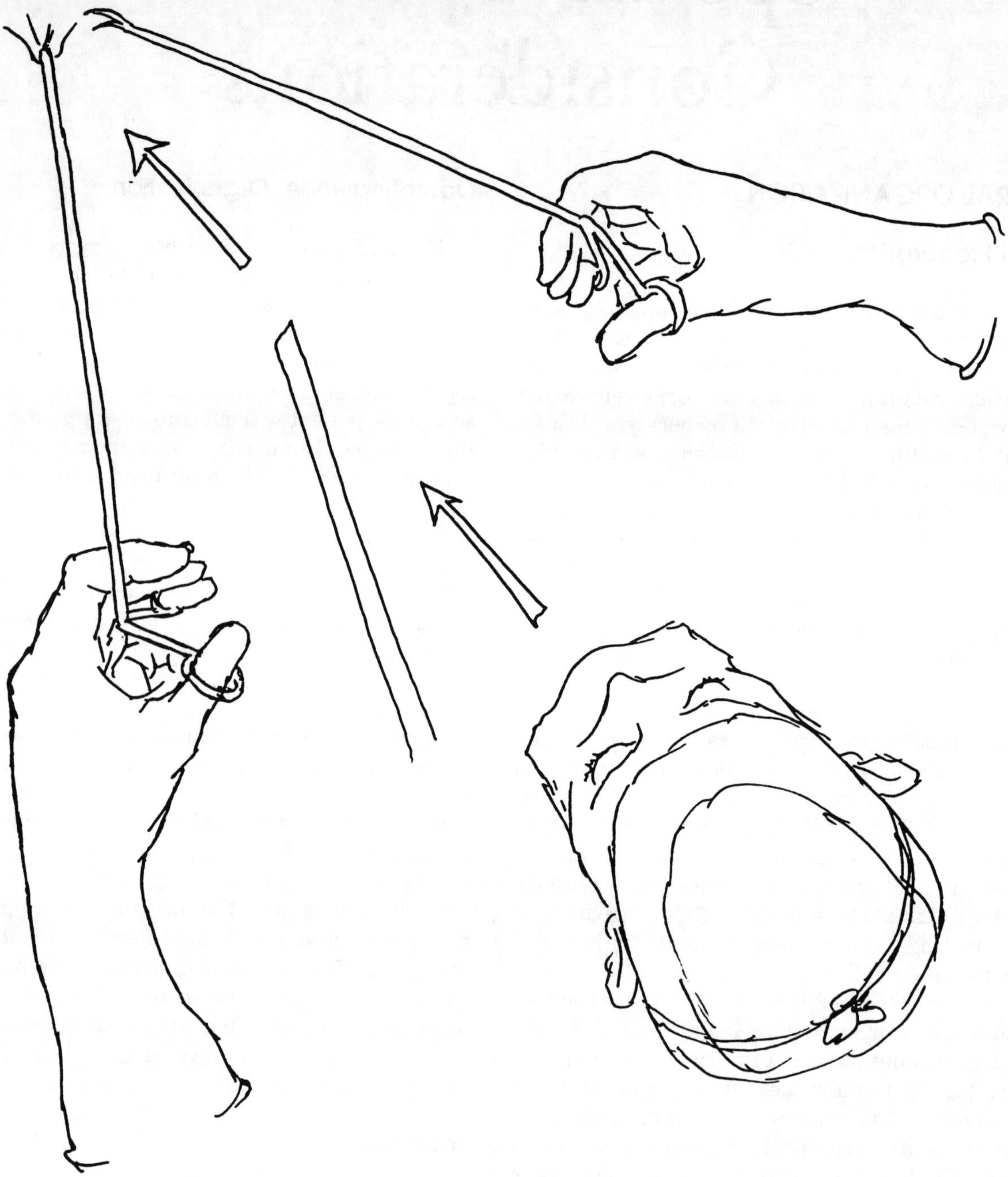

Fig. 1.1

ENTERING THE ABDOMEN

Veress Needle Placement

The position of choice for initial insufflation is the umbilicus both because of its central location and because it is the site that has the least amount of subcutaneous tissue on the abdominal wall (Fig. 1.2). In addition, the midline just below the umbilicus is a fused single fascial sheet with adherent peritoneum and no preperitoneal fat. With the patient in Trendelenburg, the abdominal wall at the umbilicus is elevated with penetrating towel clips or with the surgeon's hand. Placing the clips on either side of the umbilicus exposes the umbilical recess. Orienting the clips one below the other in the midline below the umbilicus lifts the abdominal wall 45 degrees above vertical and gives a better angle of penetration for the Veress needle (as well as two visible vampire bites). The elevation lifts the abdominal wall away from the underlying great vessels (the mobile viscera simply shift due to the peritoneal vacuum) and allows immediate entry of air into the potential peritoneal space as soon as penetration is achieved.

Through a small vertical or horizontal incision in the lower half of the umbilicus, the skin is separated from the underlying fascia with a hemostat or with the back of the knife handle. The hub of the Veress needle is filled with saline, and the valve is closed. The Veress needle is held with the thumb and forefinger along the shaft to control the depth of penetration. Alternatively, the needle can be held between the flats of the fingers and the thumb, with the heel of the hand resting on the abdomen as a

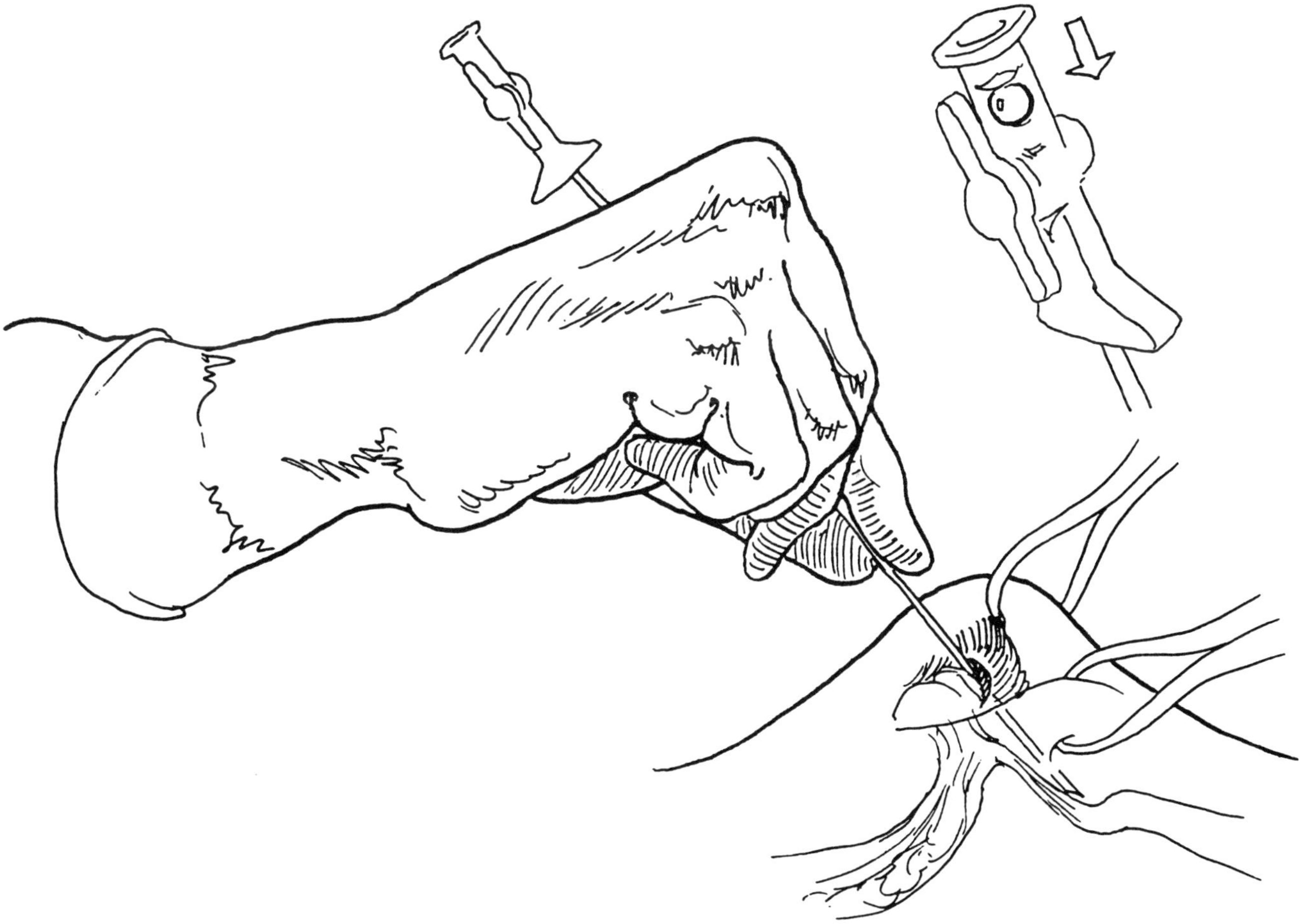

Fig. 1.2

brake (Fig. 1.3). The tip of the needle is engaged in the fascia, which requires a somewhat vertical initial orientation because of the slope of the elevated sub-umbilical fascia, especially in an obese individual. Once the needle is engaged, the valve is opened to indicate penetration when the saline drops. The needle is then directed toward the pelvis and away from the aortic bifurcation to avoid visceral injury.

The needle is advanced with firm steady pressure until two characteristic pops are felt, indicating penetration of the deep fascia and peritoneum in turn. The saline should drop cleanly when the peritoneum is entered. The needle should not be moved in a circular manner because of the damage it can cause, particularly in the presence of adhesions. A saline-filled syringe is attached, and initial aspiration should return no blood, bile, or stool. The full syringe should then be injected. There should be no resistance and little or no return on aspiration if the fluid has diffused into the free peritoneal cavity as it should.

The insufflator is set to a maximum pressure of 15 mm Hg, the line is attached, and the carbon dioxide is turned on. The maximum flow possible through the small bore Veress needle is 2 L/min. Initial pressure should be low, around 5 mm of Hg. High initial pressure indicates that the needle tip is in the wrong place or is obstructed. The needle should be removed and reinserted. All quadrants of the abdomen are percussed for tympany during insufflation to check that the gas is distributing evenly.

Passage of gas by the patient above (through the nasogastric tube) or below indicates penetration of the GI tract and insufflation should be immediately stopped. Penetration of the urinary system will be manifested by air in the urine collection bag. Major vascular injury is usually manifested by a sudden decrease in blood pressure. Bleeding may not be initially evident, especially if the injury is retroperitoneal. If there is a sudden decrease in pressure, assume that the cause is bleeding. Carbon dioxide embolus is rare but life-threatening. Cardiovascular collapse due to embolus is accompanied by the characteristic precordial mill-wheel murmur. The patient is placed in a head-down left lateral decubitus position. Other causes of hypotension during insufflation are vaso-vagal response to rapid insufflation (as is possible with the Hasson technique) and high abdominal pressure (>15 mm Hg), reducing venous return. Later in the procedure, vasodilatation due to CO_2 accumulation can reduce venous return and cardiac output. Hypoxia in the course of a long procedure can reduce cardiac output in patients with cardiac disease.

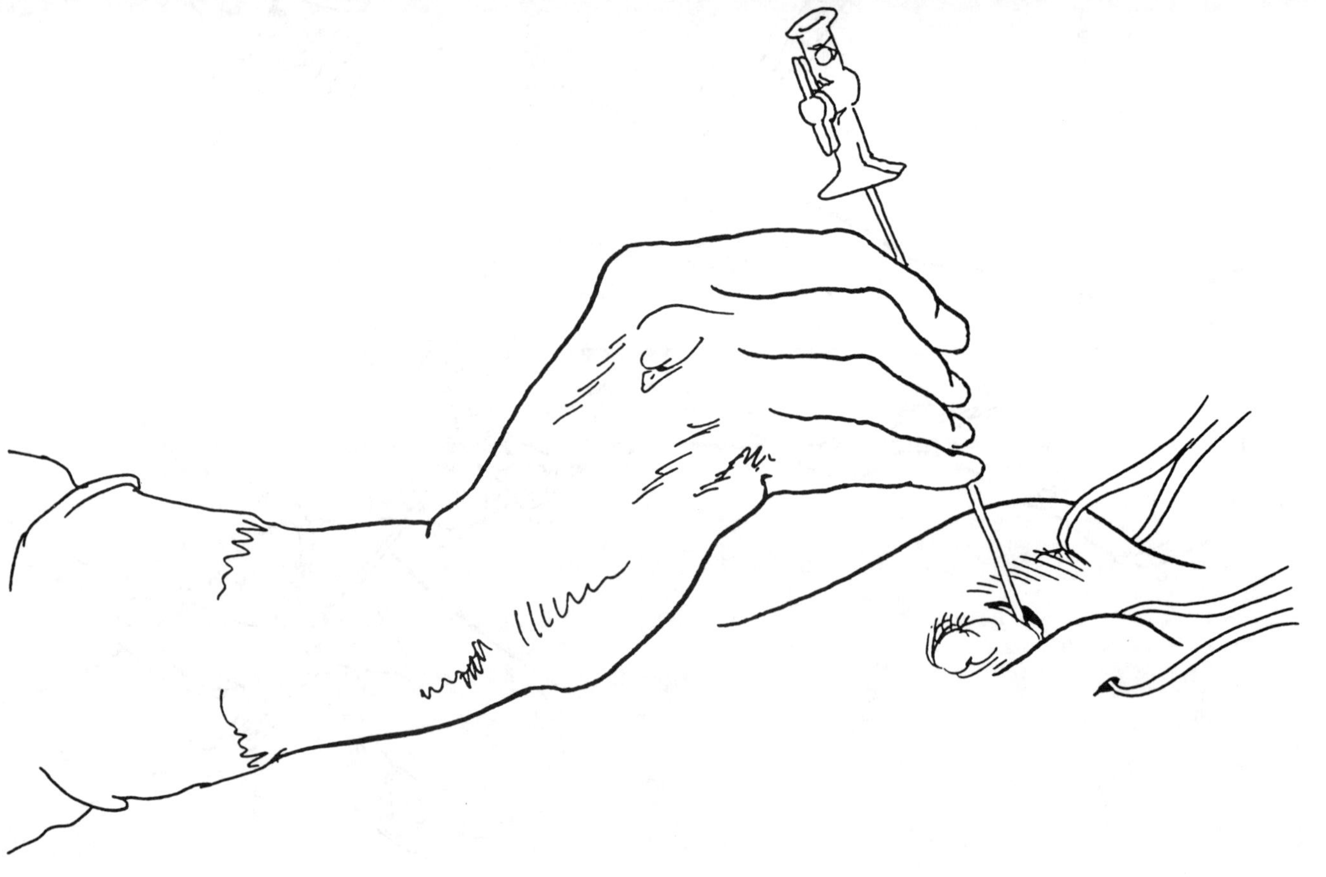

Fig. 1.3

If insufflation is successful, the pressure should approach 15 after about 6 L of gas have been delivered. In patients with increased intraabdominal volume such as pregnancy, ascites or intestinal obstruction, the volume will be less. The Veress needle is removed, and a trochar is introduced through the umbilical incision (Fig. 1.4). The incision should have been made large enough to allow passage of the shaft of the trochar without undue resistance. Forcing the trochar against a tight skin opening can end in disastrous results when the skin gives. The depth of penetration is again controlled by a finger along the shaft or by the other hand holding the shaft. There should be a feeling of clean penetration and a rush of gas on removing the stylette. The gas is reattached, and the pressure should again be 15 mm or below. A

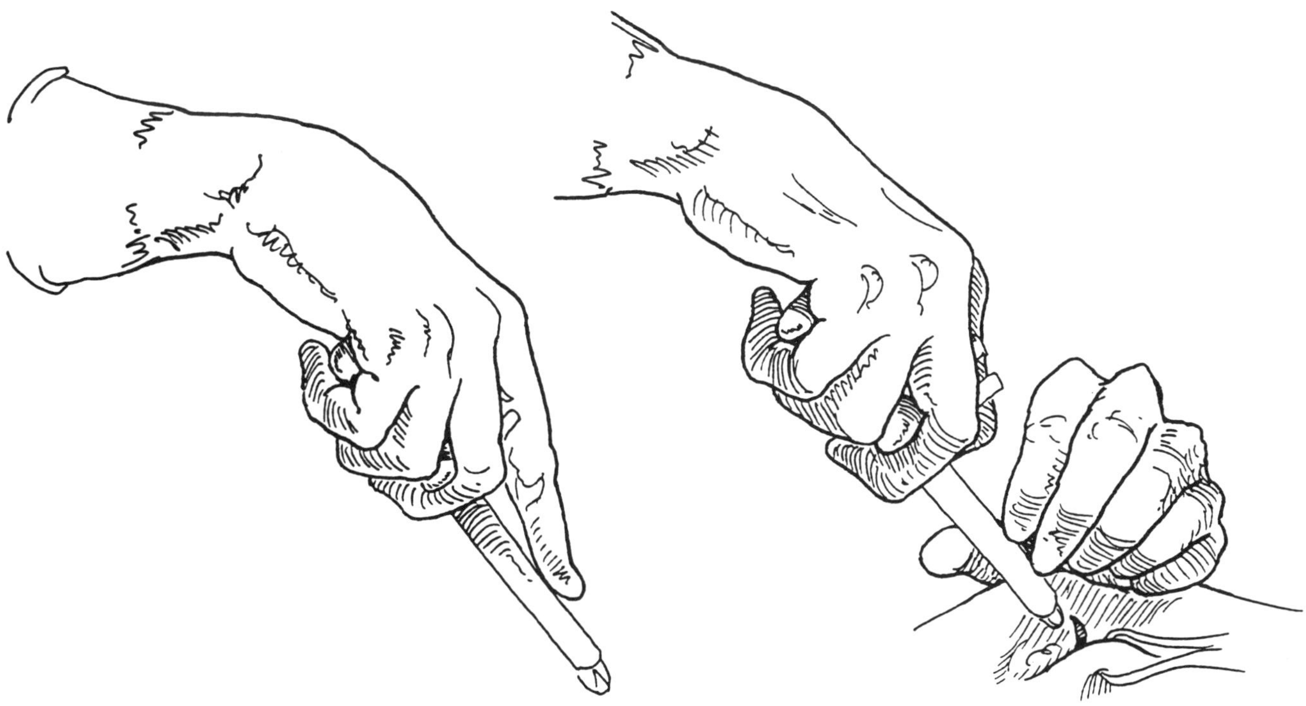

Fig. 1.4

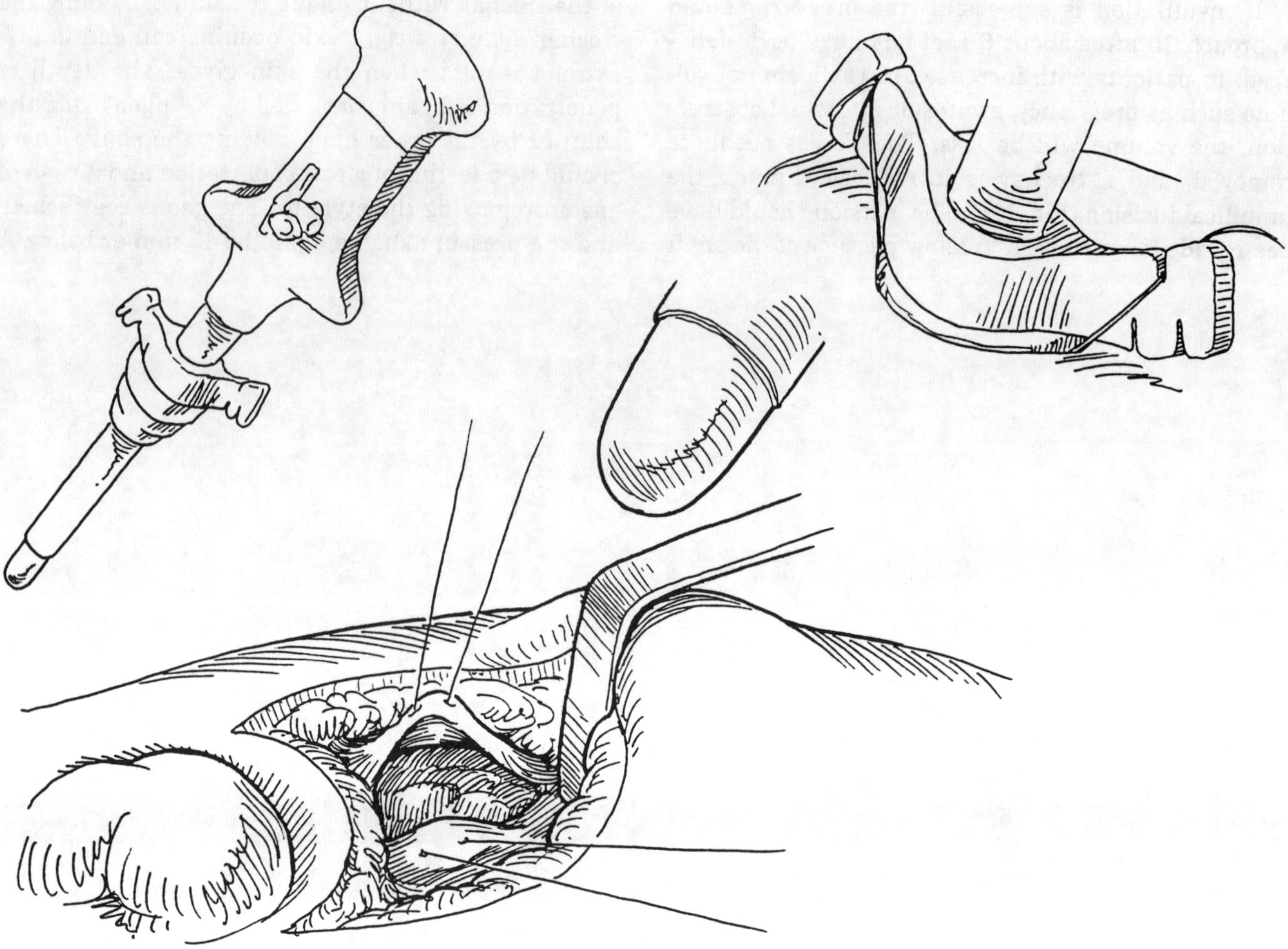

Fig. 1.5

pre-warmed telescope is introduced to check for free entry and for any local injury. A full examination of the abdominal cavity is then performed.

If the Veress technique is unsuccessful or if the patient is suspected to have significant adhesions, the open Hasson technique is used (Fig. 1.5). Through a slightly larger skin incision, sturdy stay sutures are placed in the fascia on either side of the midline and fascia and peritoneum are opened under direct vision. The canula is introduced so the cone-shaped collar is firmly seated against the fascia, and the wings are secured with the stay sutures.

In the previously operated abdomen, other sites than the umbilicus may be chosen for initial penetration. The use of ultrasound (looking for areas of freely moving viscera) has been tried successfully. The use of a small (5 mm) trochar and scope may also be a prudent first step to introduce a larger scope under direct vision at the umbilicus or elsewhere. A mini-scope the size of the Veress needle is also available.

All subsequent trochars are placed under direct vision. After the second trochar is placed, an open grasper can be used to apply upward pressure around the next incoming stylette for added safety (Fig. 1.6). If adhesions are present, they are sharply dissected with cautery scissors in preparation for placement of other trochars (Fig. 1.7). Transillumination of the abdominal wall helps identify

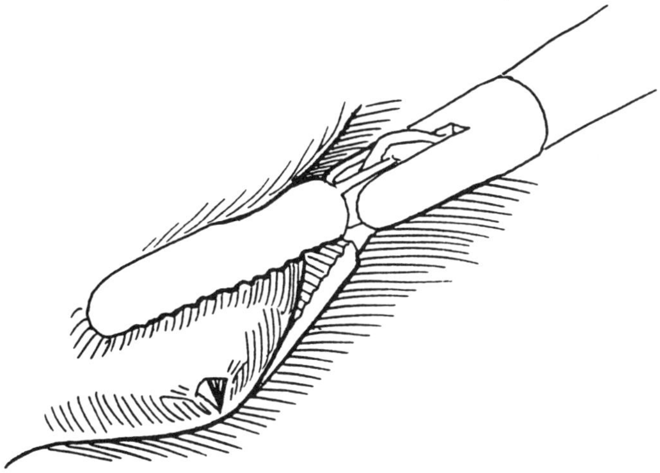

Fig. 1.6

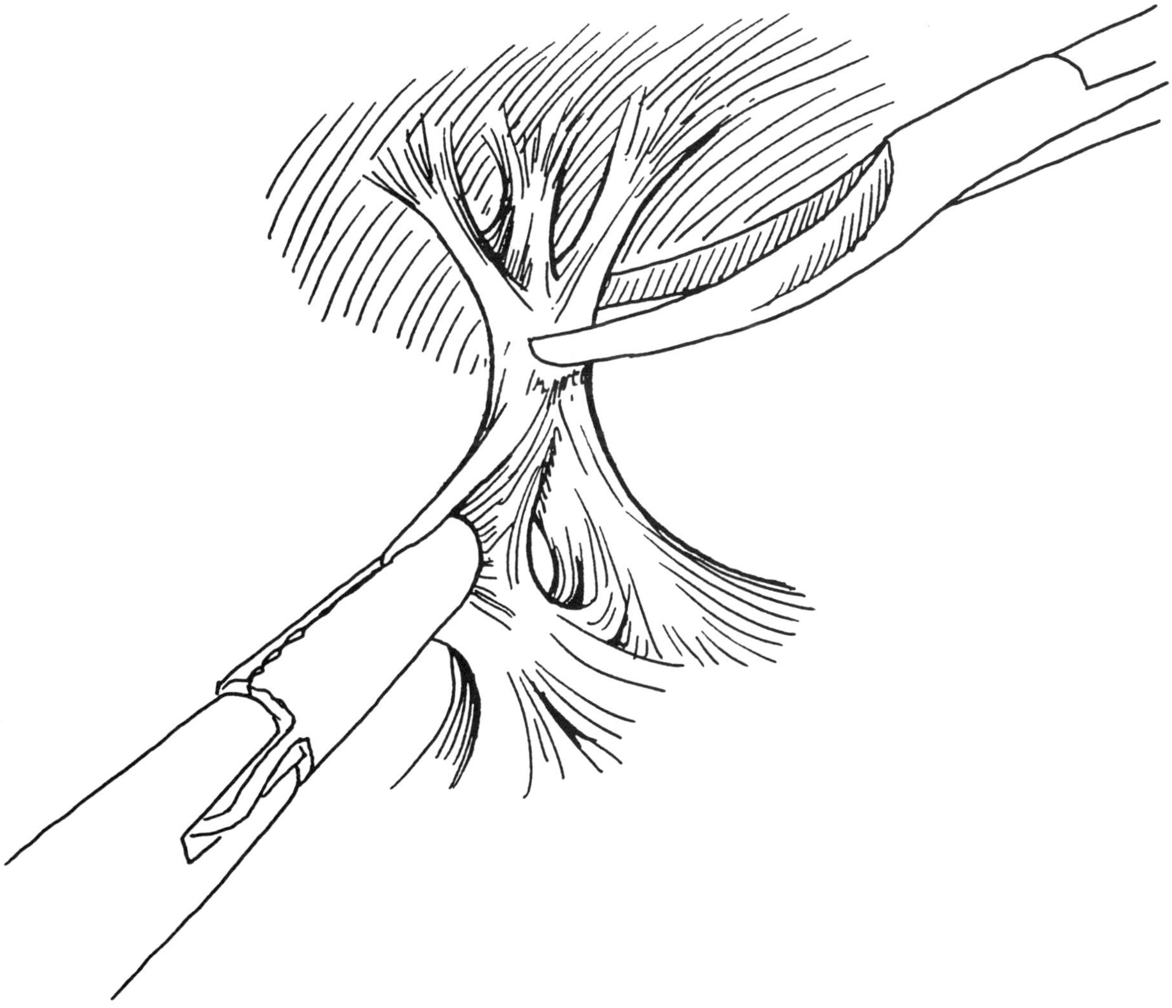

Fig. 1.7

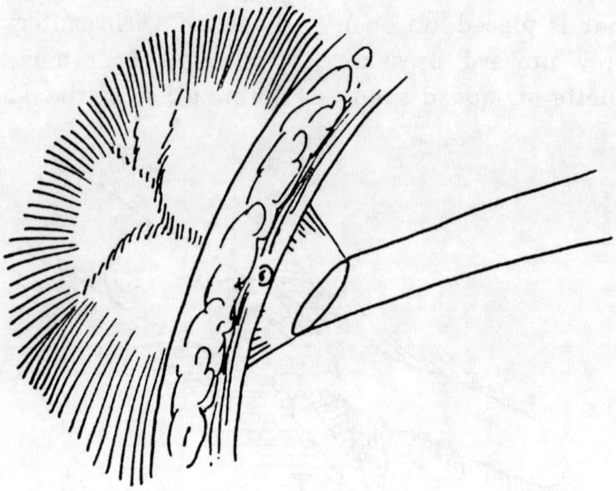

Fig. 1.8

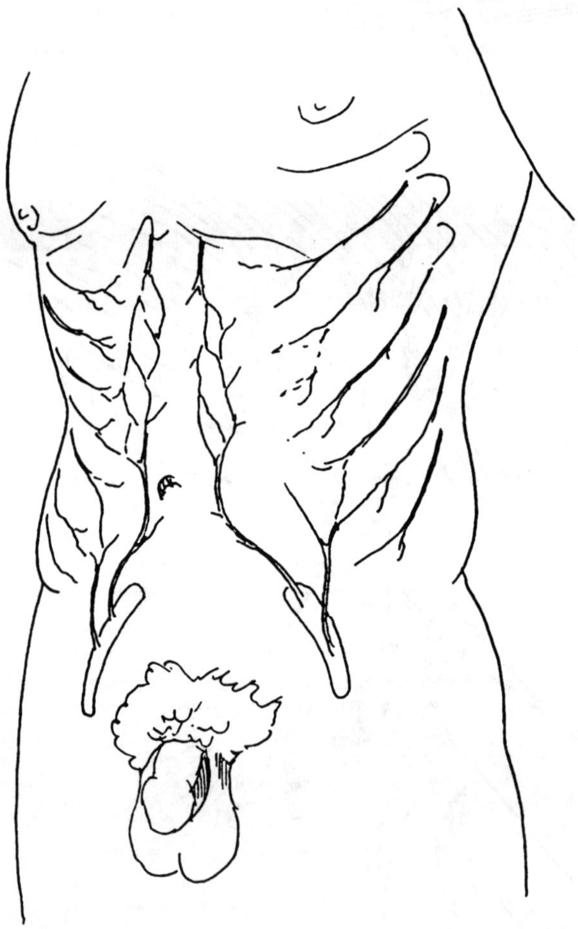

Fig. 1.9

and avoid vessels (Fig. 1.8). The major abdominal wall vessels are the inferior and superficial epigastric vessels in the lower abdomen, the superior epigastric vessels in the upper abdomen, and the intercostal vessels running around the flanks (Fig. 1.9).

Trochar Positioning

The principle guiding the placement of trochars is the "eyes, hands, camera" axis. There should be no working port between the camera port and the operative field, and adjacent ports should be far enough apart so that they do not interfere with one another. The operating trochars are arranged in a semicircle opposite the pathology, with the surgeon centered in the arc. The surgeon must be able to operate bimanually within an arc of 45-90 degrees. Ports for assistants may be outside or even opposite the surgeon's arc. The axis of the camera should ideally be between the surgeon's hands. If that is not possible, the camera should deviate by no more than 30 degrees, in which case, the lens bevel of the 30 or 45 degree scope can still be positioned and directed to give the surgeon a straight line of sight (see Fig. 1.1). The camera always remains oriented so that the image is upright and level. The bevel of the telescope lens rotates independent of the camera to visualize structures optimally from an oblique, upward, or downward view.

When retraction is necessary, the retractor should come in at a 90-degree angle to the camera. Ten millimeter and larger trochars should always be placed through the rectus muscle and not lateral to avoid herniation.

IN THE ABDOMEN

Exposure

Whether an operative procedure flows smoothly or entails a monumental struggle depends to a large degree on exposure, and exposure depends on several interrelated factors: preoperative assessment and planning to identify potential anatomical problems, anomalies, resectability, operative approach, and surgical options; proper equipment and the disposition of that equipment; position of the patient; positions of the operating team members; optimal trochar size, number, and position; maintenance of optimal inflation pressure; coordination of movements between the surgeon operating bimanually, the assistant and the camera operator; and skillful use of the proper instruments for manipulation, retraction, hemostasis, irrigation, and suction.

Bimanual operation provides the surgeon with optimal assistance and helps compensate for lack of depth perception. Bimanual manipulation is necessary for intracorporeal knot tying. It is the ideal for all procedures, but is particularly critical for advanced procedures.

The camera operator plays a critical role in compensating for the limited ability to move tissue around and see behind structures. By rotating the lens angle within the constraints of the eye/hand/camera principle, the camera operator provides the needed visualization. Visualization of instruments as they are introduced protects against injury. The close-up magnification allows for fine precise surgery.

The interaction of surgeon and assistant in laparoscopy weighs more heavily on the side of the surgeon having an active roll and the assistant a more passive one than is the case in open surgery. The surgeon positions the assistant's retractors initially and should use fixed retractors whenever possible.

Tissue Factors

Several features of handling tissues laparoscopically are different from open surgery. The increased intraabdominal pressure affects tissue; there is a diminished feel of the tissue and control of major bleeding and rapid access to vascular injury can be problematic.

Capsular tears of solid organs sustained in a high-pressure environment have a tendency to extend. The inability to apply broad pressure and surface hemostatic agents effectively hinders control of such injuries. It is important to retract solid organs with instruments that spread the pressure over the broadest possible surface area to prevent tears.

Increased pressure also collapses veins and may make manipulation more difficult. In addition, the lack of venous filling may leave the surgeon unaware that there is a venous opening that can later bleed and through which carbon dioxide can enter the venous system and embolize.

Tissue feel is compromised by the friction of the instrument shaft within the cannula, particularly if there is a rubber collar in place. Until there is a friction-free system available, the surgeon should use visual clues to determine the amount of force being applied and use the least traumatic instruments possible.

Bowel should be manipulated as little as possible to avoid ileus, a major inherent benefit of laparoscopy, and to prevent perforation. Debilitated patients with depleted stores of submucosal collagen are particularly prone to perforation. The bowel should be grasped only with atraumatic clamps and only on the antemesenteric border. Damage to the small blood vessels on the mesenteric border can lead to necrosis and perforation in the first few days after surgery. Bowel that is to be removed should be held in preference to bowel that will remain in place. Unrecognized thermal injury, either directly or through inductive coupling can also lead to delayed perforation.

Hemostasis

Hemostasis is achieved by identifying and securing blood vessels before they are divided, and by accurately and judiciously using cautery when necessary. A knowledge of vascular anomalies helps avert misadventures. Abdominal wall bleeding from a trochar injury may be controlled by cautery, but may require a through-and-through stitch to apply pressure until the vessel seals. A Foley catheter balloon may be pulled up against an abdominal wall bleeder to tamponade it and allow a clot to form.

Adherence to basic surgical principles of hemostasis is essential: never cut what you cannot see, keep the points of your scissors clearly visible, dissect under tension, skeletonize and gain distal and proximal control before dividing vessels, use pressure to control bleeding and suction to identify anatomy before applying definitive measures, use the appropriate size clips for the vessel, add a ligature for security on major vessels, and avoid mass ligature. As soon as a significant bleeder is encountered, the camera should be retracted to avoid fouling of the lens and the delay required for cleaning. Irrigate to clear away blood and clots to visualize anatomy clearly. Irrigation solution should contain 5000U of heparin per liter to prevent clot formation and help wash out clots.

Bipolar cautery is safer than monopolar because there is no transmission of current, which can cause distal injury. Bipolar coagulation may be sufficient for small or medium vessels (e.g., inferior epigastrics). In such a case, the vessel should be cauterized proximally, distally, and at the site of transection. The bipolar tip may be applied open near surface bleeders for a field effect. Never activate the cautery until the tissue is grasped and elevated away from surrounding tissue. Use the minimal effective power setting.

When unipolar cautery is used, it should be in the spray mode to give local and surface coagulation without deep penetration. A coagulation unit that detects current leaks is preferable. A combination suction/irrigation device with a cautery tip provides exposure and control. Avoid coagulating near sensitive structures like bile ducts. A coagulating scissors should be used to sharply divide adhesions. Blunt dissection of adhesions will lead to tears and broad areas of bleeding.

The tip of the Metzenbaum scissors may be held .5 mm from a point bleeding source. For a wider ooze, the broad surface of the back of the scissors may be applied at the same distance one or several times. For surface bleeding of solid organs, the spray coagulation mode or the argon beam coagulator should be used.

Smoke accumulation from cautery must be evacuated to maintain visualization. The valve of a port near the site of cautery may be partially opened or a gas scavenger system may be used. In either case, a high volume insufflator is necessary to maintain a steady state.

Topical hemostatic agents may be used alone or in combination with coagulation modes. These agents need to be held in place for several minutes and applying broad pressure is difficult. Suction is used to keep the area dry and visualized while waiting.

Hemostatic clips should be the proper size for the vessel. Double clips should be placed on the proximal side of an artery and a loop ligature should be added for larger vessels. Clips are easily dislodged by subsequent manipulation. Check both sides of a divided vessel for hemostasis.

When using the vascular staples in a linear stapling device, always check the staple line. Hemostasis is not guaranteed and an additional stitch may be necessary.

A combination of these methods may be necessary in highly vascular areas like the retroperitoneum and pelvis. After hemostasis is achieved, irrigate and check the area, and do it again before closing.

EXITING THE ABDOMEN

After copious irrigation with normal saline at body temperature to remove all clots and debris, all sites of dissection should be checked visually for hemostasis. A 10-mm cannula with high-volume irrigation may help evacuate large clots.

Anastomoses should be checked for competence. Upper bowel anastomoses can be checked by injecting methylene blue through the NG tube and observing for leaks. Low colon anastomoses can be checked by flooding the pelvis with saline and injecting air through the rectum.

If continued fluid accumulation is anticipated, a closed drain can be placed (see Fig. 2.48). The indications for a drain decrease with the increasing experience of the surgeon.

Trochars are always removed under direct vision to check for bleeders that were tamponaded by the sheath and to check that no bowel is pulled out. All trochar sites 10 mm and larger are closed at the fascial level as well as the skin. Several devices are available to place fascial sutures while the abdomen is still inflated before removing the trochars. These facilitate the closure and make it safer and more accurate.

The patient is placed in the horizontal position before removing the trochars to allow complete evacuation of subdiaphragmatic carbon dioxide. The last cannula is removed over the laparoscope to ensure no bowel is trapped. The patient is hyperventilated for a few breaths to aid in complete decompression and avoid postoperative shoulder pain.

If there is an anticipated need to return for a second look in the immediate postoperative period, the skin fixation collars of the camera port and two grasper ports may be left in place, packed with cellulose hemostatic agent to prevent herniation, and taped over the top to use for reentry.

2

The Biliary System

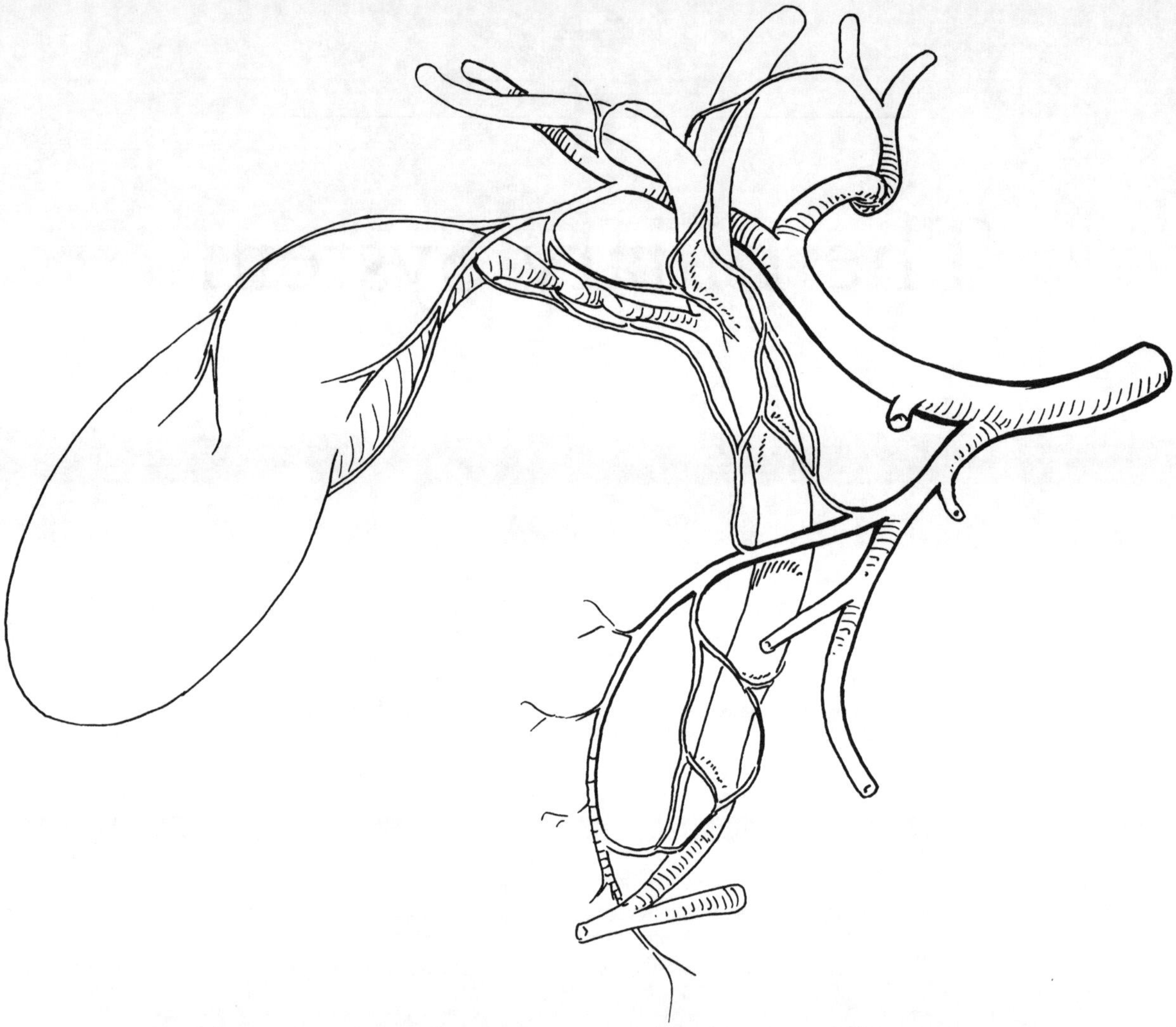

2

The Biliary System

EMBRYOLOGY

Liver and Bile Ducts

The first 8 weeks of gestation are collectively called the embryonic period to differentiate it from the subsequent fetal period. The second half of the embryonic period, weeks four through eight, is a time of dramatic evolution of organ systems. During this time, the rapid growth of a primitive pattern is immediately followed by extensive remodeling and modification. By the conclusion of the embryonic period, the mature anatomic pattern has been established in many cases.

The variations from "normal" anatomy seen in adult life often have their origin in the developmental growth pattern. The word normal is applied to the most common anatomic arrangement seen in a population and on average accounts for about 70% of individuals. The percentage varies from structure to structure. Variations in the extrahepatic bile ducts and arteries, for example, are common.

At the beginning of week four (Fig. 2.1A), the mid portion of the primitive gut is widely open to the yolk sac beneath the developing heart. The body wall partition between the heart and the gut is called the septum transversarum and is lined with gut endoderm on the intestinal side. The gut endoderm grows into the septum transversarum and forms the liver bud or diverticulum. The cephalad end of the diverticulum consists of multiple cords of cells that will form the liver parenchyma. Bifurcation of the cephalad portion of the bud at this stage results in duplication of the common bile duct. A bud on the side of the hepatic diverticulum will become the gallbladder. The stalks of these structures will become the extrahepatic biliary ducts. A secondary outpouching of the hepatic pedicle appears on the elongating stalk and will become the ventral pancreatic bud.

By the beginning of the fifth week (Fig. 2.1B), the midgut has progressively closed below the liver bud to form the future duodenum, and the growing liver mass is protruding into the abdominal cavity in the ventral mesentery formed by gut closure. The gallbladder and hepatic, cystic, common and pancreatic ducts are well demarcated at this time. Gallbladder and extrahepatic ductal variations derive from developmental anomalies occurring during the fourth week. During the fifth week there is florid proliferation of liver cells and elongation of the extrahepatic ductal structures. The lumens of the extrahepatic ducts and the duodenum become filled with cells by the end of the fifth week.

At the beginning of week six (Fig. 2.1C), the liver mass protrudes into the abdomen, retaining a portion of connection to the cephalad portion of the septum transversarum. The area of contact within the reflections of peritoneum will be known as the bare area of the liver. The extrahepatic bile ducts recanalize from the duodenal end toward the liver during the sixth week. Incomplete recanalization of the common duct results in septation. Ductal atresia is considered to be an acquired, not a developmental condition. Usually there is a dominant right and left hepatic duct at the end of growth and remodeling, and they unite outside the liver substance 90% of the time. Additional residual connections are not uncommon and most frequently they are on the right side. The gallbladder remains solid until well into the fetal period.

Toward the end of the embryonic period (Fig. 2.1D), weeks six to eight, the right side of the liver increases in size and the left side undergoes peripheral

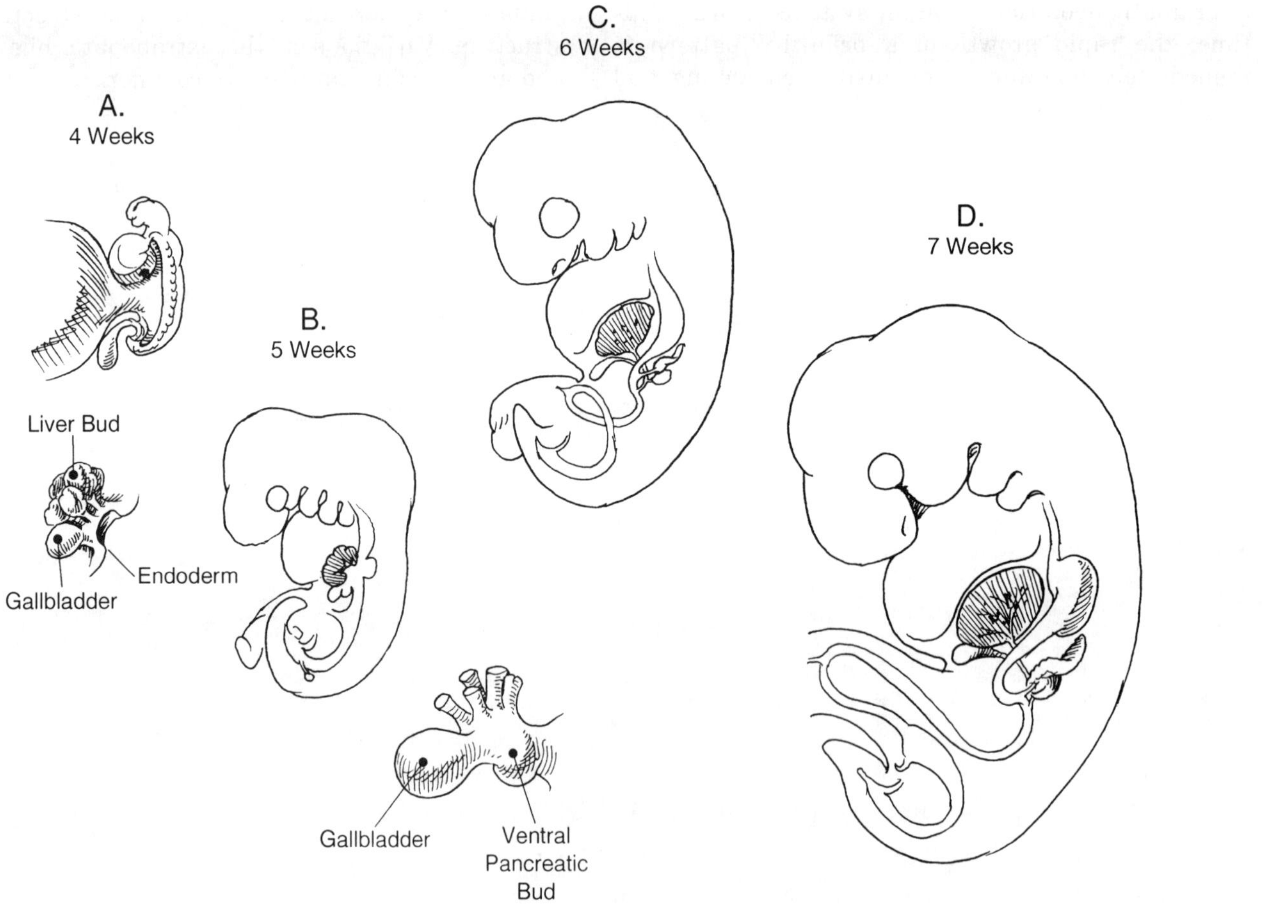

Fig. 2.1

regression. By the end of week eight, the liver accounts for 10% of body mass, but by birth it is 5%.

While the intrinsic structural changes are going on, positional changes are also occurring. The initial ventral position of the proximal biliary structures (Fig. 2.2A) is altered by a shift of the duodenum. By differential duodenal wall growth and/or rotation, the duodenal end of the bile duct and the ventral pancreatic anlage are shifted posteriorly and to the left (Fig. 2.2B). This brings the ventral pancreas into contact with the dorsal bud, which formed from the opposite duodenal wall slightly cephalad to the liver bud. Fusion of the pancreatic masses enwraps the distal common duct to a variable extent (Fig. 2.2C). The ductal systems of the two buds anastomose, with the dorsal duct forming the major distal pancreatic portion and the ventral duct forming the proximal duct in the head.

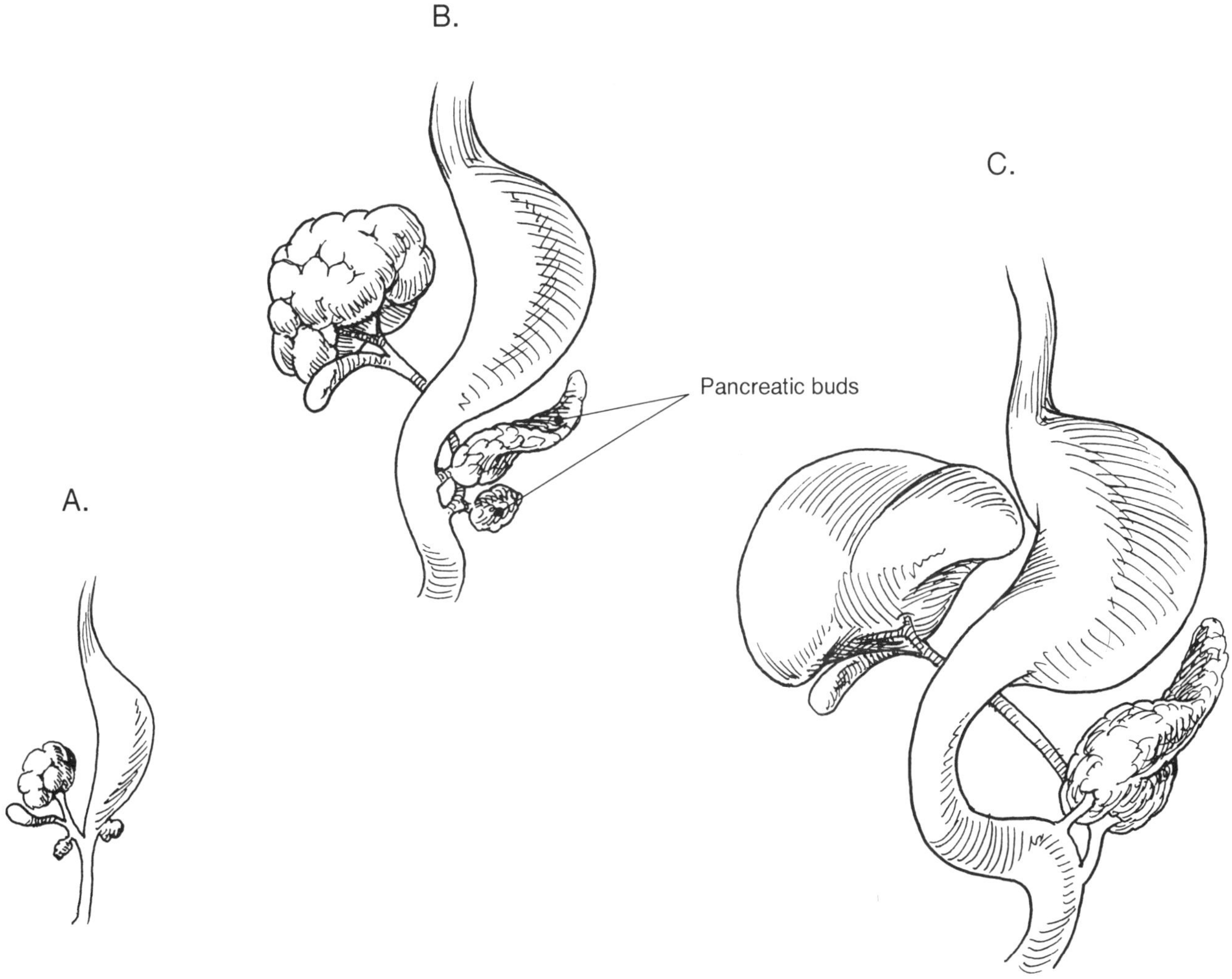

Fig. 2.2

VASCULATURE

The early paired dorsal aortae of the third week fuse distally resulting in paired dorsal somatic and lateral splanchnic branches (Fig. 2.3). The multiple vitelline vessels, which went to the yolk sac from the paired aortae, become midline vessels in the course of fusion. They lie in the gut mesentery and supply the intestinal structures. The ventral mesentery between the gut and the closing body wall eventually regresses except for the part between stomach and liver (later the gastrohepatic omentum and hepatoduode-

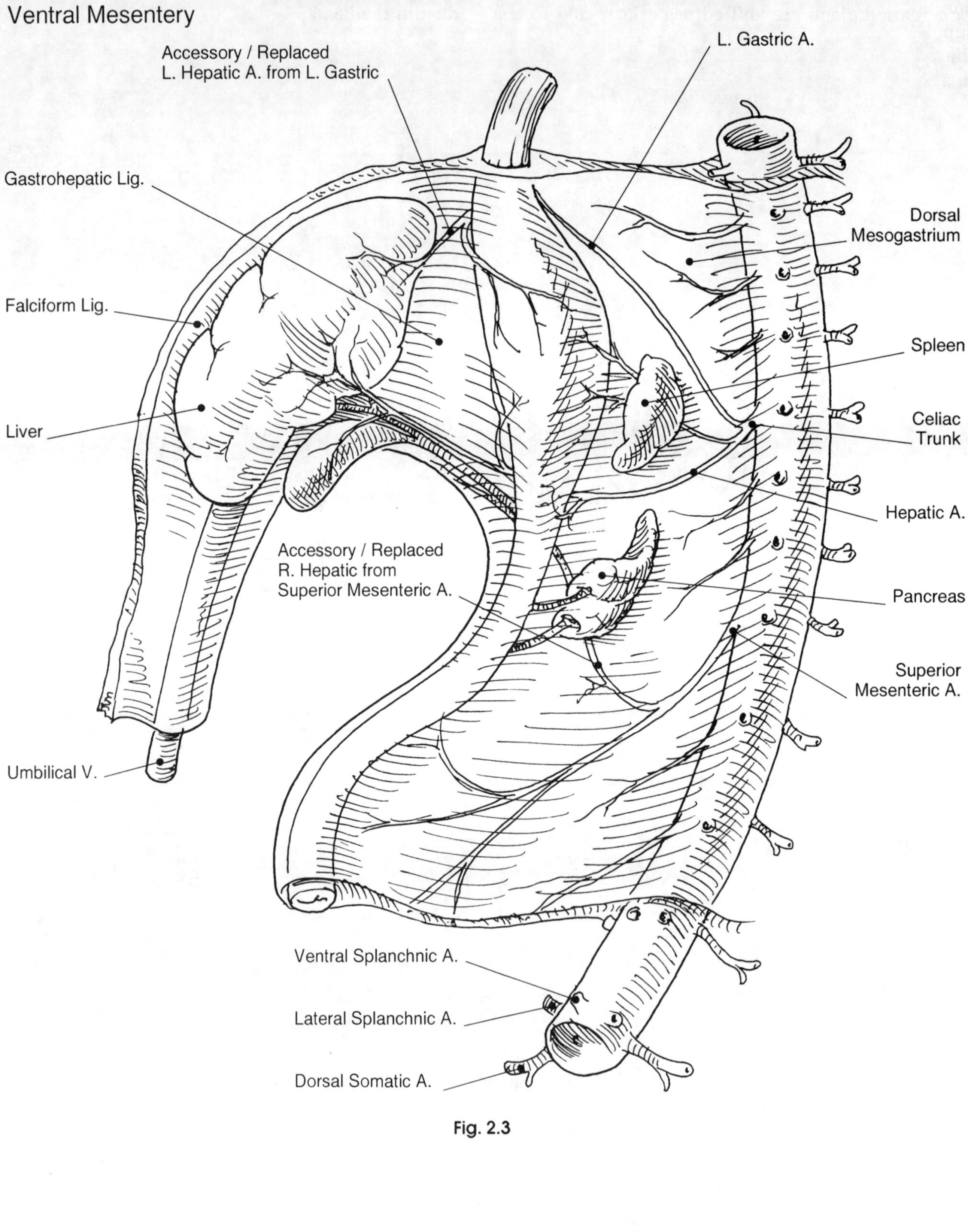

Fig. 2.3

nal ligament) and the connection between liver and body wall (the coronary and falciform ligaments). A few of the mesenteric vessels become dominant trunks, taking over the distribution networks of the adjacent vessels through anastomosis and regression of the adjacent stems. In most cases, the celiac, superior mesenteric, and inferior mesenteric arteries remain. One branch of the celiac, the hepatic artery, normally continues into the ventral gut mesentery to supply the liver and biliary system. Continuation to the liver of the left gastric branch of the celiac results in an additional artery to the left lobe of the liver. If the hepatic artery branches normally into left and right limbs, the aberrant vessel is said to be accessory. If there if no normal left branch, the vessel is called a replaced left hepatic artery. A continuation branch from the superior mesenteric artery can form an accessory or replaced right hepatic artery. There is a high degree of variability in the extrahepatic arteries. The intrahepatic branches parallel the segmental pattern of the biliary ducts and portal vein.

The development of hepatic venous channels is complex. In the 4-week embryo (Fig. 2.4A), the vitelline and umbilical veins pass through the sep-

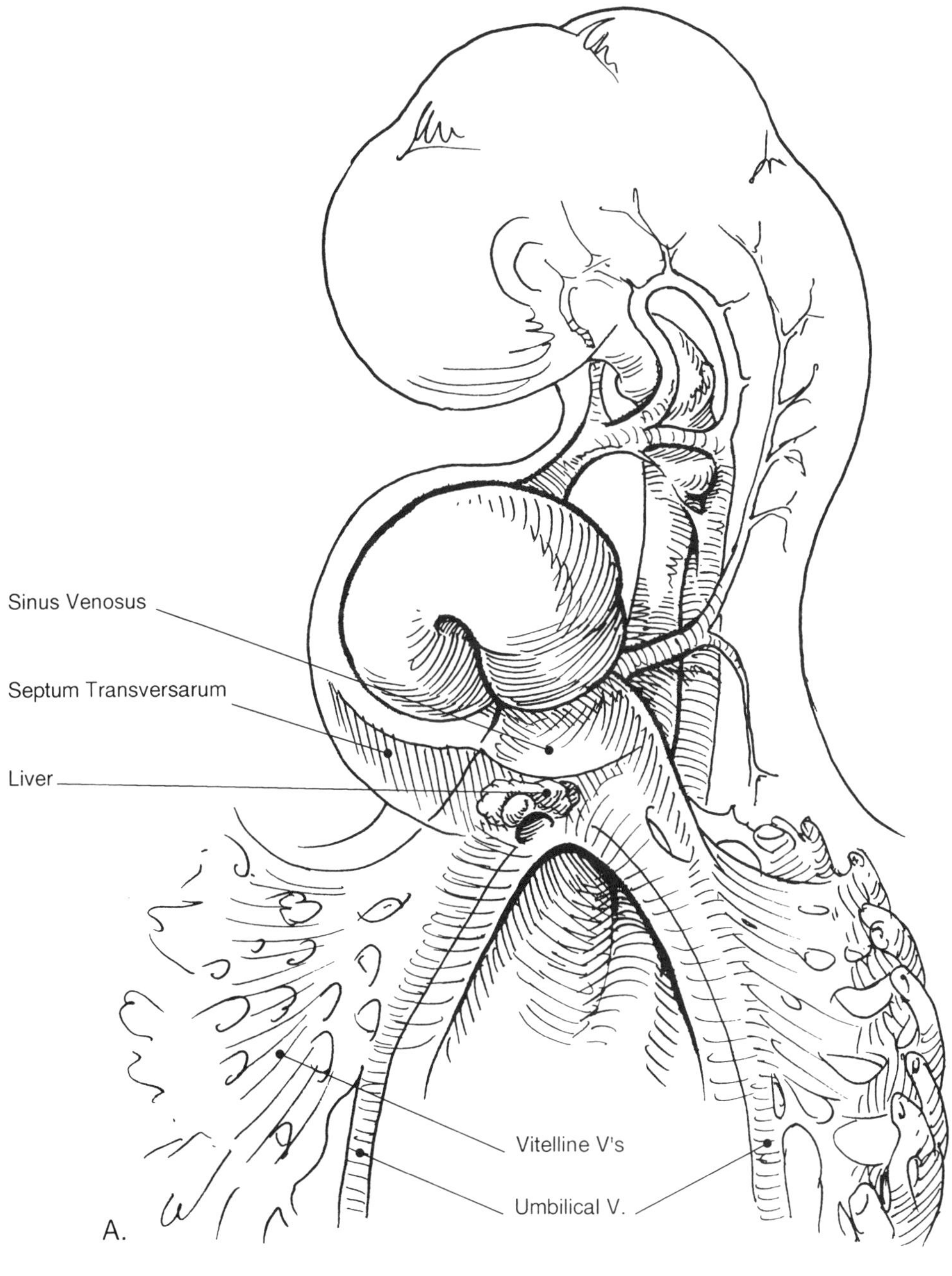

Fig. 2.4A

tum transversarum to reach the sinus venosus at the caudal end of the heart. As the body wall folds together closing the midgut, the vitelline vessels intermingle with the proliferating hepatic cells and anastomose with each other and with developing hepatic sinusoids to form a rich hepatic venous plexus (Fig. 2.4B). The left-sided connection between this plexus and the sinus venosus regresses. The large dominant right dorsal hepatocardiac vein is later joined by the right subcardinal vein forming the intrahepatic portion of the inferior vena cava. The extrahepatic vitelline veins interconnect around the developing duodenum, selectively regress and form a single channel, the portal vein, passing behind the duodenum. The right umbilical vein regresses and the left anastomoses with the hepatic venous plexus, losing its connection to the sinus venosus.

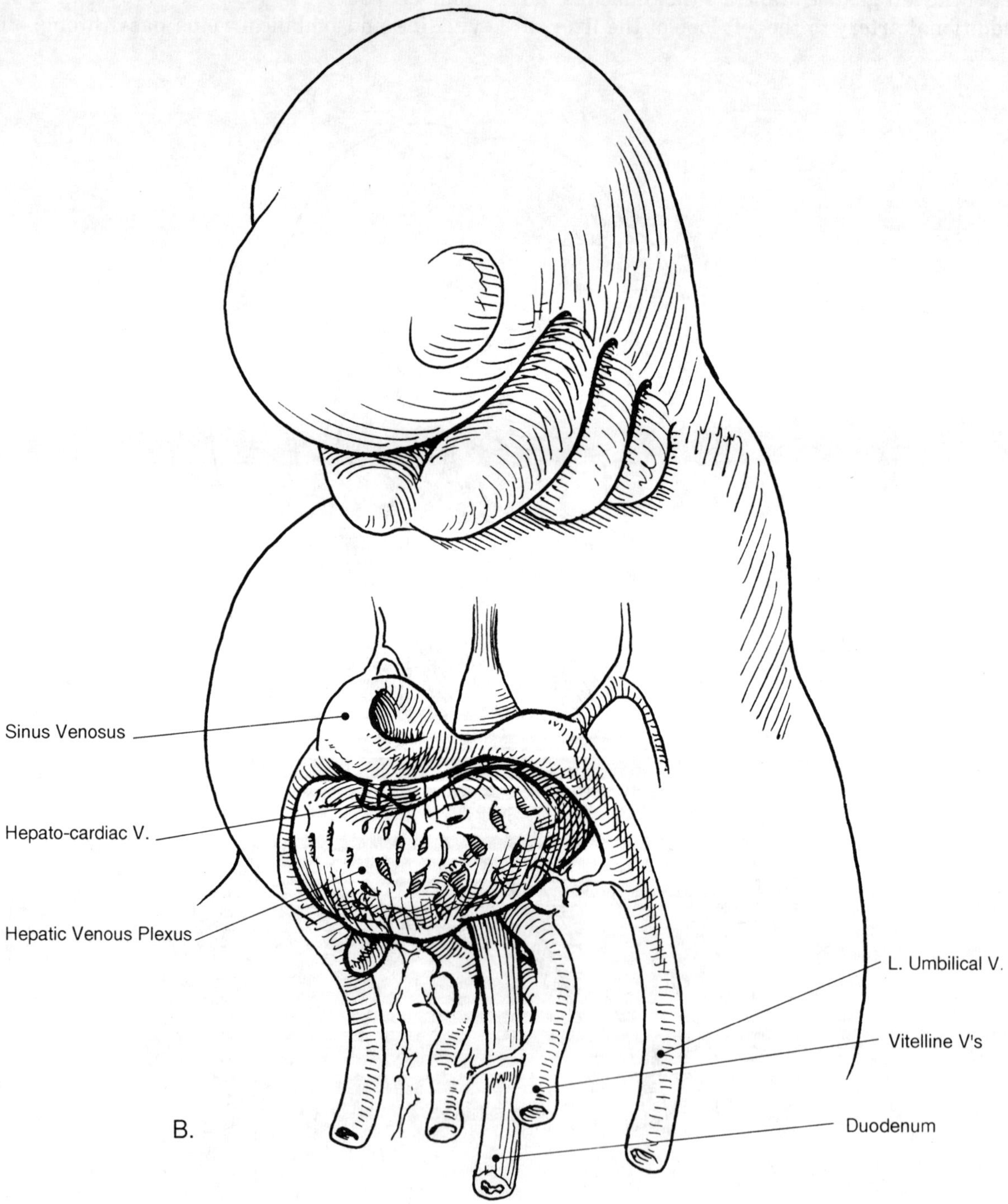

Fig. 2.4B

The increased flow of umbilical blood finds a hemodynamically preferred path through the hepatic plexus and forms a dominant channel, the ductus venosus (Fig. 2.4C). The ductus venosus lies in the hepatic attachment of the gastrohepatic omentum and drains into the differentiating right atrium along with the hepatic portion of the inferior vena cava. The ductus drains through the portion of the hepatic venous plexus that will become the distribution of the left portal vein. The vestiges of the umbilical vein remain connected to the left portal vein as the round ligament of the liver in the edge of the residual ventral mesentery (falciform ligament) caudally, and the ductus venosus remnant remains as the ligamentum venosum running in the cephalad direction from the left portal to the inferior vena cava. The portal inflow follows a segmental pattern, while the veins on the other side of the liver lobules coalesce into larger channels that lie between liver segments.

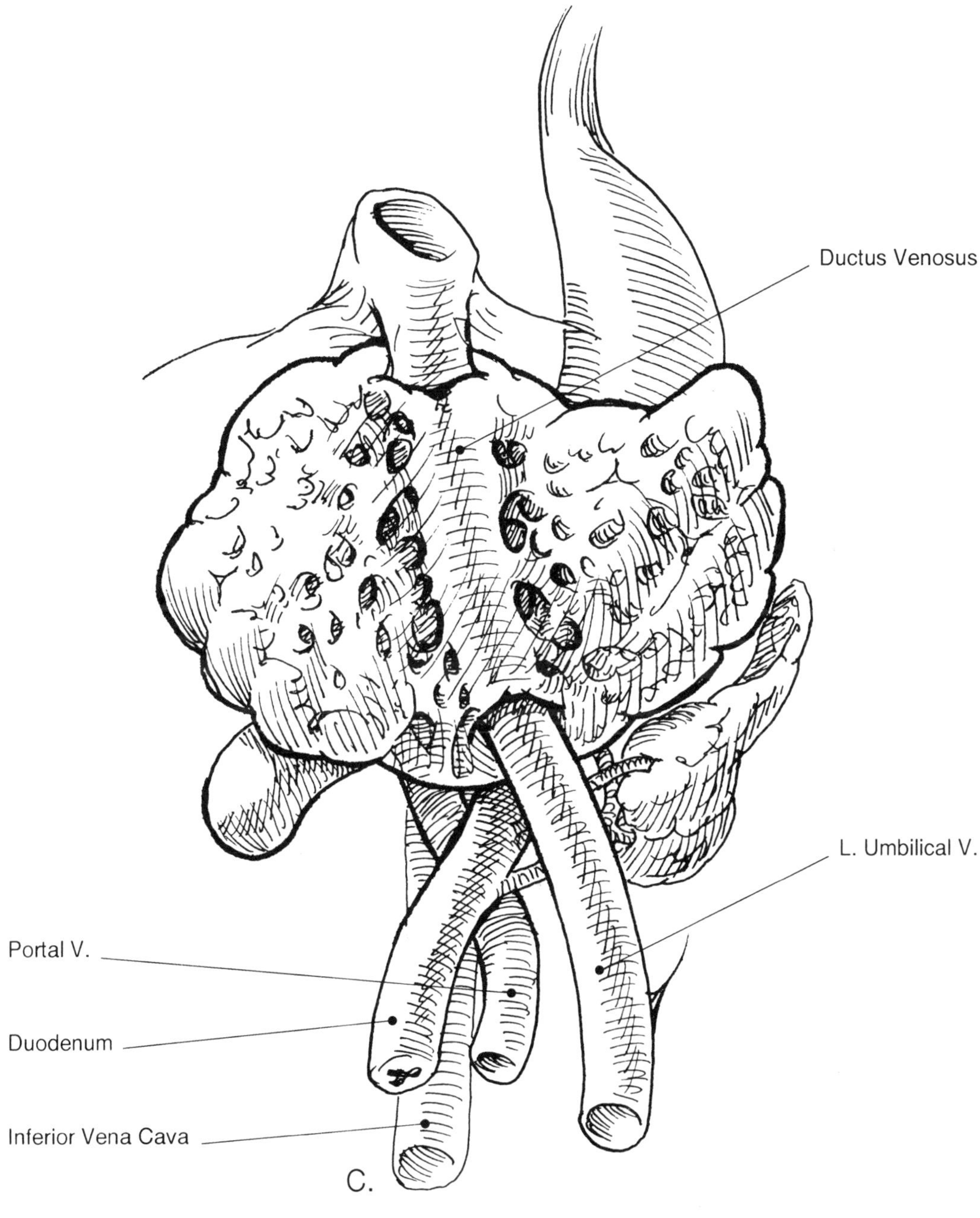

Fig. 2.4C

ANATOMY

The Liver

The bulk of the liver fills the dome of the right hemidiaphragm and extends across the midline beneath the heart (Fig. 2.5A). The most common variation of anterior surface shape, decreased size of the segment to the left of the falciform ligament, is beneficial for laparoscopic access to the extrahepatic biliary structures. A fibrous extension from the tip of the lateral segment of the left lobe may persist as a reminder of its embryonic size (Fig. 2.5B). Less common is downward extension of the right lobe, which can cause access problems (Fig. 2.5C). The liver edge runs from upper left to lower right, leaving the anterior wall of the gastric body and antrum exposed on the left and the proximal transverse colon exposed to the right of the greater omentum. The tip of the noninflamed gallbladder may peek out between the right lower liver edge and the colon.

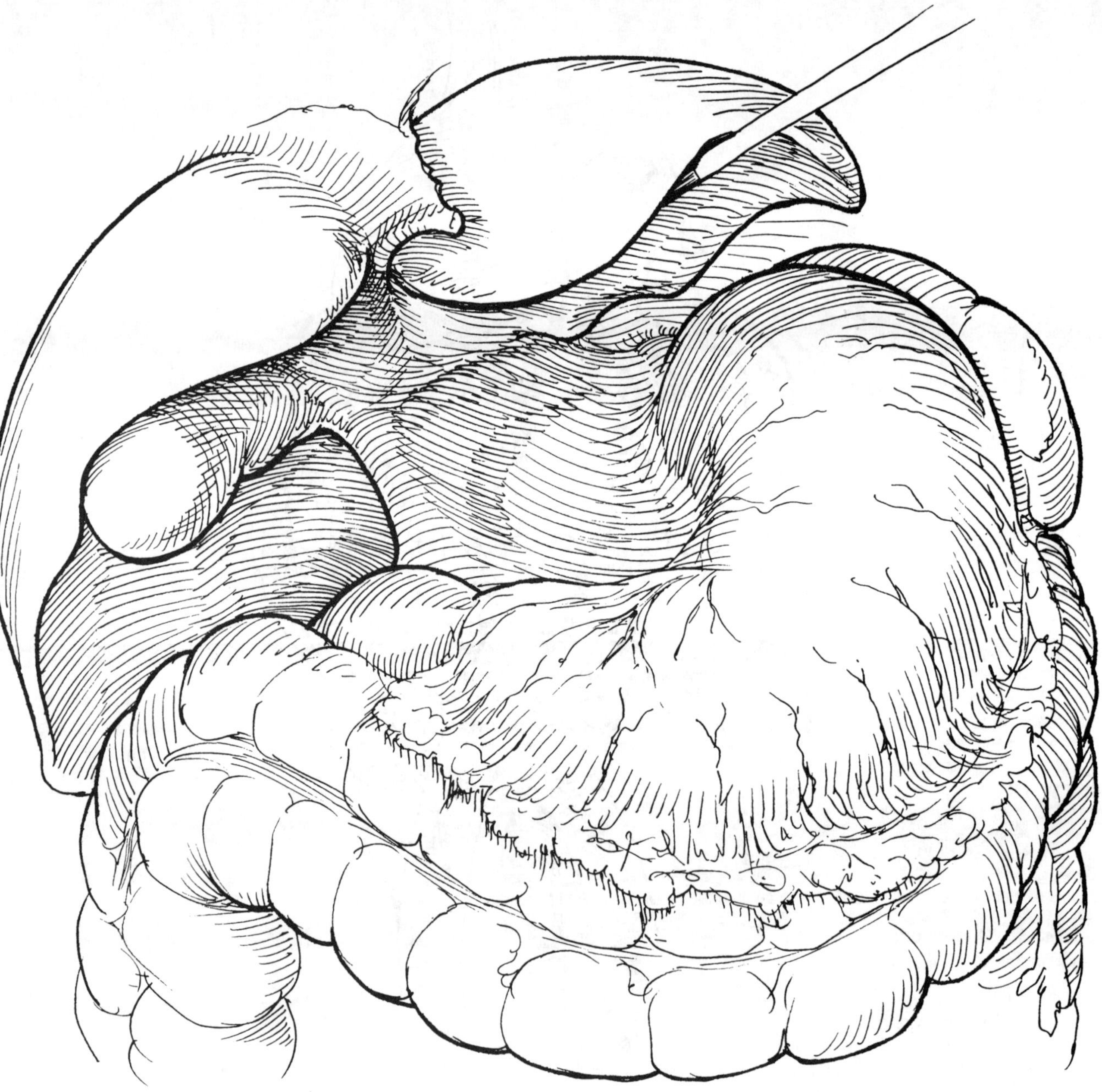

Fig. 2.5A

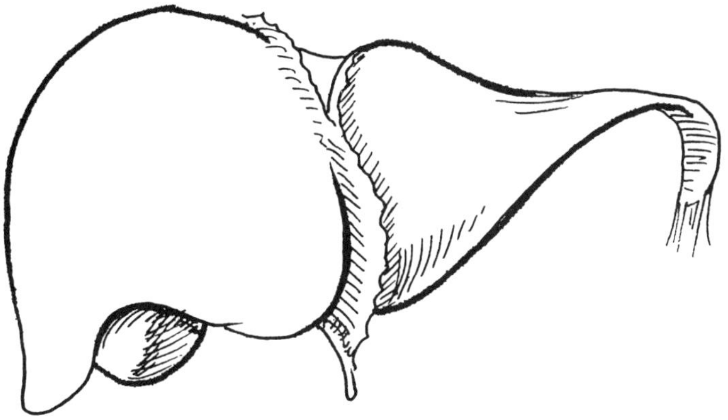

Fig. 2.5B

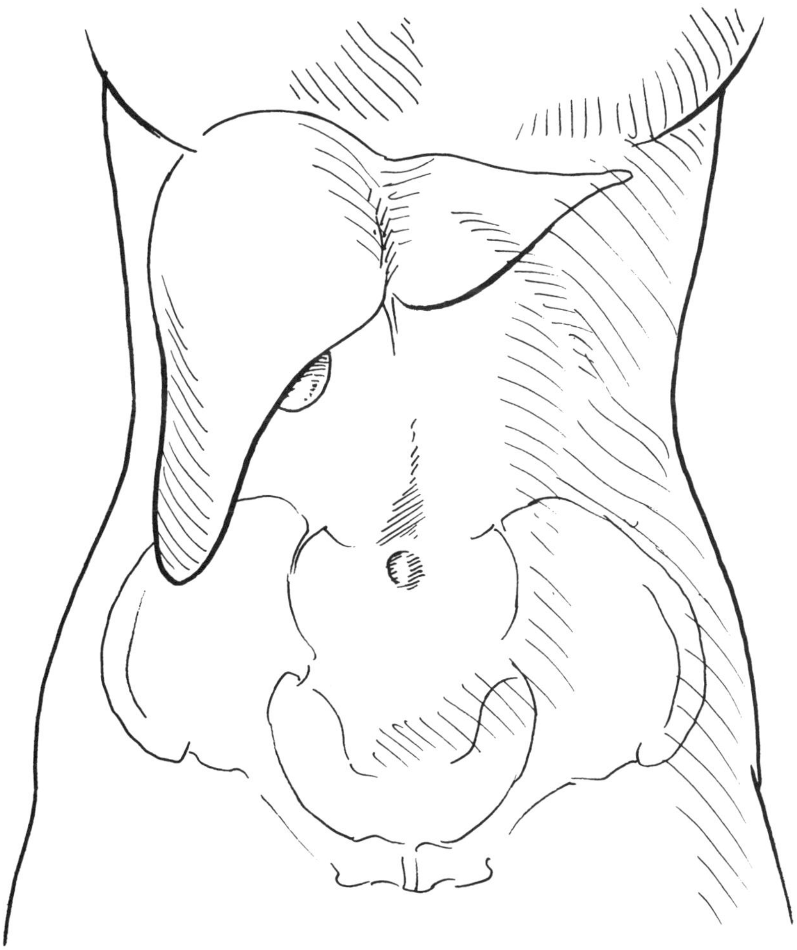

Fig. 2.5C

To visualize the liver anatomically in three dimensions, it is necessary to place it in the context of the abdominal cavity and surrounding organs. The residual direct apposition of the liver to the diaphragm arises from the common origin of these two structures in the embryonic septum transversarum (Fig. 2.6A). This bare area is delimited by the reflection of the parietal peritoneum from the under side of the diaphragm onto the liver. The peritoneal reflection forms a diamond-shaped ring or crown over the liver, hence the name coronary ligament.

The boundary of "ligaments" is far superior and posterior on the dome of the liver, leaving a deep suprahepatic recess on the right. In the center of this area is the inferior vena cava at its junction with the major hepatic veins. The anterior border of the peritoneal reflection is continuous with the falciform ligament, the cephalad part of the ventral mesentery. The right and left borders also narrow to acute corners, the triangular ligaments. When dividing the left triangular ligament to mobilize the lateral segment of the left lobe of the liver, the surgeon must be aware of

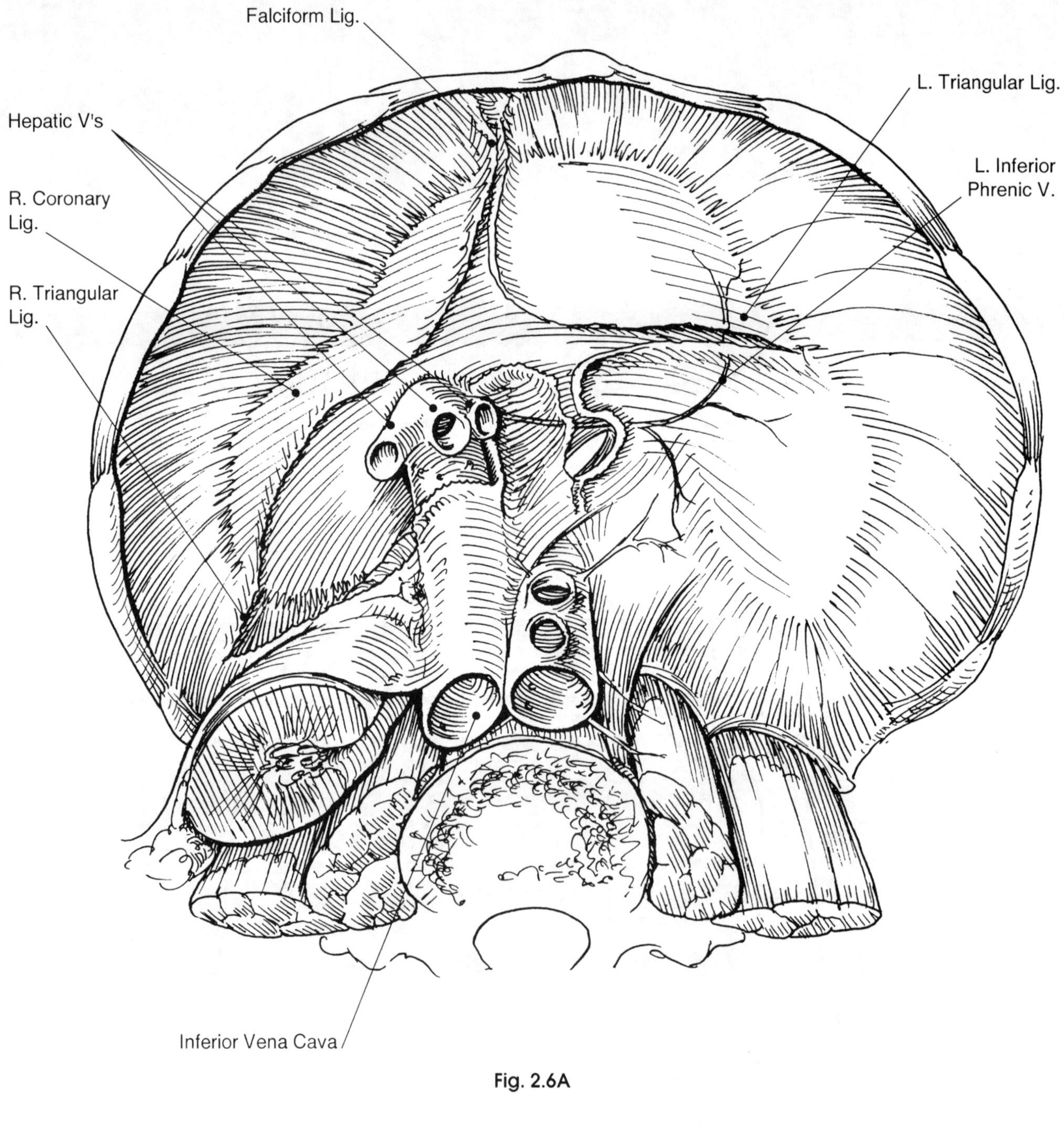

Fig. 2.6A

the proximity of the hepatic veins and inferior vena cava. Access to a venous injury at this high posterior location requires heroic measures. Small veins draining from the posterior surface of the liver directly into the vena cava reflect the evolution of the cava from the dorsal part of the hepatic venous plexus. Note the left inferior phrenic vein crossing the anterior lip of the esophageal hiatus, a fairly constant relationship.

The upper abdominal organs lie in a broad inverted U or kidney bean shape when viewed from a laparoscopic or CT scan perspective (Fig. 2.6B). The spine and great vessels indent the posterior contour, and the organs rest posterolaterally in the diaphragmatic recesses on either side. The most posterior organs are the kidneys.

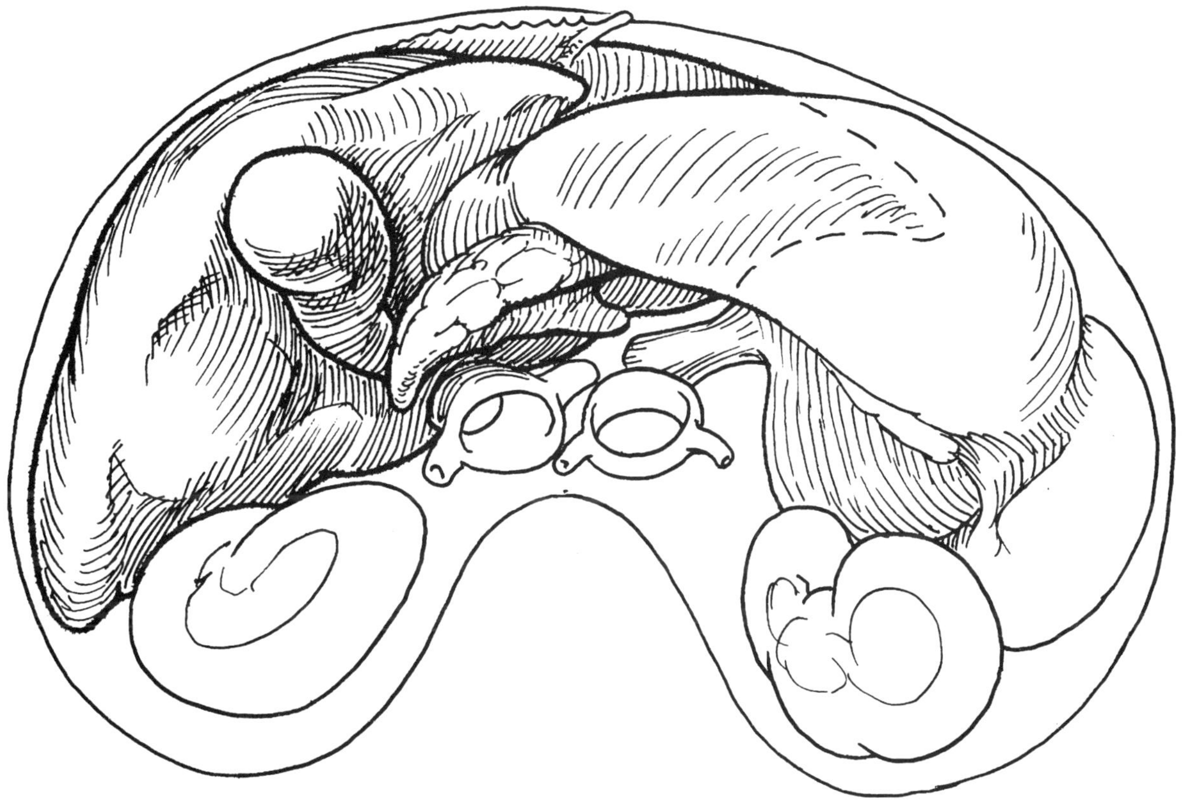

Fig. 2.6B

Viewed in sagittal section (Fig. 2.7), the profile of the abdominal cavity is wedge shaped owing to the slope of the lumbar vertebrae and the bordering psoas muscles. The hepatorenal recess (Morrison's pouch) is the deepest part of the peritoneal cavity. On the right, the bulge of the kidney and perirenal fat indents the undersurface of the liver posteriorly, and the hepatic flexure of the colon is in contact with the anterior part of the undersurface.

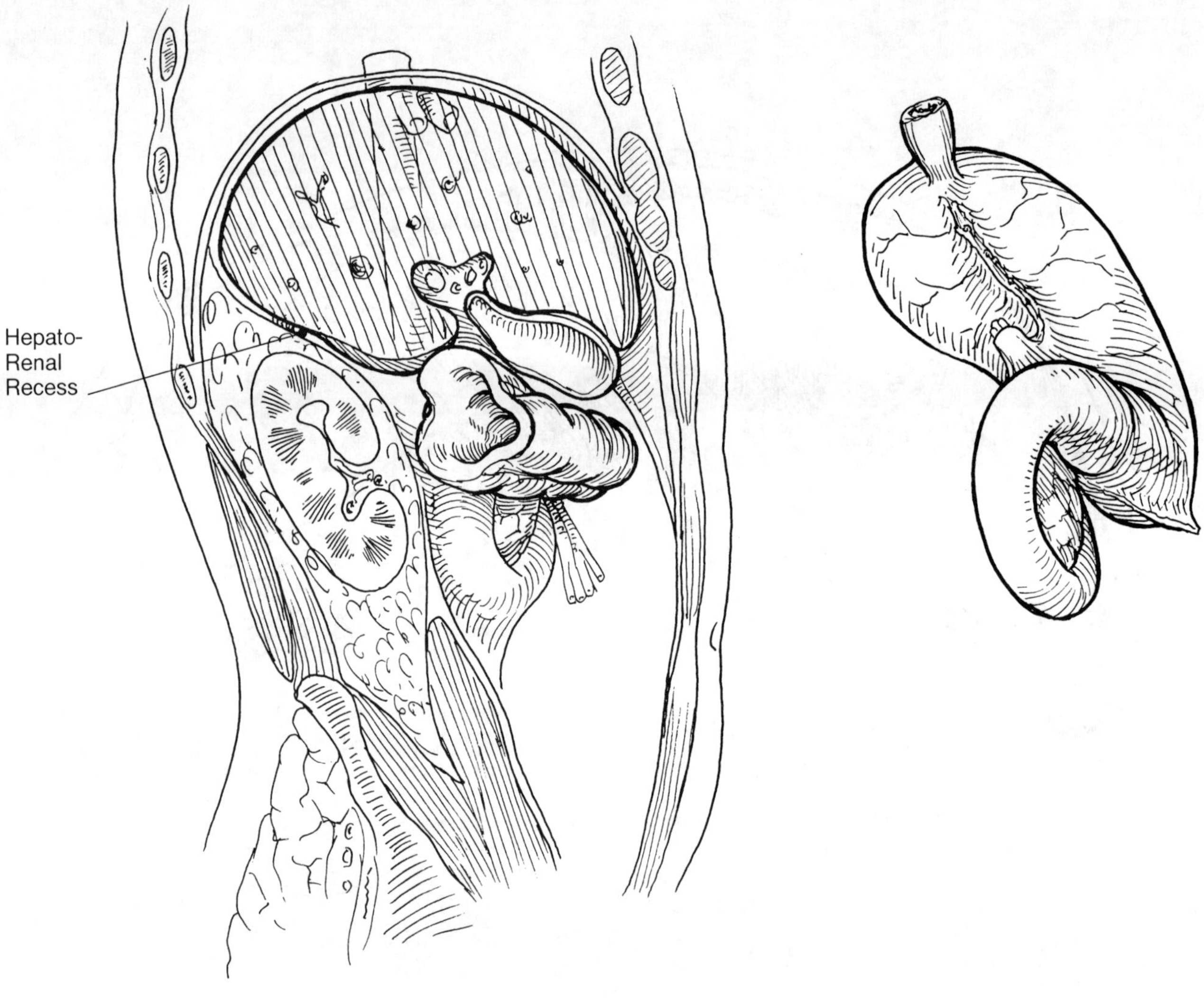

Fig. 2.7

In sagittal reconstructions of the right upper quadrant (Fig. 2.8), the inferior vena cava is centrally located in the abdomen and the hepatic portal structures in the hepatoduodenal ligament lie just anterior to it. In the anterior view seen in a cholangiogram, the common bile duct often overlies the right border

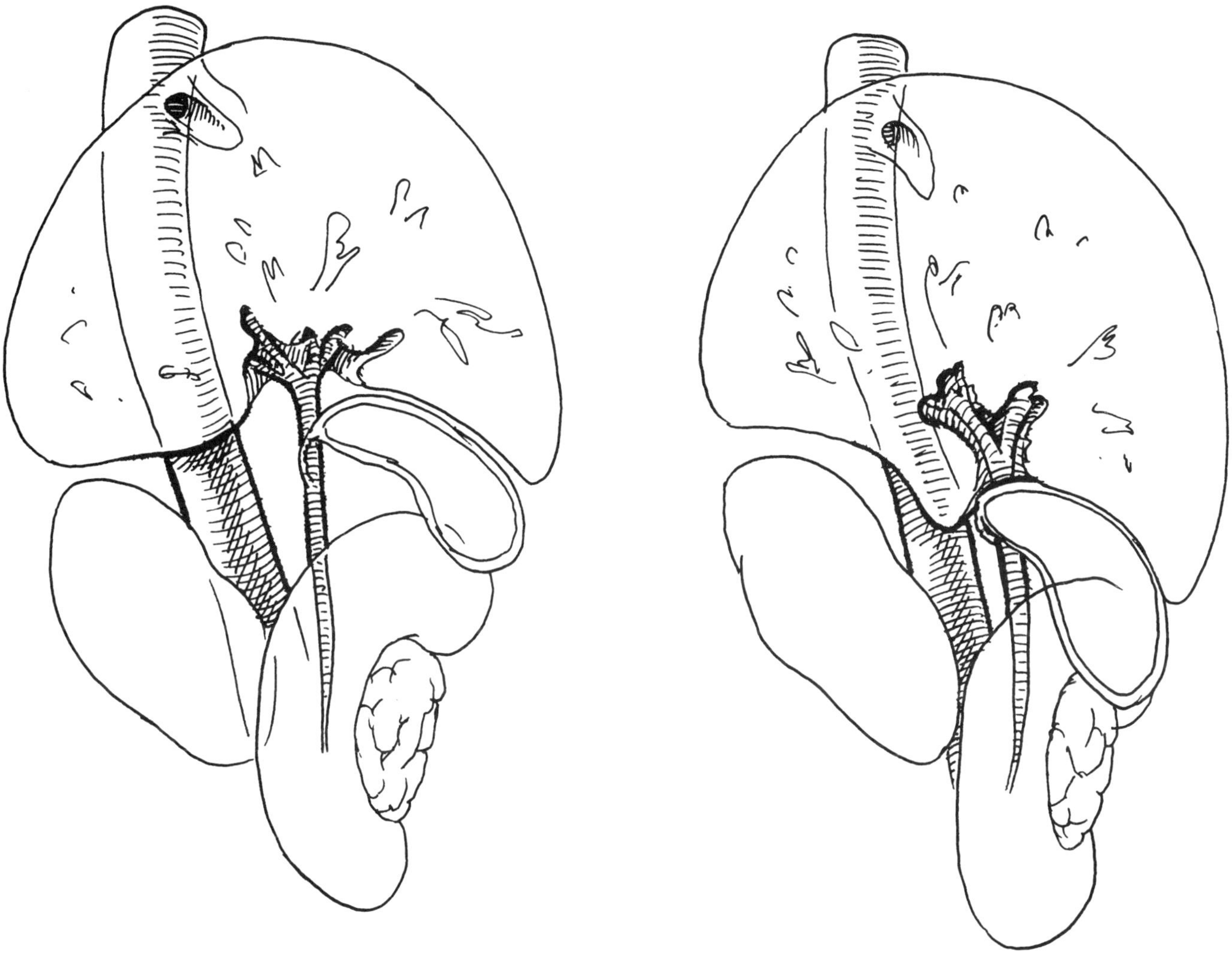

Fig. 2.8

of the lumbar vertebral bodies. Rotate the patient slightly to the right to see subtle defects without background interference (Fig. 2.9).

Elevating the liver reveals the gastrohepatic omentum, the other remnant of the ventral mesentery, running from the lesser curve of the stomach to

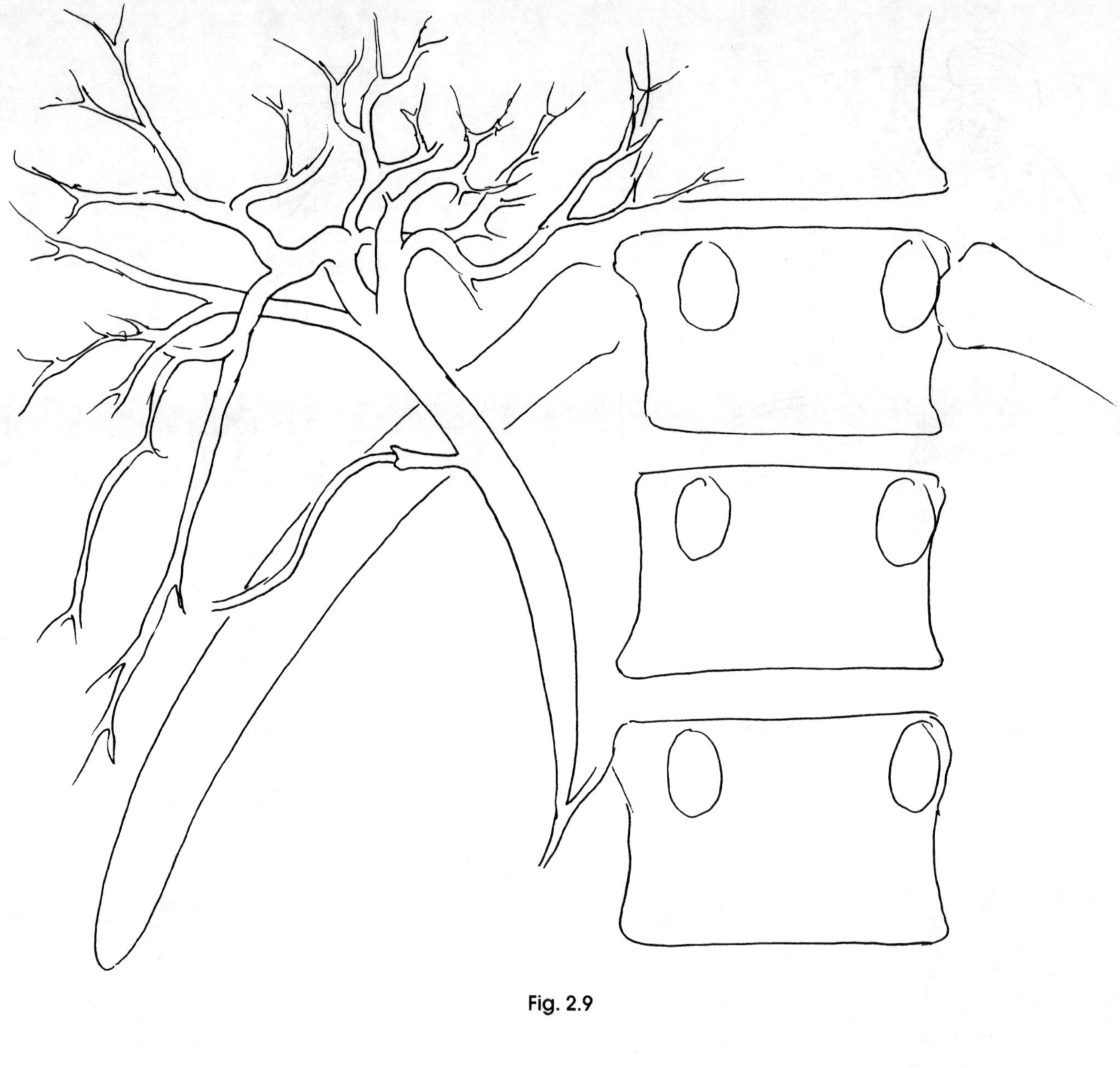

Fig. 2.9

the groove for the ligamentum venosum and to the liver hilus (Fig. 2.10). The free edge of this membrane wraps around the hilar structures and is called the hepatoduodenal ligament. The plane of contact between the anterior surface of the gastric fundus and the undersurface of the lateral segment of the left lobe of the liver can now be seen. The first part of the duodenum, previously obscured by the liver edge, is now exposed and its relationship to the underside of the quadrate lobe and to the body of the gallbladder is evident. Finally, on the right, the relationship of the hepatic flexure of the colon to the underside of the right lobe and to the gallbladder is exposed.

Removing the stomach and colon reveals the root

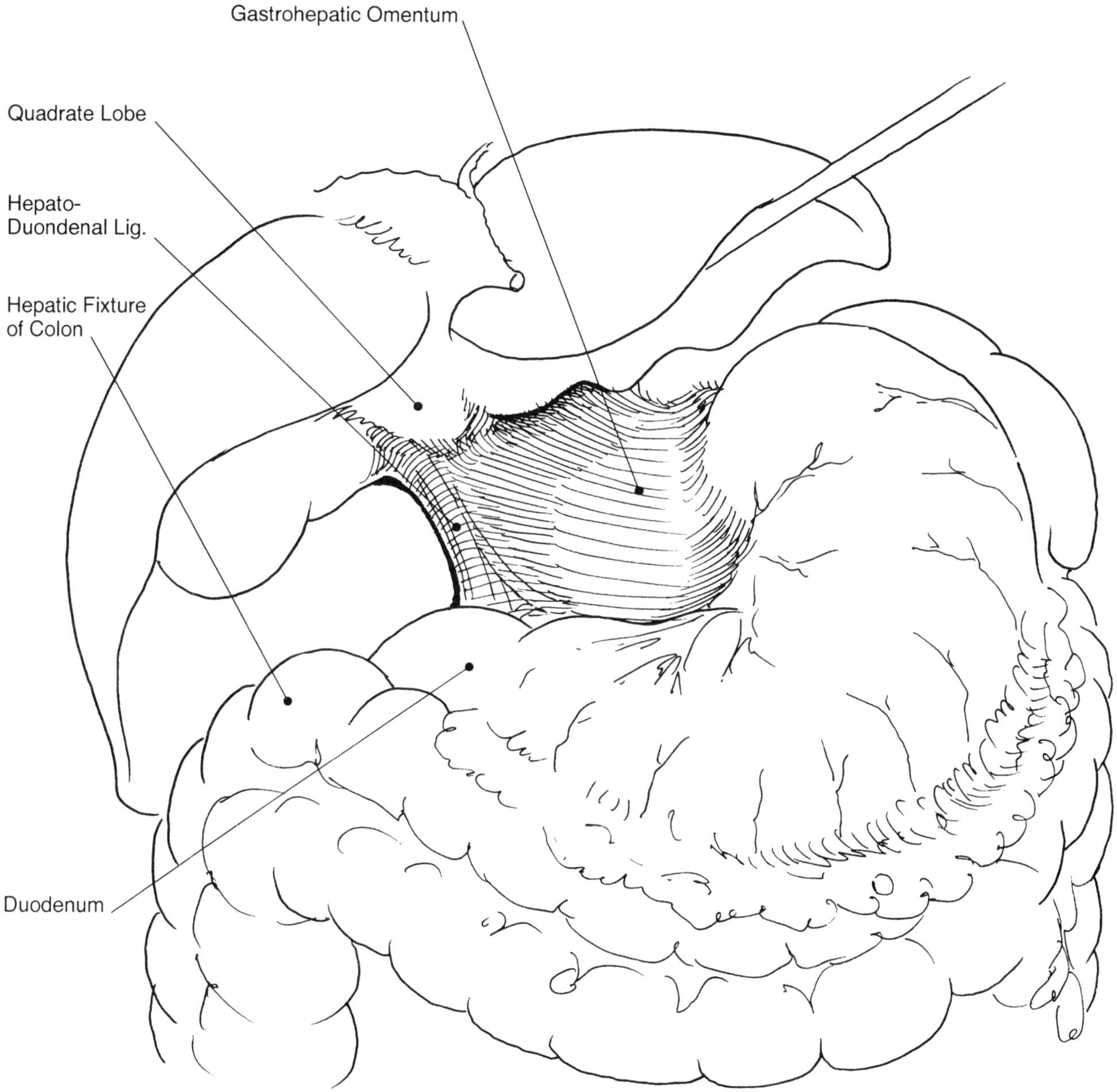

Fig. 2.10

of the transverse mesocolon and the boundaries of the omental bursa beneath the lesser omentum (Fig. 2.11). The caudate lobe of the liver, seen in the upper recess of the bursa, is often large. The hepatopancreatic fold is seen as the ridge formed by the hepatic artery as it turns from the retroperitoneum of the omental bursa into the hepatoduodenal ligament.

Stripping the remainder of the posterior parietal peritoneum exposes the structures of the hepatic hilum and their relationships to the pan-

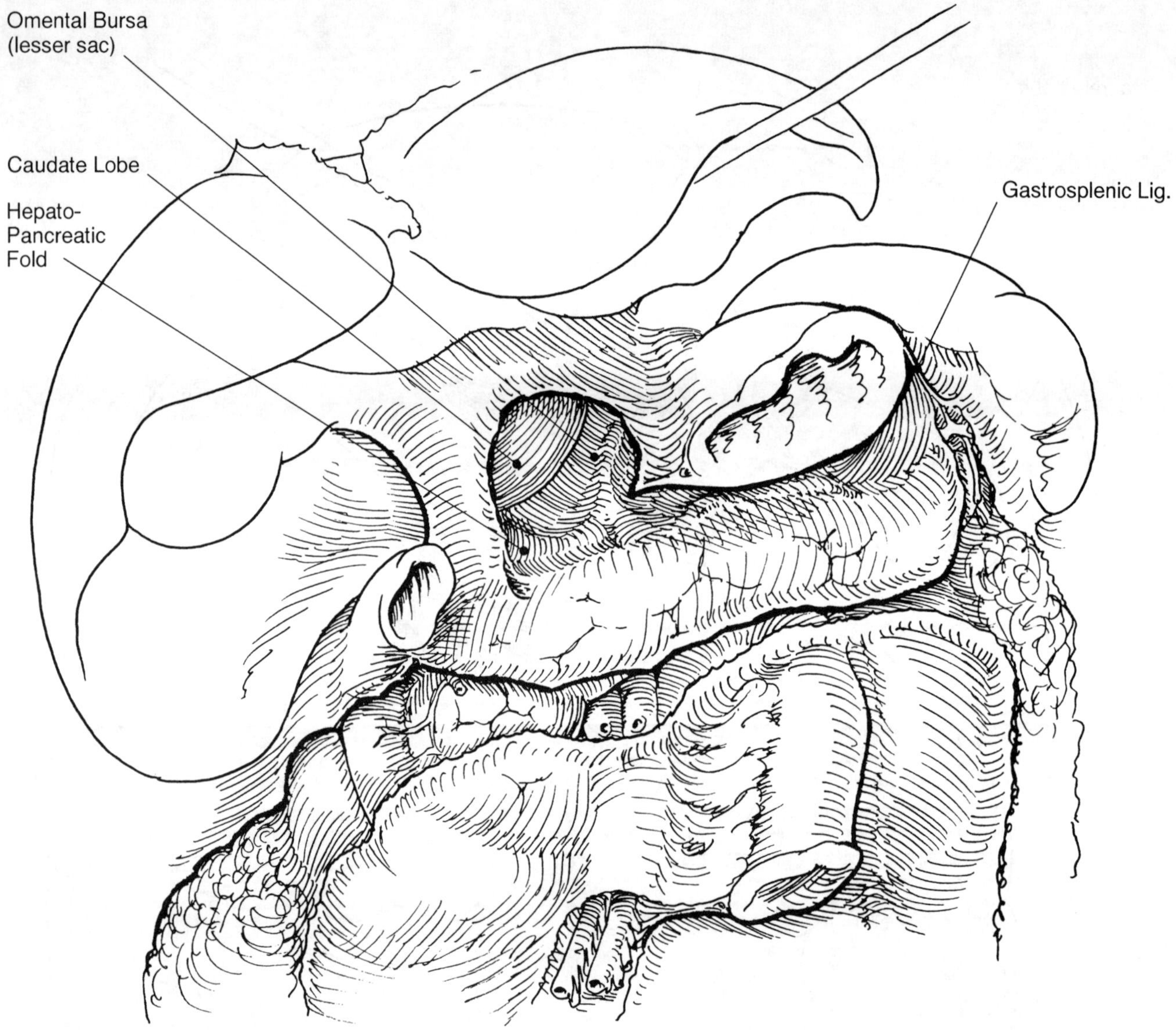

Fig. 2.11

creas (Fig. 2.12). In its common three-branched form, the celiac trunk gives rise to the left gastric, splenic, and hepatic branches.

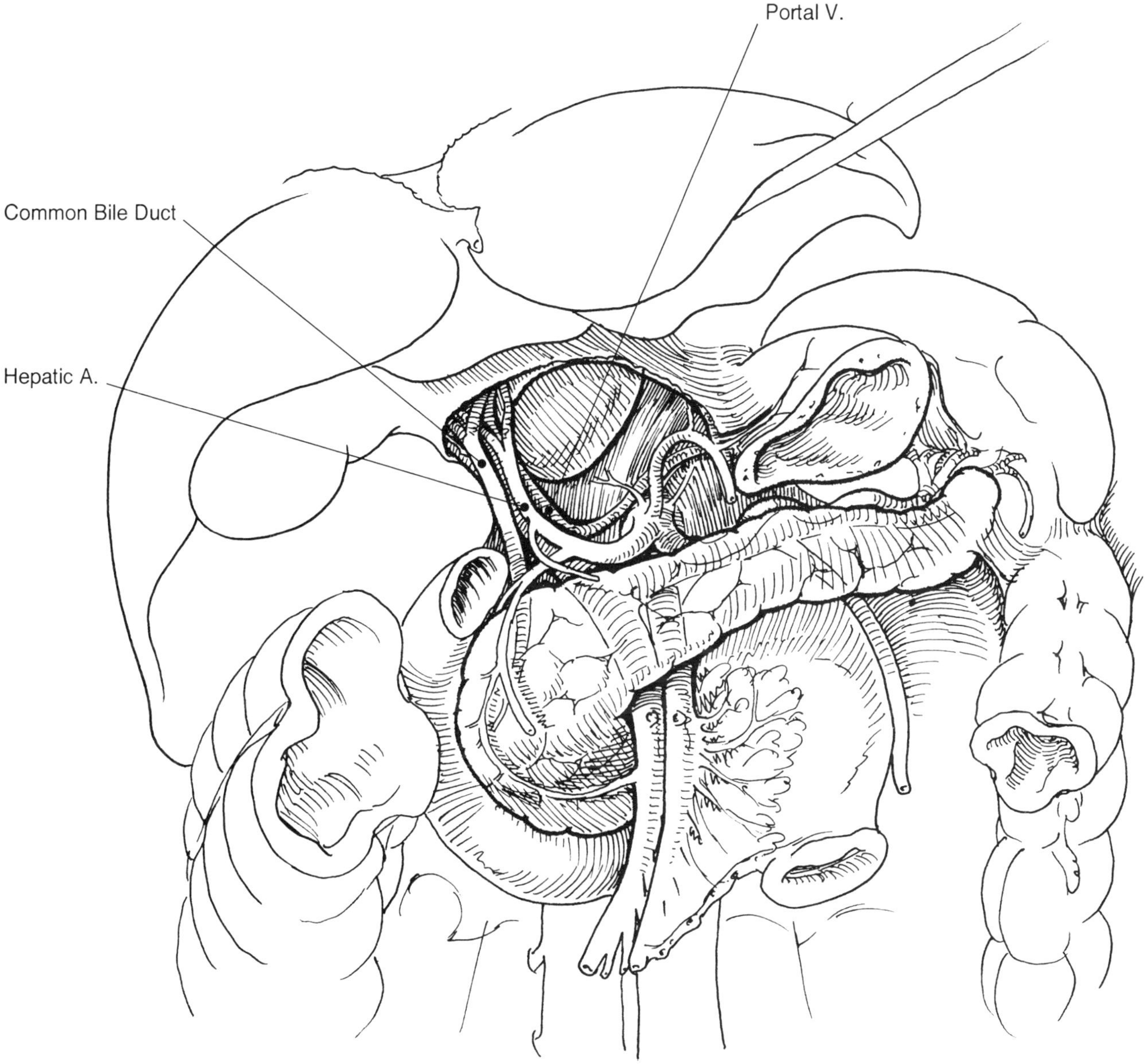

Fig. 2.12

The upper abdominal organs viewed from behind complete the three-dimensional concept of the region (Fig. 2.13). The right lobe of the liver projects back over the upper pole of the kidney, with the right adrenal wedged between the kidney, the liver, and the inferior vena cava. The inferior vena cava lies embedded to a greater or lesser extent in the fossa demarcating the right and left liver lobes. To the left of the vena cava is the caudate lobe of the liver. The gastrohepatic omentum runs from the lesser curve of the stomach to the groove of the ligamentum venosum and the liver hilum. The esophagus lies just to the left of the quadrate lobe between the lower thoracic aorta posteriorly (behind the crus of the diaphragm) and the lateral segment of the left lobe anteriorly. The tapering margin of the left lobe peeks above the cardia of the stomach adjacent to the anterior border of the spleen. The fourth portion of the duodenum rises up between the (removed) body of the pancreas anteriorly and the (removed) aorta posteriorly.

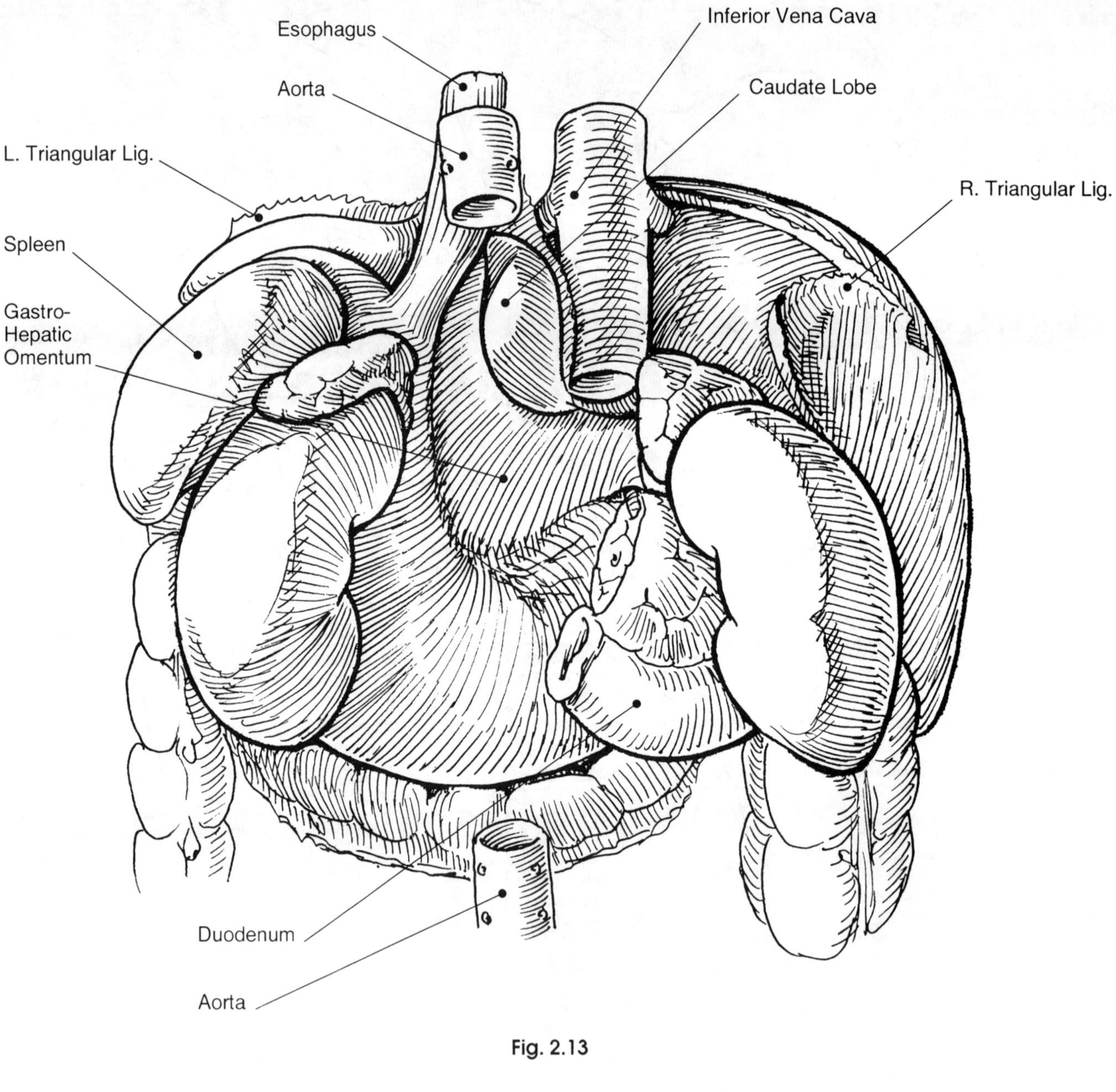

Fig. 2.13

On the underside of the liver the hilum forms a deep transverse central fissure (Fig. 2.14). The main hilar structures, the common hepatic duct, hepatic artery, and portal vein are offset to the right side of the fissure, leaving longer extrahepatic portions of the left branches of each. The plane along the gallbladder fossa and the inferior vena cava basically separates the right lobe from the left (the caudate lobe has some bilobar relationships). At the left end of the hilar fossa, an often incomplete groove contains the round ligament of the liver, the remnant of the umbilical vein. The extrahepatic portion of the round ligament below the umbilical notch lies in the free edge of the falciform ligament. Extending diagonally back from the left end of the hilum is the groove for the ligamentum venosum, which runs from the left branch of the portal vein to the inferior vena cava at the diaphragm. The gastrohepatic omentum also attaches in this groove and continues across the hilum to enfold the main hilar structures as the hepatoduodenal ligament. The caudate lobe lies between the inferior vena cava and the gastrohepatic omentum. It is connected to the right lobe by a narrow isthmus, the caudate process, lying between the hilum and the vena cava. The caudate process is the roof of the epiploic foramen, the passage between the omental bursa and the greater peritoneal cavity. The hepatoduodenal ligament is the anterior margin of the foramen, and the vena cava is the posterior margin. The inferior peritoneal reflection of parietal peritoneum onto the liver passes across the inferior vena cava just below the liver and extends over part of the adrenal indentation on the adjacent right lobe.

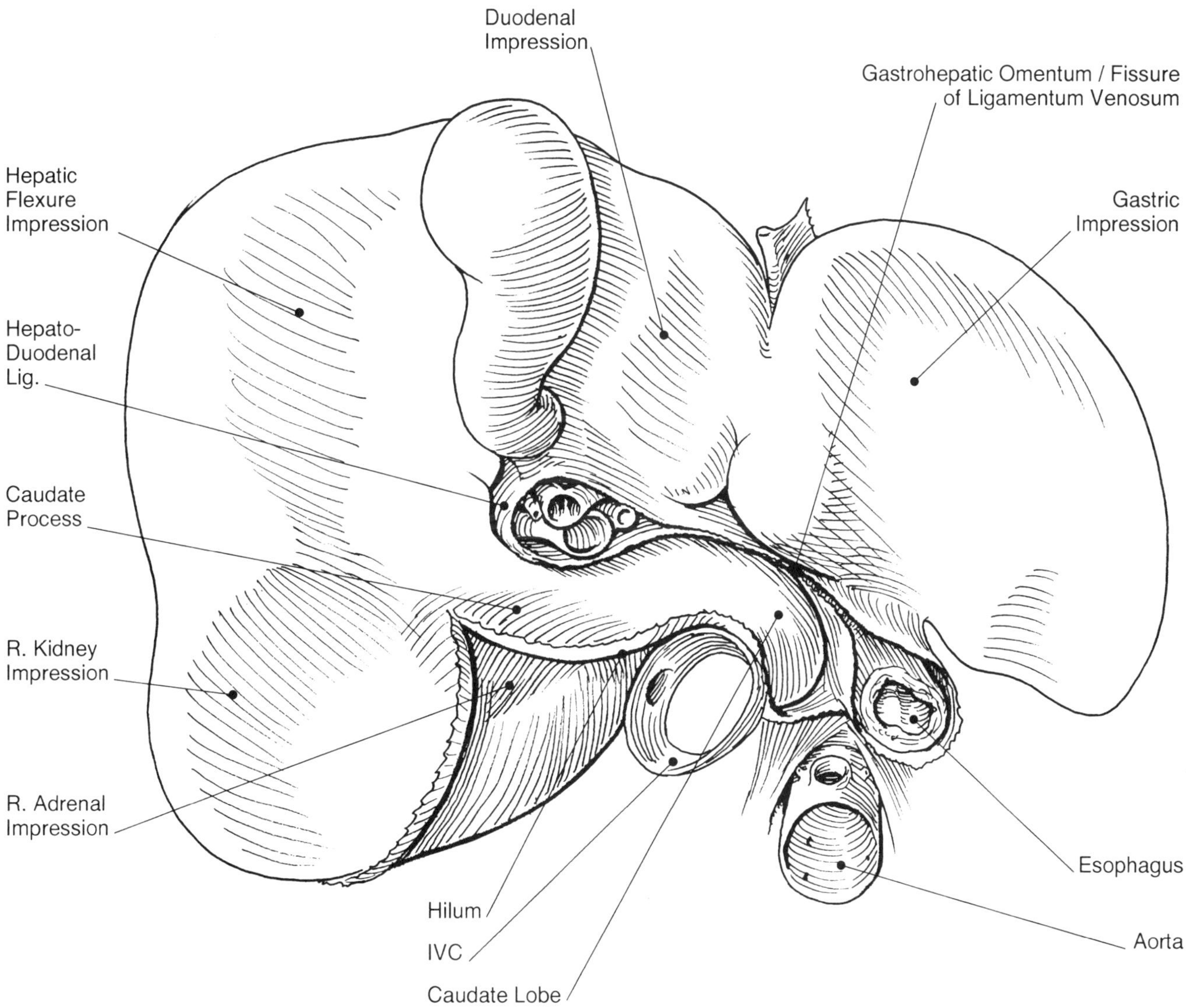

Fig. 2.14

Segmental liver anatomy (shown from an oblique caudal view, Fig. 2.15) is important to the laparoscopic surgeon. Knowledge of the normal bile duct pattern (seen in about 70% of individuals) is necessary for recognition of anomalous patterns, allows recognition of non-visualizing branches on cholangiogram due to obstruction or injury, and alerts the surgeon to structures that can be injured in and around the gallbladder bed. The bile ducts, portal vein branches, and hepatic arterial branches follow a similar pattern of distribution to hepatic segments. The hepatic veins run between segments.

The right and left lobes of the liver are separated by a plane through the gallbladder bed and the inferior vena cava fossa, and each lobe is divided into two segments. The middle hepatic vein lies in this interface between the two lobes. The right lobe is divided into an anterior and posterior segment by an oblique transverse plane which houses the right hepatic vein. The left lobe is divided into medial and lateral segments, with the left hepatic vein lying between. Each of these major segments has a superior and inferior division. The small caudate lobe, behind the superior part of the medial segment, is variably associated with both lobes. The terminal branches of the hepatic arteries and portal vein communicate with the hepatic veins at the level of the hepatic lobules. The portal vessels and ducts enter and exit each segment from the centrally located porta hepatis. The inferior parts of the right anterior and left medial segments

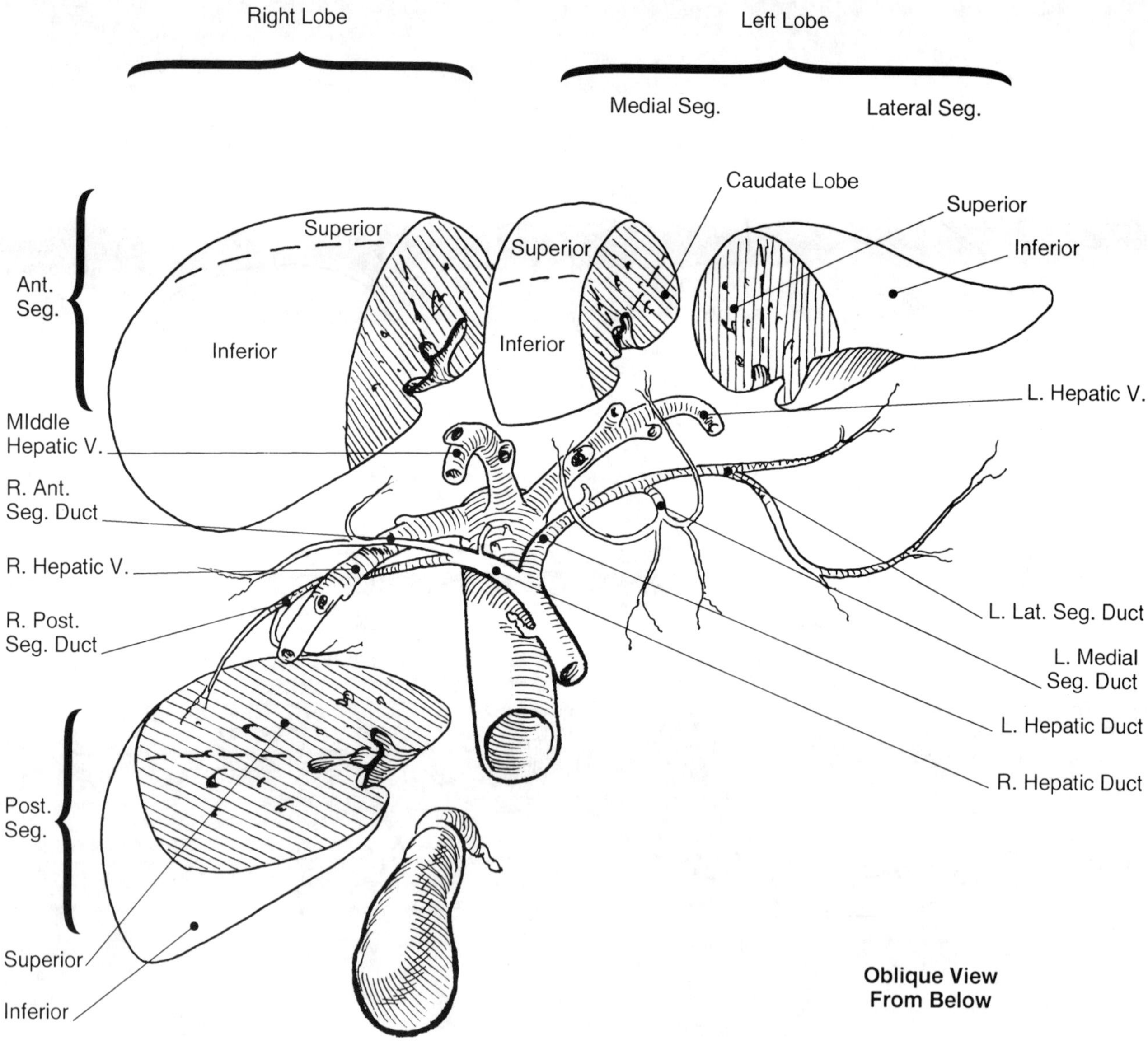

Fig. 2.15

make up the gallbladder bed and the segmental channels of these areas are subject to injury during cholecystectomy.

The usual bile duct pattern seen on cholangiogram (Fig. 2.16A) shows the confluence of the right and left hepatic ducts forming the common hepatic duct at the hilum (90% of the time outside the liver substance). The right hepatic duct is formed by the union of the anterior and posterior segmental ducts, usually close (~1 cm) to the confluence of right and left hepatic ducts. The right anterior segmental duct is shorter and more caudal in position than the posterior segmental duct. In the frontal plane on cholangiogram it appears to bifurcate more medially than the posterior. In about one third of individuals, a subvesical duct exists, lying superficially in the gallbladder bed and draining into the right anterior duct. Unlike other bile ducts, it is not accompanied by a branch of the portal vein. It does not communicate with the gallbladder but is vulnerable to injury during cholecystectomy.

The confluence of the left lateral superior and inferior ducts is usually at or to the right of the left segmental fissure. The superior branch is long and thin and drains the apex of the left lobe, including the fibrous appendix representing regressed embryonic liver tissue. In a small percent of individuals (~5%), bile ducts may persist in this fibrous band and cause bile leak when this band is transected in dividing the left triangular ligament of the liver.

The superior and inferior portions of the medial segment of the left lobe are drained by four small ducts. The junction of the medial segmental duct with the lateral forms the left hepatic duct toward the center of the liver hilus. The caudate portion of the medial segment (see Fig. 2.14) drains in three parts. The caudate process, farthest to the right, usually drains into the right ductal system, the left side

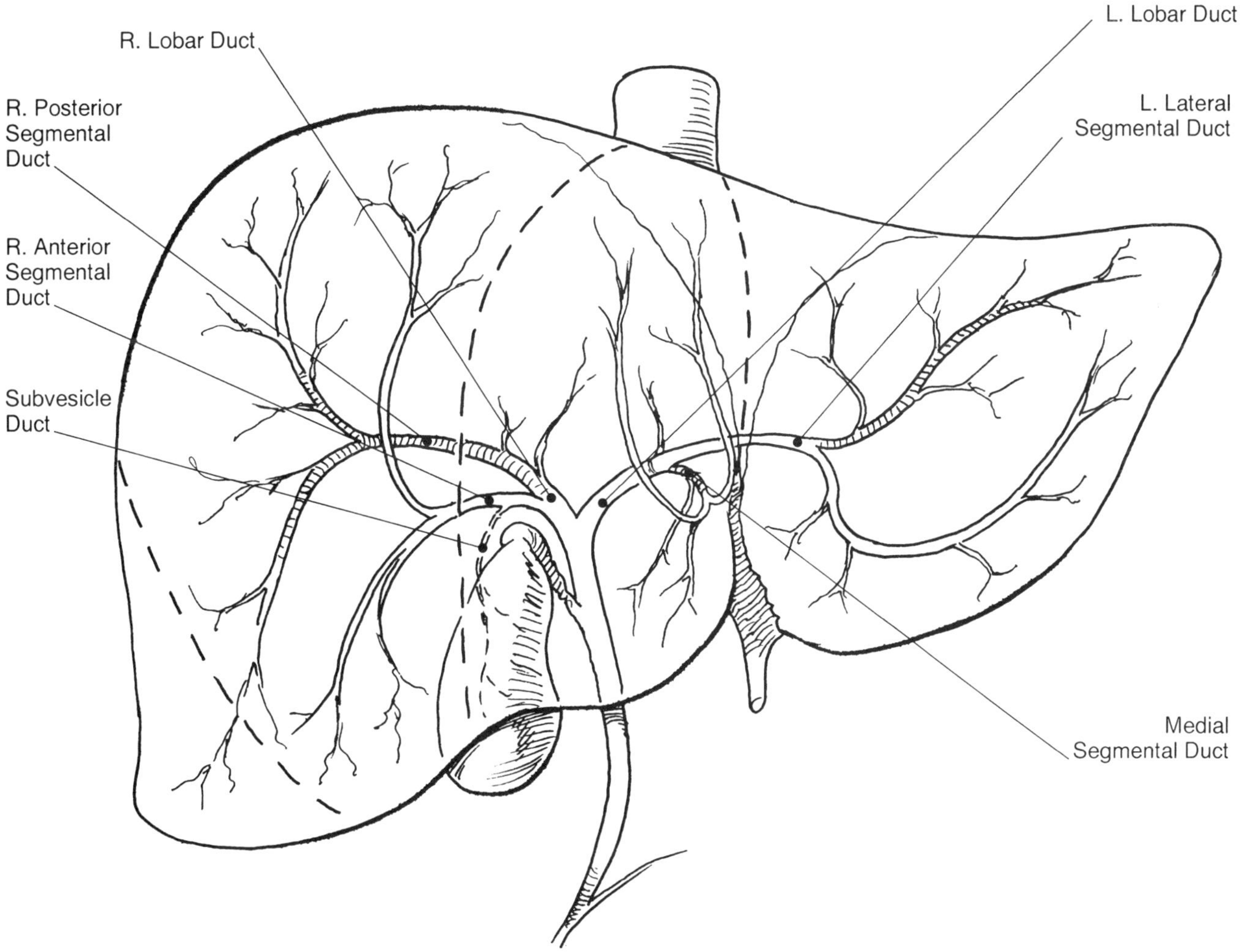

Fig. 2.16A

of the caudate lobe usually drains to the left system and the right portion of the caudate lobe between the two is equally likely to drain into either.

There is a moderate amount of variation in the intrahepatic bile duct pattern. Centrally, the main right and left hepatic ducts usually converge in the liver hilum (10% of the time within the liver substance). In about 22% of individuals, the right posterior segmental duct may cross the lobar fissure and drain into the left hepatic duct (Fig. 2.16B). In 6% of cases, the right anterior segmental duct crosses to the left (Fig. 2.16C). Separate drainage of the right segmental ducts leads to confusion and injury during cholecystectomy. These ducts are properly called aberrant rather than accessory since they drain normal liver regions and are not supplemental. On the left side, the medial segmental duct drains into the inferior division of the lateral segmental duct about a quarter of the time (Fig. 2.16D).

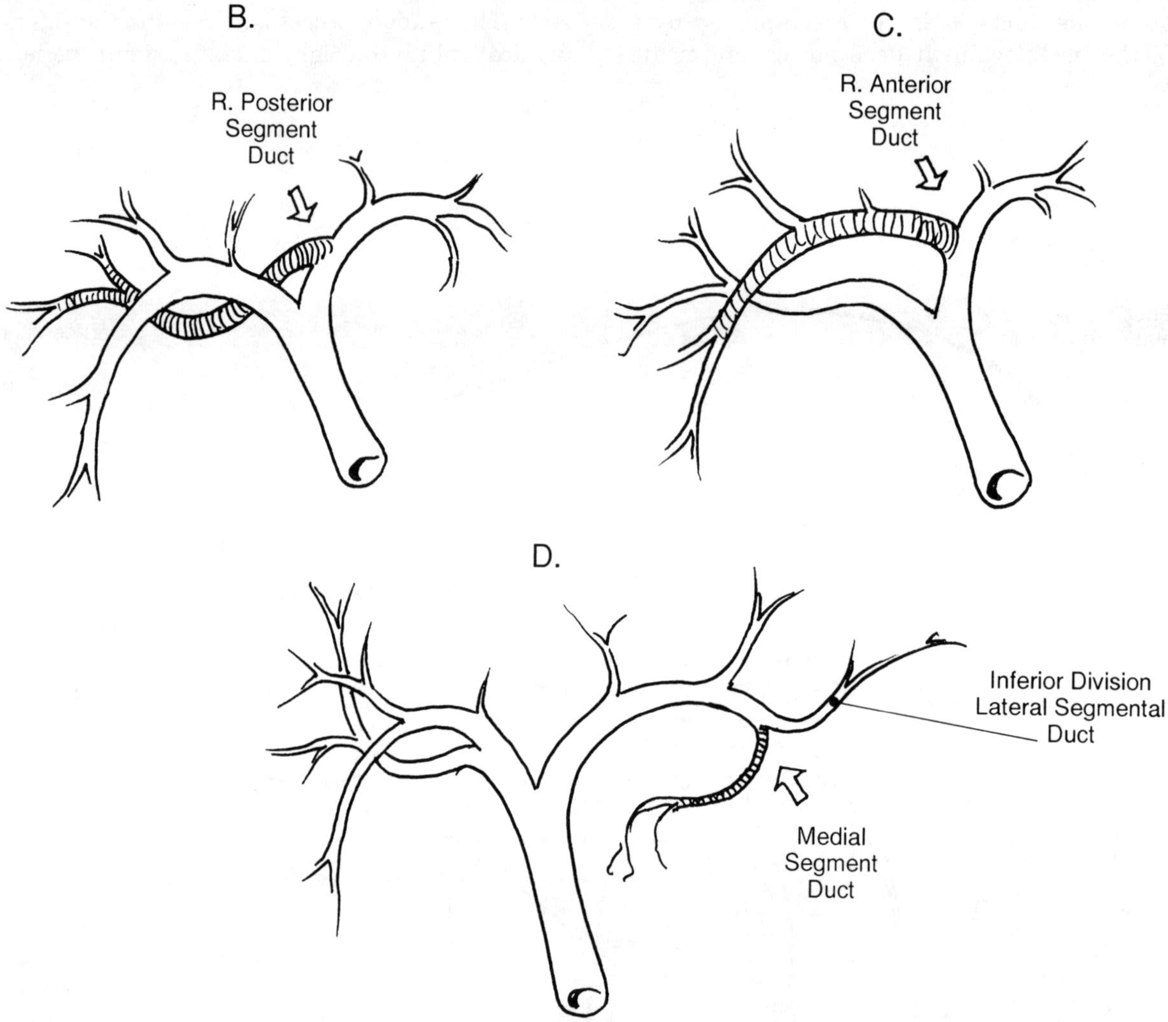

Fig. 2.16 B, C, D

Of the peripheral branches, the right posterior superior branch is the most constant. The other subsegmental branches drain into alternate channels about 20% of the time.

The portal vein distribution viewed from below (Fig. 2.17), reflects the segmental anatomy of the liver. The portal vein divides outside the liver toward the right side of the hilum, leaving a longer segment of the left branch in the portal fissure. The right branch lies close beneath the folded over infundibulum of the gallbladder where it is vulnerable to injury. The right division usually divides into anterior and posterior branches to the two major segments of the right lobe, which are oriented anterior-superior and posterior-inferior. The two branches occasionally originate at the main portal division, creating a trifurcation. During cholecystectomy, the right branch of the portal vein is subject to injury near the liver hilum.

The left branch of the portal vein arches anteriorly into the liver substance at the groove for the round ligament. It divides into branches to the medial and lateral segments of the left lobe. Each segmental branch supplies the superior and inferior parts of that segment. Proximal branches of the main right and left portal veins supply the caudate lobe. Some venous drainage from the gallbladder goes to the right branch of the portal vein, but a significant amount drains directly into the liver bed.

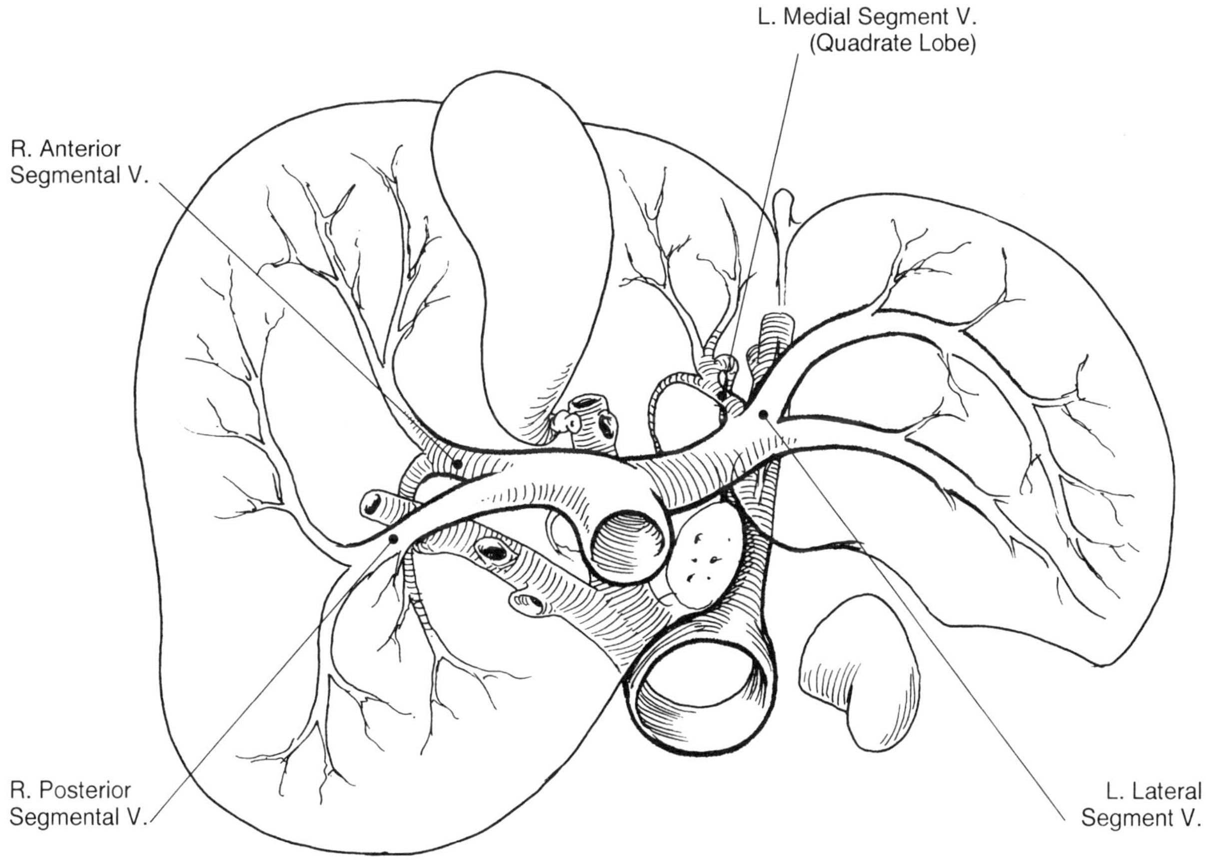

Fig. 2.17

The Gallbladder

The origin of the gallbladder as the caudal component of the hepatic diverticulum, and its progression through solid and revacuolization stages results in many variations, each occurring a small percentage of the time (Fig. 2.18). Duplications result from early appearance of more than one gallbladder bud (Fig. 2.18A). Usually both gallbladders lie to the right of the falciform ligament, but at least one instance of bilobar position has been reported. A bilobed gallbladder on a single stem or a diverticulum occurs when the early bud grows in a lobulated manner (Fig. 2.18B).

The final position and freedom of the gallbladder depends on its relationship to the developing liver mass. The gallbladder may occasionally be found beneath the lateral division of the left lobe to the left of the falciform ligament or may be flipped posteriorly (Fig. 2.18C). The gallbladder may be largely surrounded by liver substance or even totally embedded (Fig. 2.18D). At the opposite extreme, it may hang free with a partial or complete mesentery. Instances of a gallbladder in the falciform ligament and herniated into the epiploic foramen have been reported.

The shape and internal structure of the gallbladder may vary (Fig. 2.18E). Constrictions may occur along the length of the organ. A proximal constriction may be mistaken for the cystic duct, resulting in a gallbladder remnant being left after surgery. Internal septations result from incomplete vacuolization which happens late in biliary development. Such septae may be longitudinal or transverse. The latter often result in a folded appearance at the fundus, the Phrygian cap. The proximal end of the gallbladder, the infundibulum, is often dilated (Hartman's pouch) and folded in a sigmoid shape. Carefully dissect and unfold this bend to safely identify the underlying cystic duct.

The length, diameter, and junction points of the cystic duct may vary (Fig. 2.18F). The long duct provides an extra margin of safety, whereas the short duct is more hazardous for the laparoscopist. Rarely, there is virtually no duct, with a broad-based attachment. Very rarely, there may be two separate cystic ducts from a single gallbladder. The critical reference point in laparoscopic cholecystectomy, the transition between infundibulum and cystic duct, may be abrupt and sharp or may taper gradually (Fig. 2.18G).

Much controversy has occurred over the frequency or even existence of direct connections (ducts of Lushka) between the gallbladder and intrahepatic ducts in the adult (Fig. 2.18H). Although such connections are occasionally reported (more prominent

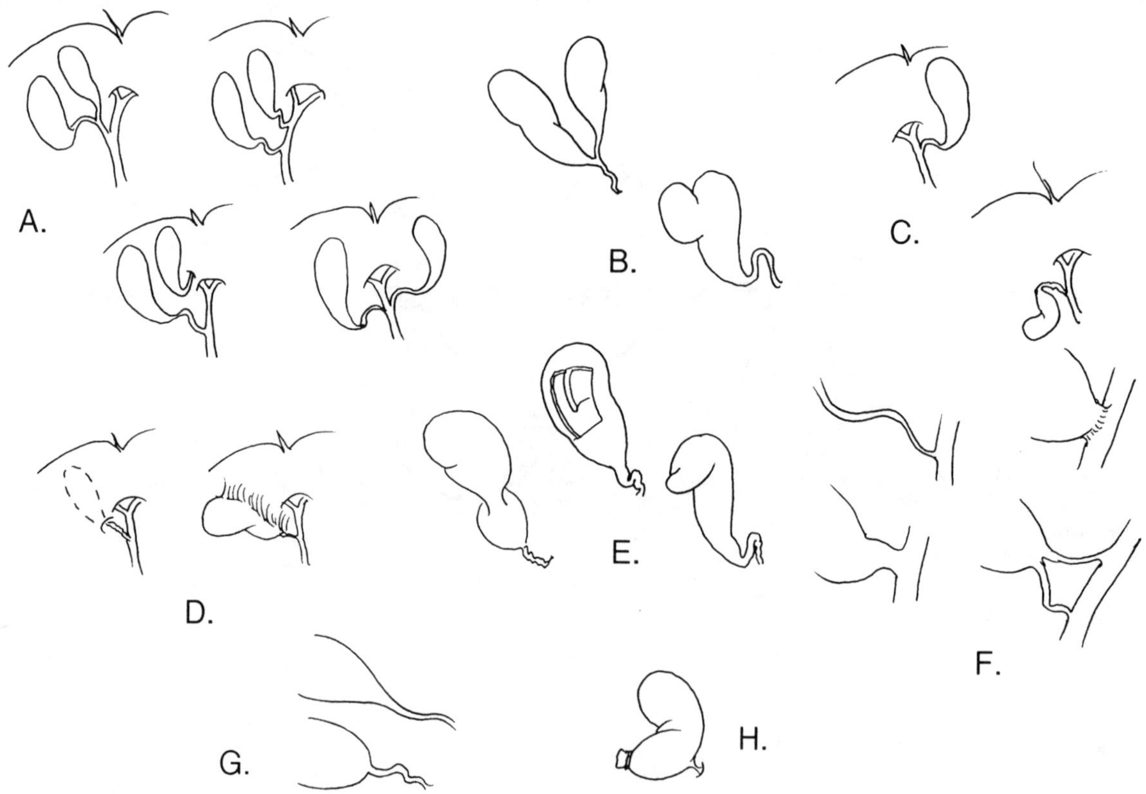

Fig. 2.18

in infants), most significant bile leaks from the gallbladder bed result from injury to underlying segmental hepatic ducts, especially the subvesical duct seen in one third of individuals..

Although the two or three most common variant anatomic patterns usually account for 90-95% of instances the surgeon will encounter, rare and unexpected anomalies should be kept in mind and lead the surgeon to proceed with caution, especially around the biliary system. For example, there is a case report (Kihne) of right and left hepatic ducts draining into the body of the gallbladder in the liver bed with a blindly ending hepatic duct stump. Only a preoperative ERCP or a preemptive operative cholangiogram through the gallbladder could have identified the anomaly before dissection began, and there was no apparent reason for doing either. Routine cholaniography may avert complete transection in such a case.

The presence of a large stone may cause inflammation and pressure necrosis leading to fistula formation between the gallbladder and an adjacent structure (Fig. 2.19). A stone in the fundus may erode and pass into the duodenum producing intermittent bouts of obstruction over a few-day period (gallstone ileus). A cholecysto-colonic fistula may also form. In both cases, air may be seen in the biliary tree. A stone impacted in Hartmann's pouch, either one that is folded next to the common duct or one that is close by virtue of a short or absent cystic duct, may erode into the common duct causing obstructive jaundice (Mirizzi's syndrome).

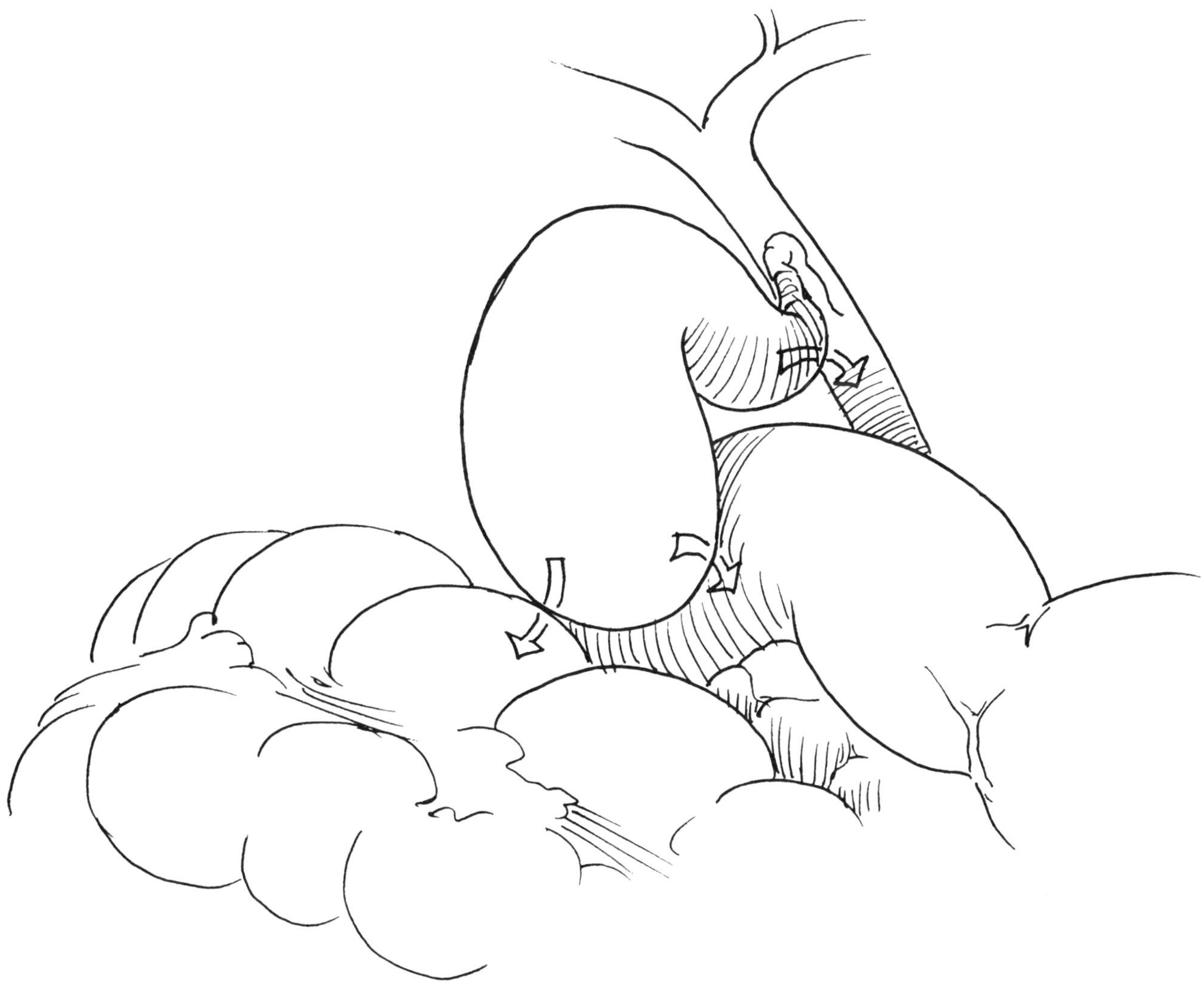

Fig. 2.19

Extrahepatic Bile Ducts

The right and left hepatic ducts normally unite toward the right side of the portal fissure to form the common hepatic duct (Fig. 2.20). The common hepatic duct lies anterior and to the right in the portal triad of bile duct, hepatic artery, and portal vein. The common hepatic duct usually receives the cystic duct and is called the common duct from that point distally.

The junction of cystic and common hepatic duct forms a distinct angle in two thirds to three quarters

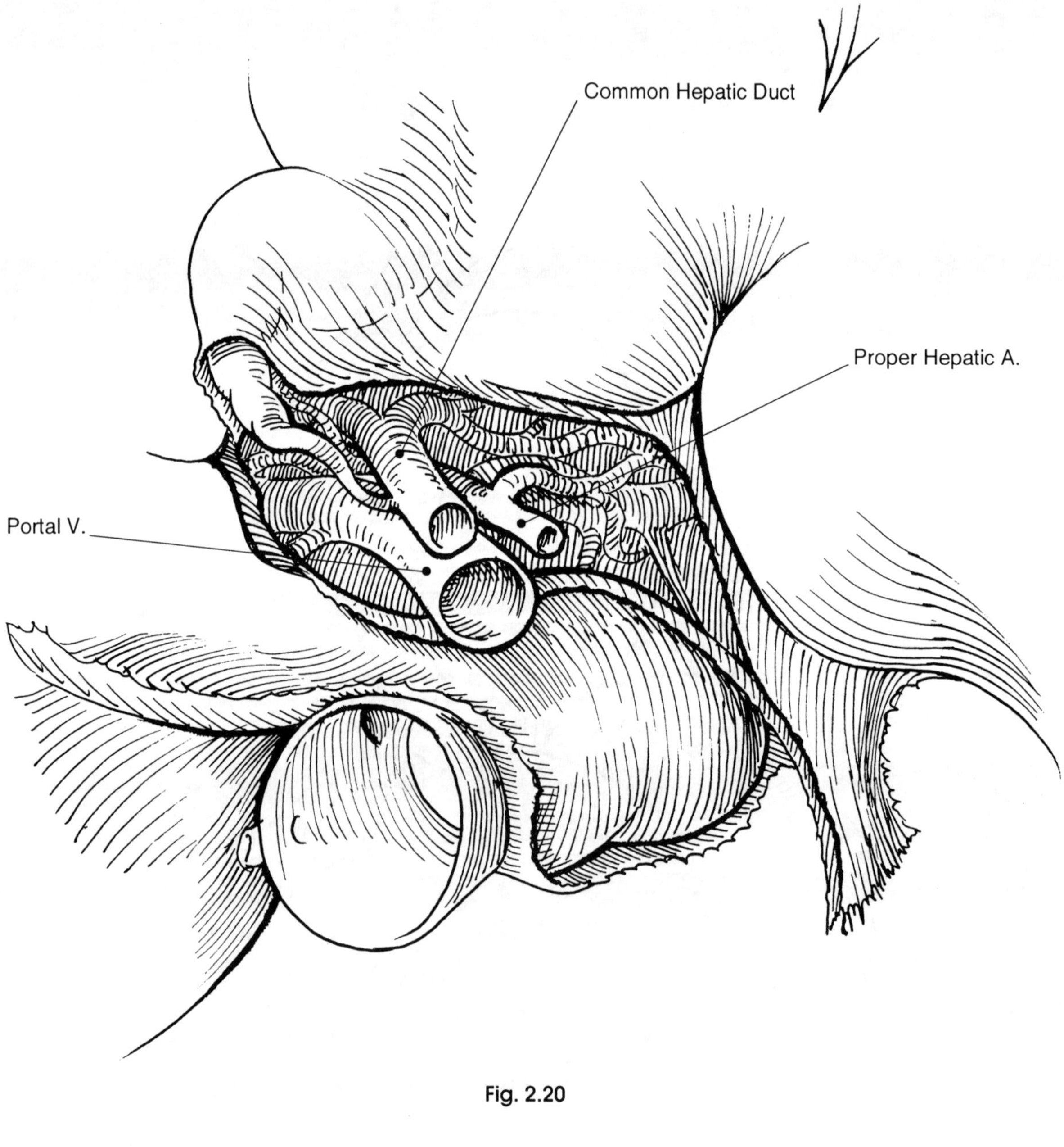

Fig. 2.20

of individuals (Fig. 2.21A), the rest having a parallel course for a variable distance (Fig. 2.21B). The parallel segment of cystic duct is often bound so that identification is difficult. In most cases the opening lies above the duodenum. If the gallbladder is used for biliary bypass, confirm by cholangiogram that the cystic duct orifice is well above the obstruction. The cystic duct often enters the posterior (Fig. 2.21C) or left side (Fig. 2.21D) of the common duct. In the latter case, it most frequently passes behind the common duct. The cystic duct may join the biliary tree anywhere from the liver hilum to the duodenum (Fig. 2.21E) and may join one of the hepatic ducts, usually the right. It may also join an aberrant right hepatic duct or a division of the right hepatic duct, usually the posterior (Fig. 2.21F).

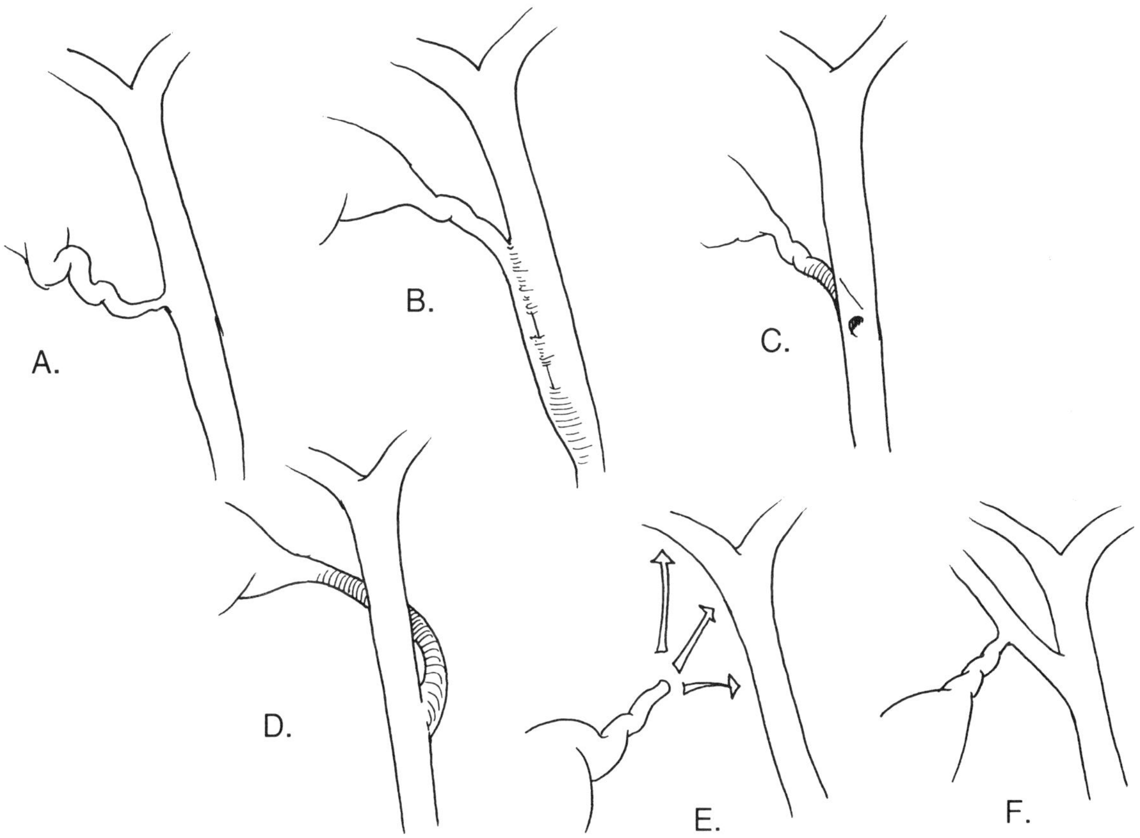

Fig. 2.21

The common bile duct has a short supraduodenal course in the hepatoduodenal ligament, a retroduodenal and a pancreatic portion (Fig. 2.22). In three quarters of individuals, the tapering distal end of the common duct enters the mid portion of the descending doudenum (second portion) on its medial wall. The rest most often enter more distally, rarely more proximally.

The pancreatic portion of the common duct may be totally enclosed in pancreatic substance, or may lie in a groove of variable length depending on the amount of duct surrounded by the dorsal anlage during

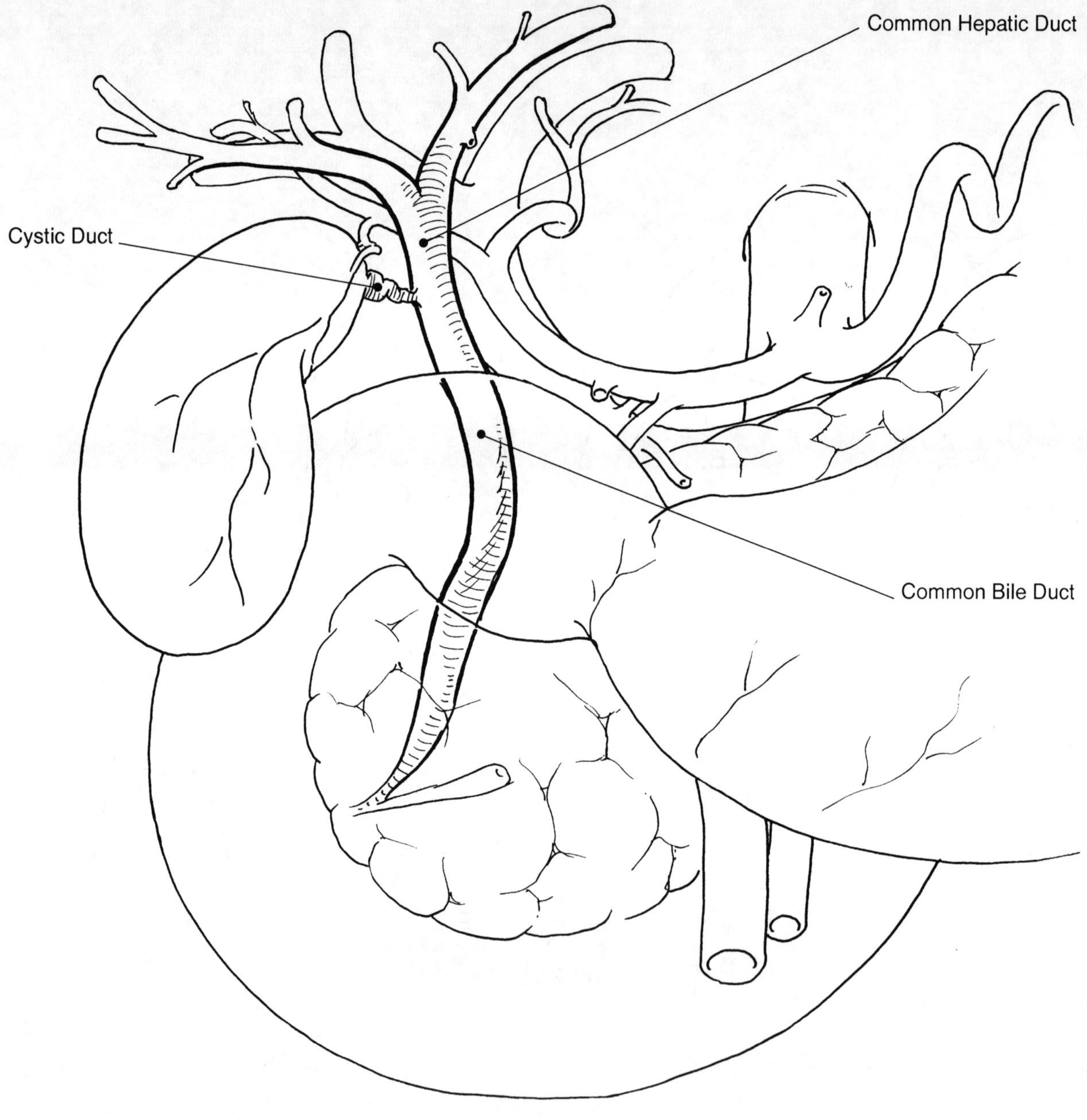

Fig. 2.22

embryonic fusion (Fig. 2.23). The junction of common and pancreatic ducts reflects the origin of the ventral pancreatic bud from the embryonic bile duct. The length of common ampullary channel in most individuals is about one third the length of the ducts' parallel course. Most of the remainder have complete septation and separate duodenal entrance of common and pancreatic ducts.

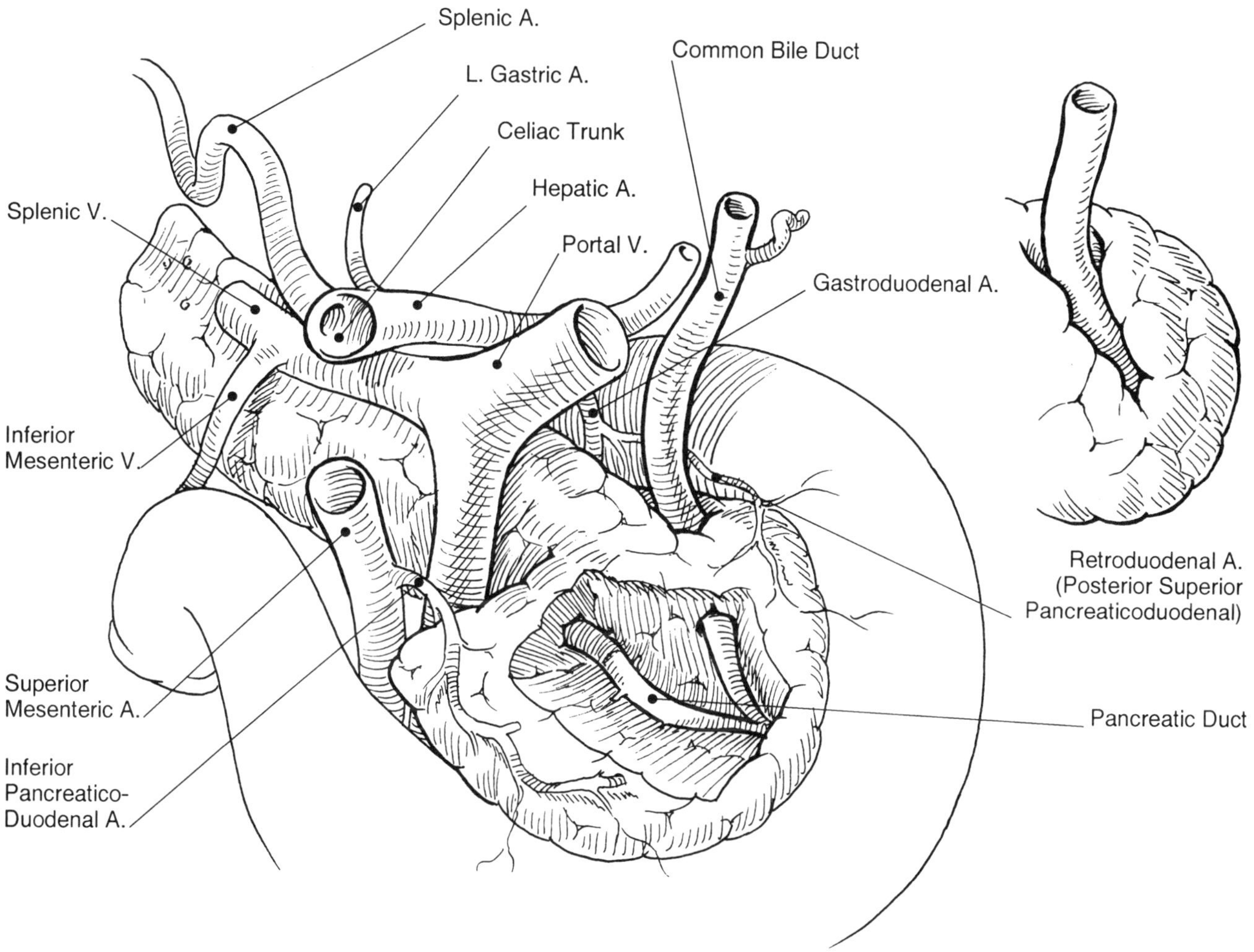

Fig. 2.23

Anomalous bile duct drainage at the liver hilus is not uncommon (~12%) and usually involves right-sided ducts (Fig. 2.24A). They may join the ductal system, including the cystic duct, anywhere along its course. Rare anomalies of the bile ducts as noted above should always be kept in mind.

The location of the cystic duct junction determines the length of the common hepatic duct. When the junction is at the bifurcation of right and left hepatic ducts, there is by definition no common hepatic duct (Fig. 2.24B)

Duplication of the common hepatic/common duct are rare and result from the persistence of two main stems of the hepatic bud (Fig. 2.24C). The cystic duct usually connects to the independent right duct while the left duct connects with the pancreatic duct. There may be cross connections.

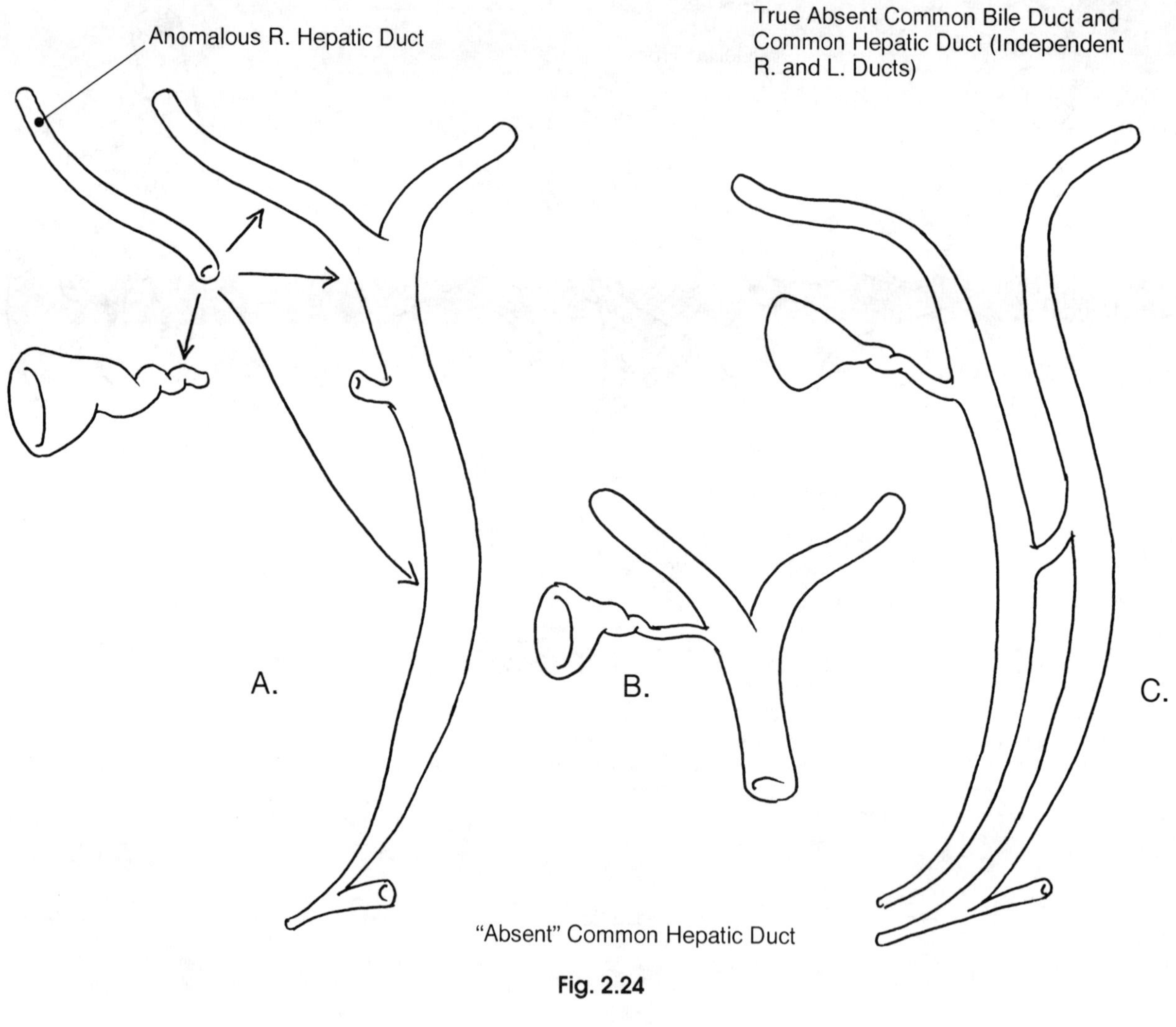

Fig. 2.24

Hepatobiliary Arterial Supply

The biliary arterial blood supply is even more variable than the bile ducts. This is in contrast to the constancy of the portal venous system which supplies 60-70% of hepatic blood flow and significant amounts of oxygen. A common hepatic artery arises from the celiac trunk about 80% of the time (Fig. 2.25) with a small percent (5-8%) arising directly from the aorta or from the superior mesenteric artery. Only 55% of the time is this vessel the sole artery to the liver, however. In 12% of individuals, there is no common trunk giving rise to right and left hepatic branches but rather separate right and left hepatic arteries from one of several sites. They may arise separately from the celiac trunk, from its branches, from the aorta or from the superior mesenteric artery.

Beneath the posterior peritoneum of the lesser sac, the common hepatic artery runs a short distance to the right along the superior border of the pancreas, raising the hepatopancreatic fold in the peritoneum at the caudal margin of the epiploic foramen. There it gives off the gastroduodenal artery, which descends on the pancreatic head behind the first portion of the duodenum. The continuation of the main vessel is called the proper hepatic artery. It gives off the right gastric artery and turns up into the hepatoduodenal ligament, the free edge of the gastrohepatic omentum. The proper hepatic artery ascends to the left and anterior in the portal triad and bifurcates into right and left branches near the liver hilum. The right branch usually passes dorsal to the common hepatic duct to enter the hepatocystic triangle (cystic duct, hepatic duct, and underside of the liver).

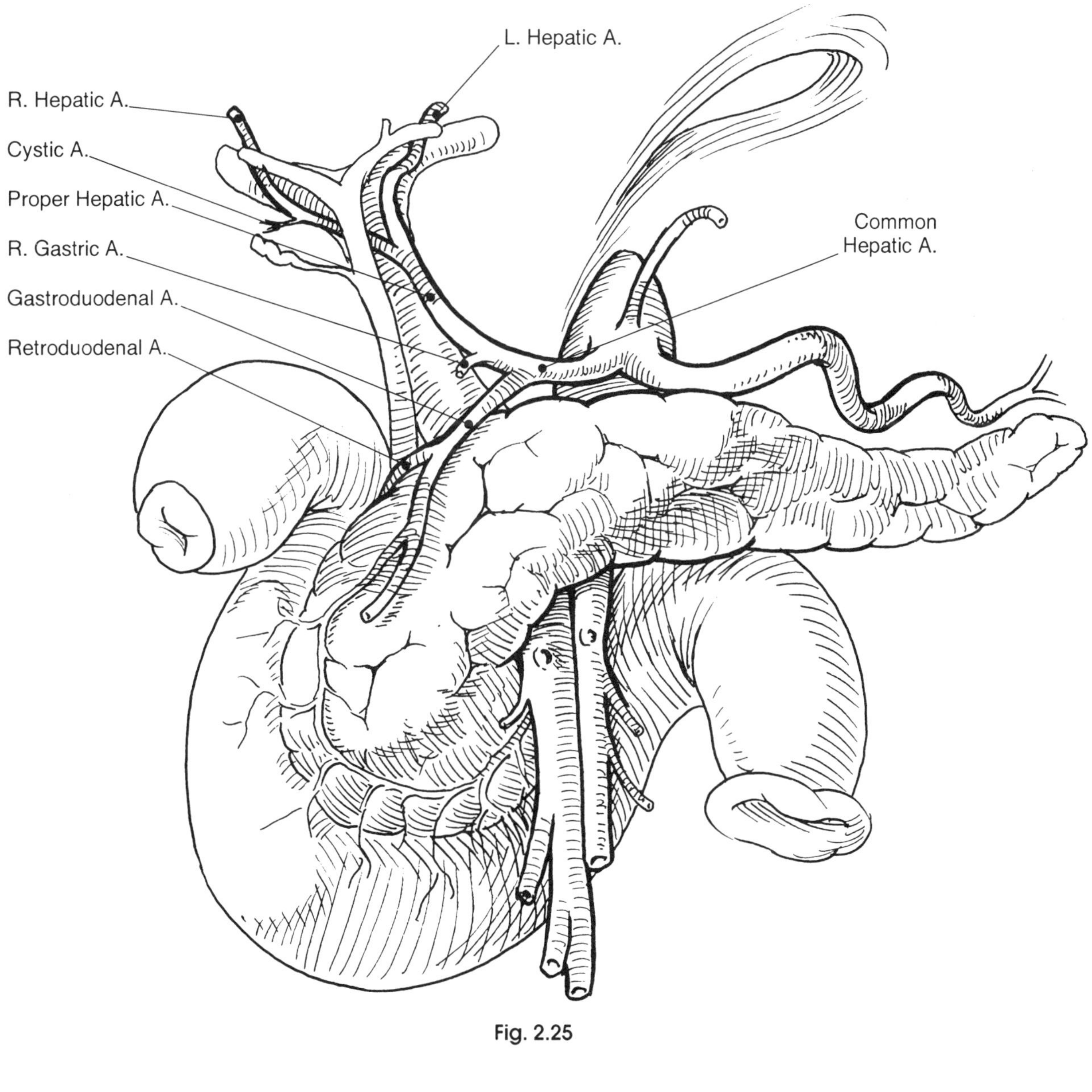

Fig. 2.25

The right hepatic artery arising from a normal proper hepatic passes posterior to the common hepatic duct in three quarters of the population and anterior in the rest (Fig. 2.26A, B). In many cases (15%)

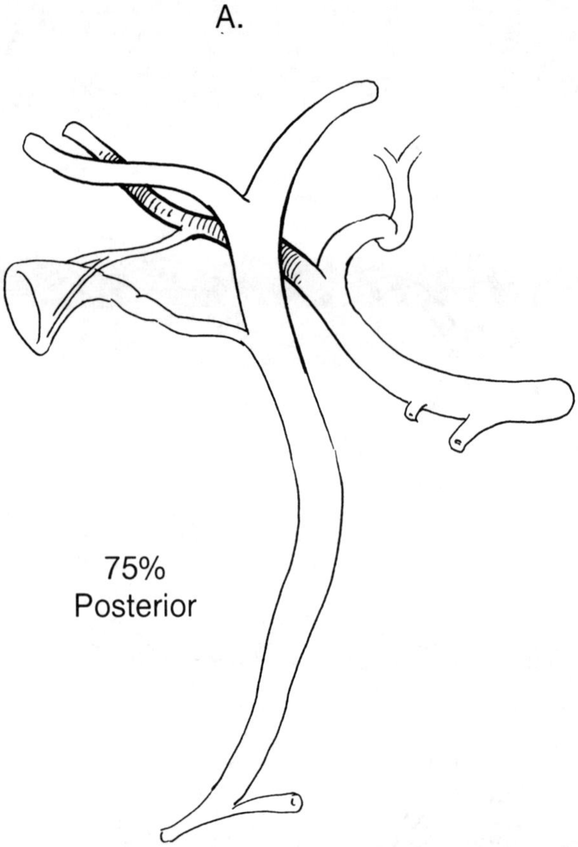

Fig. 2.26 A, B

the right hepatic artery bows close to the cystic duct, a "caterpillar hump" configuration (Fig. 2.26C), that puts the vessel in jeopardy during cholecystectomy.

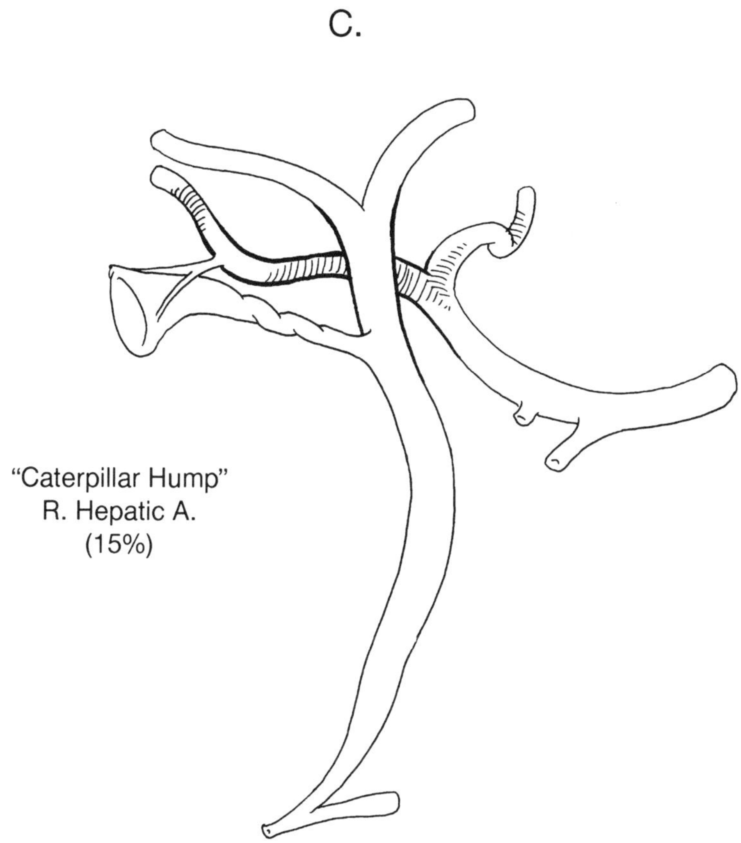

Fig. 2.26C

The anomalous right and left hepatic arteries each occur close to 20% of the time (Fig. 2.27A). Slightly more than half of such vessels replace the branch that would normally appear on the proper hepatic, and the rest are accessory to the corresponding branch. The anomalous left hepatic commonly arises from the arch of the left gastric artery and passes through the cephalad part of the gastrohepatic omentum to the left lobe of the liver. The anomalous right branch commonly arises from the proximal superior mesenteric artery behind the neck of the pancreas (Fig. 2.27B). It crosses deep to the superior mesenteric vein and the common duct and ascends to the right. It usually passes deep to the cystic duct and enters the hepatocystic triangle where it is subject to injury.

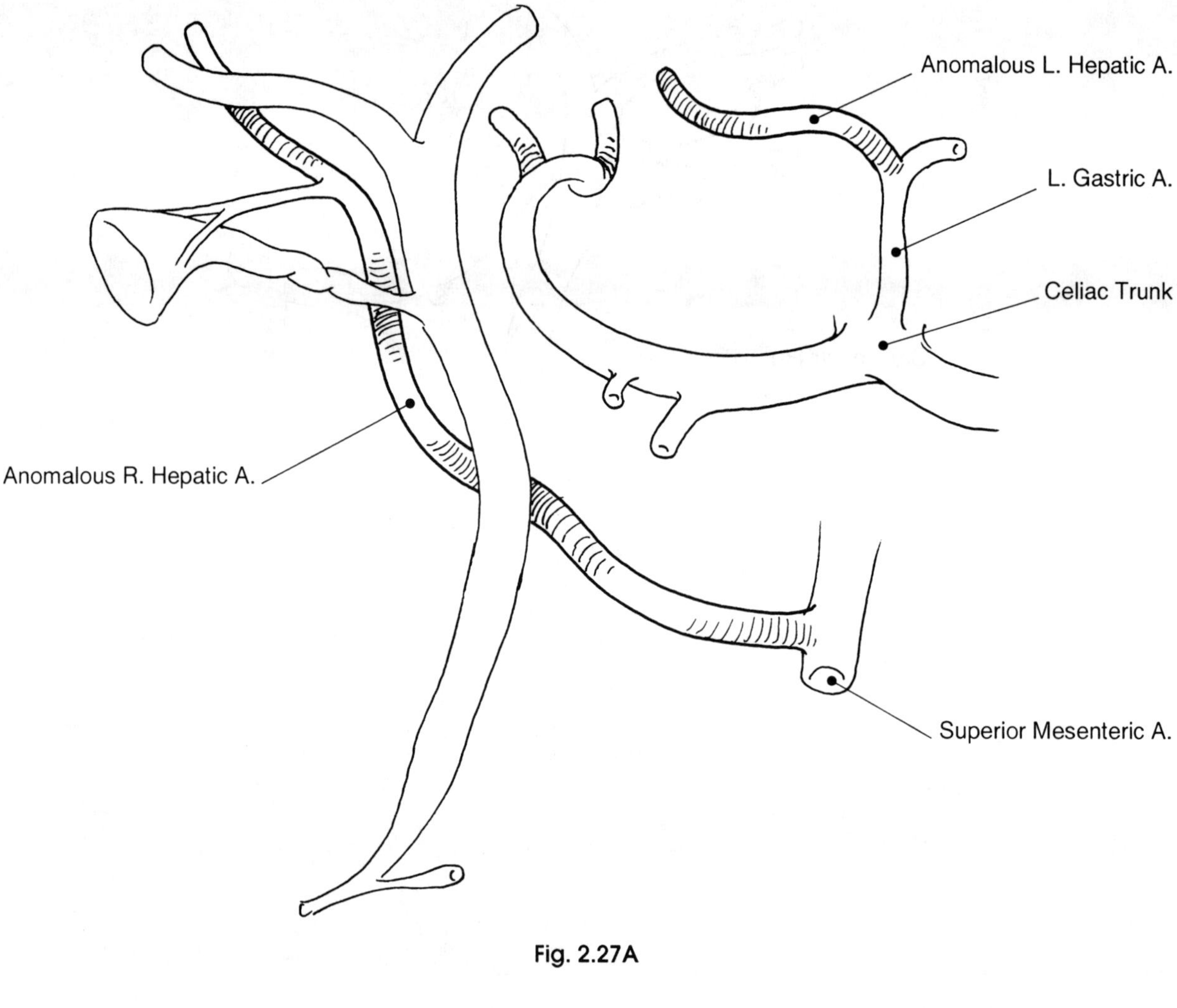

Fig. 2.27A

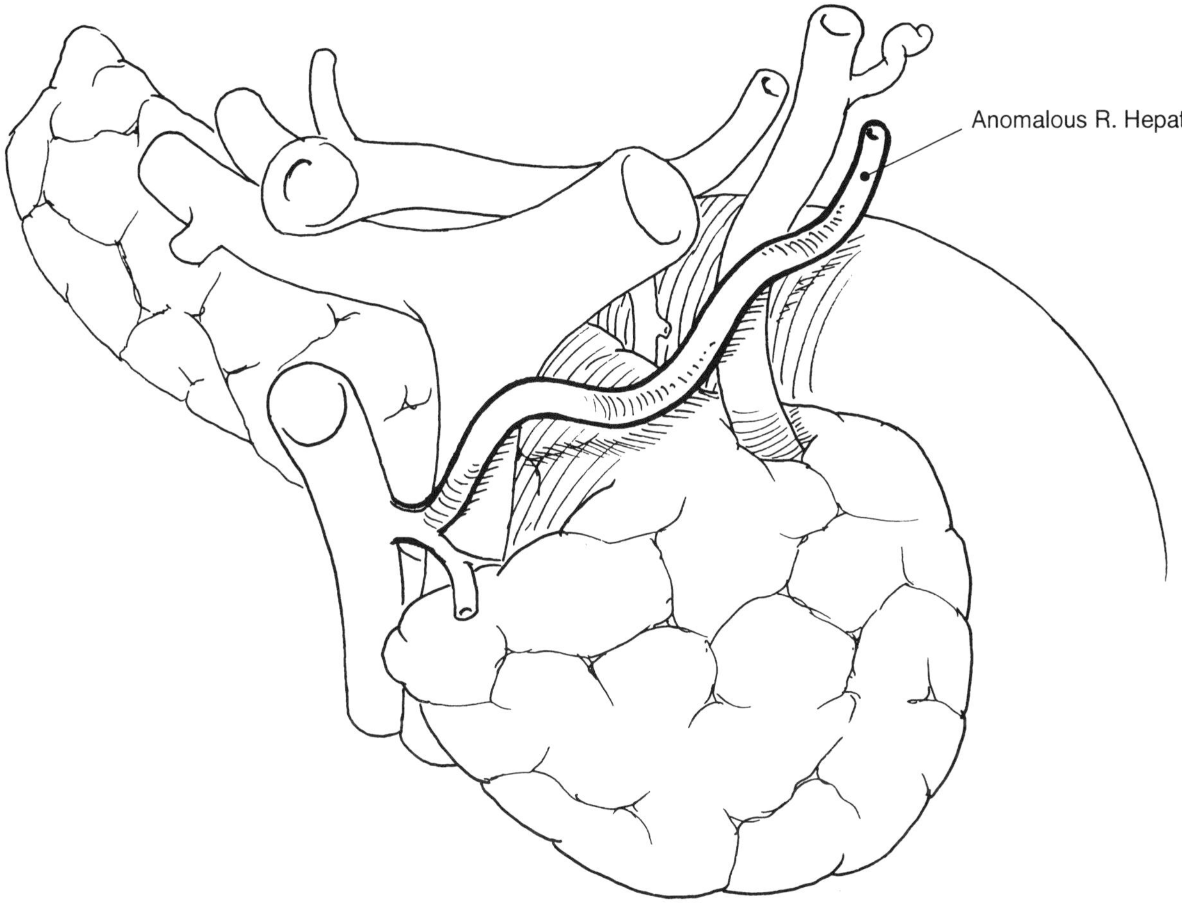

Fig. 2.27B

Three quarters of the time, the cystic artery arises from the usual posterior right hepatic artery to form the triangle of Calot (Fig. 2.28). It is usually marked by a sentinel lymph node. As the artery approaches the neck of the gallbladder, it gives off a small cystic duct branch and divides into deep and superficial branches. The deep branch lies between the gallbladder and the liver bed. The artery may bifurcate early. If only the superficial branch is ligated, the deep branch can cause troublesome bleeding.

One quarter of the time, the cystic artery arises outside of the hepatocystic triangle from any of the neighboring vessels. Such cystic vessels invariably pass anterior to the common hepatic or common duct. Occasionally the cystic artery is double, both branches usually coming from the right hepatic artery. When a cystic artery bifurcation is not identified, the presence of a second cystic vessel should be suspected.

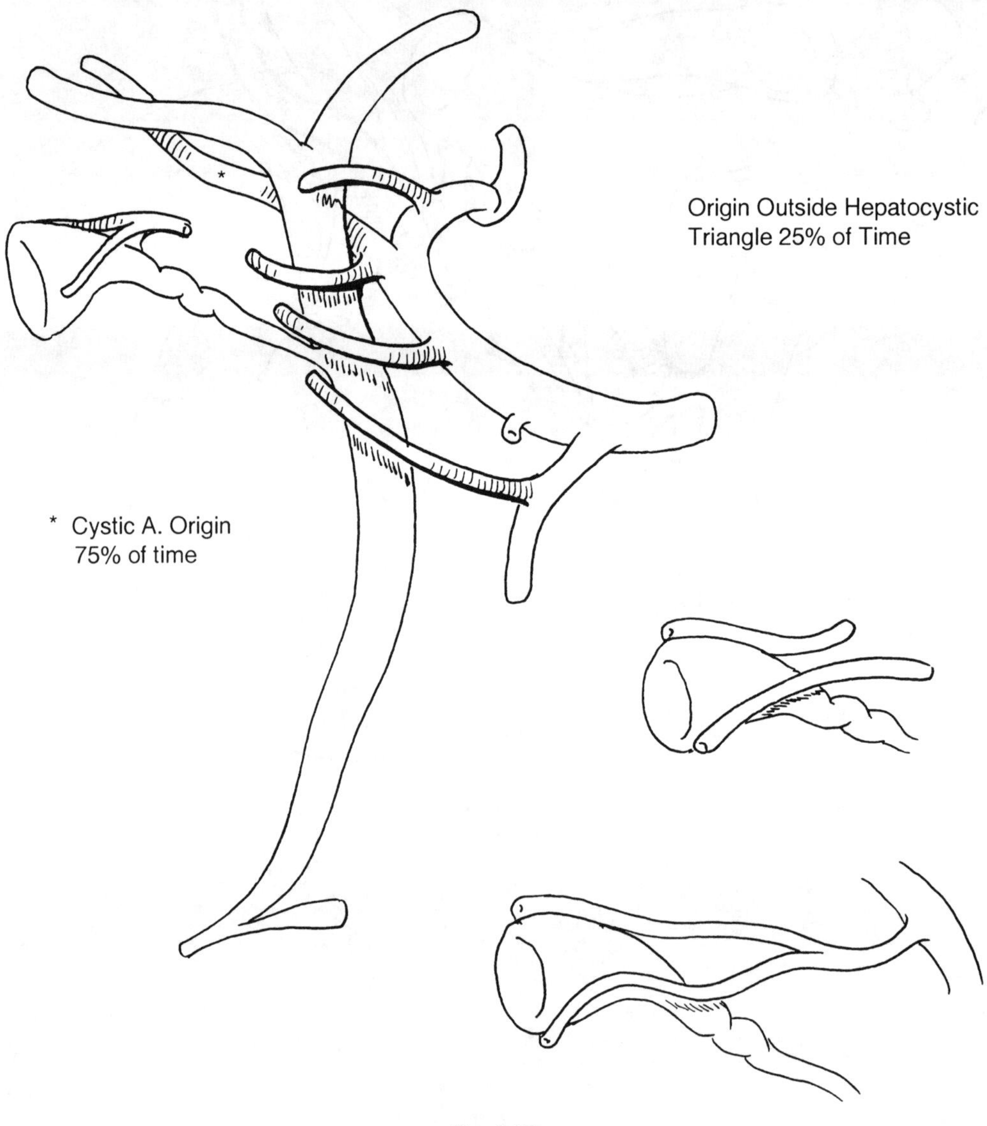

Fig. 2.28

The extrahepatic bile ducts are surrounded by a delicate network of vessels called the epicholedochal plexus (Fig. 2.29). This plexus receives feeder vessels from the hepatic and cystic arteries above and from the gastroduodenal and its retroduodenal branch from below. Variation in hepatic artery patterns modifies the source vessels to some extent. The tiny (0.3 mm) vessels on the duct surface often coalesce into axial vessels running medially and laterally along the superduodenal portion of the common duct. The dominant blood supply to this watershed area comes from below. It is the most vulnerable area for ischemic compromise and the most common site of post operative strictures. Mechanical stripping of the plexus, crush injury, and direct and indirect thermal injury (especially with monopolar cautery) are potential mechanisms of damage.

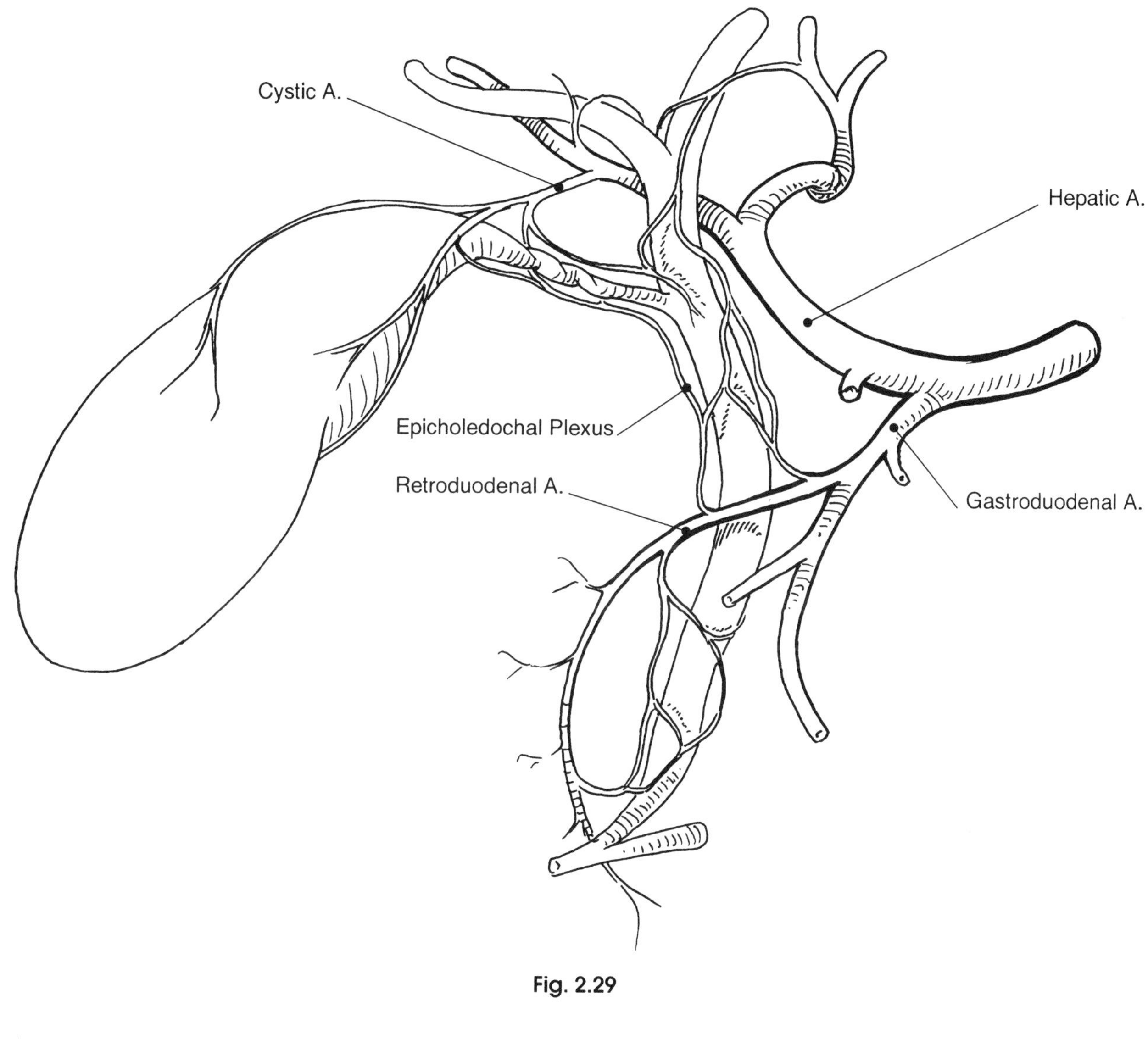

Fig. 2.29

LAPAROSCOPIC BILIARY SURGERY

Background

Open cholecystectomy has been performed for a hundred years and is the standard against which the morbidity and mortality of laparoscopic cholecystectomy must be compared. Laparoscopic cholecystectomy was first performed in France in 1987 and in the United States in 1988. The relearning period is now over for most trained surgeons and morbidity and mortality have stabilized at a level comparable to open surgery. The incidence of major bile duct injury by laparoscopy, although still a small percent (.2-.6%), is two to three times the rate with open (.07-.1). The potential devastating nature of these injuries and the large number of cholecystectomies performed makes prevention of these injuries a major concern. The laparoscopic technique is now a routine part of residency training. Because the great majority of cholecystectomies are now performed laparoscopically, residency training must include open technique for those occasions when it is needed.

Many patients with gallstones are asymptomatic and are not surgical candidates since complications are invariably preceded by symptoms. Exceptions are those patients in whom the risk of gallbladder cancer is increased (porcelain gallbladder, solitary polyp larger than one cm., anomalous pancreatic/bile duct junction, age over 65 with longstanding symptoms, and a stone larger than 3 cm). For patients with symptomatic gallstones or documented biliary dyskinesia (less than 30% ejection 20 minutes after cholecystokinin stimulation), laparoscopic cholecystectomy is the procedure of choice. As of February 1993, it was estimated that 80% of the 600,000 cholecystectomies done in the United States annually were being done laparoscopically. There have been significant benefits in shortened patient recovery time and decreased discomfort. Challenges currently being addressed are the management of choledocholithiasis and of acute and complicated presentations.

Contraindications to laparoscopic cholecystectomy are clear in some situations and are being challenged in others. Patients with acute peritonitis, cholangitis and sepsis, acute pancreatitis, end-stage cirrhosis with portal hypertension, suspected carcinoma, and biliary-enteric fistulas are not candidates. Systemic medical risk factors such as coagulopathy and anesthesia risk must be weighed as for any surgery. Late (third-trimester) pregnancy presents mechanical risks to the gravid uterus. Factors that make laparoscopic surgery more difficult such as morbid obesity and prior upper abdominal surgery are also important. The patient with acute cholecystitis is now being cautiously approached laparoscopically. The presence of a mass in 15-20% of acute situations may decrease the chance of a successful laparoscopic outcome if the omentum hides a pericholecystic abscess or gangrenous gallbladder. In addition to the thickened gallbladder wall making grasping and retraction difficult, edema of the porta hepatis and hepatoduodenal ligament obscure the vital anatomy and make dissection hazardous.

The surgeon who tackles difficult cases must be skilled at both open and laparoscopic techniques, and mature enough to recognize when to convert to open cholecystectomy (7-33% in acute vs. 5% in elective) to avert disaster. The performance of laparoscopic cholecystectomy at the standard of open operation requires awareness of anatomic variation and clear visualization of the anatomy to minimize dissection related injury.

Setup

The patient may be placed in the supine position with the legs together or spread, the latter being favored in Europe (Fig. 2.30). With the legs together, the surgeon stands to the patient's left, the assistant stands to the patient's right and the camera operator stands on the patient's left toward the feet. With the patient's legs spread, the surgeon stands between the patient's legs, the assistant stands to the patient's right and the camera operator stands to the patient's left. A third option is for the camera operator to stand between the legs with the surgeon initially on the patient's left. The surgeon and camera operator can then change places if common duct exploration is indicated. The spread leg position avoids crowding between the surgeon and camera operator. The stomach and bladder are decompressed before insufflation and cannula placement.

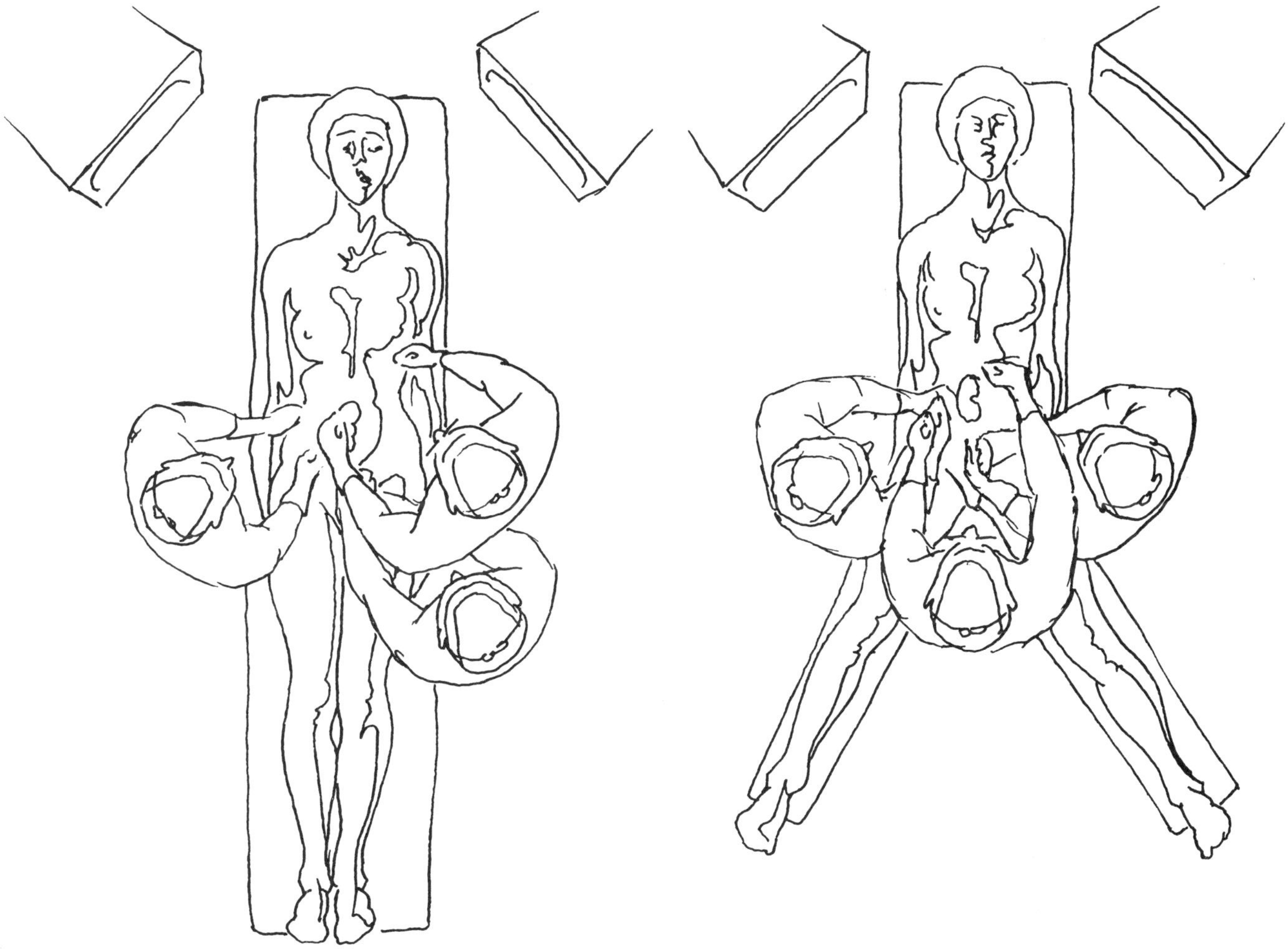

Fig. 2.30

Four cannulas are placed: a large umbilical camera port, a large epigastric port and small right midclavicular port for the surgeon, and a right anterior axillary line port for the assistant (Fig. 2.31). The first cannula (11 mm) is placed in the sub-umbilical position after insufflation by the Veress technique or directly by the Hasson technique. If periumbilical adhesions are suspected, the first port can be placed in the right midclavicular line. In a very large patient, a supra-umbilical position gives a reach advantage. The laparoscope is introduced and a general exploration for adhesions, trochar injury and other pathology is performed. The patient is placed in twenty degrees of reverse Trendelenburg position to slide the viscera out of the right upper quadrant. Rotation of the patient to the left also aids exposure. The remaining cannulas are placed under direct vision.

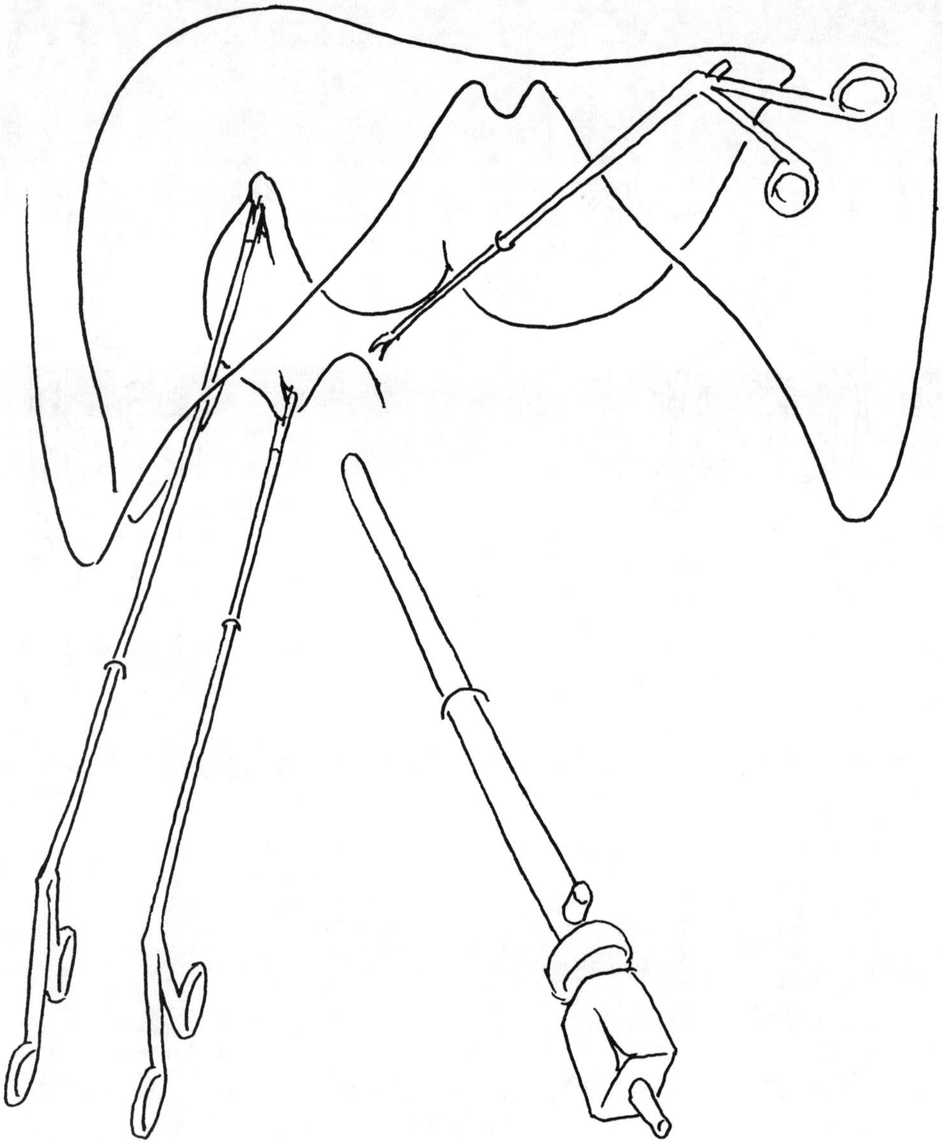

Fig. 2.31

A second 11-mm cannula is placed in the upper midline just caudal to the liver edge. It is directed toward the right to enter the abdomen at the junction of the falciform ligament and the abdominal wall. The third is a 5-mm cannula placed in the right anterior axillary line two finger breadths below the costal margin. A second 5-mm cannula is placed between the right flank cannula and the umbilical cannula, leaving enough distance to the gallbladder for unrestricted movement. An additional optional cannula site is in the mid-clavicular line on the patient's left (Fig. 2.32). An instrument placed through this port is passed beneath the falciform ligament to retract a stiff, firm or enlarged liver, or to retract the duodenum and hepatic flexure downward.

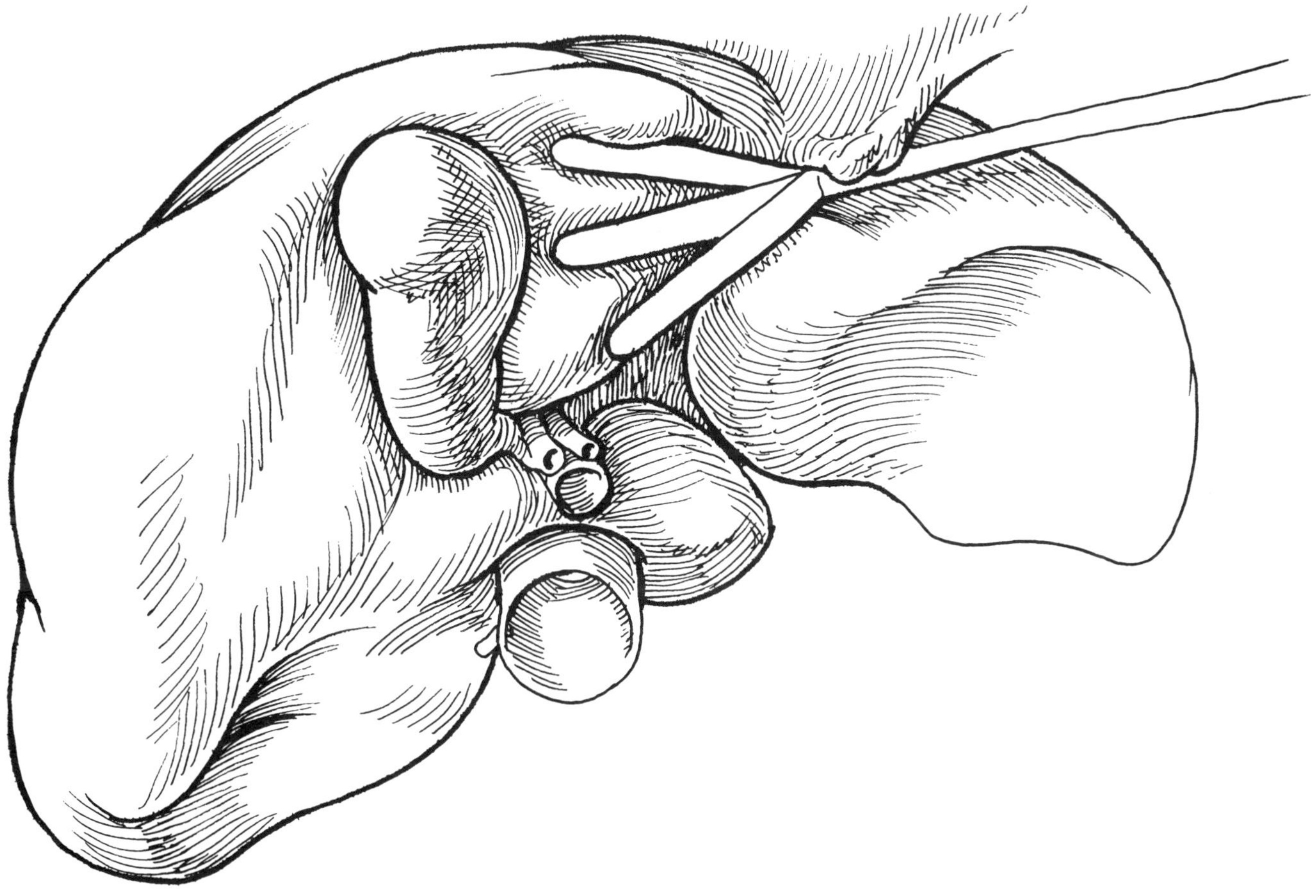

Fig. 2.32

Technique

If the gallbladder and liver are pliable, the assistant, using a locking grasper, grasps the fundus of the gallbladder through the flank cannula and gently elevates it toward the right upper quadrant (Fig. 2.33). A tensely distended gallbladder may need to be aspirated to obtain a purchase with a grasper which is then placed over the puncture site (Fig. 2.34). Routine aspiration decreases spillage in the event of perforation and facilitates dissection and extraction by decreasing the bulk of the gallbladder. Needle aspiration may be difficult when the bile is thick or the gallbladder is packed with stones, and a larger (5 mm) suction cannula may be necessary.

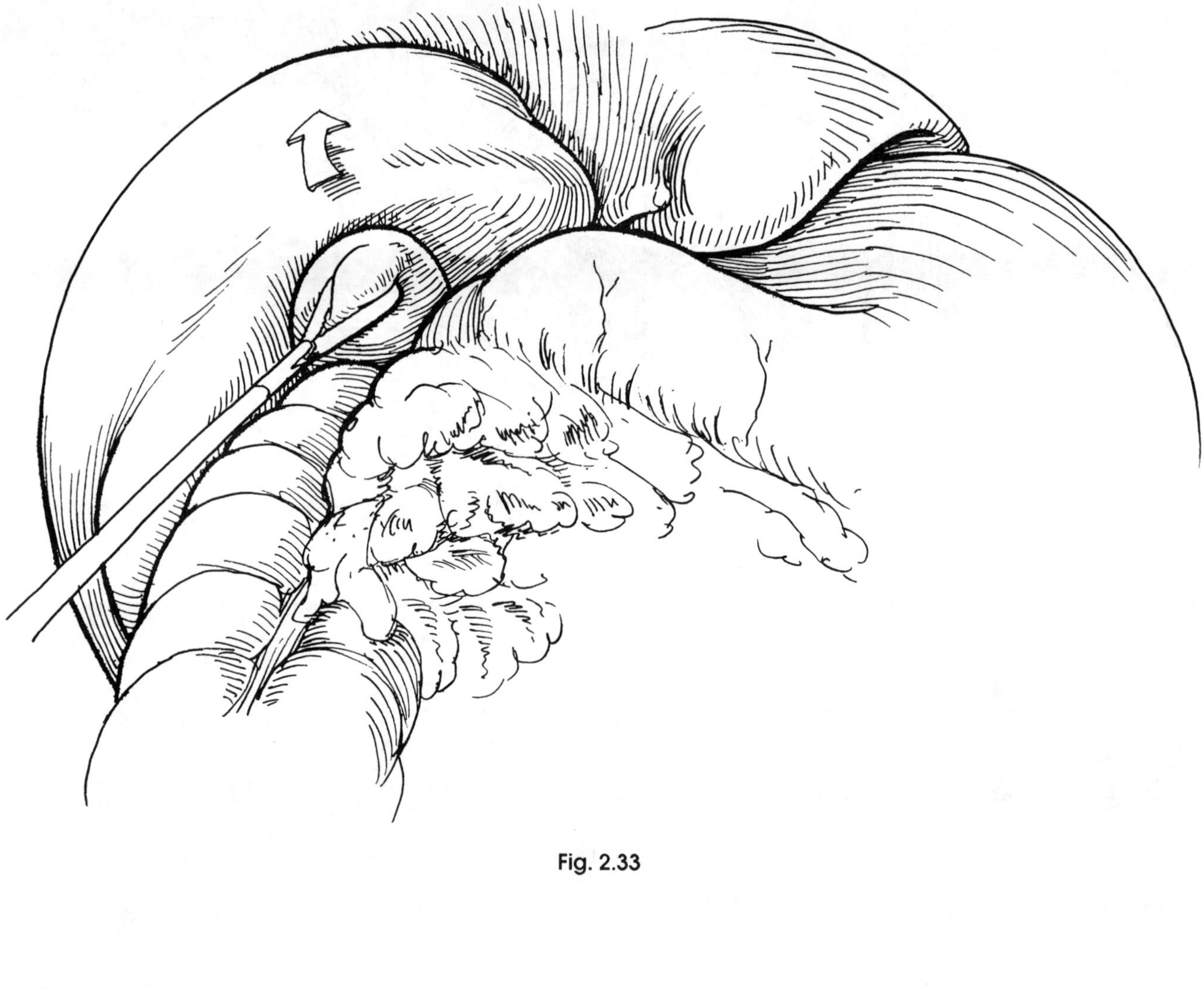

Fig. 2.33

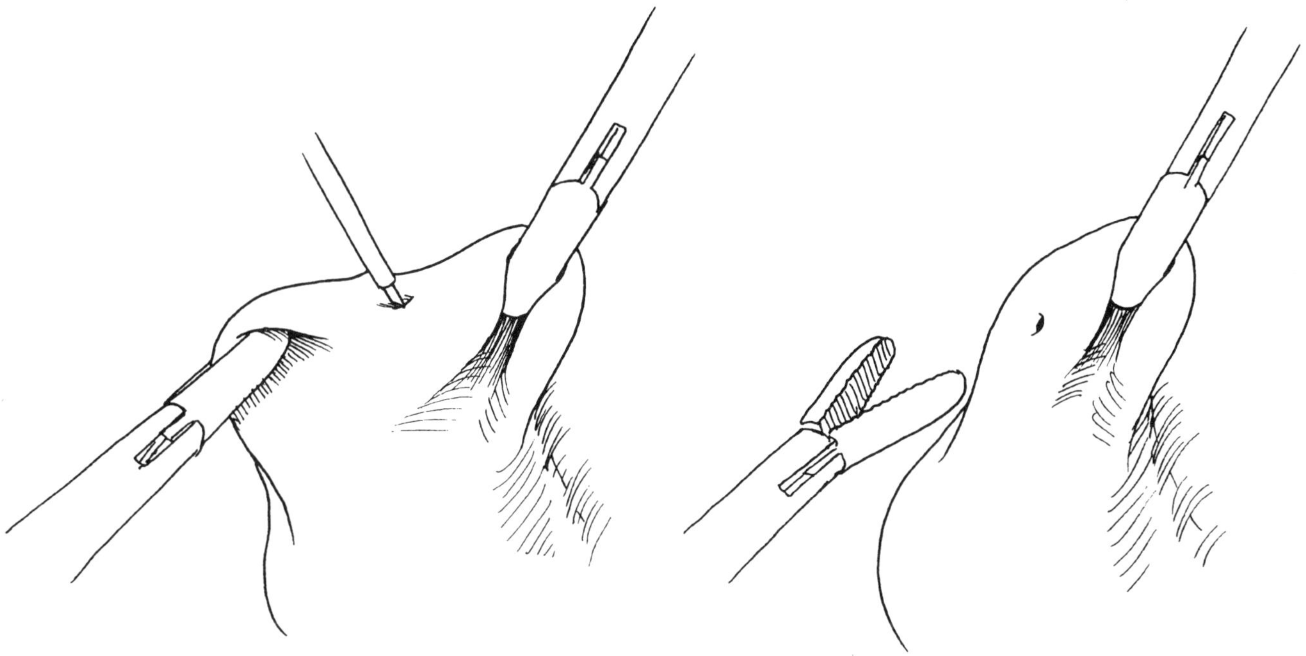

Fig. 2.34

An option at the time of aspiration is to inject contrast and perform a cholangiogram through the gallbladder. Especially when there is significant inflammation and edema, this has the advantage of demonstrating the anatomy before dissecting in the hepatocystic triangle. Successful imaging is almost universal in non-acute cases. Even with the high percentage of impacted stones in acute cholecystitis, contrast passes in two thirds of cases. If clear mucous (mucocele/hydrops) or pus is aspirated, the gallbladder is emptied and a cystic duct cholangiogram can still be tried. If successful, the morbidity, technical difficulties and time expenditure of cystic duct cholangiography are avoided by cholecystocholangiography. The injection of a volume equal to the aspirate (~30cc) should be followed by 10-20 seconds of gallbladder compression by a blunt probe. If injection is observed by fluoroscopy, the flow may be stopped when adequate filling is observed and a smaller amount of contrast may be used. Occasionally a larger amount (up to 60cc) is required. A double balloon catheter has been devised to minimize spillage. A potential disadvantage is overlap of the infundibulum obscuring the cystic duct. There are also less false positive results with this method because air remains in the fundus. The gallbladder is again aspirated after the cholangiogram.

Next, adhesions between the gallbladder and adjacent structures (omentum, colon and duodenum) are separated by the surgeon (Fig. 2.35). Sharp scissors/cautery dissection should be used to divide adhesions to the liver to avoid avulsing the capsule. As the

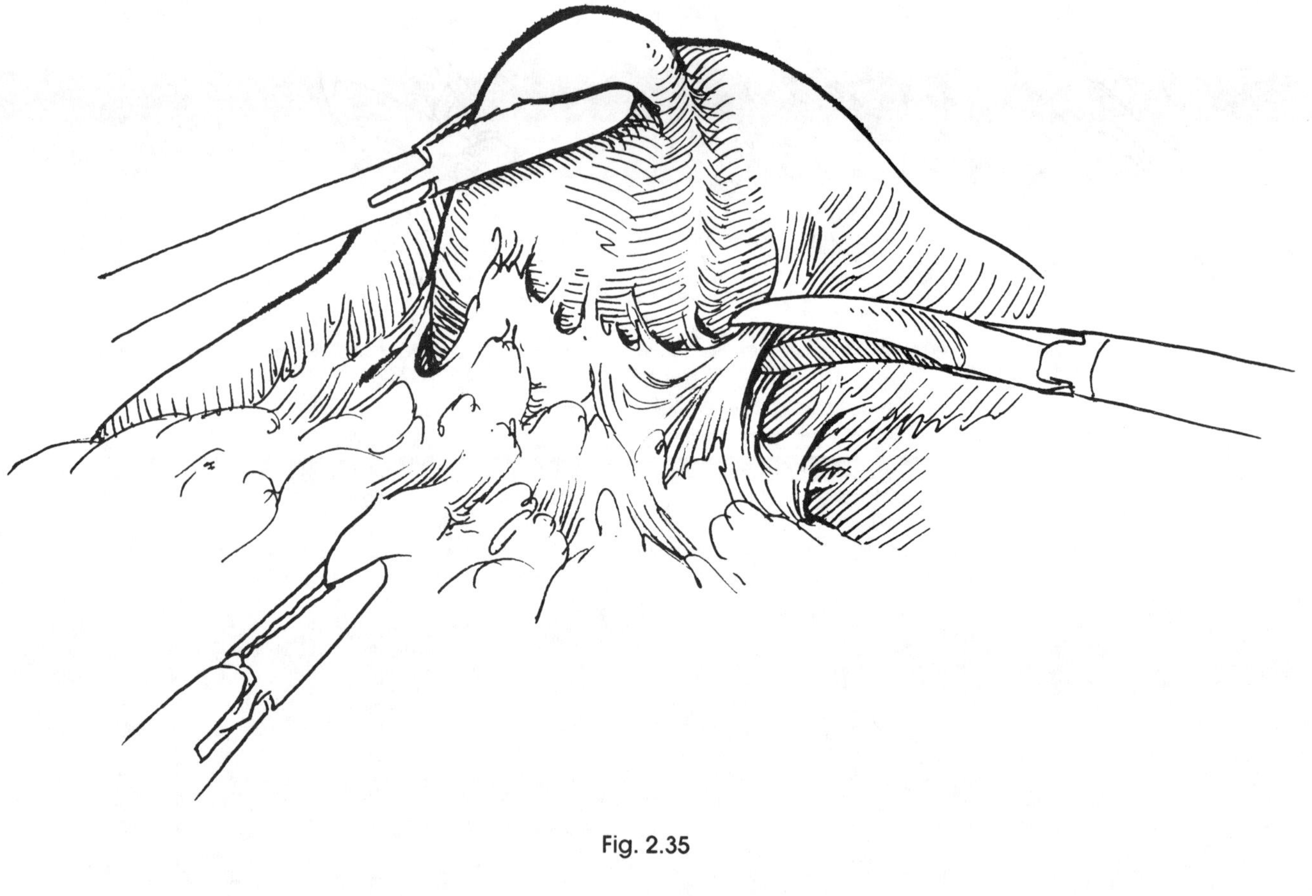

Fig. 2.35

gallbladder is progressively freed down to the neck, the fundus is pushed up as high as possible over the edge of the liver beneath the dome of the diaphragm to uncoil Hartmann's pouch (Fig. 2.36).

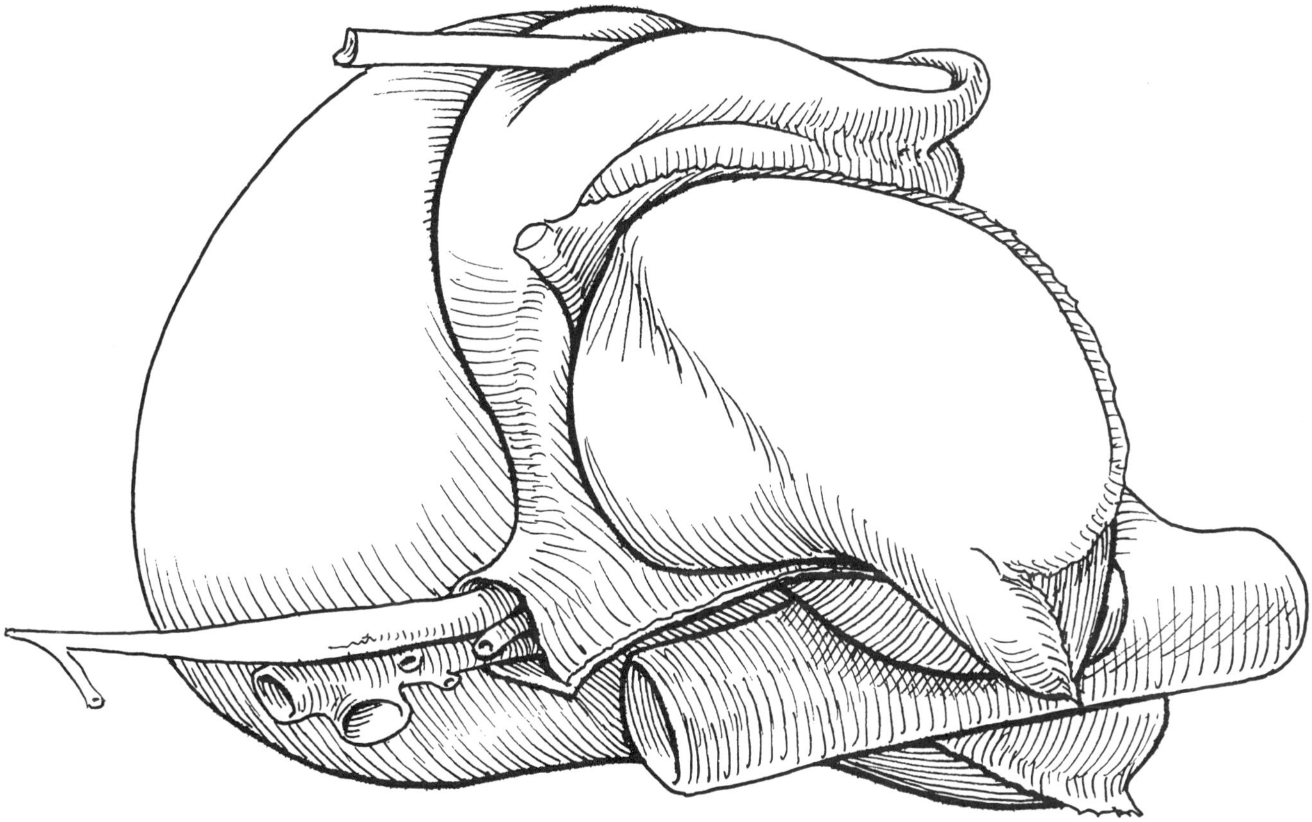

Fig. 2.36

To begin the dissection in the hepatocystic triangle, the surgeon, grasps the infundibulum (Hartmann's pouch) with the left hand instrument, and retracts it inferolaterally (Fig. 2.37). It should not be retracted

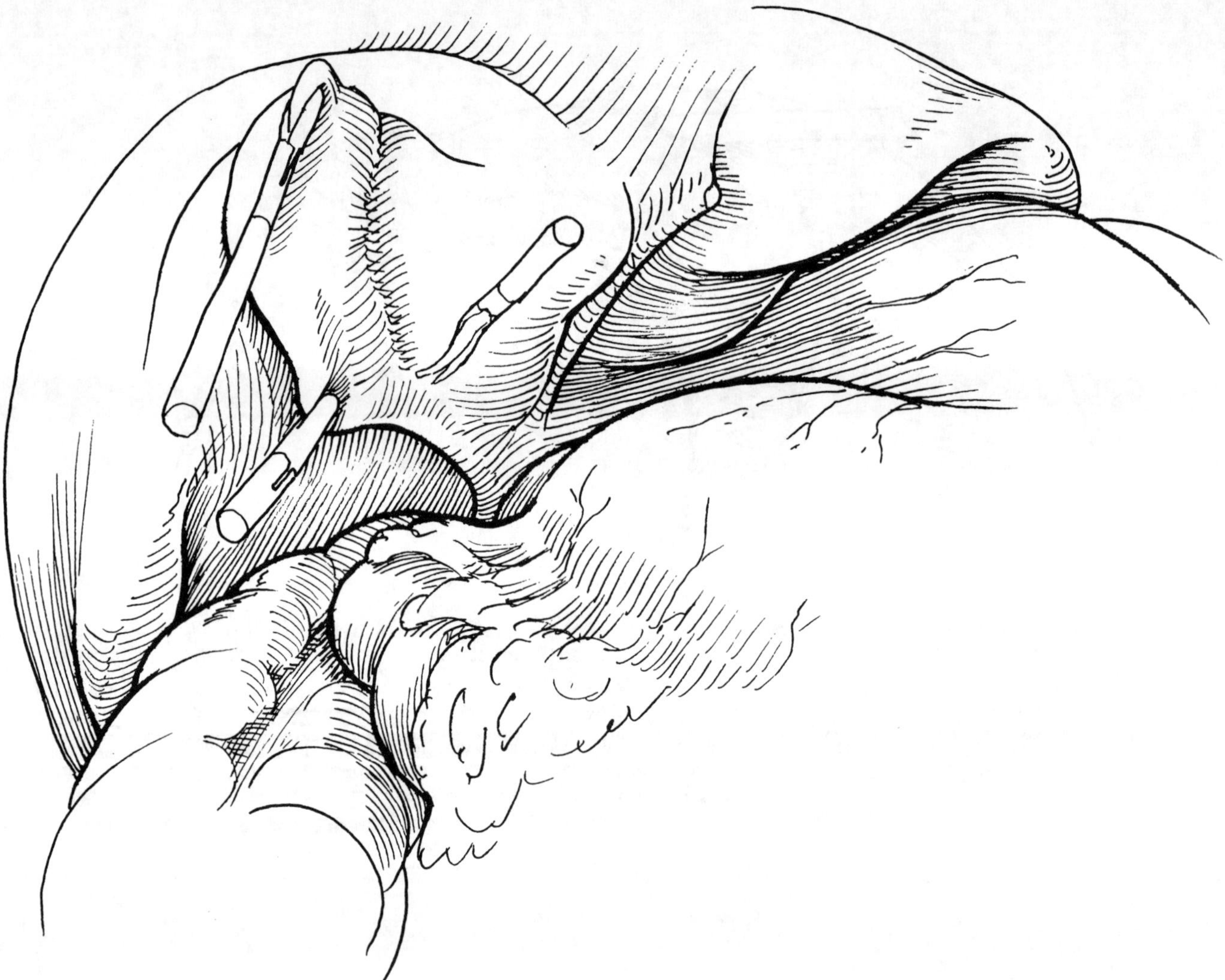

Fig. 2.37

cephalad because this narrows the cholecystohepatic triangle and brings the cystic and common hepatic ducts into dangerously close apposition (Fig. 2.38). It also straightens the angle between the cystic duct and the common duct so that the latter may be mistaken for the former. If there is a large stone in the infundibulum an attempt may be made to milk it out. If this cannot be accomplished, a retractor may be used to move the pouch to the right.

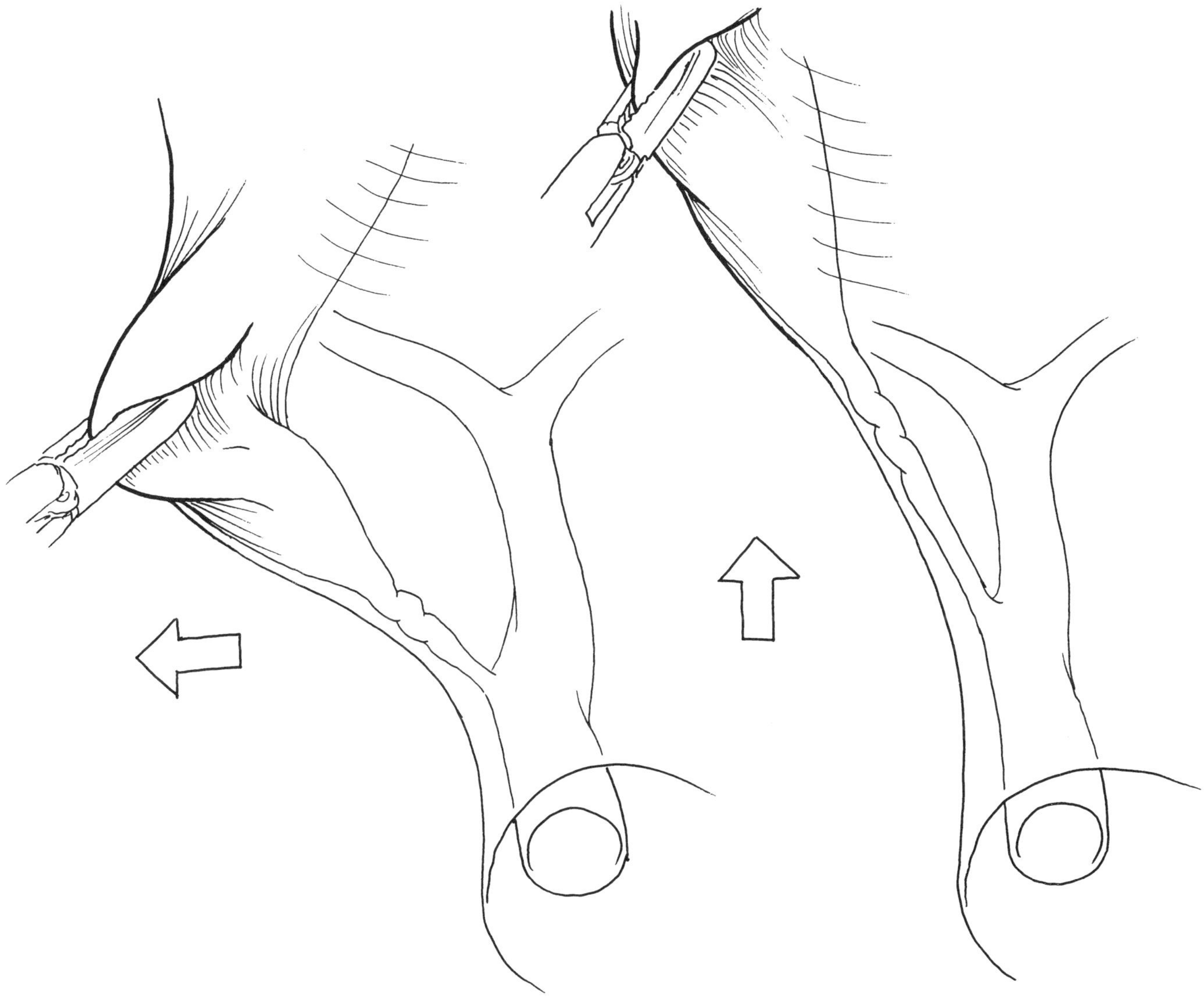

Fig. 2.38

The surgeon next proceeds to carefully dissect and identify the structures in the hepatobiliary triangle. Clear visual identification is absolutely necessary for safety and depends on adequate exposure and meticulous hemostasis. Even a small amount of blood can obscure a critical relationship. Dissection of the edge of the hepatoduodenal ligament begins high and lateral near the neck of the gallbladder while Hartmann's pouch is retracted to the patient's left (Fig. 2.39). An aberrant right hepatic artery, present about 17% of the time, may be the closest structure to the right edge of the hepatoduodenal ligament. The variations in the clarity of the transition from gallbladder neck to cystic duct, the duct length, and possible modes of insertion, must be kept in mind when looking for the cystic duct.

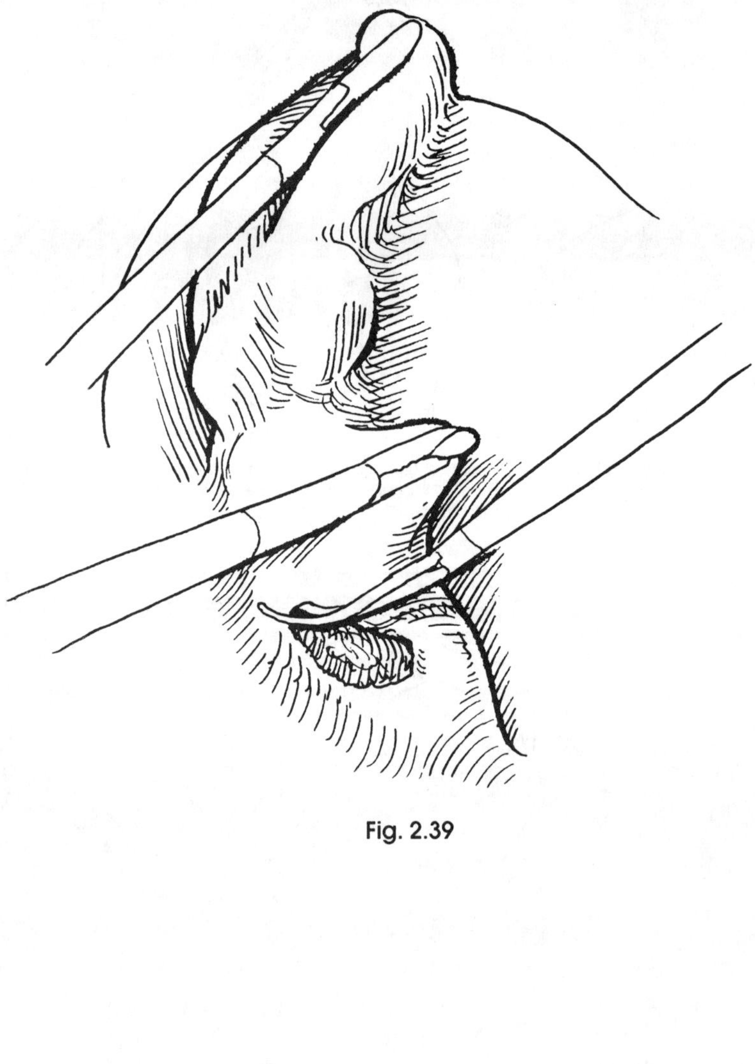

Fig. 2.39

The ampulla is next retracted to the patient's left, the peritoneum is opened around the edge of the cystic duct junction and the peritoneal incision continued toward the left side of the hepatocystic triangle (Fig. 2.40). Cautery should not be used in the hepatocystic triangle. The cystic artery, often marked by the cystic duct node (of Calot), is carefully isolated at the posterior part of the triangle. The cystic duct branch of the cystic artery should be noted.

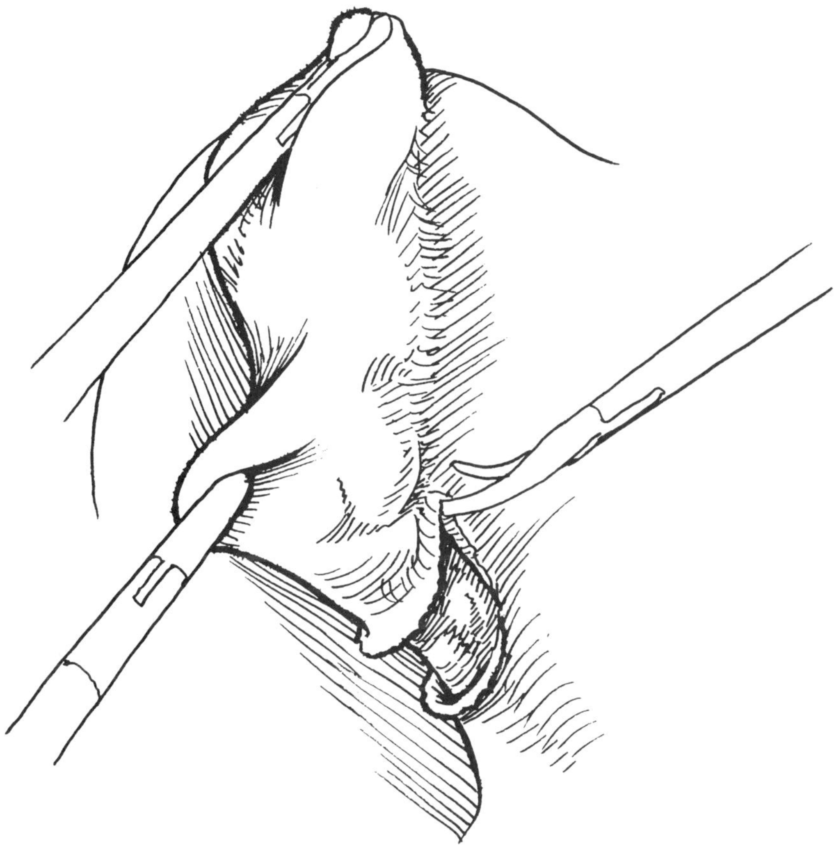

Fig. 2.40

Dissection at the junction of infundibulum and cystic duct should be visualized at all times by varying the angle of the scope to give a clear view (Fig. 2.41). The cystic duct and neck of the gallbladder should be completely freed circumferentially and the junction point clearly visualized (Fig. 2.42). The completion of dissection should demonstrate what has been called the "critical view" (Fig. 2.43). The cystic

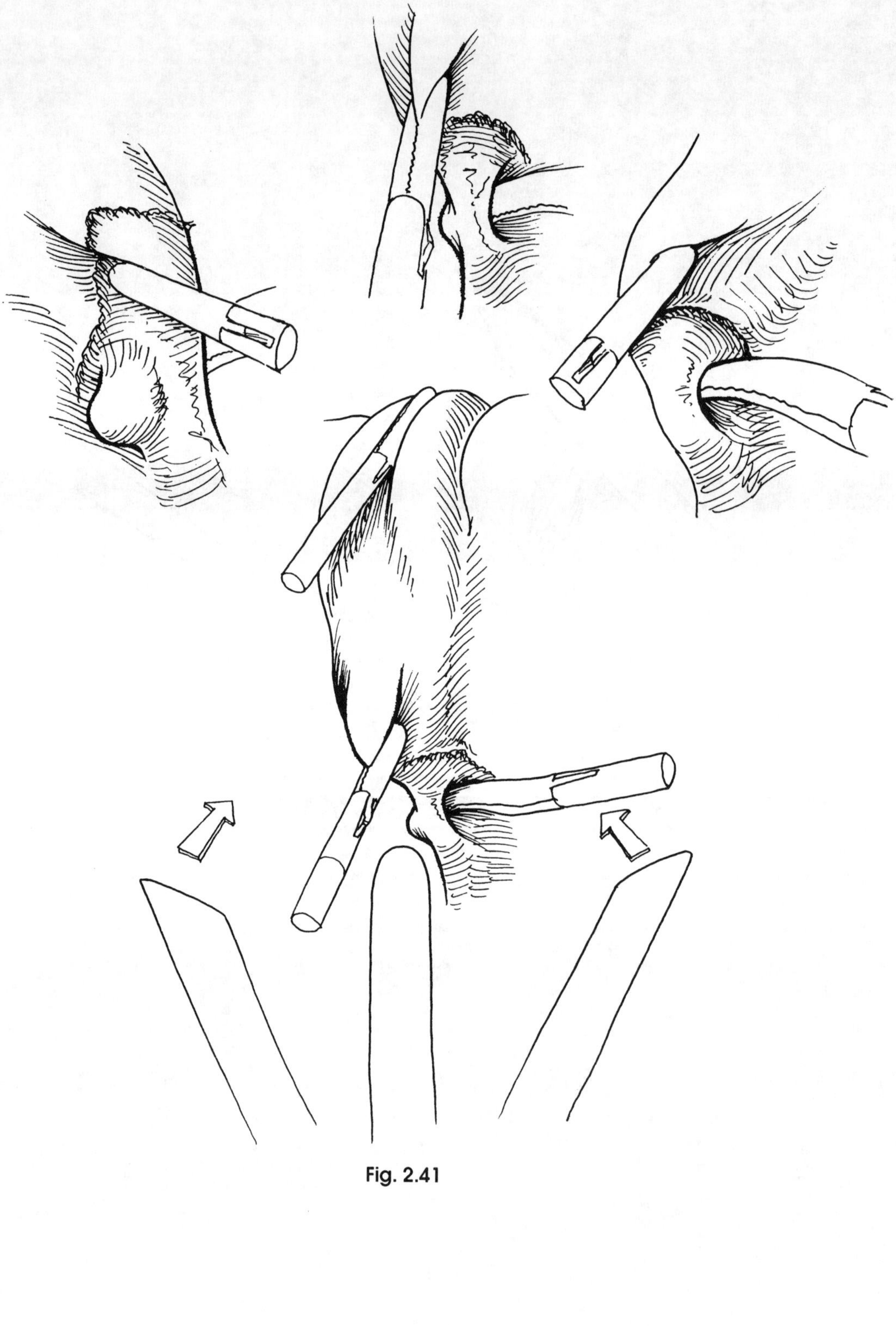

Fig. 2.41

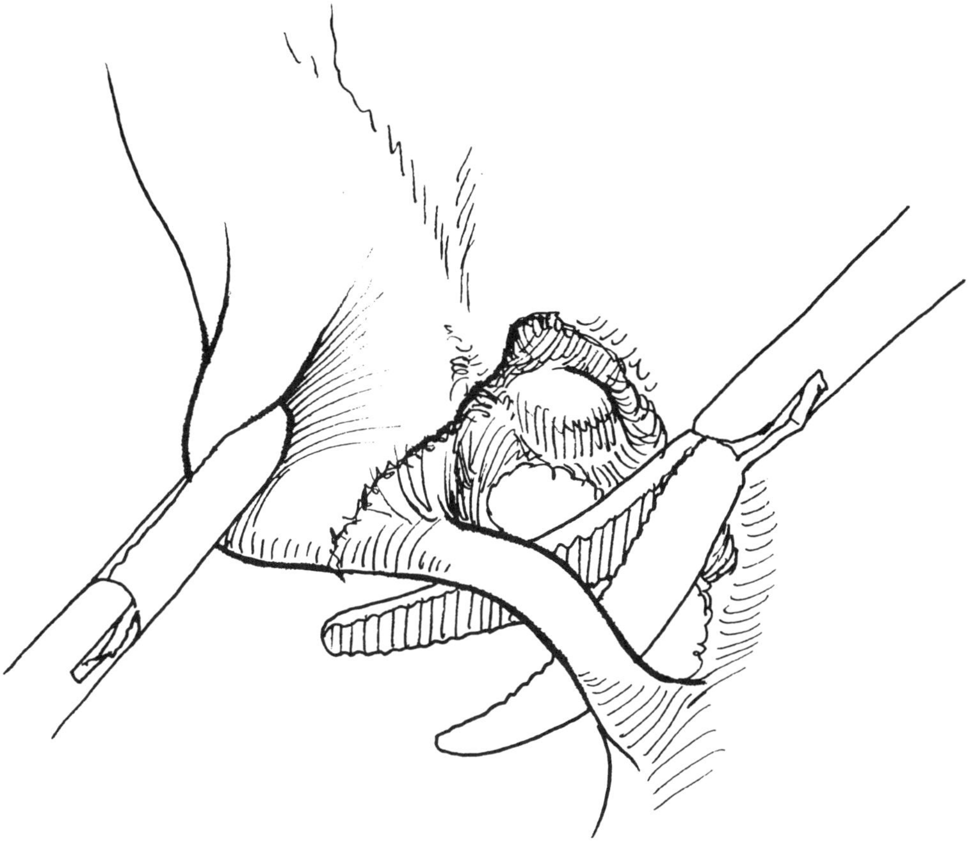

Fig. 2.42

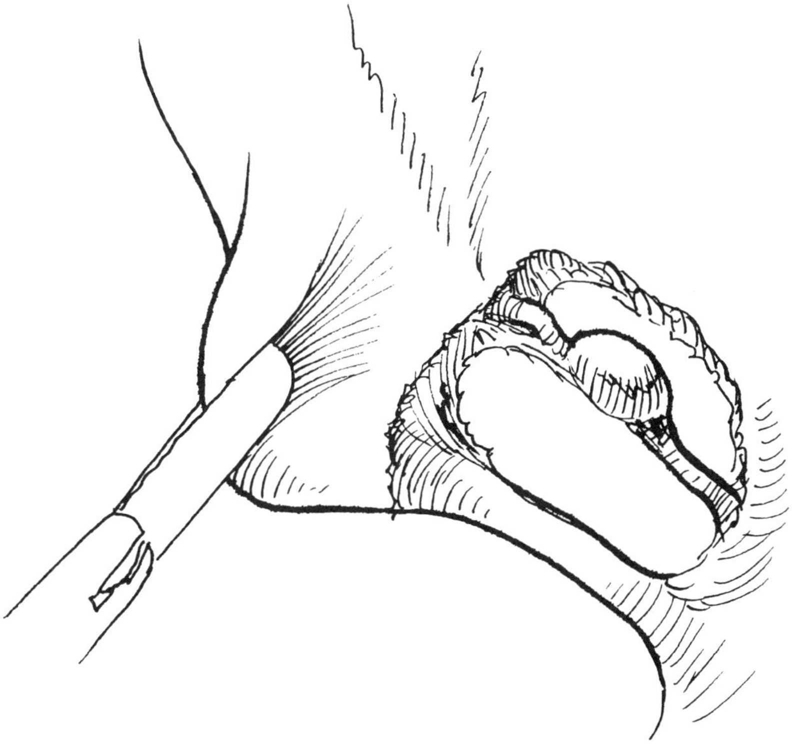

Fig. 2.43

artery and cystic duct should be free of surrounding tissue and seen to clearly terminate at the gallbladder, and the infundibulum of the gallbladder should be free from the liver bed. The cystic artery branches should be seen passing onto the wall of the gallbladder and not turning back into the liver ("caterpillar hump" right hepatic artery). A large artery should raise suspicion that the vessel in question is a right hepatic branch. A small or single artery should raise suspicion of an additional cystic artery branch that is not yet visible, either because of an early bifurcation or duplication. The critical view should be seen before any structure is clipped.

The cystic artery is then secured with two clips proximally and one distally and divided (Fig. 2.44). Both points of the clips and scissors should be visible

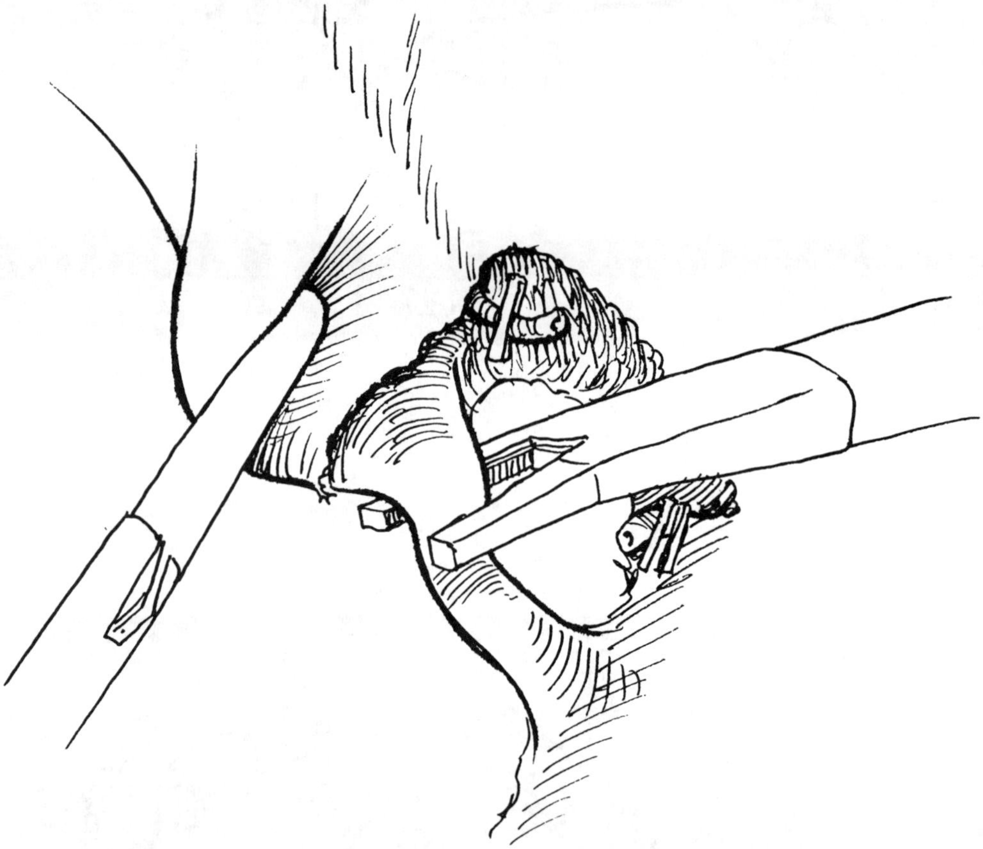

Fig. 2.44

before closing. A clip is placed at the junction of the cystic duct and the gallbladder neck. If no cholangiogram is to be done, a second clip is then placed on the cystic duct a comfortable distance away from the common duct (Fig. 2.45) while the infundibulum is being held to the right with minimal traction. Traction is then released and the position of the clip inspected to ensure that there is no tenting of the common duct. A third clip is placed adjacent to the second on the gallbladder side of the duct.

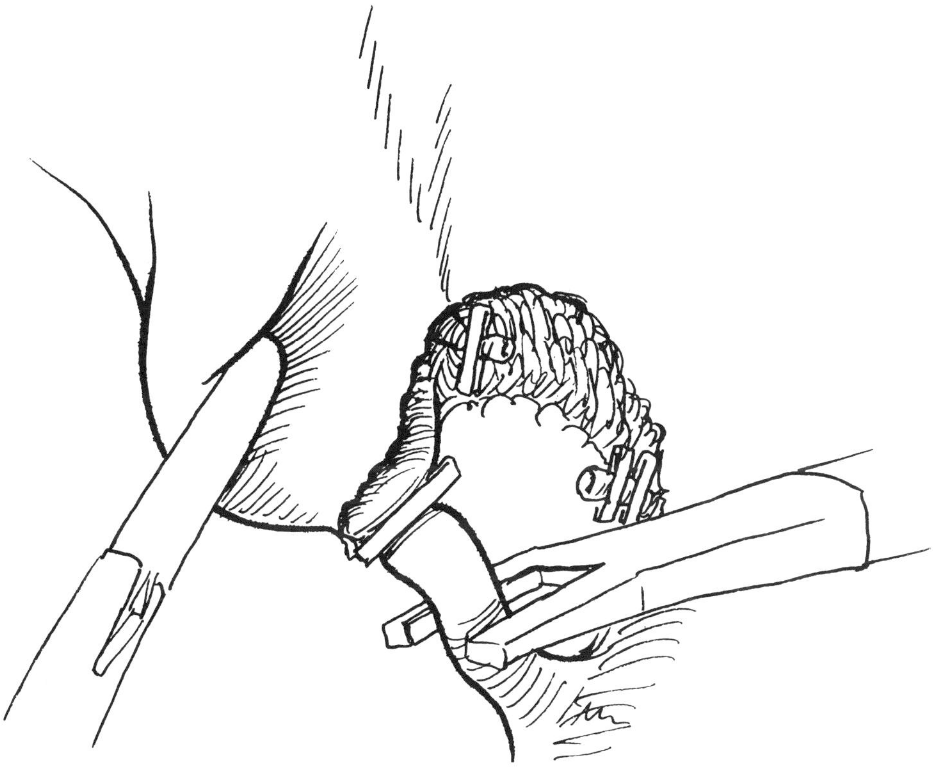

Fig. 2.45

A cholangiogram can be performed after the clip at the gallbladder neck is placed. There is continuing debate whether to do cholangiogram routinely or selectively. It should be done if choledocholithiasis is suspected or if there is any uncertainty about the anatomic relationships. Most surgeons use cholangiography selectively if risk factors for common duct stones are present. Without risk factors, the incidence of unsuspected stones (4%) is equal to the false positive cholangiogram rate. Most small common duct stones pass spontaneously if no intervention is performed. Weighing that fact against the morbidity of cystic duct cholangiography and of unnecessary common duct exploration and the success rate of stone extraction by ERCP (95% in experienced hands) favors a selective approach. Fluoroscopy shows promise of improving the accuracy and reducing the time for cholangiography.

To perform a cholangiogram, a small transverse nick is made in the cystic duct proximal to the clip using a fine dissecting scissors (Fig. 2.46A). A cholangiogram catheter is passed into the duct and grasped, most conveniently using the instrument (Olsen clamp) designed for this purpose. Introducing the catheter past the spiral valves of a small cystic duct can be tricky. Slight dilatation of the opening may be beneficial. A jiggling movement on advancing the catheter increases the chances of finding the channel, and irrigating with saline as the catheter is advanced helps open the lumen. The catheter tip should be advanced only far enough to be secured in the mid cystic duct (Fig. 2.46B). If advanced further, the tip often abuts the opposite wall of the common duct and obstructs flow or angles down the common duct and gives a distal picture only (Fig. 2.46C). It may also perforate the opposite wall of the common duct (Fig. 2.46D). Forceful advancement may perforate or avulse the cystic duct (Fig. 2.46E). Some contrast should be injected under direct vision in case the catheter becomes dislodged when the instruments are relaxed. When releasing the instruments before the cholangiogram, tension should be relaxed slowly to prevent dislodgment. The patient is rotated 15 degrees to the right to prevent overlap of the common duct and spinal column. Fluoroscopy is performed or one or two radiographs are taken using 7-10cc of dilute (50% contrast diluted another 50% with saline) iodinated contrast.

If the cholangiogram is normal (no filling defects, filling of proximal and distal ducts, flow into the duodenum), the catheter is removed and two clips are placed on the proximal cystic duct well away from the common duct. The cystic duct should not be under tension when the clips are placed and should be relaxed and checked after placement to avoid tenting and injuring the common duct. The cystic duct is then divided. An inadequately secured cystic duct is a major culprit in postoperative bile leak. If there is any doubt, a loop ligature may be added, again staying far from the common duct.

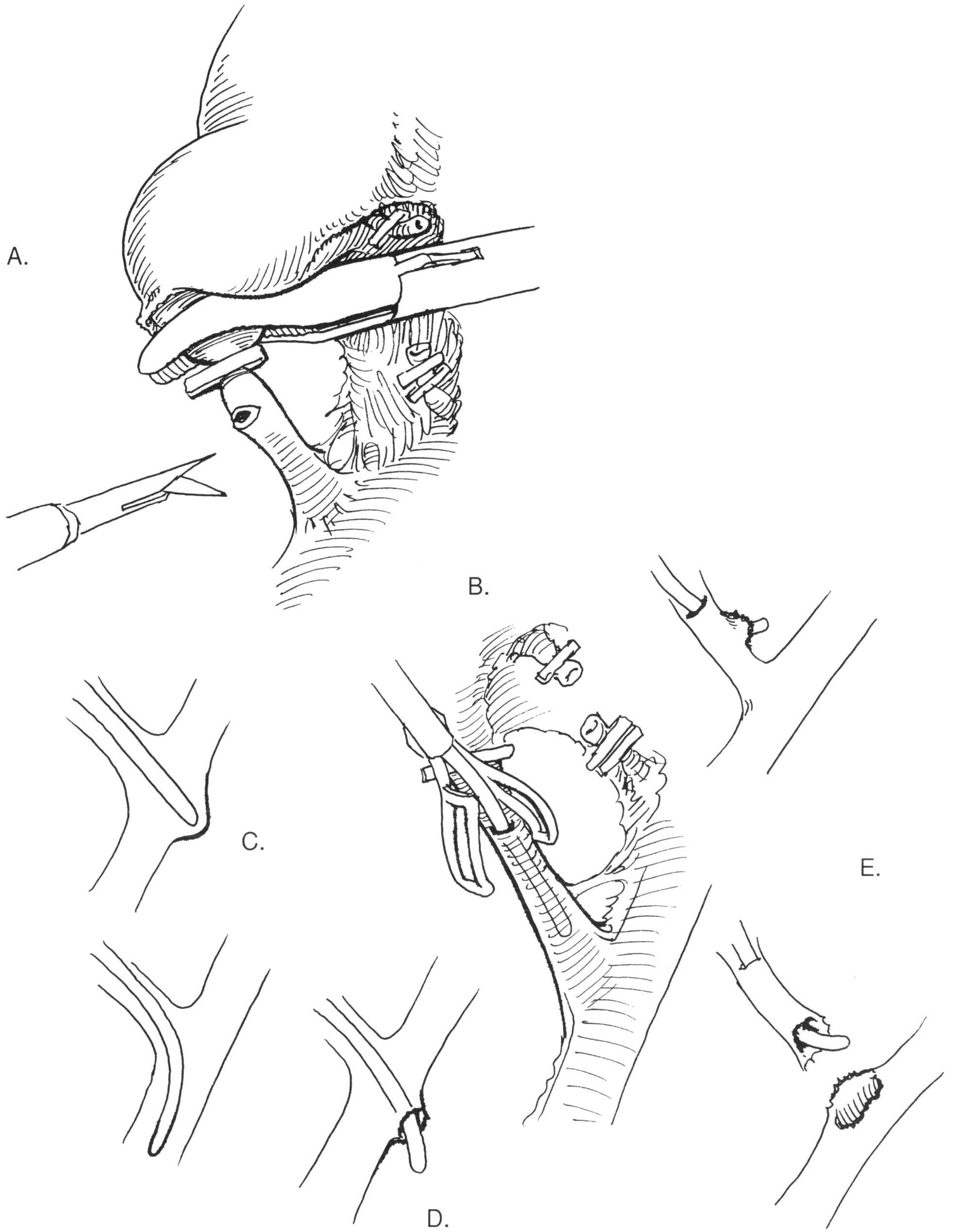

Fig. 2.46

Grasping the neck of the gallbladder, the surgeon proceeds to dissect the gallbladder out of the liver bed, staying in the subserosal plane to avoid bleeding and injury to underlying bile ducts, a second major cause of postoperative bile leak (Fig. 2.47). The gallbladder is manipulated by surgeon and assistant to maintain constant traction as the cautery scissors or spatula divides the tensed tissue. Perforation of the gallbladder can be controlled with an endoloop ligature if the wall is pliable. A major tear in a gallbladder filled with stones can be handled by catching the stones in a bag for later retrieval. A bleeding point in

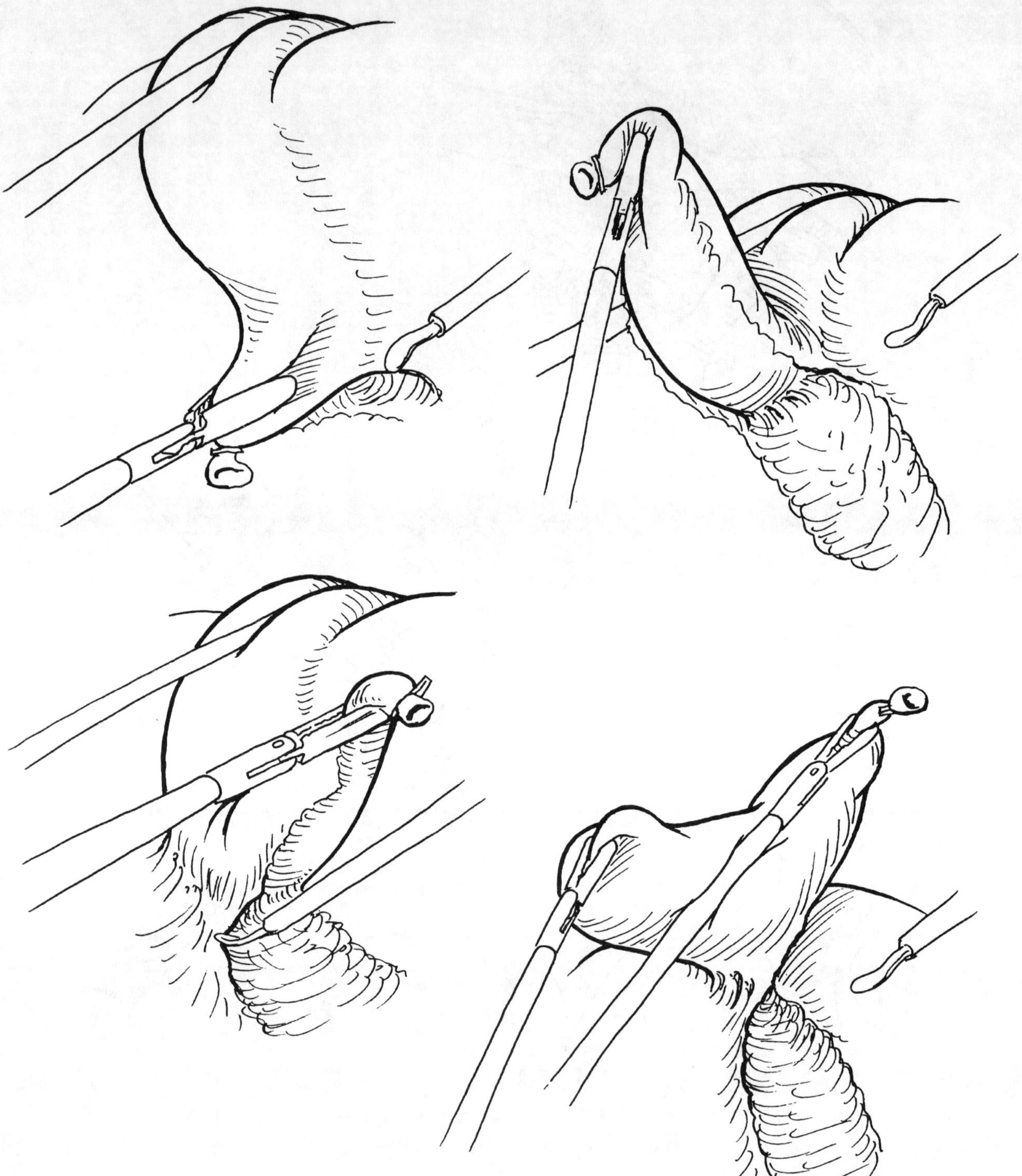

Fig. 2.47

the gallbladder bed that is hard to control should be exposed by dissecting surrounding gallbladder wall. Topical hemostatic agents or argon beam coagulation can be used when monopolar cautery fails to control the bleeding point. When the gallbladder is mobilized up to the fundus, traction is maintained to expose the liver bed, irrigate and achieve hemostasis. The last attachment is then divided.

The hepatorenal recess (Morrison's pouch) and the subphrenic gutter lateral to the liver are irrigated and suctioned. The gallbladder may be removed through either the large epigastric or umbilical port site. The epigastric site has a smaller potential for hernia formation, the camera does not have to move and it is not necessary to work at a reverse angle. If the gallbladder is removed without a plastic sac, there is more potential for infection, particularly at the epigastric site because there is more surrounding fat than at the umbilical site. If there is a significant mass of stones and/or bile, it is safest to place the gallbladder in a strong sac for removal and the fascial opening can be enlarged with a Mayo scissors under direct vision. If the gallbladder mass will still not come through intact, the neck of the sac can be opened and the stones crushed and extracted with ring forceps to decompress the sac.

If there is concern about the potential for bile leak or oozing (e.g., acute gallbladder, coagulopathy) a closed suction drain can be placed by drawing it in through a large port (Fig. 2.48). A grasper is passed retrograde through a large port from a facing port site and the tubing of the drain is pulled through.

The large port sites should be closed at the fascial level. This can be done under laparoscopic visualization with one of several devices now available, or it can be done externally. The latter is often difficult, especially in an obese patient.

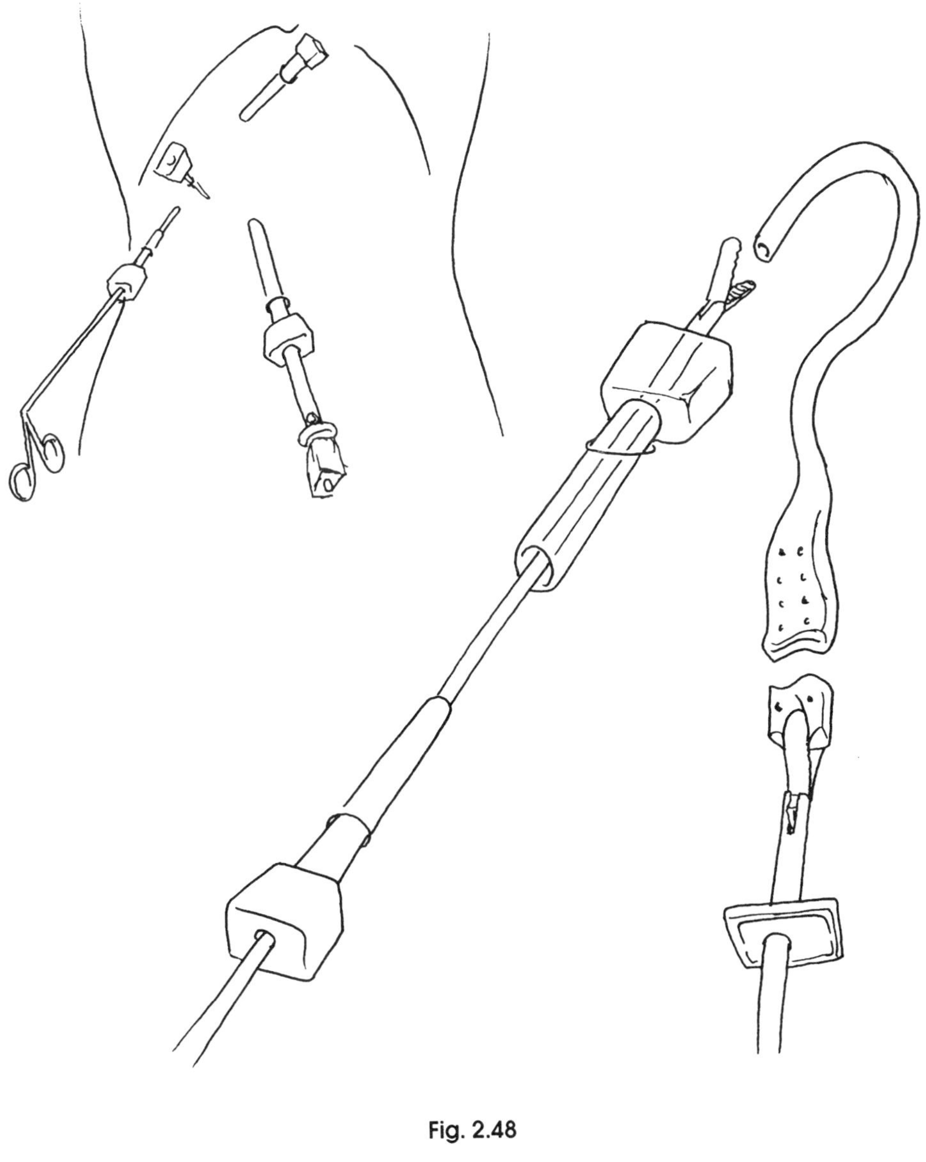

Fig. 2.48

The Difficult Gallbladder

The anatomic and pathologic features of a particular case often present technical difficulties. As a surgeon becomes more skilled in laparoscopic surgery, it is reasonable to tackle more challenging cases. However, the more difficult the exposure and dissection, the greater is the danger of injury to the patient and the surgeon must honestly judge his of her abilities and limitations. Knowing when to desist and convert to open is the best strategy to avert disaster. Adhesions and acute cholecystitis are two major factors in conversion and the rate of conversion in acute cholecystitis is about four times that in elective cholecystectomy.

There are a few pathological and constitutional factors that should preclude a laparoscopic approach. These include a recognized cholecysto-enteric fistula, carcinoma of the gallbladder, pericholecystic abscess, significant portal hypertension, acute pancreatitis, generalized peritonitis, cholangitis, and septic shock. Other factors raise the level of difficulty and should lower the threshold for conversion to open operation. These can be divided into problems of access to the biliary tree and problems manipulating diseased structures.

The morbidly obese patient presents problems in reaching the peritoneum to insufflate, problems insufflating adequately at safe pressures, problems reaching the operative site, and exposure problems from a bulky omentum and mesenteries (Fig. 2.49). Longer instruments and additional ports for retraction of a fatty liver and omentum may be necessary to overcome these obstacles.

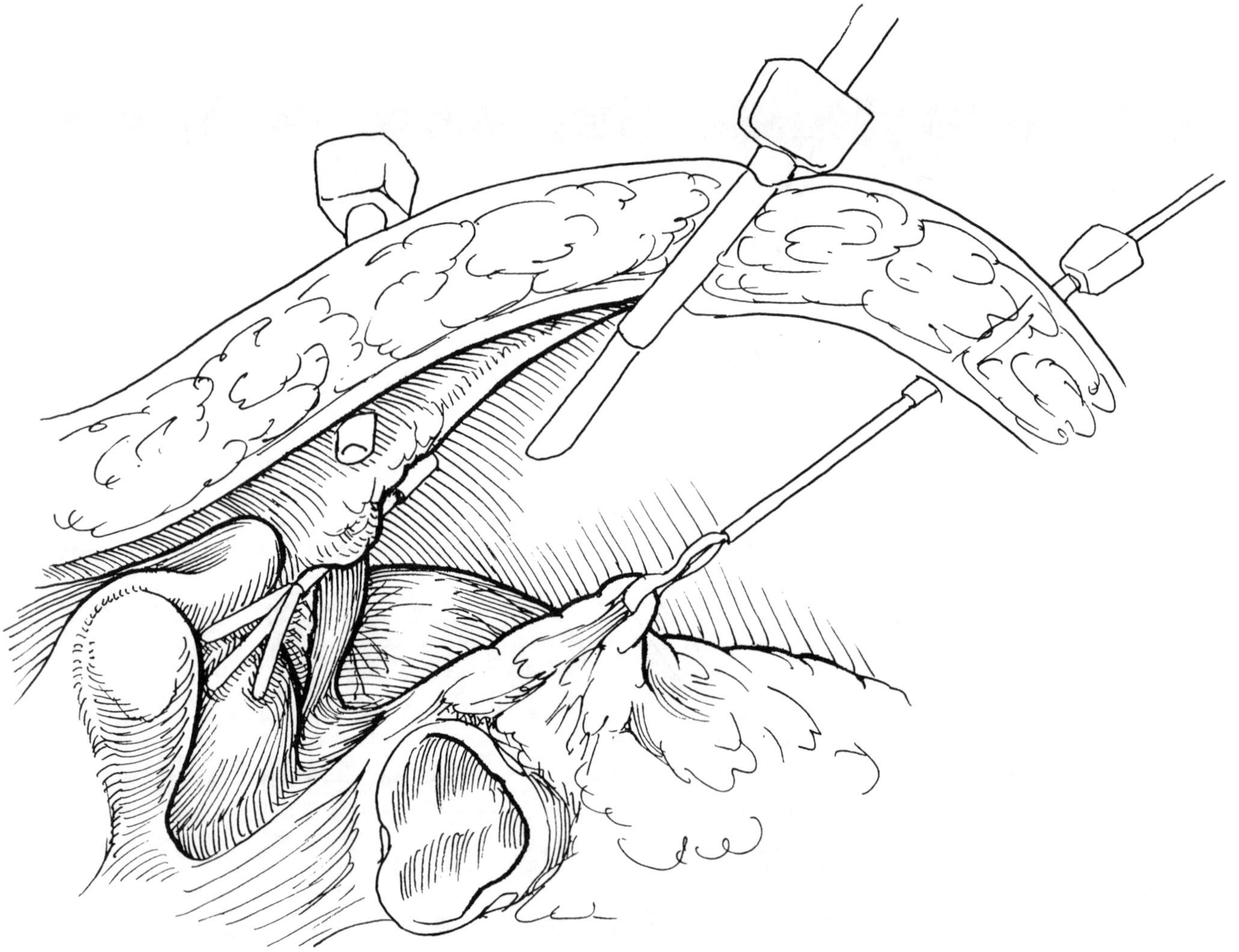

Fig. 2.49

Patients who have had prior upper abdominal surgery may have extensive adhesions (Fig. 2.50). Ultrasound has been used successfully by some to map adhesions and identify a safe initial entry site where the underlying viscera are mobile. Open technique with a Hasson cannula is the safest approach. A small right upper quadrant (mid-clavicular line) or upper midline entry port can also allow use of a 5-mm scope to observe the umbilical site during introduction of a large port. Adhesions close to the entry site can be gently pushed aside with the tip of the telescope until there is adequate room to place additional ports. Once additional instruments can be introduced, filmy adhesions can be bluntly dissected and firmer bands, particularly those attached to liver, can be divided with cautery scissors to avoid bleeding from avulsion of liver capsule.

Hemostasis must be especially meticulous in cases where the bleeding risk is increased such as correctable coagulopathies, acute cholecystitis, and early portal hypertension. The presence of blood increases the risk of collateral damage in two ways. It obscures vital structures and absorbs light, reducing visibility. Diathermy should be used cautiously only at low settings and in the spray mode until the anatomy is clearly identified.

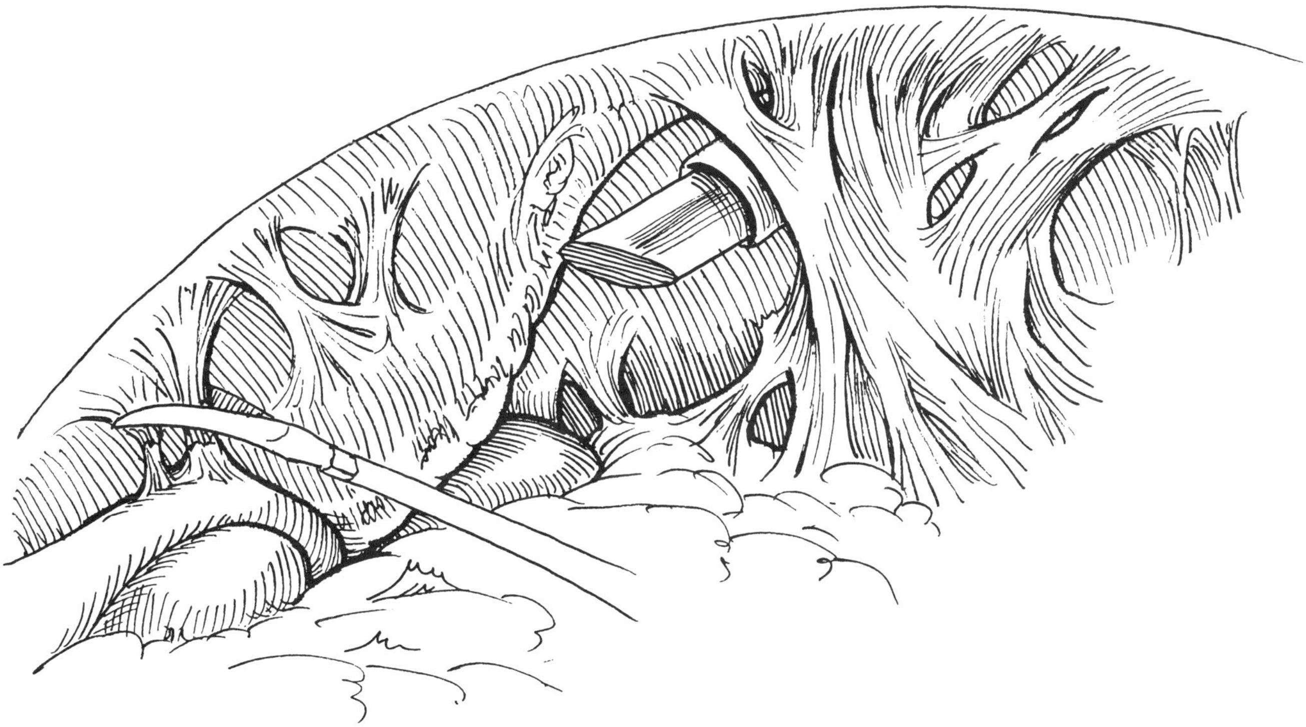

Fig. 2.50

If the liver is bulky from fatty infiltration, enlarged lobe or polycystic disease, alternate means of retraction will be required (Fig. 2.51). Inflexible shrunken livers from cirrhosis present a similar challenge to exposure.

An acutely inflamed gallbladder will often be encased in omentum (Fig. 2.52A). The plane between omentum and gallbladder wall must be carefully opened with blunt dissection to expose enough fundus to grasp or aspirate if necessary. Aquadissection

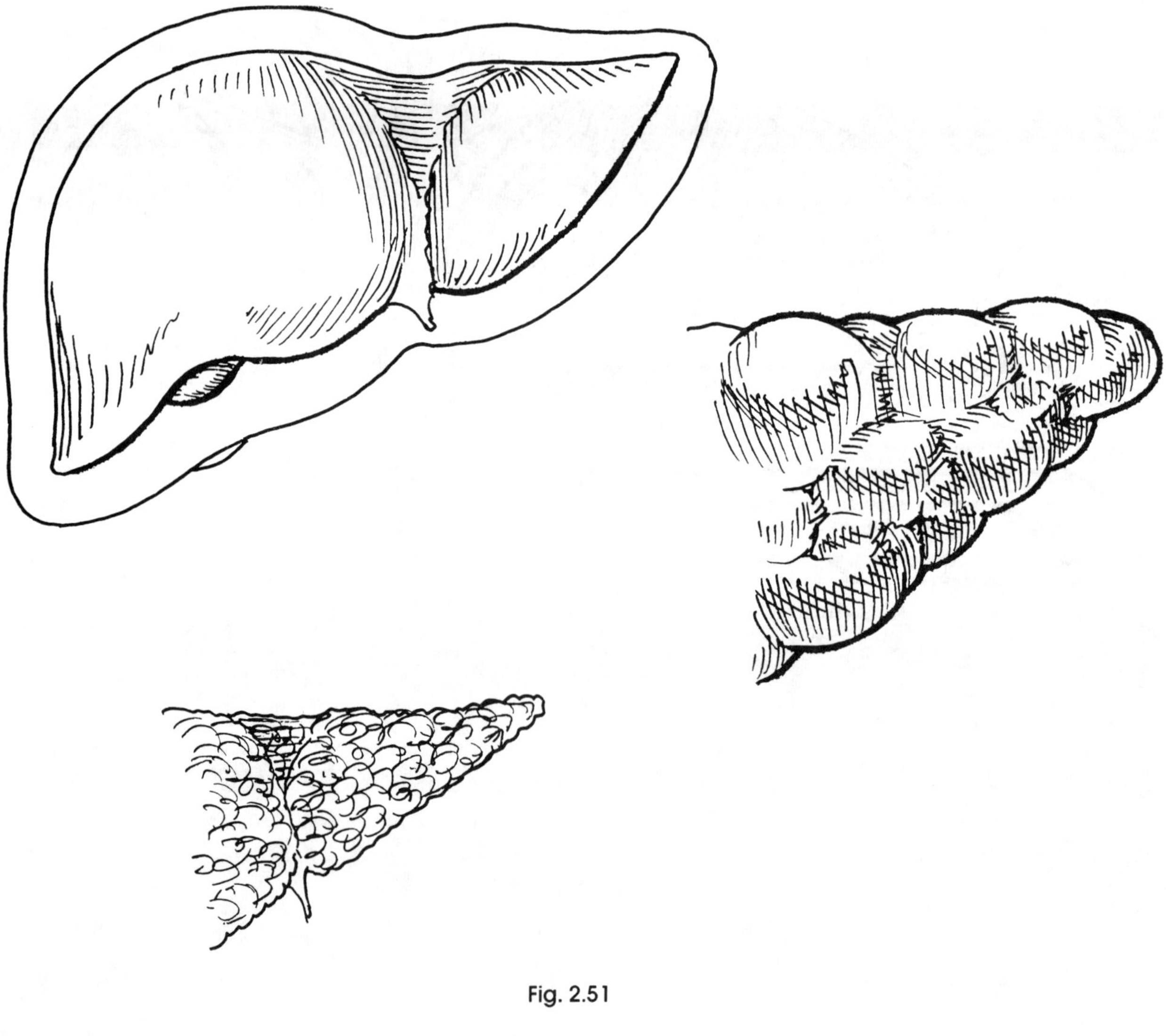

Fig. 2.51

should be used early and liberally. If a pericholecystic abscess or gangrenous gallbladder (Fig. 2.52B) is present, the procedure might best be converted to open. The friable gangrenous gallbladder wall may be difficult to dissect from the liver bed. In such a case, the back wall can be left in place and the mucosa ablated with cautery (Fig. 2.52C).

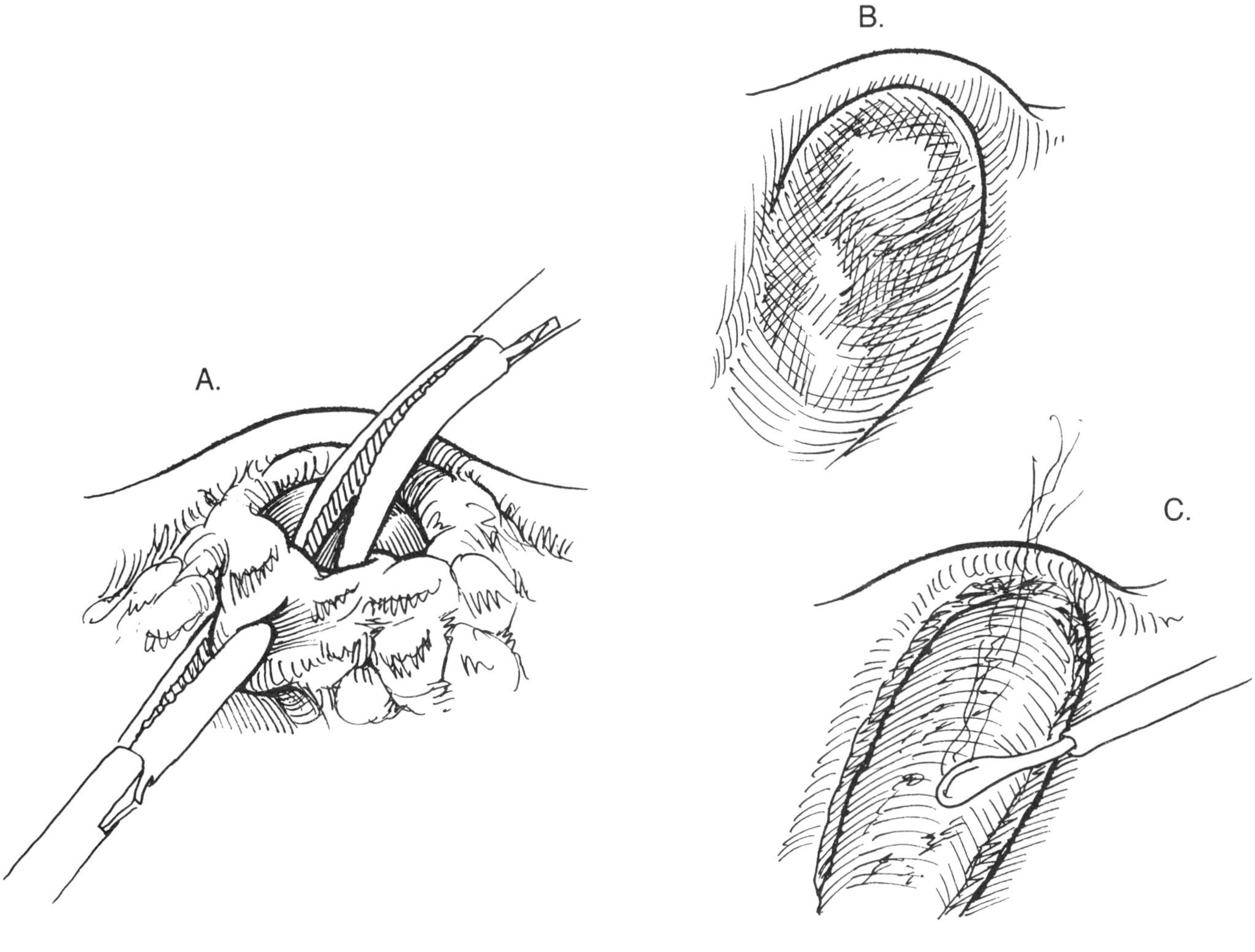

Fig. 2.52

A tensely distended gallbladder should be aspirated as soon as the fundus is exposed (Fig. 2.53). A large aspirating needle is inserted and the gallbladder contents milked upward as the sac collapses. The presence of thick bile and sludge may require the use of a larger aspirating cannula. If the gallbladder wall is pliable, a small hole can be closed with the grasper. A larger hole may require suture or a loop ligature.

If the gallbladder is packed with bulky stones, it can be opened and emptied into an adjacent plastic

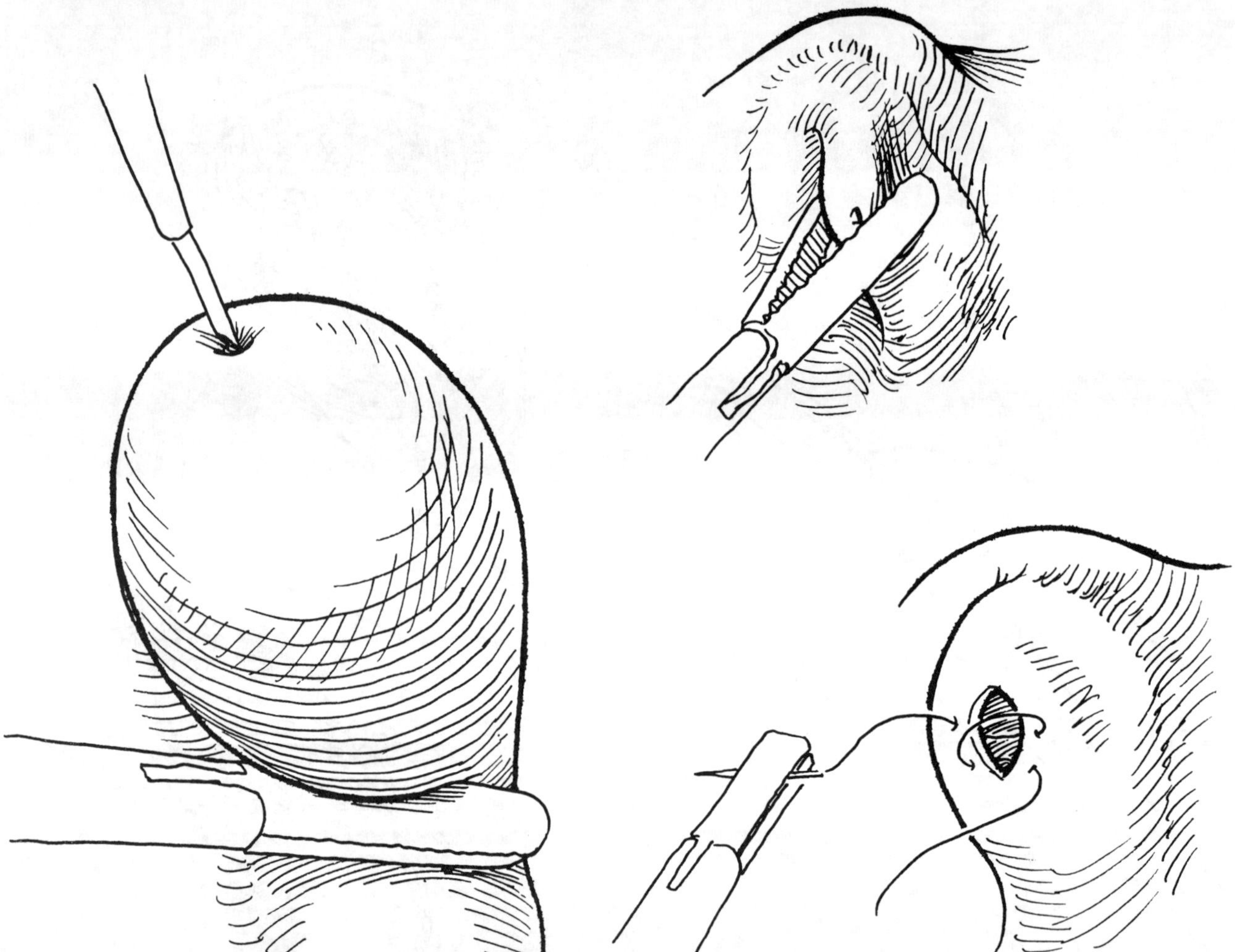

Fig. 2.53

sac (Fig. 2.54). The sac is secured by its purse string and left above the liver until the end of the case. The opening in the gallbladder wall can be sutured. It may not be possible to disimpact a large stone in Hartmann's pouch. Such a stone must be bluntly manipulated during dissection.

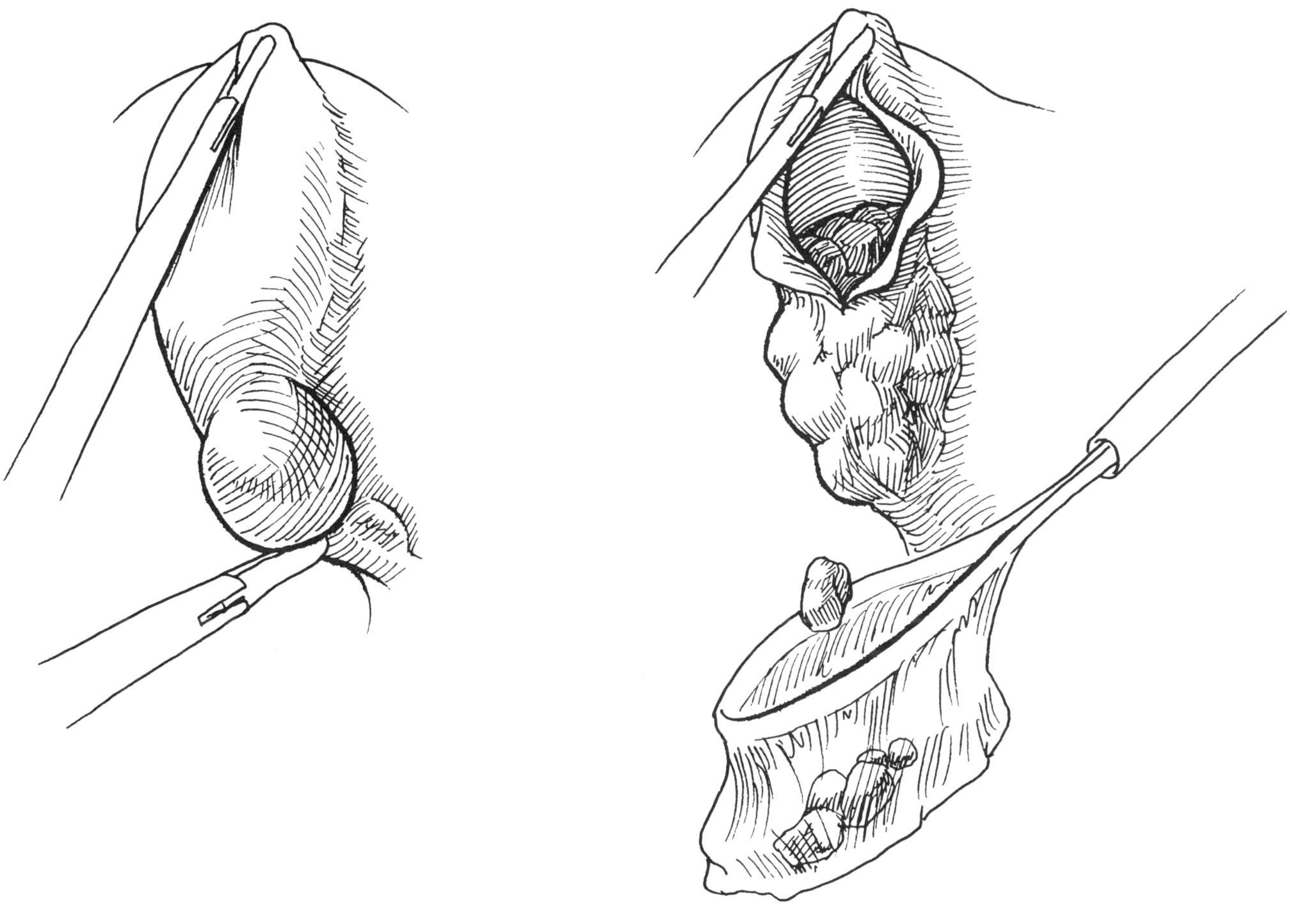

Fig. 2.54

The gallbladder wall may be thickened in acute cholecystitis, rigid and calcified (porcelain) or firm and shrunken (scleroatrophic) (Fig. 2.55). If purchase with a grasper is not possible, mobilization of the fundus may be started with blunt dissection. Once an adequate length of fundus is freed, it can be surrounded with a loop ligature for retraction. Another option that works well if there is a large stone impacted in the fundus, is to hold up the fundus with the open jaws of an atraumatic grasper. Retrograde (from the fundus to the neck) dissection can be continued if the cystohepatic triangle is edematous and thickened as it often is in the acute situation. Bleeding from the intact cystic artery compounds the difficulty in such cases.

On reaching the infundibulum the surgeon must determine if the cystic duct can be safely identified. Cholangiogram, which can be performed through the ampulla, is worthwhile doing routinely to identify the anatomy in acute cholecystitis. An overriding

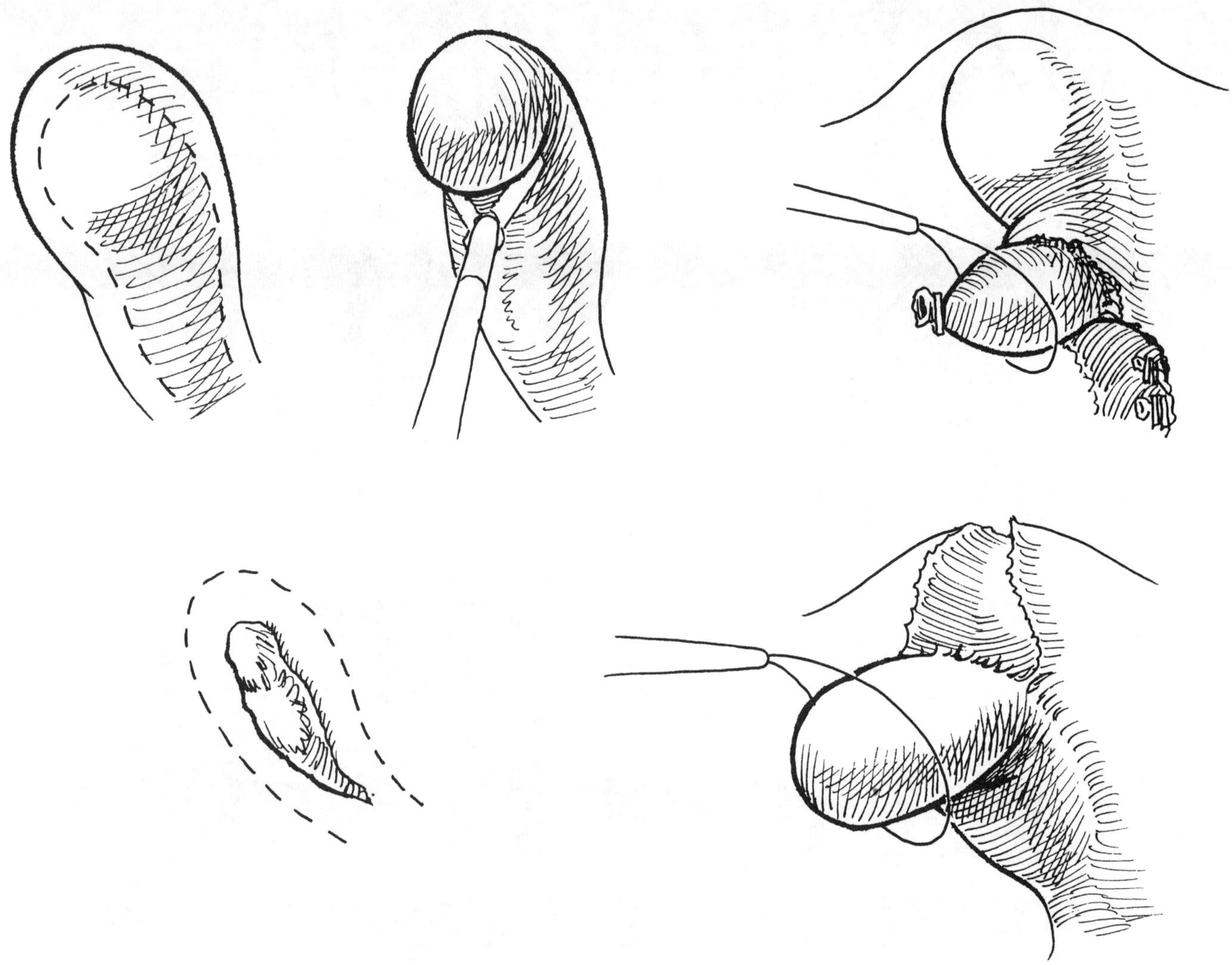

Fig. 2.55

Hartmann's pouch may obscure a short cystic duct or a fistula between Hartmann's pouch and the common duct (Mirizzi's syndrome) (Fig. 2.56A). The short duct may be successfully exposed and divided, using either a clip placed without tension on the common duct (Fig. 2.56B) and/or a loop ligature. A cholangiogram should be performed if the anatomy is unclear. A long wide cystic duct may need to be stapled for secure closure (Fig. 2.56C). A running suture or 8-mm clip can also be used to close such a duct.

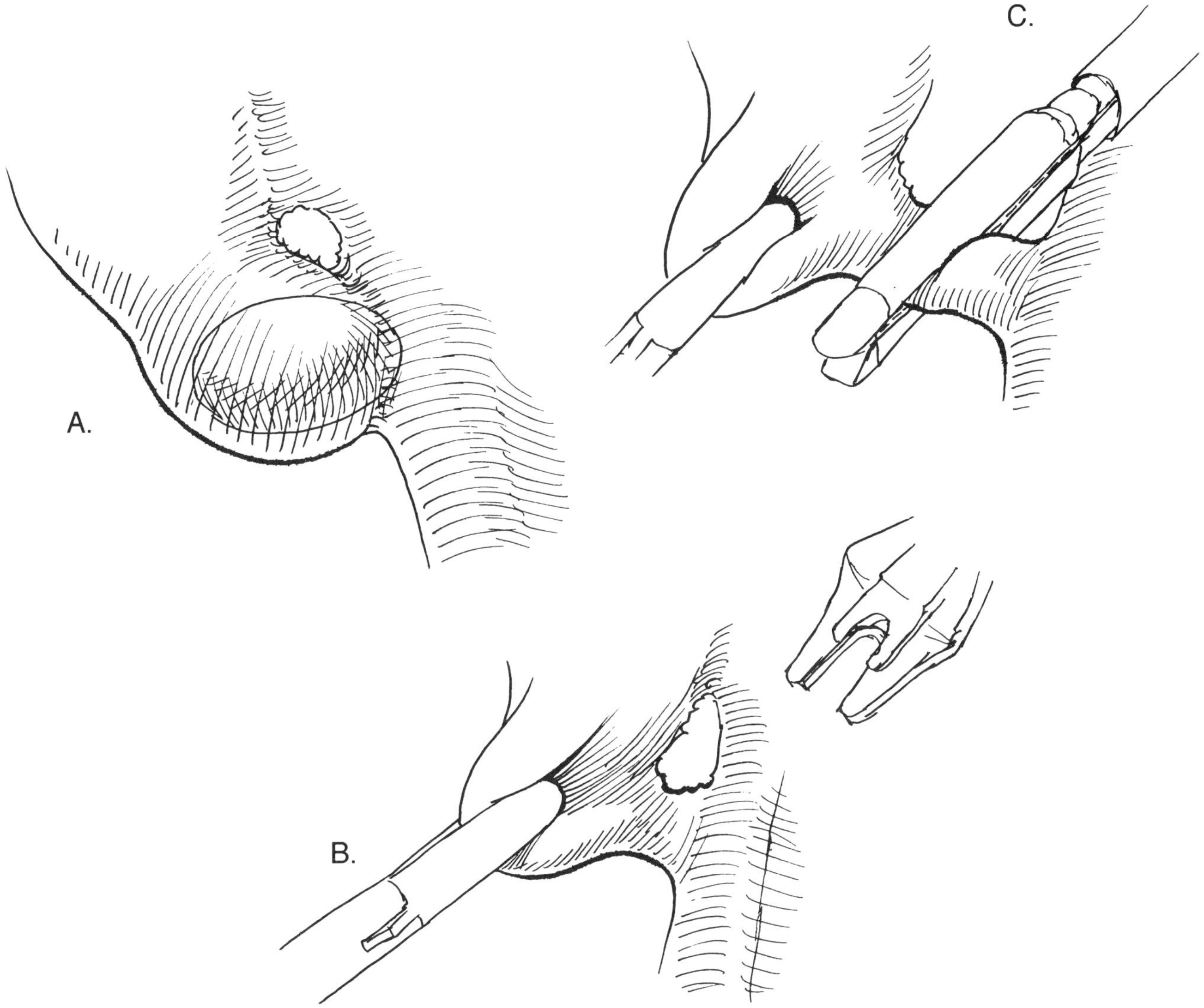

Fig. 2.56

Complications

In addition to the general risks of laparoscopy, biliary laparoscopy may be complicated by bile collections and bile duct injury. The majority of postoperative bile collections are subclinical, occur in up to 30% of cases, and resolve spontaneously. Clinically significant bile leakage after laparoscopy occurs with about the same incidence as after open cholecystectomy (0.3-0.6%). About half of these leaks come from the cystic duct (Fig. 2.57). The mechanisms include insecure clipping, a tear proximal to the clip (dissection injury, catheter perforation), avulsion injury or inadvertent cautery applied to the clip (which desiccates the duct and allows the clip to fall off). A quarter of the leaks come from the gallbladder bed, usually from injury to underlying segmental hepatic ducts rather than from cholecystohepatic (Lushka) ducts. The remainder of leaks, and by far the most serious, come from major injury to extrahepatic ducts. Operator inexperience, inflammation and aberrant anatomy lead to misidentification of bile ducts and technical errors.

The first sign of a significant bile collection is failure to improve rapidly after surgery. This may be followed by increasing abdominal pain with requirement for more pain medication, anorexia, nausea and vomiting, ileus, distention, tenderness, low grade fever and mild leukocytosis. Jaundice may follow. Delay in making the diagnosis is not uncommon. If there is no major duct injury and no distal obstruction, percutaneous drainage may be sufficient treatment. Major injury must be ruled out by ultrasound, CT scan, liver scan (for evidence of ongoing leak), ERCP and/or percutaneous transhepatic cholangiography.

Major bile duct injury due to mechanical occlusion or disruption manifests early. Stricture due to dissection or thermal injury to the pericholedochal plexus is thought to result from ischemia and occurs late. Mechanical injuries most often result from the common duct being misidentified as cystic duct. If intraoperative cholangiogram is done, 80% of such injuries

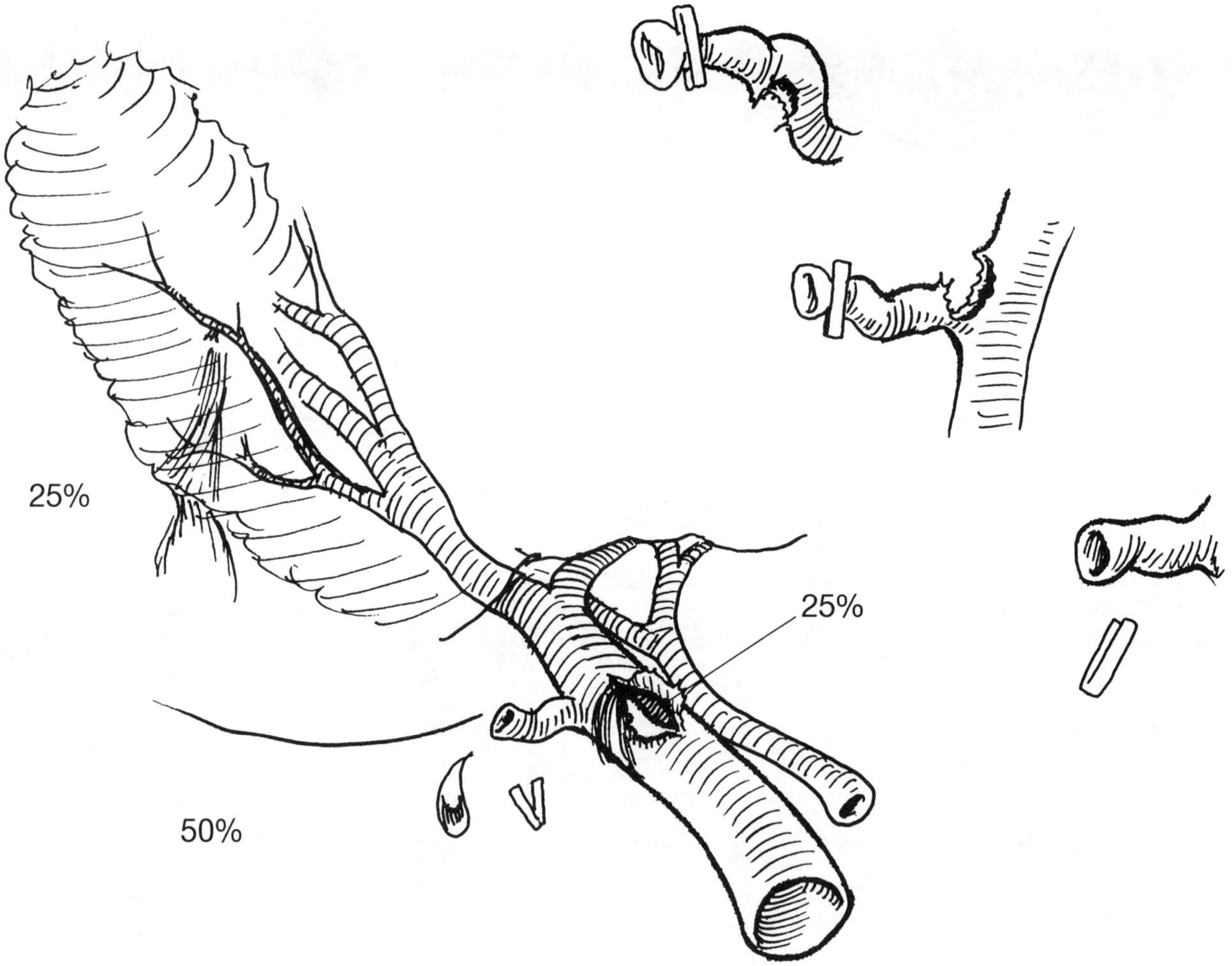

Fig. 2.57

can be identified at the time of surgery, while only 27% are recognized without cholangiogram. Even with cholangiogram, there is often failure to recognize the lack of filling of a right segmental duct (Fig. 2.58). The proximal ducts must be visualized. Failure to fill the proximal ducts can be a sign of common duct cannulation, and transection may result if not recognized.

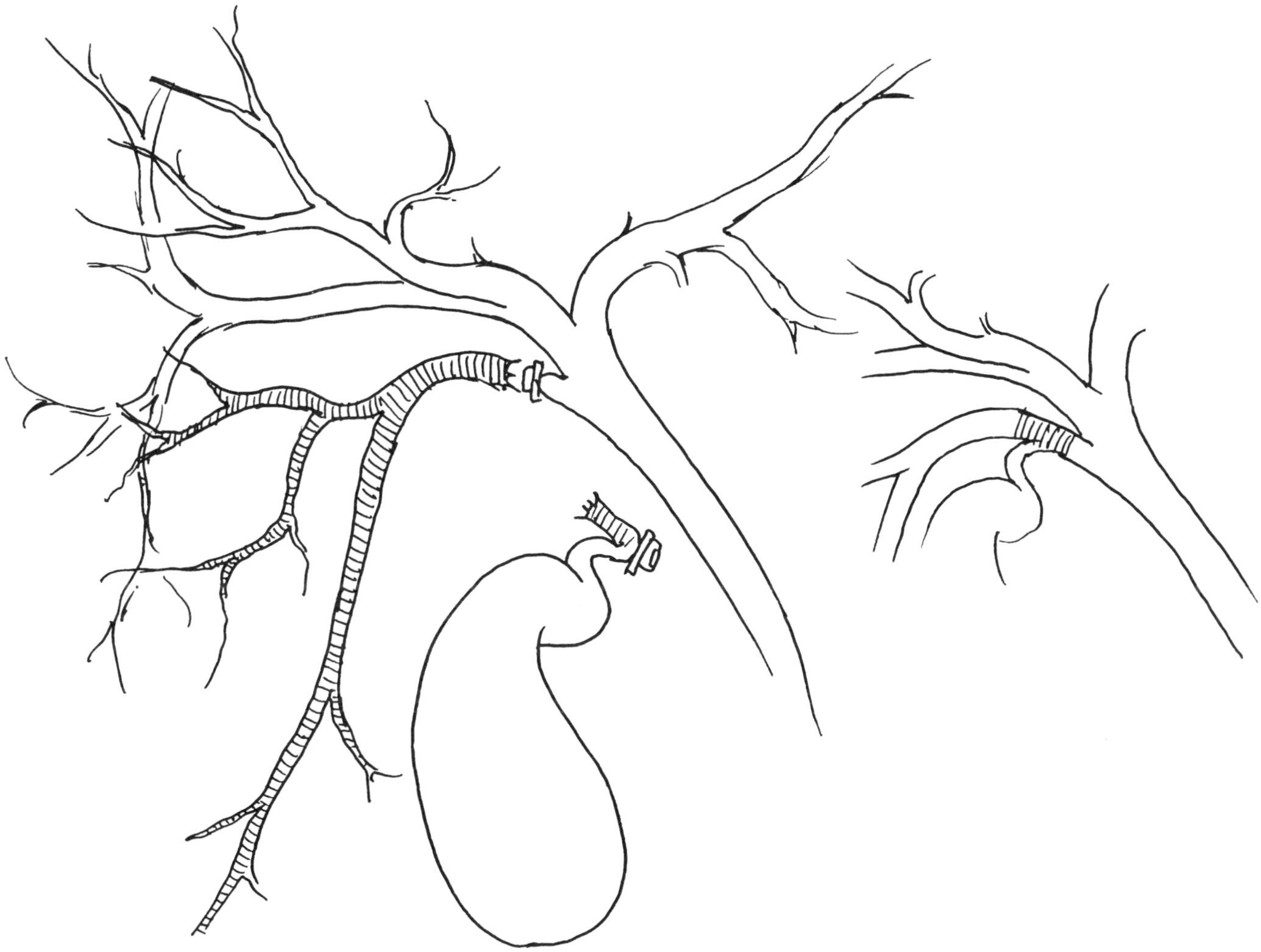

Fig. 2.58

The increased risk factors associated with the difficult gallbladder predispose to injury by causing misidentification, tenting, overbite when clipping in a pool of blood etc. The severity of the injury depends on how close to the bifurcation it is and how much of the duct is excised (Fig. 2.59).

Simple laceration or transection is best managed in expert hands by opening the abdomen and doing primary repair with fine absorbable suture over a stent such as a T-tube limb. Circumferential repair is subject to late ischemic stricture. A short stenosis of the duct may be managed by an endoscopic or percutaneously placed stent. Complete occlusion, transection and excisional injuries are treated by hepaticojejunostomy with mucosa to mucosa anastomosis. If the injury is recognized early, immediate surgery is the treatment of choice, preferably by experts in hepatobiliary surgery. If late, the leak is controlled by drainage and a period of several weeks is allowed to pass before surgery so that the inflammation can subside.

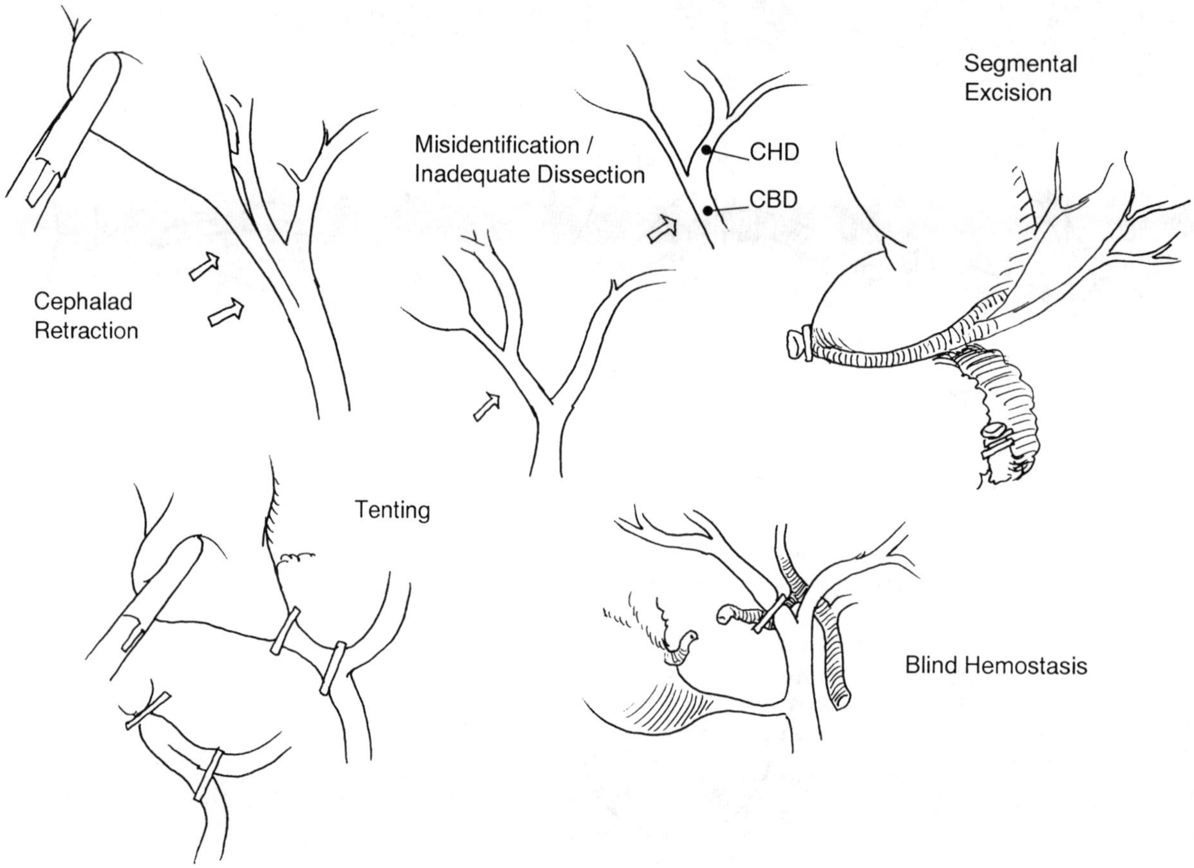

Fig. 2.59

Management of Common Duct Stones

The operative management of common duct stones must be tempered by two factors at the present time. One is the high success rate of ERCP with sphincterotomy in expert hands in clearing the common duct of stones (95%). The other is the high degree of technical expertise required for laparoscopic common duct stone removal. These factors make many surgeons choose postoperative ERCP over laparoscopic choledochotomy.

Many are routinely using pre-operative ERCP for all patients with elevated liver enzymes. However, only one third of such patients have a common duct stone at the time of endoscopy, and the procedure does have significant morbidity (~10%) and mortality (~1%). Two additional negative factors associated with ERCP are cost and the long-term sequelae of sphincterotomy, which is routinely done to extract stones. For the one third found to have stones, the cost factor may be balanced against the increased operative time and morbidity of common duct exploration, especially in older patients. The late stricture rate following sphincterotomy makes the procedure more worrisome in young patients.

On the other hand, only two thirds of patients with common duct stones have elevated enzymes and/or a dilated common duct. The other one third may therefore require intraoperative or postoperative common duct stone removal.

The decision whether to do prophylactic preoperative ERCP or to wait for the intraoperative cholangiogram must also be balanced against the fact that the majority of common duct stones are small and pass spontaneously. This is supported by historical clinical experience and by the likelihood that the majority of those with a history of elevated enzymes and negative ERCP most likely passed a stone. This is also supported by the fact that many of those who in the past had a stone demonstrated on intravenous cholangiogram, subsequently had a negative exploration. Add to that the possibility that another stone will pass through the cystic duct before cholecystectomy. In that case, a prior ERCP with sphincterotomy will have made the passage of the new stone easier, but the patient would have lost nothing by having the ERCP after surgery. On the other hand, in a center where expertise for laparoscopic common duct exploration exists, the 5% of pre-op ERCP failures have a second chance. Once a significant size stone is demonstrated on cholangiogram, the choice between intraoperative and postoperative intervention must be made.

There are several options for intraoperative common duct stone removal (Fig. 2.60). The two that are currently favored by advanced laparoscopic surgeons are laparoscopic common duct exploration, and cystic duct dilatation with trans-cystic duct stone extraction by choledochoscopy. The size of the stone affects the management strategy. Stones less than 4 mm in size can be left with the expectation that they will pass spontaneously. Stones between 4 and 8 mm can be extracted by laparoscopic transcystic choledochoscopy or ERCP. Stones between 8 mm and 1.4 cm can be treated by either ERCP or laparoscopic com-

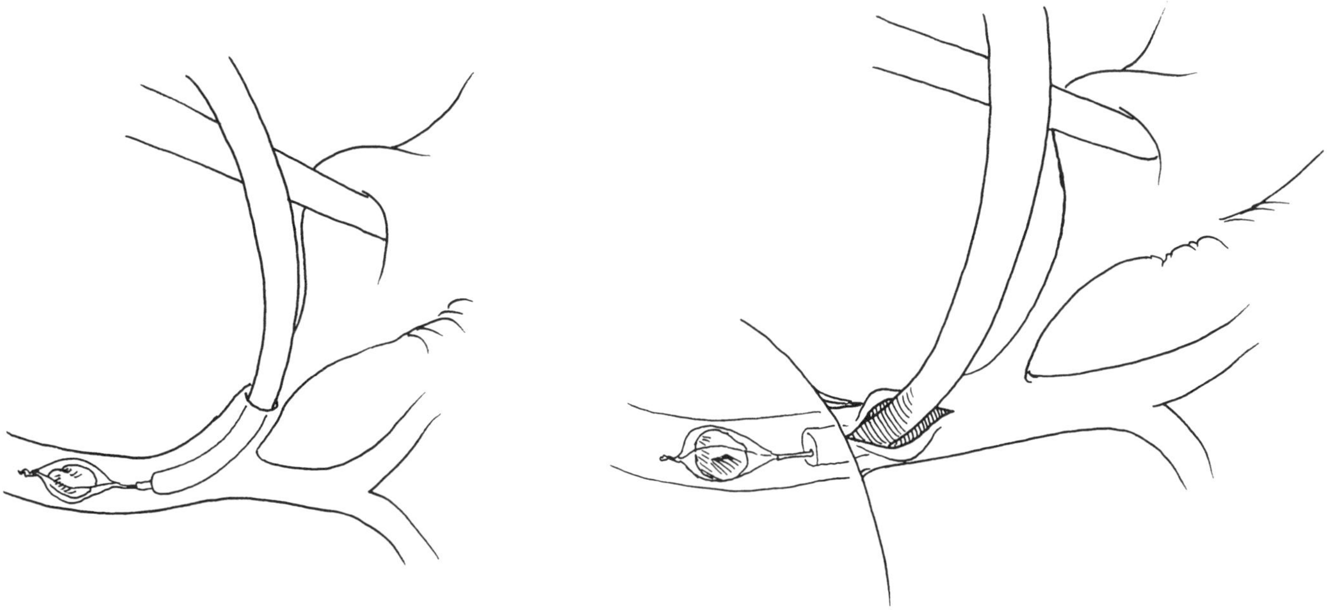

Fig. 2.60

mon bile duct exploration. Stones larger than 1.4 cm can be extracted by laparoscopic common duct exploration because they are too large to be removed by ERCP, or lithotripsy may be done with either procedure to fragment and remove the stone..

Laparoscopic common duct exploration requires considerable expertise. It is advisable only when the common duct is dilated and is indicated when there is a large stone (>1 cm), multiple stones or impacted stones. It is contraindicated with a small duct where there is a significant risk of stricture. Choledochotomy allows the use of an 8-mm scope with good optics and a large manipulation channel. The procedure is much the same as open exploration although stay sutures are not generally needed. The choledochotomy is made above the upper border of the duodenum and is made equal in length to the size of the largest stone. Placement of the T-tube, stent, or trans-cystic drain and duct closure are advanced laparoscopic skills.

Recent interest has focused on trans-cystic duct stone extraction for stones between 4 and 8 mm in size. An opening is made in the cystic duct where it is widest near the common duct. A pressure-controlled balloon is used to slowly dilate the cystic duct to a diameter that is less than the inner diameter of the common duct (7 mm is usually possible), but as large as the largest calculus. The majority of cystic ducts (80-90%) can be successfully dilated, however there is a risk of damage to the cystic duct-common duct junction and to the common duct itself. The balloon (or ureteral dilators) is passed into the cystic duct over a guidewire and the cystic duct is observed for tearing as dilatation proceeds. A smaller flexible choledochoscope is passed. The closest stone is trapped first with a balloon or basket, removed with the scope, and the procedure repeated. High success rate has been reported with this technique. A large volume of irrigation is ultimately used so it must be warm. A drawback is that it is only possible to get into the proximal ducts 10% of the time. If the trans-cystic route is unsuccessful, it can be followed by laparoscopic choledochotomy.

SUMMARY

Safe laparoscopic biliary surgery starts with solid understanding of normal and variant anatomy. Every procedure on the biliary tract should be approached with healthy respect and caution in view of the devastating consequences of error. Each surgeon should honestly assess his or her limitations and not exceed them. Any uncertainty should be resolved by cholangiogram. There should never be any embarrassment about falling back on a safer, more conservative, alternative.

Chapter 2: The Biliary System

EMBRYOLOGY

O'Rahilly R, Muller F. Human Embryology and Teratology. New York:Wiley-Liss, 1992:139-181.

Skandalakis JE, Gray SW. Embryology for Surgeons, Baltimore:Williams & Wilkins, 1984:282-333.

Wind GG, et al. Microcomputer reconstruction of pancreaticobiliary embryogenesis. Clin Anat 1989;2:225-233.

ANATOMY

Adams, DB. The importance of the extrahepatic biliary anatomy in preventing complications at laparoscopic cholecystectomy. Surg Clin North Am 1993;73:861-871.

Benson EA, Page RE. A practical reappraisal of the anatomy of the extrahepatic bile ducts and arteries. Br J Surg 1976;63:853-860.

Bergman RA, Thompson SA, Afifi AK. Compendium of Human Anatomic Variation. Baltimore:Urban & Schwarzenberg, 1988:77, 78, 167, 16.

Crist DW, Gadacz TR. Laparoscopic anatomy of the biliary tree. Surg Clin North Am 1993;73:785-797.

Dodson TF. Surgical anatomy of hepatic transplantation. Surg Clin North Am 1993;73:645-659.

Gray H, Clemente CD (ed.). Anatomy of the Human Body:Philadelphia:Lea & Febiger, 1985:1489-1502.

Hartfield PM, Wise RE. Anatomic variation in the gallbladder and bile ducts. In:P Felson B, editor. Roentgenology of the Gallbladder and Biliary Tract. New York:Grune & Stratton, 1976:15-22.

Hiatt JR, et al. Surgical anatomy of the hepatic arteries in 1000 cases. Ann Surg 1994;220:50-52.

Hugh TB, Kelly MD. Laparoscopic anatomy of the cystic duct. Am J Surg 1992;163:593-595.

Klihne MJ, et al. Persistent cholecystohepatic ducts. Arch Surg 1980;115:972-974.

Linder RM, Cady BC. Hepatic resection. Surg Clin North Am 1980;60:349-367.

McNulty JG. The anatomy of the liver, biliary tract and pancreas. In:McNulty JG, editor. Minimally invasive therapy of the liver and biliary system. New York:Thieme Medical Publishers Inc., 1994:4-24.

Northover JMA, Terblanche J. A new look at the arterial supply of the bile duct in man and its surgical implications. Br J Surg 1979;66:379-384.

SURGERY

Bezzi M. Complications after laparoscopic cholecystectomy. Surg Endosc 1995;9:29-36.

Baigrie RJ, et al. Laproscopic cholangiography through the gallbladder. J Am Coll Surg 1994;178:175-176.

Branum G, et al. Management of major complications after laparoscopic cholecystectomy. Ann Surg 1993;217:532-541.

Cuschieri A, Berci G. Laparoscopic Biliary Surgery. Oxford:Blackwell Scientific Publications, 1992:69-141.

Heinerman M. Endoscopic retrograde cholangiographic demonstration of a double gallbladder following laparoscopic cholecystectomy. Surg Endosc 1995;9:61-62.

Kelley WE, Jr. Laparoscopic choledochoscopy with a small-caliber endoscope. Surg Endosc 1995;9:293-296.

Kuster G, et al. Intraoperative cholangiography for laparoscopic cholecystectomy. Surg Gyn Obstet 1993;176:411-417.

Madariaga JR, et al. Corrective treatment and anatomic considerations for laparoscopic cholecystectomy injuries. J Am Coll Surg 1994;179:321-325.

Miyajima N. Experience with laparoscopic double gallbladder removal. Surg Endosc 1995;9:63-66.

Moont M. Cholecystocholangiography. (letter) Surg Endosc 1995;9:544-545. NIH Consensus Conference. Gallstones and laparoscopic cholecystectomy. JAMA 1993;269:1018-1024.

Paterson-Brown S, Garden J (eds.). Principles and Practice of Surgical Laparoscopy. London:WB Saunders Co. Ltd., 1994.

Rattner DW, et al. Factors associated with successful laparoscopic cholecystectomy for acute cholecystitis. Ann Surg 1993;217:233-236.

Rossi RL (ed). Biliary Tract Injuries Revisited. Surg Clin North Am 1994;74:755-780, 805-824, 931-966,

Schrenk P, et al. Laparoscopic cholecystectomy, cause of conversion in 1,300 patients and analysis of risk factors. Surg Endosc 1995;9:25-28.

Strasberg SM, et al. An analysis of the problem of biliary injury during laparoscopic cholecystectomy. J Am Coll Surg 1995;180:101-125.

Tierney S, et al. The current management of common duct stones. In:Cameron JL editor. Adv Surg 1995;28:271-299.

Warren, KW. Pitfalls of gallbladder surgery. Hospital Practice 1967:29-37.

Wherry DC, et al. An external audit of laparoscopic cholecystectomy performed in medical treatment facilities of the department of defense. Ann Surg 1994;220:626-634.

Zucker KA. Surgical Laparoscopy Update. St. Louis: Quality Medical Publishing, 1993:110-185.

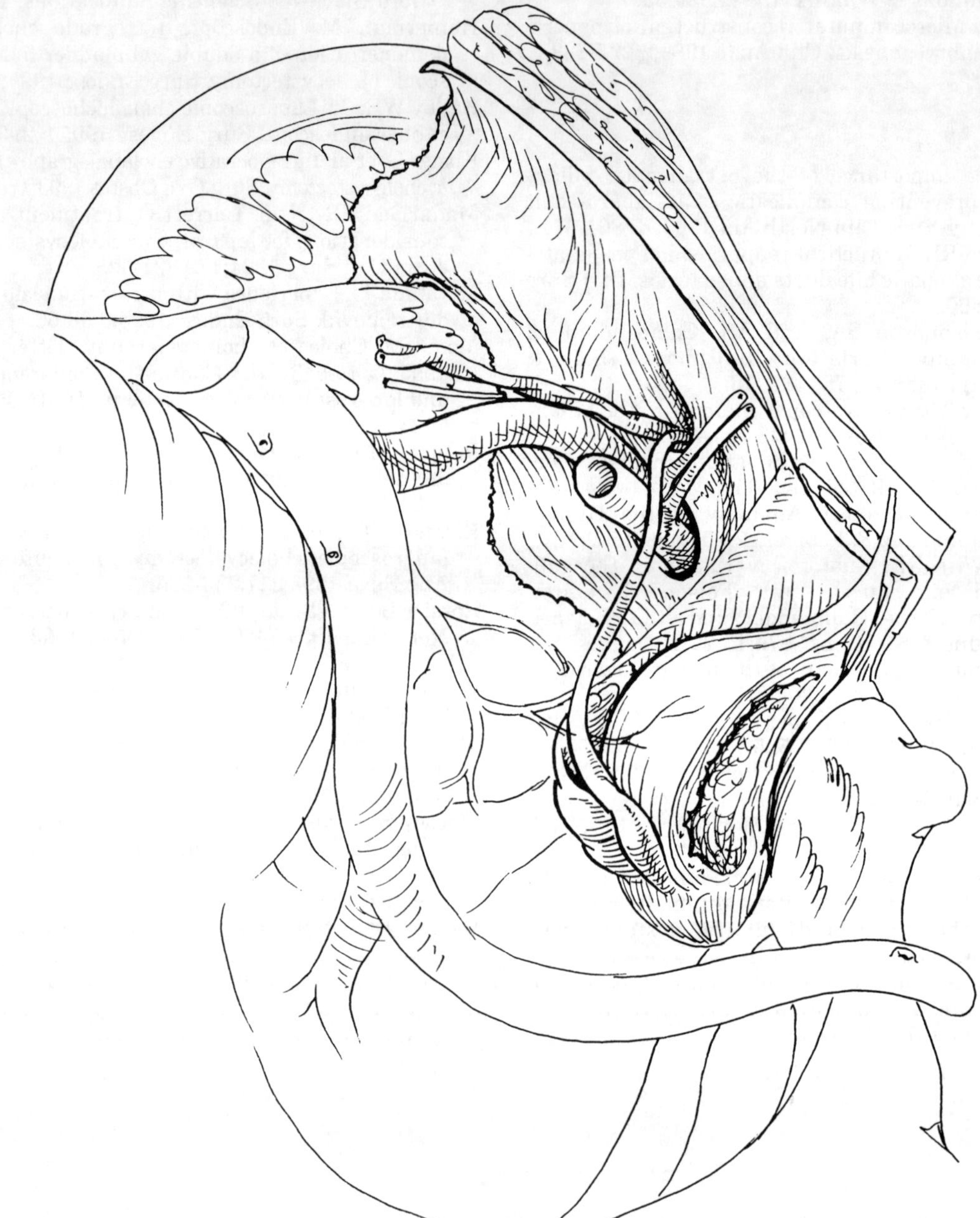

3

The Inguinal Region

Successful laparoscopic repair of groin hernia depends on complete understanding of the regional anatomy. The precedents set by successful hernia repairs of the past form the basis of evolving laparoscopic approaches. In this chapter, groin anatomy is presented from an anterior and posterior perspective, and hernia pathology is reviewed as the basis for both external and internal repair techniques. The logical starting point is the embryology of the groin.

EMBRYOLOGY

During the formation of the coelomic cavity, caudal scrotal evaginations appear in the inguinal region bilaterally (Fig. 3.1). The somatic lining of these pouches is the transversalis portion of the endoabdominal fascia, the defining membrane of the abdominal cavity. Within each of these outpouchings, a sleeve of parietal peritoneum forms an inner lining, the processus vaginalis. The

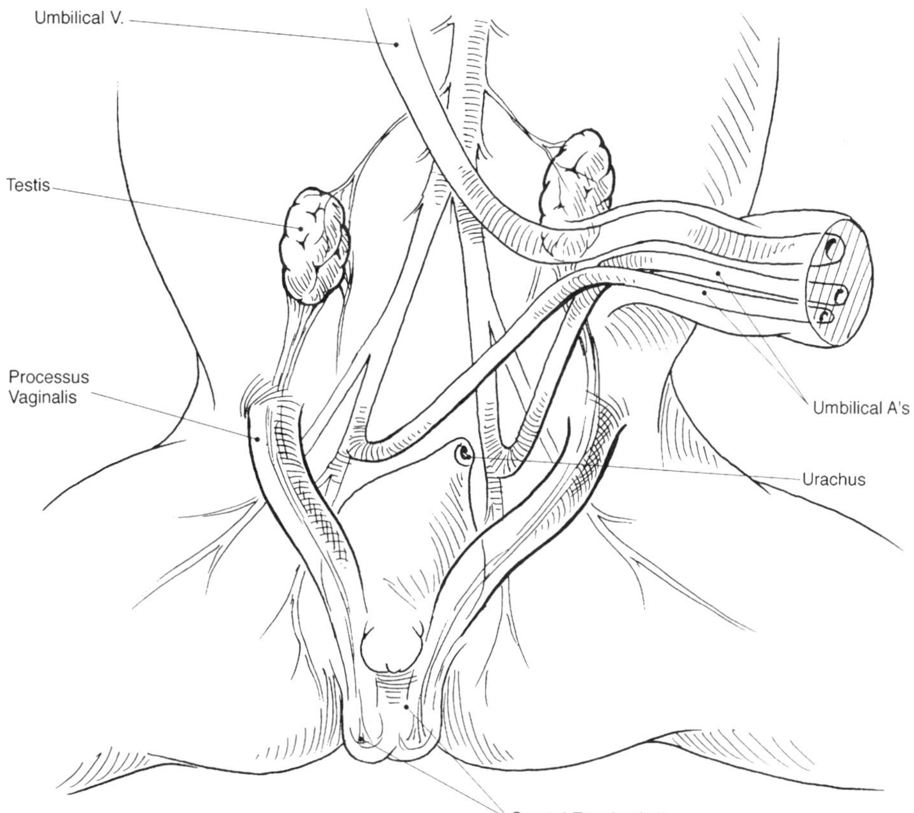

Fig. 3.1

gonads form anterior to the kidneys in the dorsal body wall of the fetus, connected to the bottom of the scrotal sac by the gubernacular ligaments (Chapters 7, 8). In the male, this anchor, combined with differential growth, result in migration of the testes into the scrotum in the third trimester of gestation.

Because the testes start in a retroperitoneal position, their path to the scrotum lies between the posterior wall of the processus vaginalis and the transversalis fascia (Fig. 3.2). The testes carry with them their abdominal blood supply, lateral aortic branches, which become the internal spermatic vessels. They also carry their ductal connection with the urinary system, the vas (ductus) deferens. After descent of the testes in the male, the evaginated transversalis fascia surrounding the spermatic cord is called internal spermatic fascia. At or shortly after birth, the processus vaginalis normally is obliterated, leaving the distal remnant as the tunica vaginalis of the testis. If this closure is incomplete, the processus remains as an indirect hernia sac in its position anterior and medial to the spermatic cord.

The ovaries in the female come to rest in the pelvis (Chapter 7). Their ligamentous distal connection to the inguinal outpouchings attach first to the cornua of the uterus and then pass through the inguinal canals as the round ligaments. A patent processus vaginalis in the female also presents as an indirect inguinal hernia.

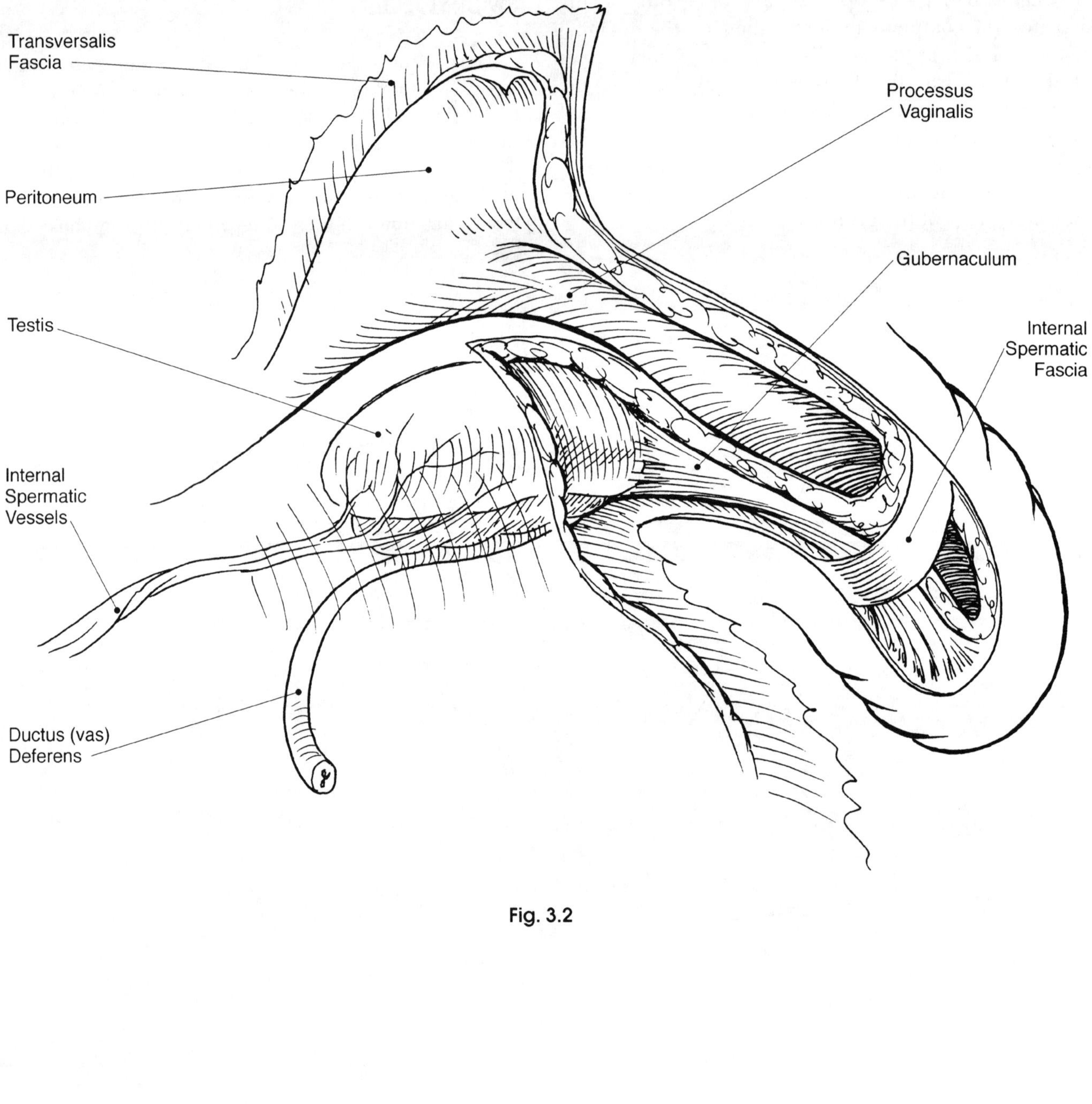

Fig. 3.2

Three extraperitoneal embryologic structures lie between the right and left inguinal areas and their remnants are seen in the laparoscopic view: the urachus and the two umbilical arteries (Fig. 3.3). The urachus connects the apex of the bladder and the embryonic allantoic membrane. Upon closure of the urachus, the remaining midline cord becomes the median umbilical ligament. The umbilical arteries, originating from the paired dorsal aortas in the third week of the embryonic period (the first 8 weeks of gestation), run toward the umbilical cord on either side of the bladder. Through vascular remodeling, their origin changes to the internal iliac vessels in the pelvis. After birth, the obliterated umbilical arteries appear as ridges beneath the anterior parietal peritoneum. They originate in the true pelvis and ascend toward the umbilicus across the medial portions of three critical inguinal structures: the pectineal ligament, the iliopubic tract, and the falx inguinalis (transversus aponeurotic arch).

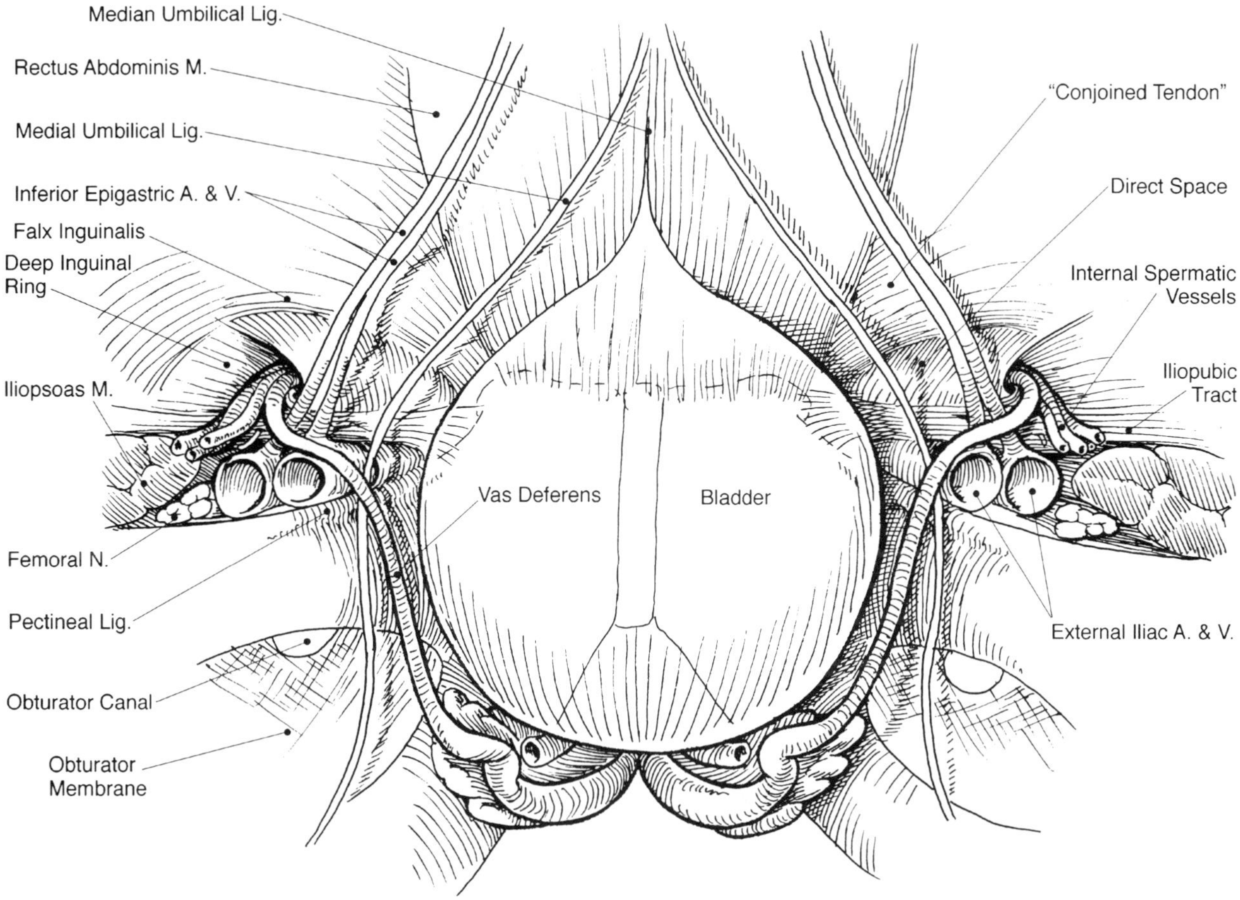

Fig. 3.3

The muscular layers of the abdominal wall originate in the posterolateral segmental myotomes and grow to encircle the abdomen. The middle of the three flank muscles, the internal oblique, provides the sheath of cremaster muscle and fascia around the spermatic cord (Fig. 3.4). Because of the lateral to medial application of this muscle layer to the exposed surfaces of the cord, the posterior aspect of the cord (covered by internal spermatic fascia) is apposed to the transversalis fascia of the posterior inguinal wall and is not covered by cremaster. The deepest muscle layer, the transversus abdominis, forms an aponeurotic arch at its caudal edge, leaving only transversalis fascia and a few aponeurotic fibers behind the cord. The superficial muscle layer, the external oblique, has a broad aponeurosis. The folded lower edge of this aponeurosis forms the inguinal ligament and the investing fascia on its outer surface extends onto the cord outside the superficial inguinal ring as the external spermatic fascia.

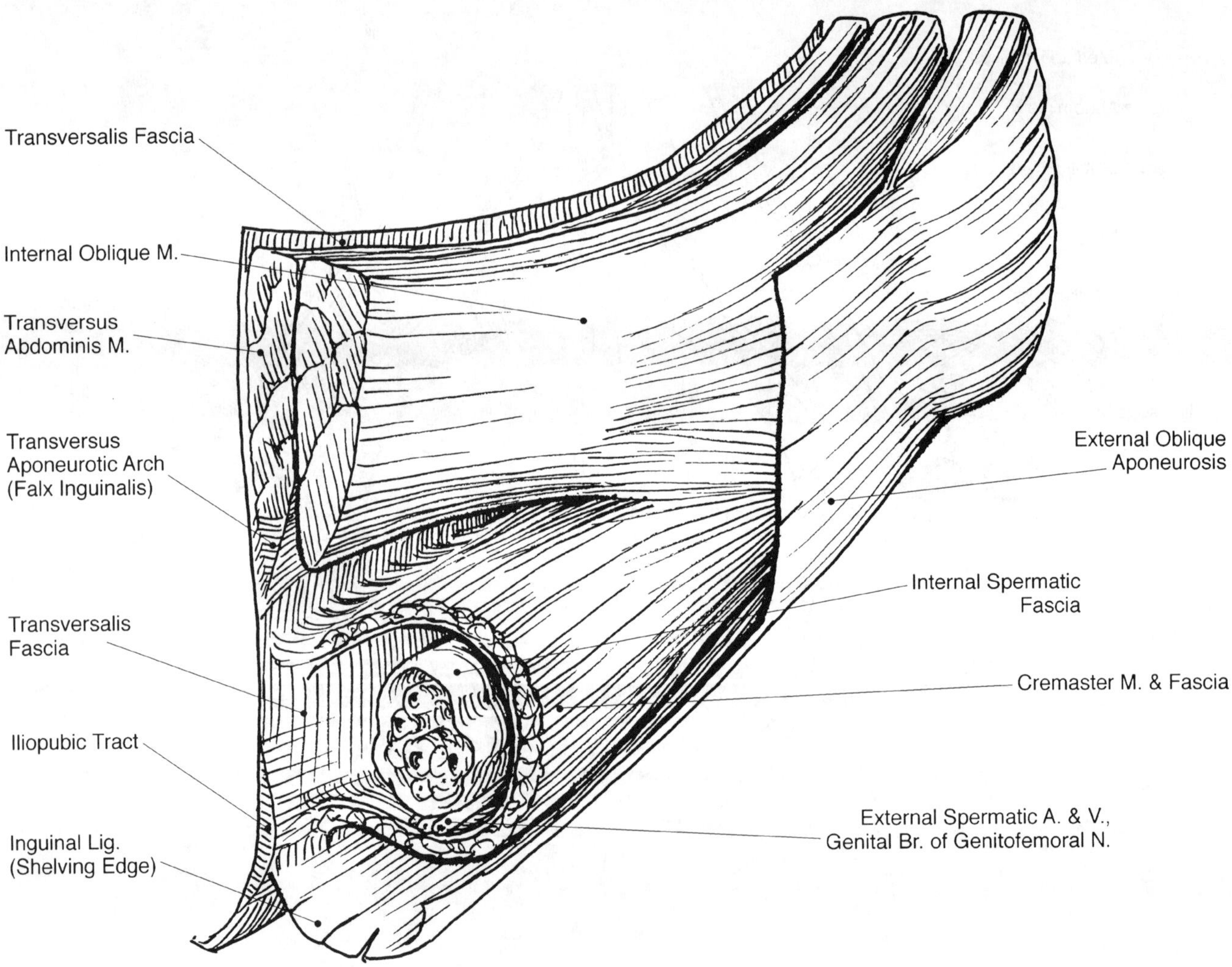

Fig. 3.4

INGUINAL ANATOMY

Overview

The caudal margin of the external oblique aponeurosis, called the inguinal ligament, spans the space between the anterior superior spine of the ilium and the pubic tubercle (Fig. 3.5). The medial fibers of the inguinal ligament fold under and reflect back to attach to the pectineal (Cooper's) ligament on the superior ramus of the pubic bone. The resulting trough in the inguinal ligament is called the shelving edge and the delta of reflected fibers is the lacunar ligament. The foramen beneath the inguinal ligament is occupied laterally by the iliopsoas muscle and medially, in order, by the femoral nerve, iliac artery and iliac vein. The lateral muscular and medial vascular space are separated by the ileopectineal fascial arch, part of the iliopsoas fascia. The medial parts of the internal oblique and transversus abdominis muscles take origin from this fascia and from the adjacent inguinal ligament.

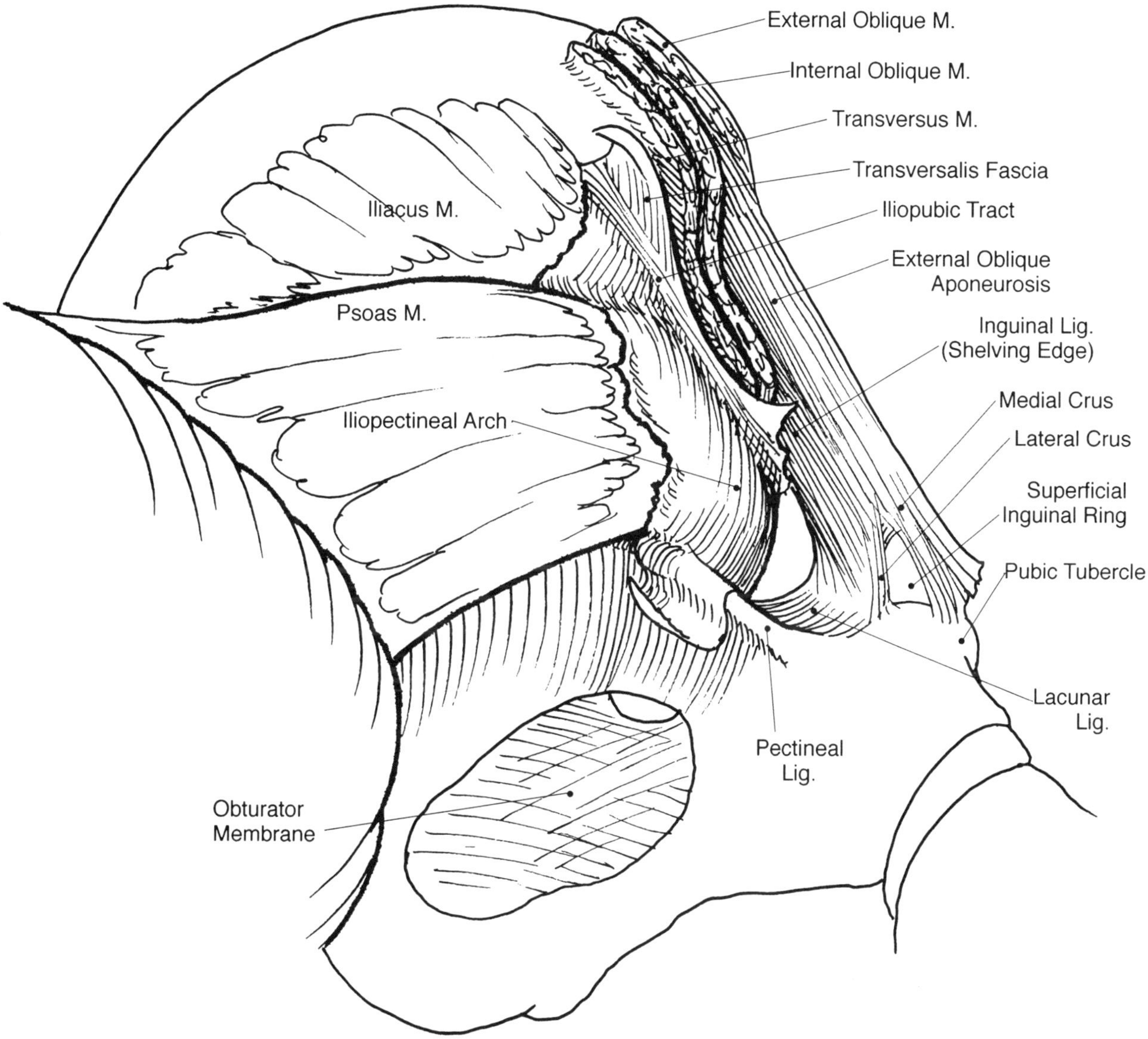

Fig. 3.5

The external iliac artery and vein follow the medial border of the iliopsoas muscle to the inguinal ligament (Fig. 3.6). The inferior epigastric vessels arise from the external iliacs just proximal to the inguinal ligament. In addition to the small pubic, external spermatic and deep circumflex iliac branches of the inferior epigastrics, the obturator artery also arises from this vessel in as many as 25% of individuals (dotted lines, inset). Its course medial to the iliacs puts it at risk during hernia repair. The vas deferens in the male arises in the pelvis and courses upward over the iliac vessels to reach the deep inguinal ring.

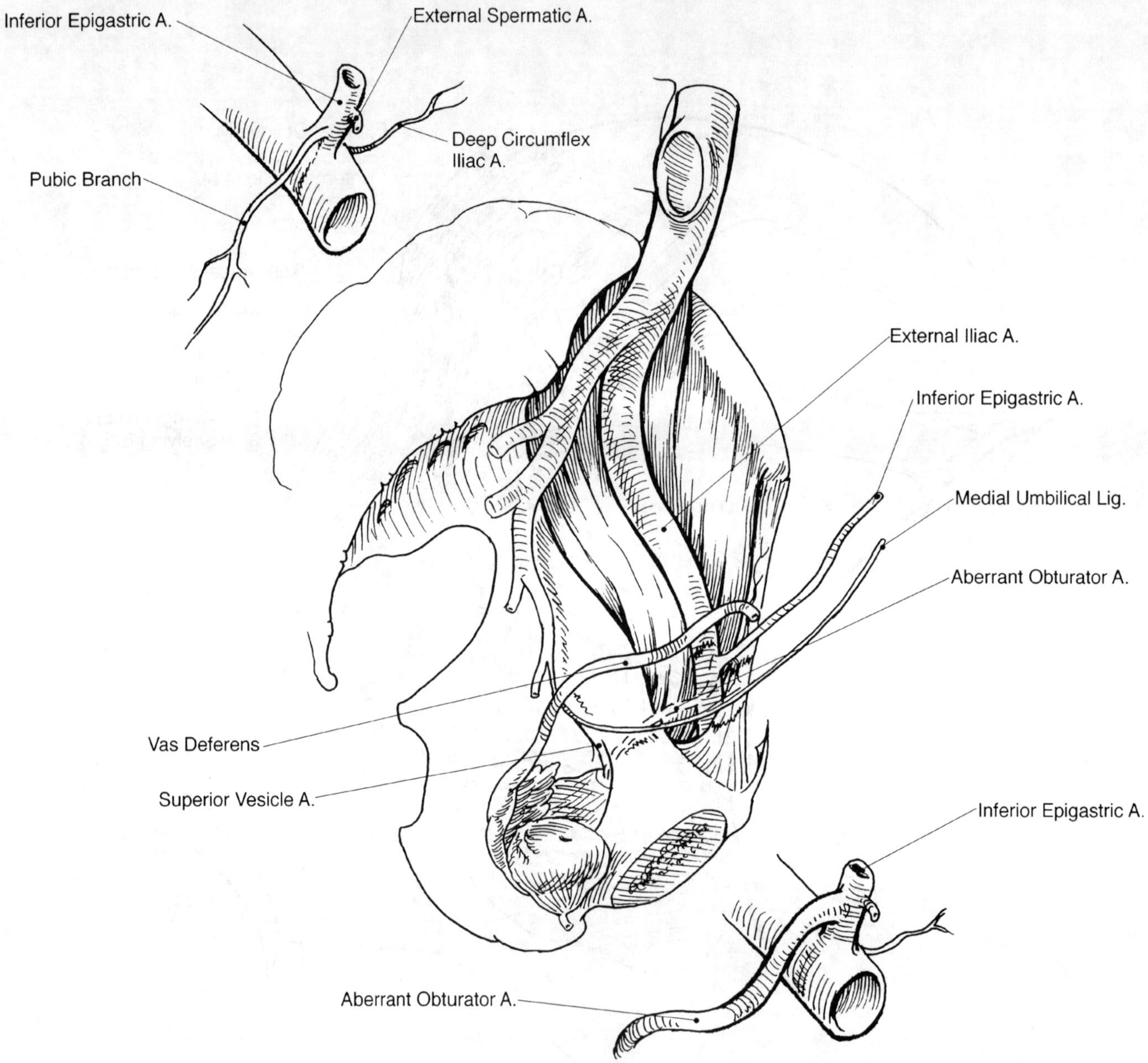

Fig. 3.6

Flank Muscles

The caudal portions of the external oblique, internal oblique and transversus abdominis muscles arise along the crest of the ilium (Fig. 3.7). The lower origins of internal oblique and transversus continue medially beyond the anterior spine and arch up from the inguinal ligament and adjacent iliopsoas fascia. At the midpoint of the inguinal ligament, the lower edge of these arching fibers form the lateral and cephalad borders of the deep inguinal ring. The muscular arches then descend toward the pubis and lateral edge of the rectus muscle (dotted line). The caudal edge of the transversus muscle, the transversus aponeurotic arch or falx (sickle shaped) inguinalis, is substantial and aponeurotic whereas that of the internal oblique is not. The falx is a critical structure in hernia repair. The medial continuations of the two sheets of muscle become aponeurotic near the edge of the rectus sheath. Only a quarter of individuals has fusion of these aponeuroses into a "conjoined tendon" at the lateral edge of the rectus near the pubis.

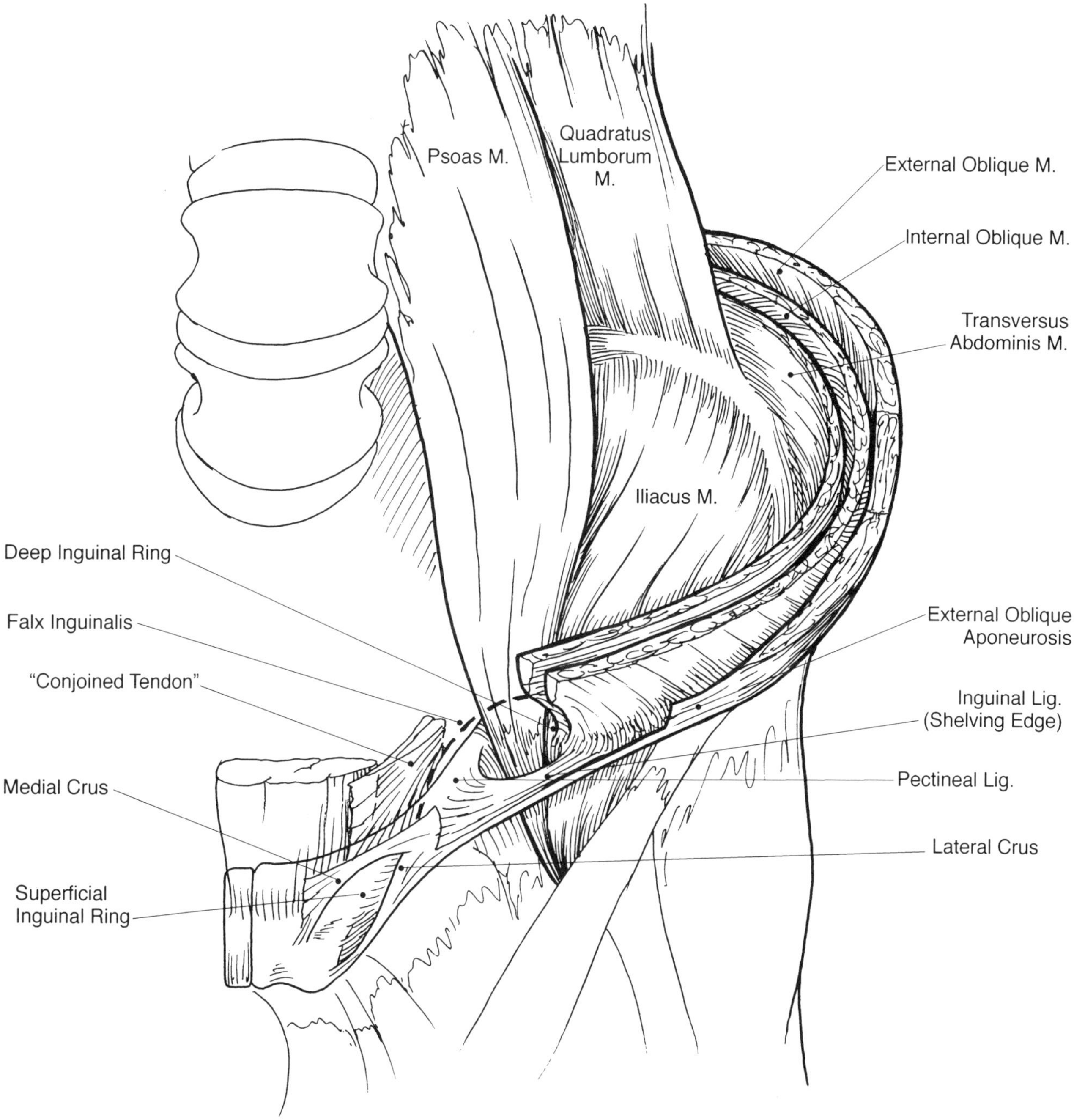

Fig. 3.7

The muscular portion of the external oblique ends at the anterior superior iliac spine and the layer continues as a broad aponeurosis. The medial ends of the lowermost external oblique aponeurosis fibers split into a medial and lateral crus which attach to the pubic tubercle and form the external inguinal ring. The attachment of the length of the external oblique aponeurosis to the anterior rectus sheath lies at the lateral border of the rectus abdominis muscle in the upper abdomen but moves progressively more medial toward the pubis so that it overlies the middle of the rectus at its lower end (Fig. 3.8). The resulting cleft affords access to the underlying fused lamina of internal oblique and transversus.

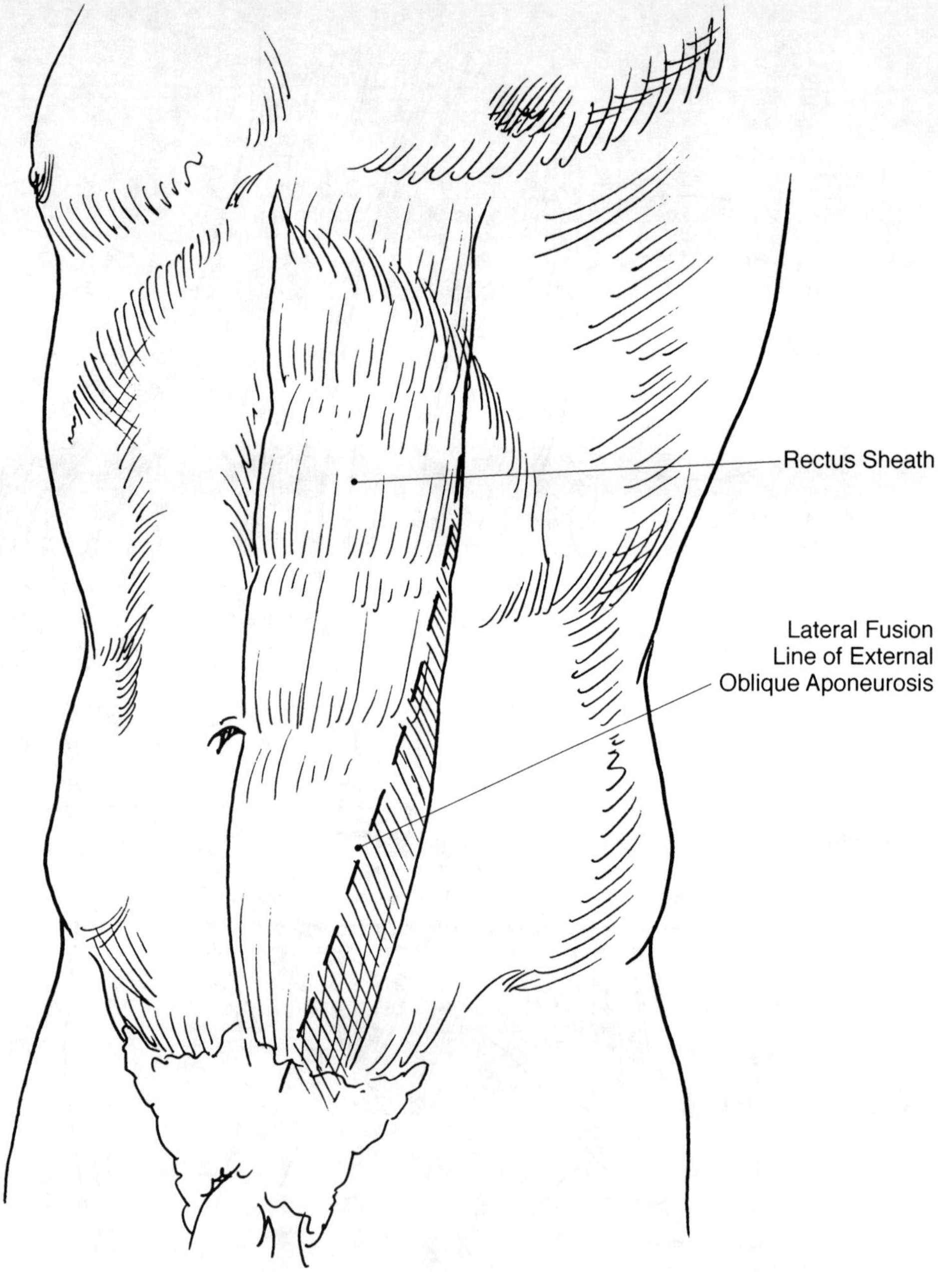

Fig. 3.8

Transversalis Fascia

The endoabdominal fascia lining the muscular walls of the abdomen is the defining outer envelope of the abdominal cavity (Fig. 3.9). The "peritoneal cavity" includes those structures "enclosed" by parietal peritoneum and is not synonymous with abdominal cavity. The structures between the endoabdominal fascia and the parietal peritoneum are called extra-, pre-, or retroperitoneal. The endoabdominal fascia is named regionally according to the underlying structures, for example the iliopsoas fascia. The fascia deep to the transversus muscle is called transversalis fascia. The fascia lining the back side of the inguinal area is part of the transversalis fascia. The transversalis fascia between the falx, the inguinal ligament, and the inferior epigastric vessels is called the direct space (Hesselbach's triangle) and forms the back wall or floor of the inguinal canal. Athough some authors describe the transversalis fascia in the groin as ending at the pectineal ligament, it is continuous over this ligament into the true pelvis as the endopelvic fascia.

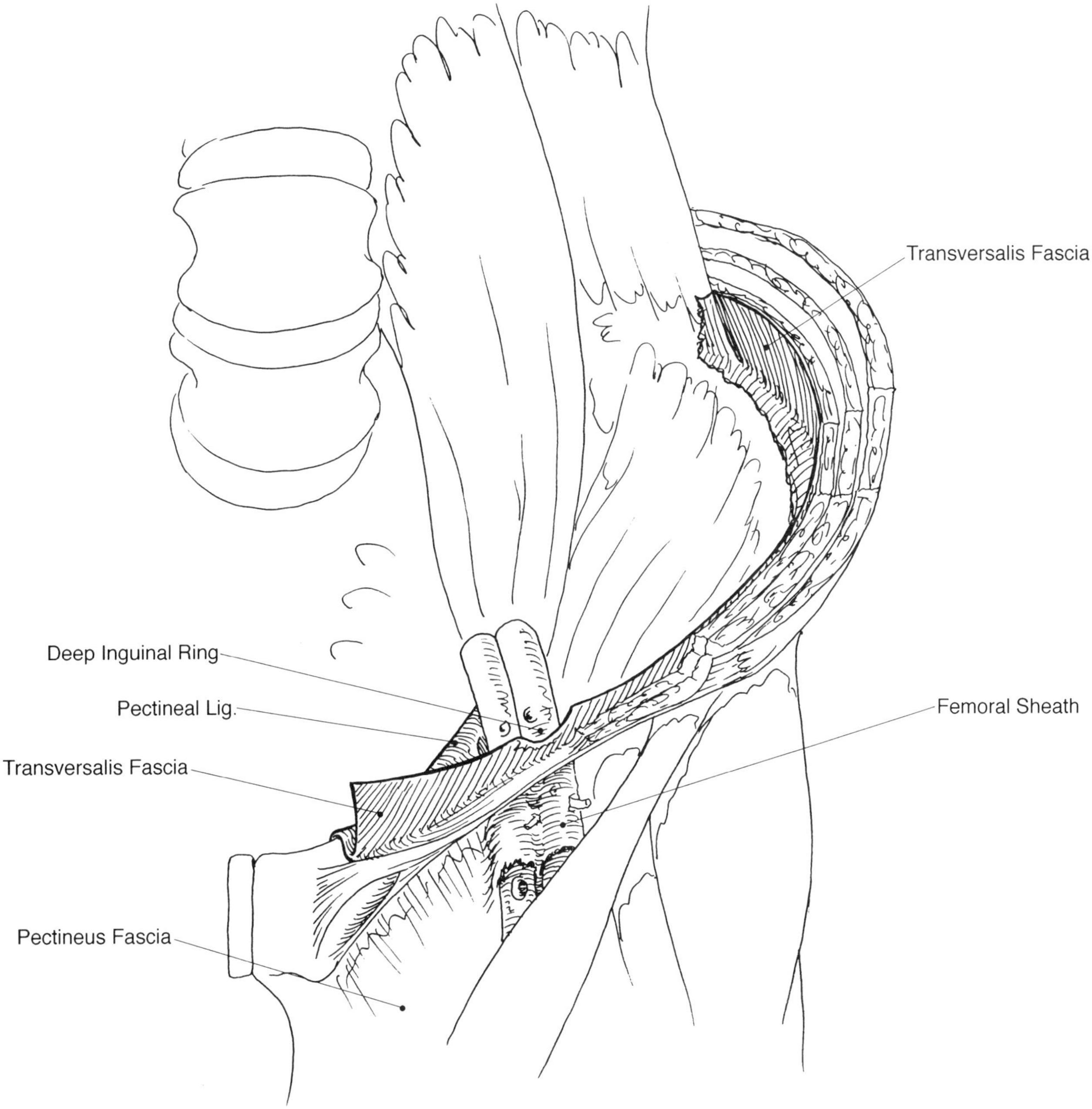

Fig. 3.9

The transversalis fascia, having lined the embryonic scrotal outpouchings, ensheathes the inguinal cords as the internal spermatic fascia and also forms the femoral sheath around the common femoral vessels as they pass into the thigh beneath the inguinal ligament (Fig. 3.10). The femoral sheath attaches to the pectineus fascia beneath the femoral vessels and forms a septum between the vessels. The top edge of this sheath medially overlies the recurved edge of the lacunar ligament. The space within the femoral sheath medial to the femoral vein is the femoral canal. Dilatation of this narrow canal results in a femoral hernia. The tight neck of such hernias predisposes to strangulation of incarcerated viscera.

The inguinal ligament is contiguous with the encircling fascia lata girdle of the thigh and the femoral sheath lies deep to the fascia lata. Thus when a femoral hernia expands the medial femoral sheath, the bulge is deep to the fascia lata. The transversalis fascia is loosely adherent to the posterior lip of the shelving edge of the inguinal ligament. The transversalis fascia spans the gap between falx and inguinal ligament forming the back wall of the inguinal canal in Hesselbach's triangle. The

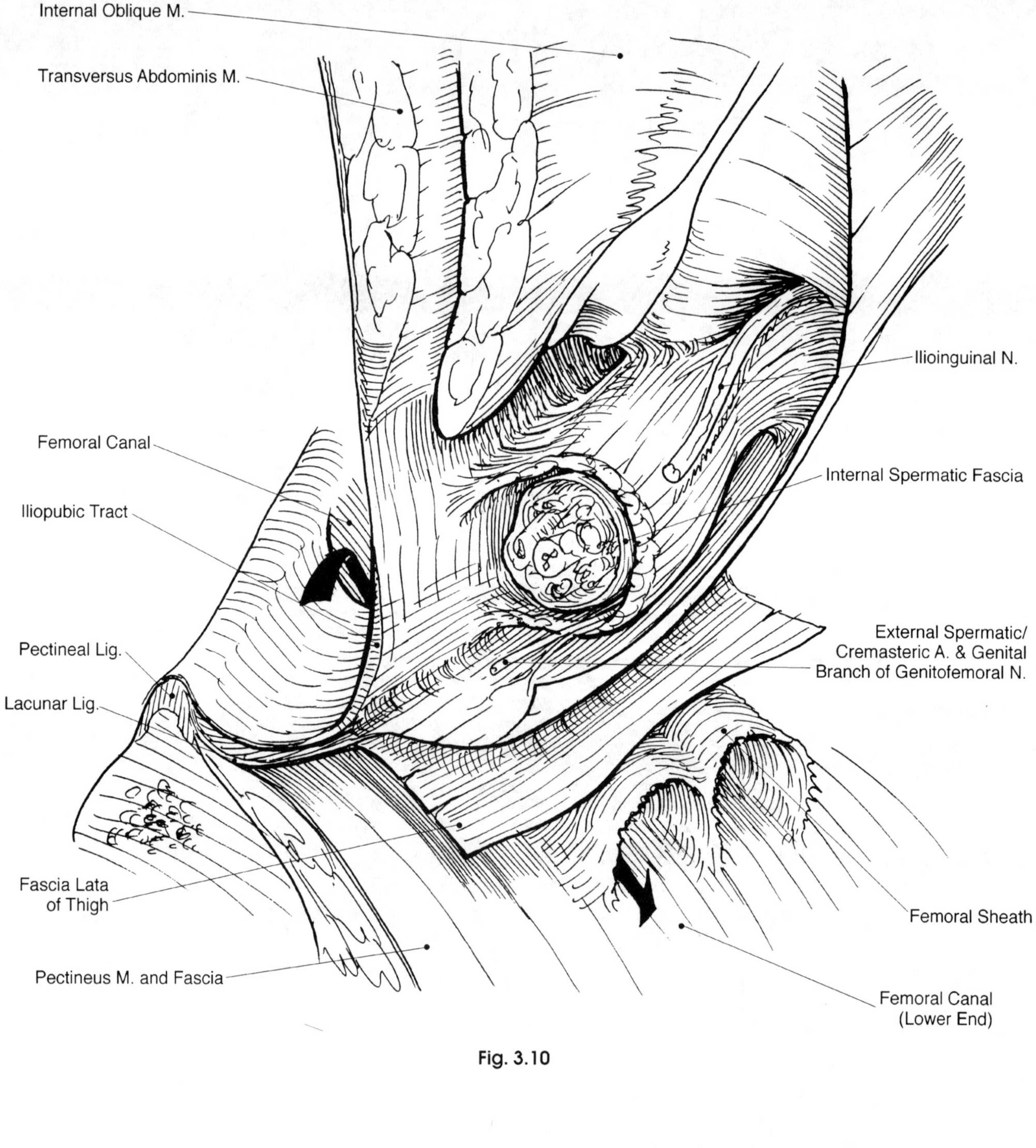

Fig. 3.10

reflection of transversalis onto the cord as internal spermatic fascia forms the deep inguinal ring. The fascia is also fused with the falx, and the combined fibrous arch forms the medial part of most non-mesh hernia repairs. Weakness and bulging of this transversalis fascial sheet is a direct hernia. A large indirect hernia may dilate the deep ring, impinging on the transversalis sheet of the direct space.

The adhesion of transversalis fascia to shelving edge results in coverage of the lacunar ligament by a sheet of transversalis (Fig. 3.11). Thus the deeper pectineal ligament is not visible anteriorly unless these lamina are sep-

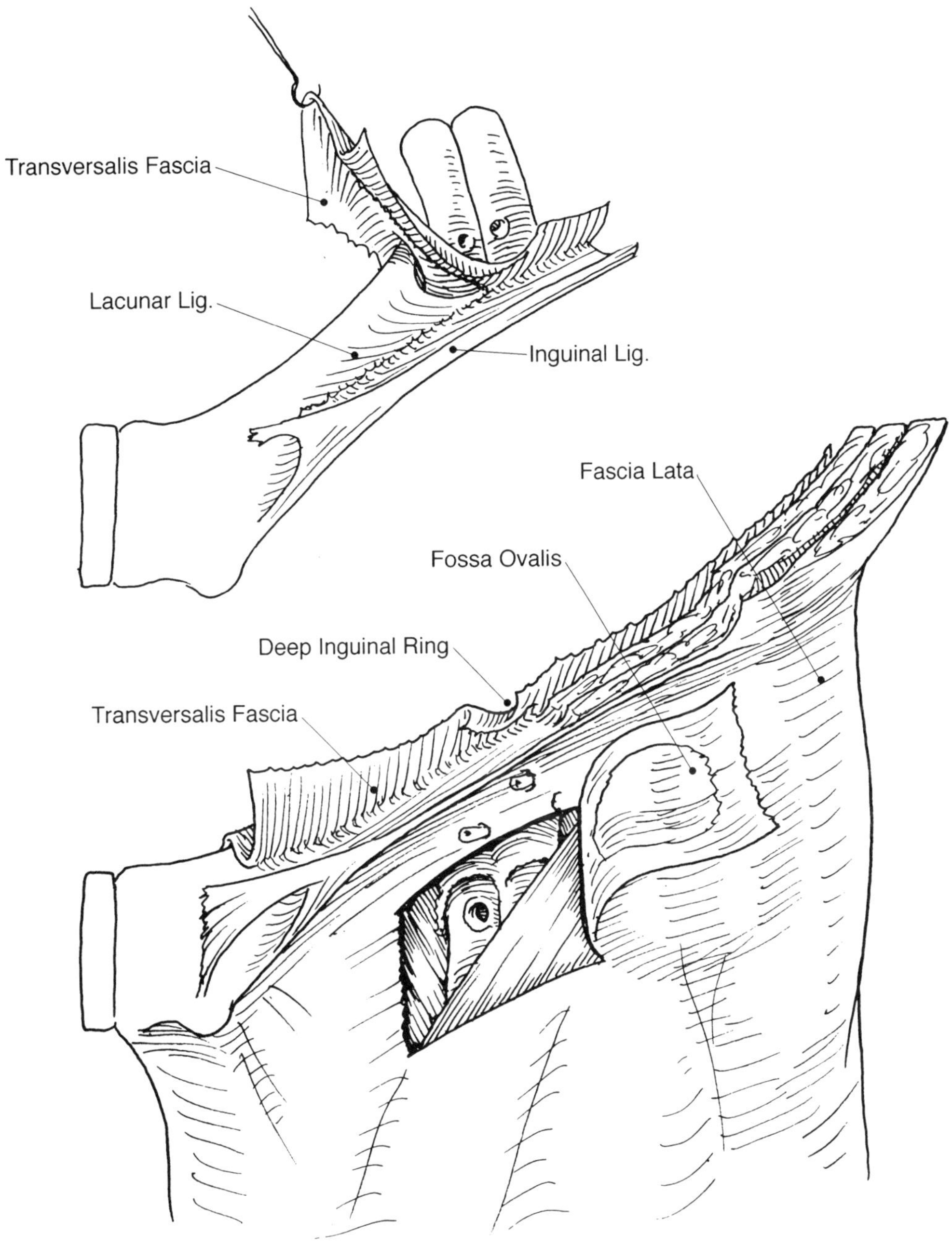

Fig. 3.11

arated or the transversalis of the direct space is opened. The transversalis immediately adjacent to the inguinal ligament is thickened to a greater or lesser degree (Fig. 3.12). This thickened band is called the iliopubic tract because it extends from the inner surface of the iliac crest to the pubis. It lies caudal to the deep ring and blends into the anterior portion of femoral sheath. This band is used as the lateral anchor in iliopubic tract type hernia repairs done from an anterior or posterior approach.

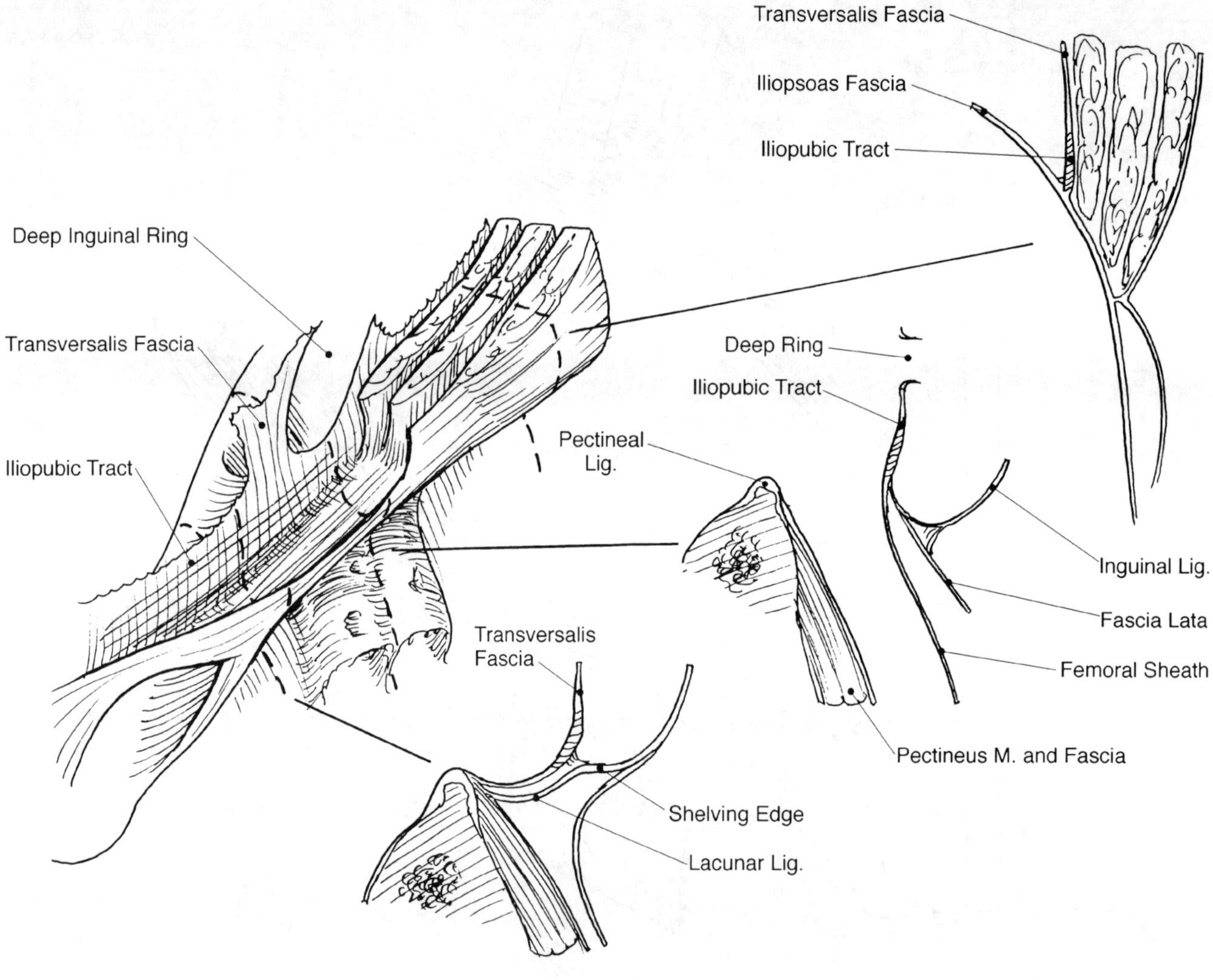

Fig. 3.12

Nerves

Several nerves pass through the inguinal region and are at risk of injury during hernia repair (Fig. 3.13). The largest of these is the femoral nerve, which emerges between psoas and iliacus muscles as they near the inguinal ligament. The nerve passes beneath iliopubic tract and inguinal ligament to emerge in the thigh. Surgeons who choose to tighten the deep inguinal ring on its lateral side must be aware of the proximity of the femoral nerve when placing the suture in the caudal margin of the ring.

Four smaller lumbar plexus nerves traverse the groin and are similarly at risk. The iliohypogastric nerve emerges from the lateral border of psoas muscle, runs diagonally across quadratus lumborum and penetrates the transversus muscle above the crest of the ilium. Its anterior branch penetrates the internal oblique muscle lateral and cephalad to the deep ring and runs medially on the internal oblique. It then penetrates the external oblique aponeurosis to innervate the area above the

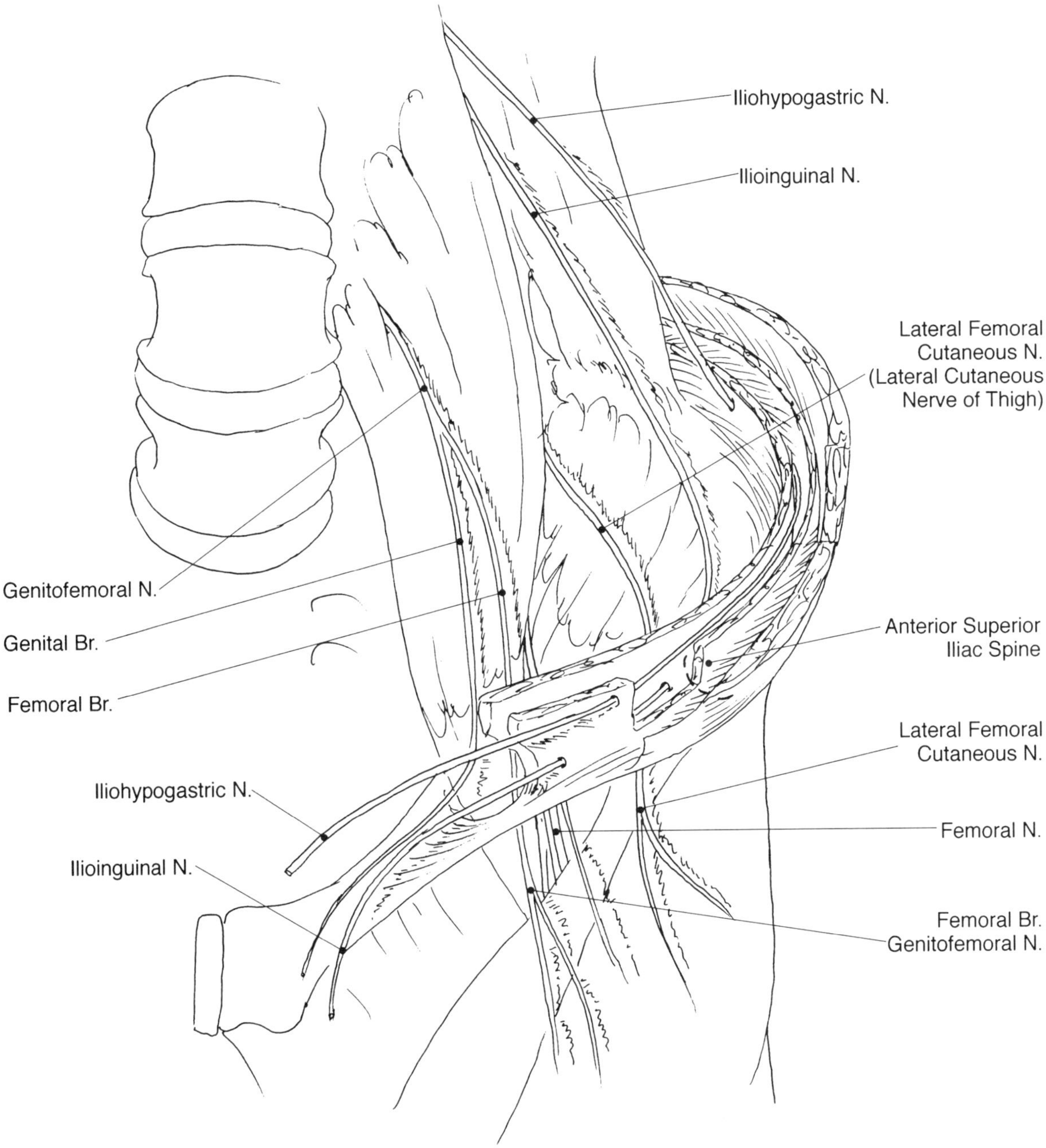

Fig. 3.13

pubis. The ilioinguinal nerve emerges from behind the psoas just below the iliohypogastric. It pierces the transversus muscle near the anterior superior iliac spine and pierces the internal oblique muscle lateral to the deep ring. Its continuation lies on the surface of the cremaster muscle and emerges at or near the superficial inguinal ring to provide sensation to the skin of the medial thigh, the root of the penis and the scrotum.

The genitofemoral nerve emerges through the body of the psoas muscle and divides into genital and femoral branches beneath the transversalis fascia. The genital branch pierces the transversalis fascia at the deep ring and runs between transversalis and cremaster fascia lateral to the cord. It is joined there by the external spermatic branches of the inferior epigastric vessels. The genital branch supplies the cremaster and the skin of the scrotum and thigh. The femoral branch passes under iliopubic tract and inguinal ligament and enters the femoral sheath lateral to the femoral artery. It supplies the proximal anterior thigh. The last nerve supplying this region is the lateral femoral cutaneous (also called the lateral cutaneous nerve of the thigh), which runs from the psoas border across the iliacus muscle. It crosses beneath the lateral end of the iliopubic tract and inguinal ligament to supply the anterolateral thigh. It lies closer to the anterior superior iliac spine than to the deep ring and is subject to injury by staples placed below the level of the iliopubic tract.

Sutures or staples placed near the deep ring endanger the femoral nerve and femoral branch of the genitofemoral. The iliohypogastric and ilioinguinal nerves are at risk from deeply placed sutures or staples cephalad and lateral to the deep ring during mesh repairs. The lateral femoral cutaneous nerve is at risk lateral to the deep ring beneath the iliopubic tract. The genital branch of the genitofemoral is at risk during internal cord mobilization and may be sacrificed when the cremaster is excised in anterior approaches.

Spermatic Cord

The spermatic cord is formed at the deep inguinal ring by the confluence of internal spermatic vessels, vas deferens, and genital branch of the genitofemoral nerve (Fig. 3.14). There is no unified cord internally proximal to this point. The internal spermatic arteries arise from

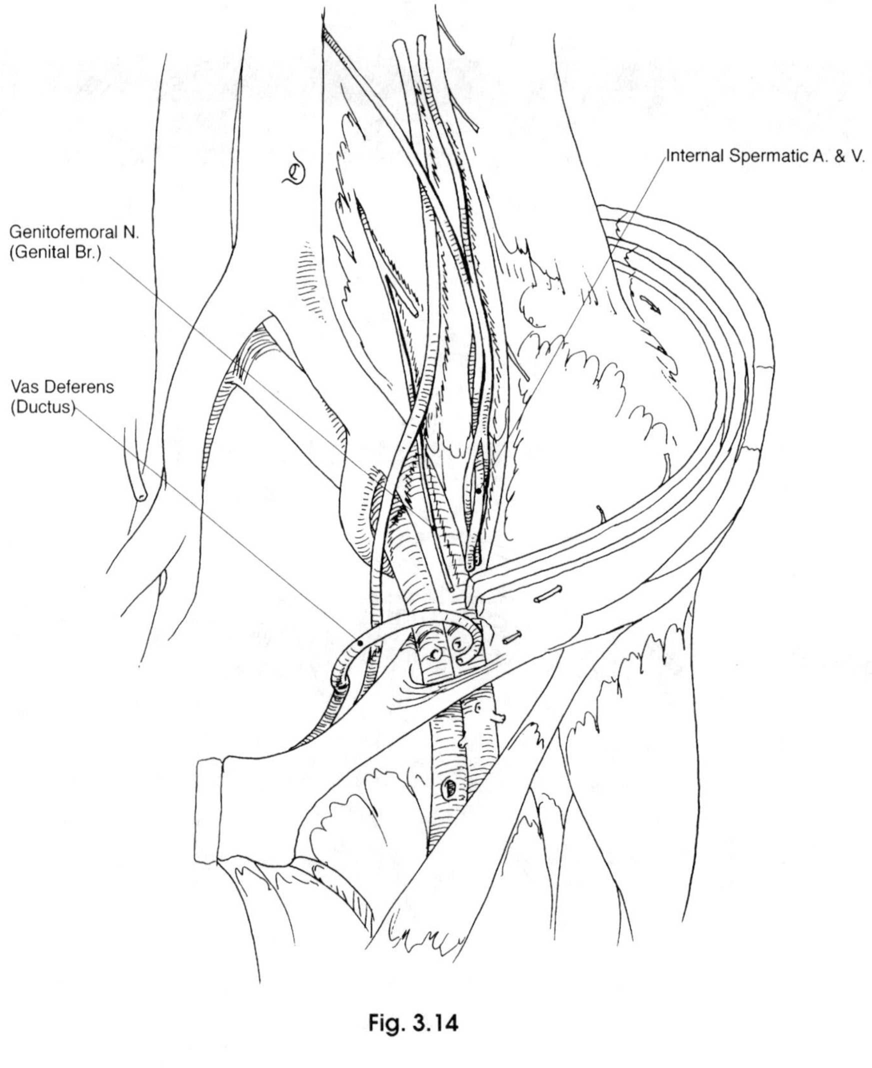

Fig. 3.14

the lateral walls of the aorta below the renals (recall the common origins of gonads and kidneys, both supplied by lateral aortic branches). The right spermatic vein (or veins) drains into the inferior vena cava (Chapter 8) while the left empties into the left renal vein.

The vas deferens arises from the pelvis, crosses the ureter and external iliac vessels to reach the deep ring (Fig. 3.15). The peritoneum over this confluence can be adherent to the underlying structures and must be stripped carefully to avoid damage. Mobilizing the delicate internal spermatic vessels (for example to encircle the "cord" with mesh) can also compromise the cord blood supply. Upon emerging into the inguinal canal through the deep ring, the vas, vessels, nerve and encircling internal spermatic fascia acquire a covering of cremaster muscle and fascia from the internal oblique muscle. The ilioinguinal nerve runs on the anterior surface of the cremaster, the genital branch of the genitofemoral within the cremaster.

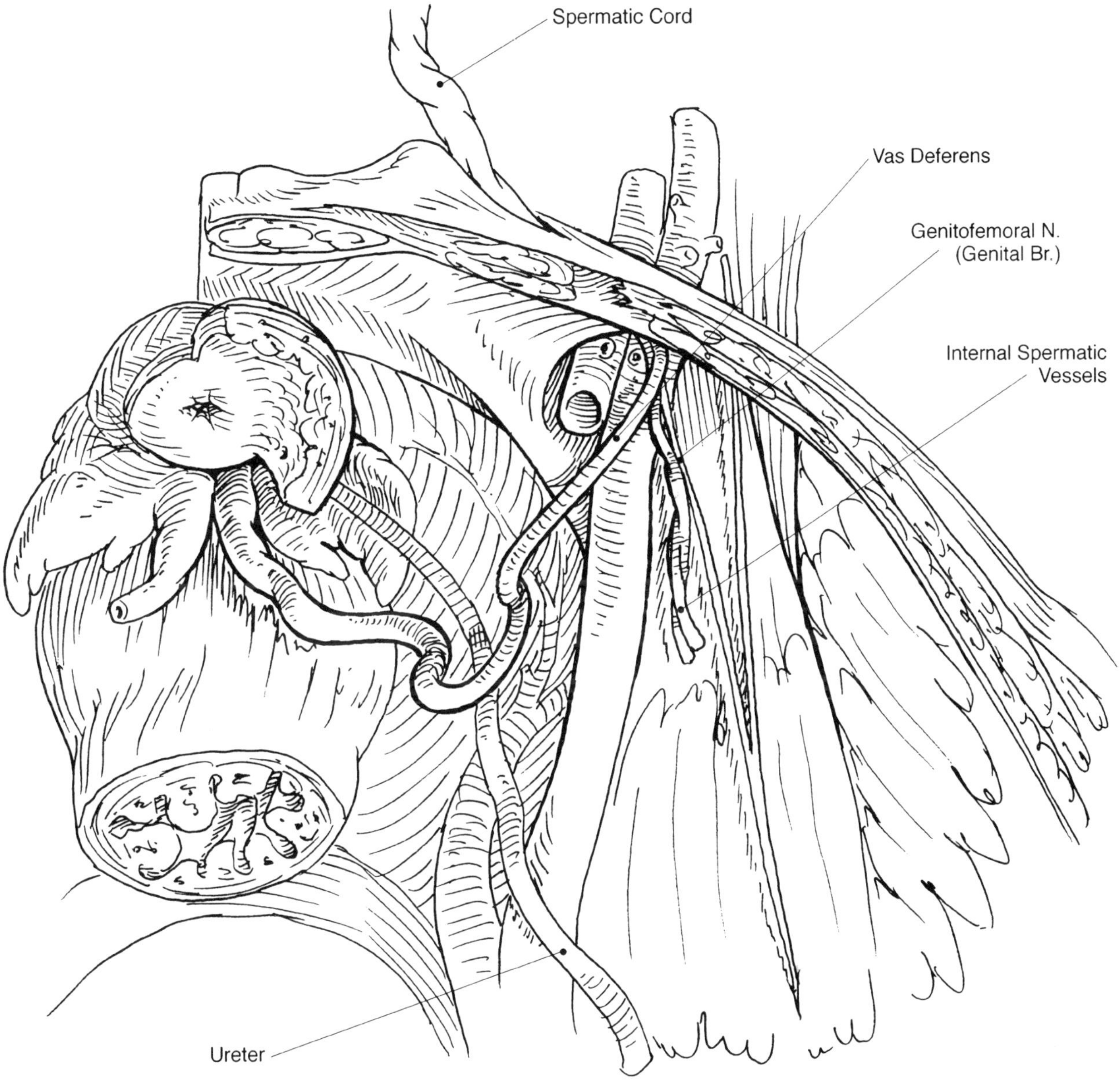

Fig. 3.15

Laparoscopic View

The accompanying series of illustrations shows the inguinal region from a cephalad and oblique view to demonstrate the anatomy with better perspective. The laparoscopic camera would be on the side of the hernia with the bevel of the scope angled to show this view from the surgeon's perspective (Fig. 3.16). The pectineal ridge on the superior pubic ramus is covered with thickened periosteum and is called pectineal ligament. It is the anchor for the medial part of one type of anterior hernia repair, for posterior mesh repairs and for posterior and inferior femoral hernia repairs.

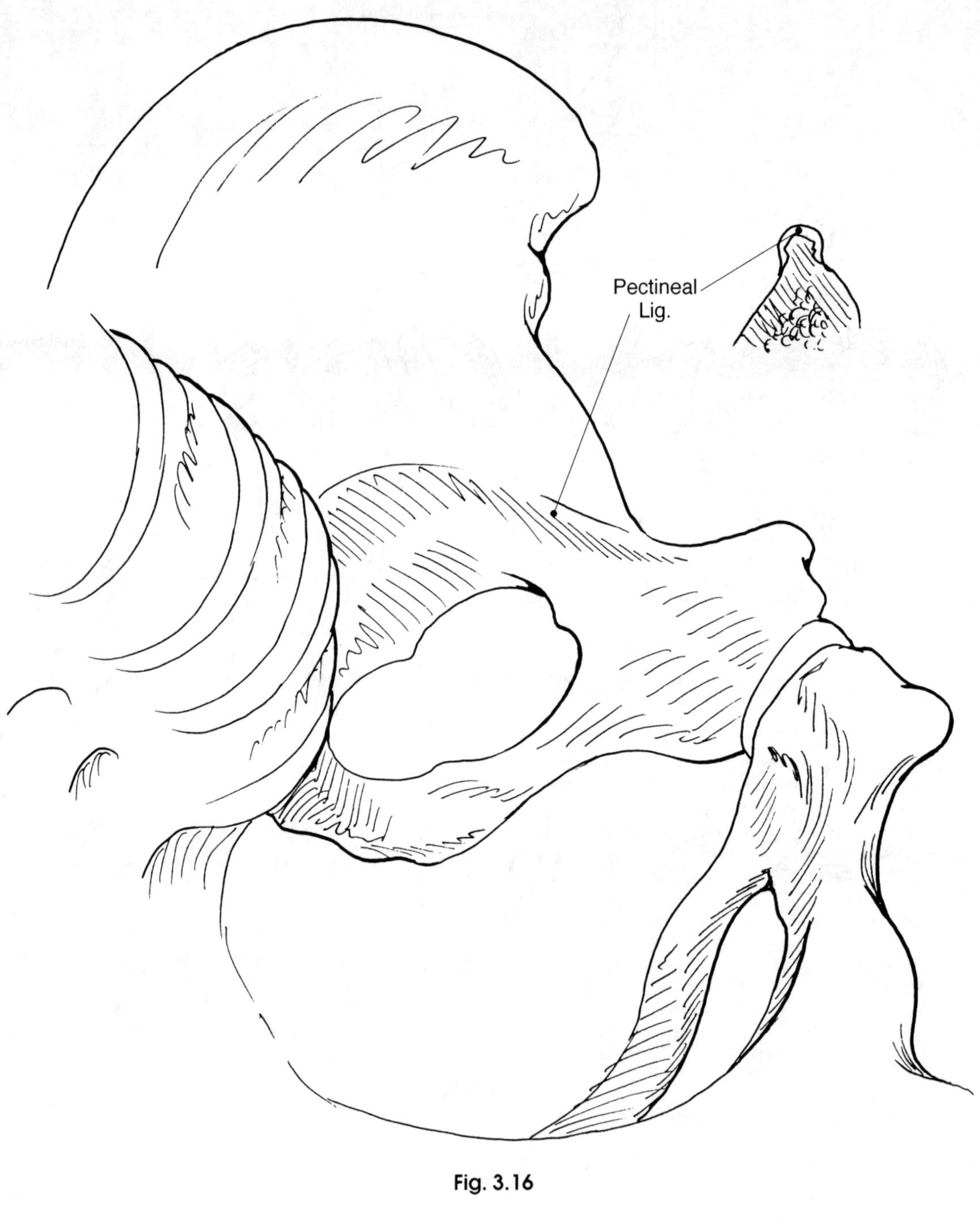

Fig. 3.16

The bony concavity between pubic tubercle and anterior iliac spine is bridged by the inguinal ligament (Fig. 3.17). The medial fibers of inguinal ligament reflect back along the pectineal ligament to form the lacunar ligament. The next most cephalad fibers attach to pubic tubercle as lateral and medial crura of the superficial inguinal ring. Note the iliopsoas muscle mass filling the lateral portion of the subinguinal space.

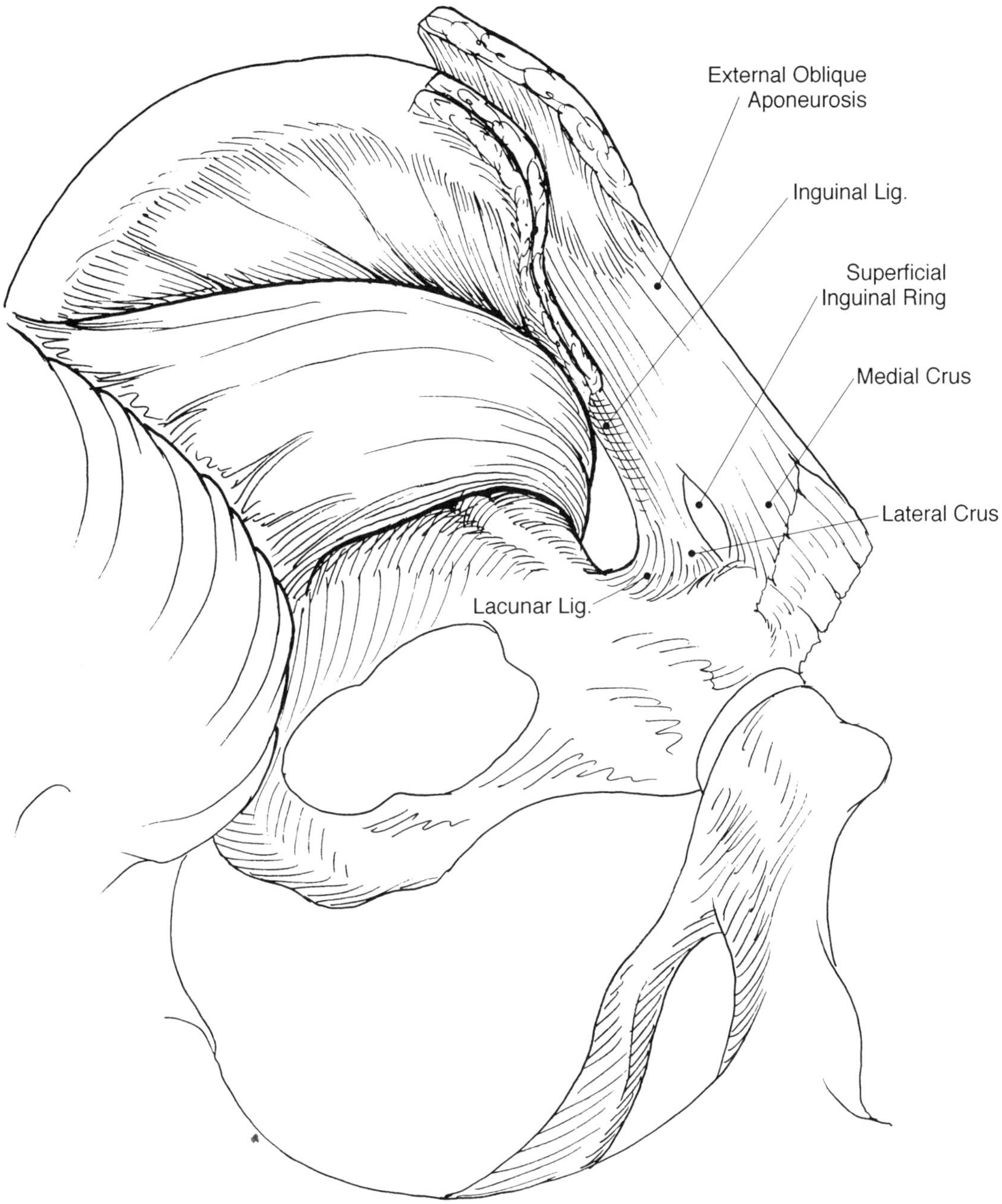

Fig. 3.17

The iliopsoas portion of the endoabdominal fascia covers the iliopsoas muscle mass (Fig. 3.18). The caudal origins of transversus and internal oblique muscles extend from the crest of the ilium onto the inguinal ligament and the adjacent iliopectineal fascia. Note the cleft between external oblique aponeurosis and the fused deeper laminae forming the rectus sheath. The arched lower borders of transversus and internal oblique muscles form the lateral and cephalad borders of the deep ring and the cephalad margin of Hesselbach's triangle. The area of these arches attaching to the pubis at the lateral edge of the rectus sheath are most commonly not fused into a conjoined tendon. It is the lower edge of the deeper arch, the falx inguinalis of the transversus muscle, that has substantial strength for anatomic hernia repair. The lower rectus sheath lies entirely anterior to the rectus muscle, leaving only transversalis fascia posteriorly.

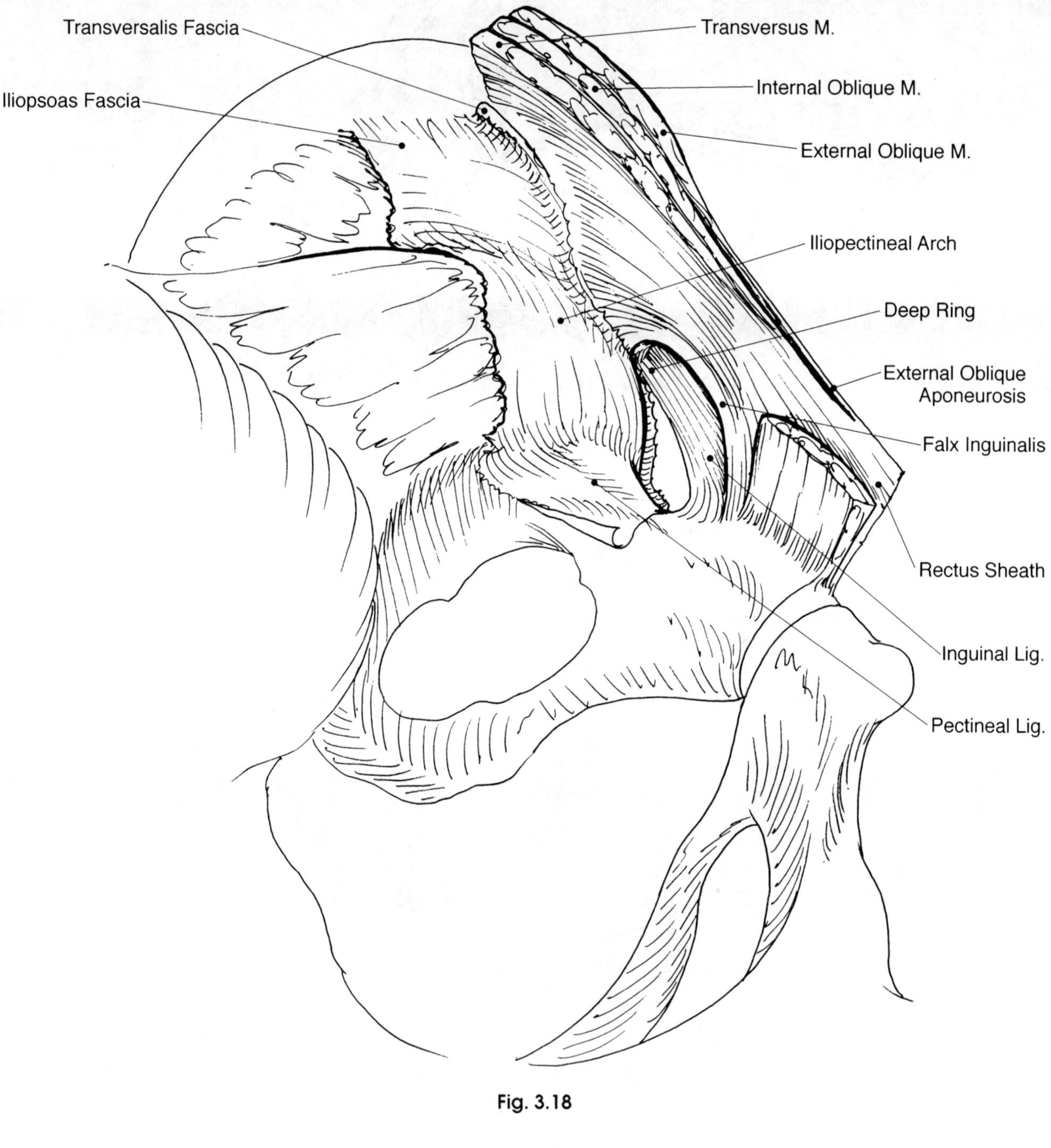

Fig. 3.18

The transversalis fascia lines the anterolateral abdominal cavity forming the back wall of the inguinal canal behind the muscular arches (Fig. 3.19). It is continuous with the iliopsoas fascia laterally and with the endopelvic fascia medially. It extends around the cord as internal spermatic fascia and around the femoral vessels as femoral sheath. The iliopubic tract is a thickened band of transversalis fascia running between iliac crest and pubis. It lies between the deep ring and the femoral sheath. The inguinal nerves lie outside transversalis fascia.

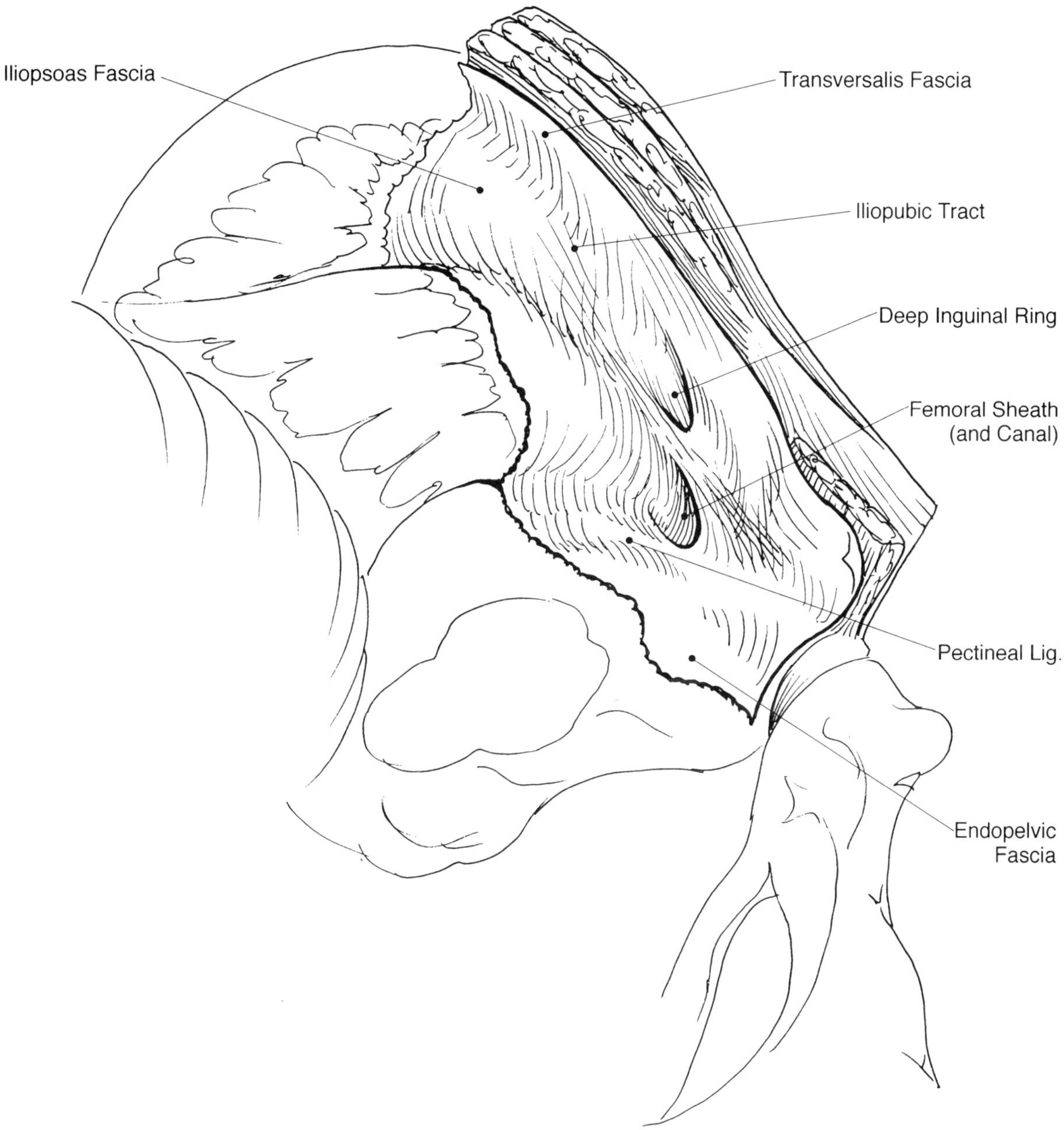

Fig. 3.19

The external iliac vessels pass between the iliopubic tract and pectineal ligament to enter the femoral sheath (Fig. 3.20). Before entering the sheath, the external iliacs give rise to the inferior epigastrics, which cross the medial border of the deep ring on their way to the rectus muscle. The internal spermatic vessels lie on iliopsoas fascia and the genital branch of the genitofemoral nerve lies deep to the fascia. These structures are joined at the deep ring by the vas deferens arching out of the pelvis.

The delta between the internal spermatic vessels and the vas has been dubbed the triangle of doom because of the iliac vessels within their boundaries. The vas crosses the pectineal ligament just medial to the femoral vein in most individuals, leaving the majority of the ligament unobstructed for hernia repair. In those individuals in whom the vas encroaches medially, it is easily mobilized.

The remnants of the obliterated umbilical arteries, the medial umbilical ligaments, arise out of the pelvis beneath the vas and forms a ridge on the transversalis fascia on either side of the bladder. They are important landmarks for avoiding injury to the bladder. On each side, they cross the pectineal ligament and Hesselbach's triangle. When mobilized medially with the bladder, they do not interfere with hernia repair. The parietal peritoneum overlying this ridge may be fatty and redundant requiring medial retraction for exposure. The bladder attachment forms a central triangle and may be part of a direct hernia bulge or a sliding part of an indirect hernia (replacing peritoneum as one wall of the sac).

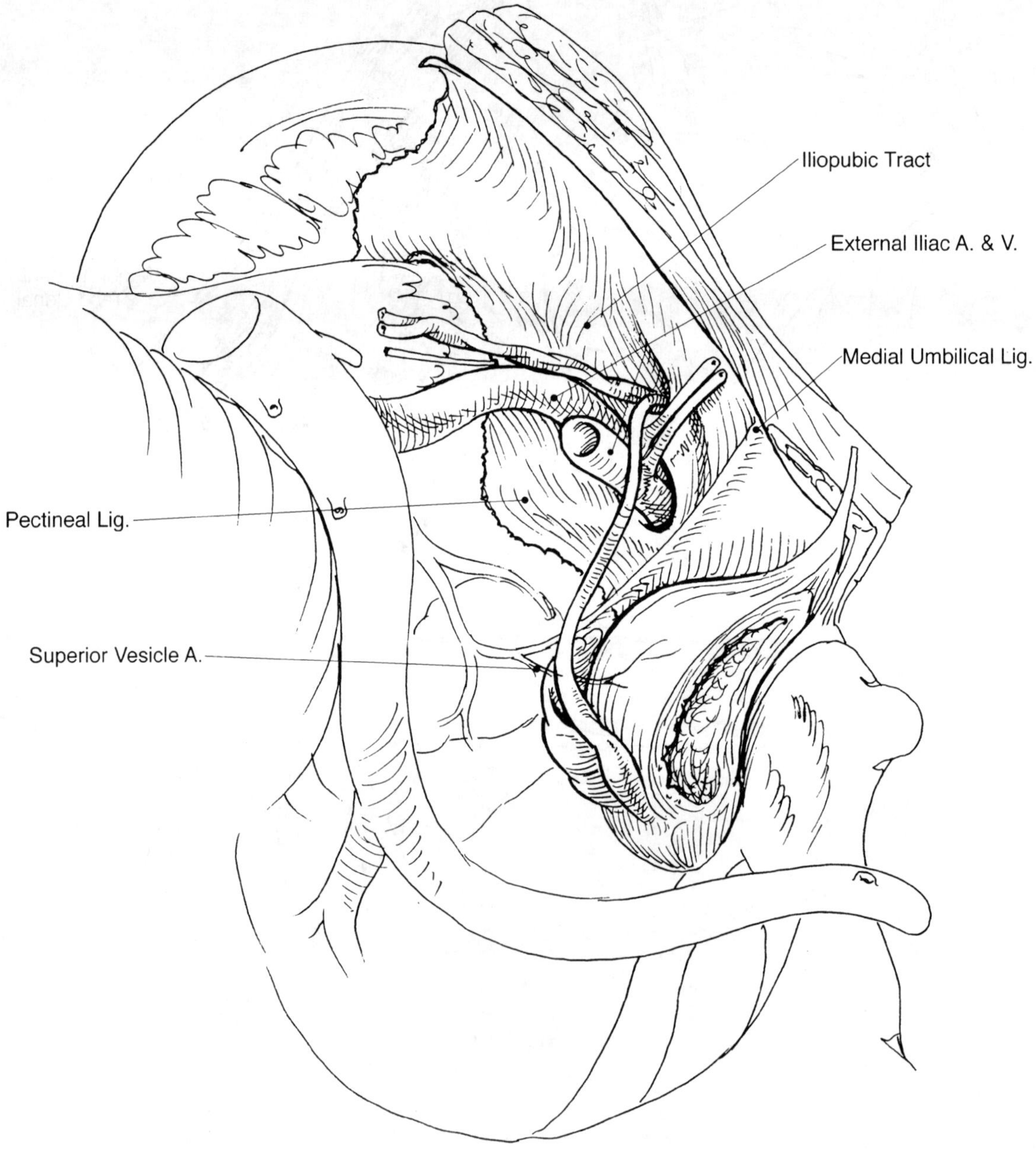

Fig. 3.20

HERNIA TYPES

Normal Inguinal Floor

In describing the "normal" relationships in the groin, two factors must be addressed: structural and functional integrity. The critical structures of the normal groin are an obliterated processus vaginalis, a firm posterior wall of transversalis fascia, a deep inguinal ring that snugly encompasses the cord structures, and a strong muscular transversus aponeurotic arch (Fig. 3.21). Failure of the processus vaginalis to fuse by the time of birth or shortly thereafter results in a "congenital" hernia, which may manifest itself in the pediatric age group or later depending on the degree of patency.

The posterior wall of the inguinal canal consists primarily of transversalis fascia with a variable and usually minimal component of aponeurotic fibers below the transversus muscle lamina. The transversalis fascia is fused to the transversus aponeurotic arch, giving it additional strength, and is bound to the shelving edge of the inguinal ligament at the thickened iliopubic tract. The evagination of transversalis fascia around the cord structures to form internal spermatic fascia marks the deep ring. This sheath is dilated and may stretch medially into the posterior wall of the inguinal canal (direct space) when an indirect hernia is present. In addition to the structural anchor the falx provides to the transversalis fascia, the muscular arch has a functional component.

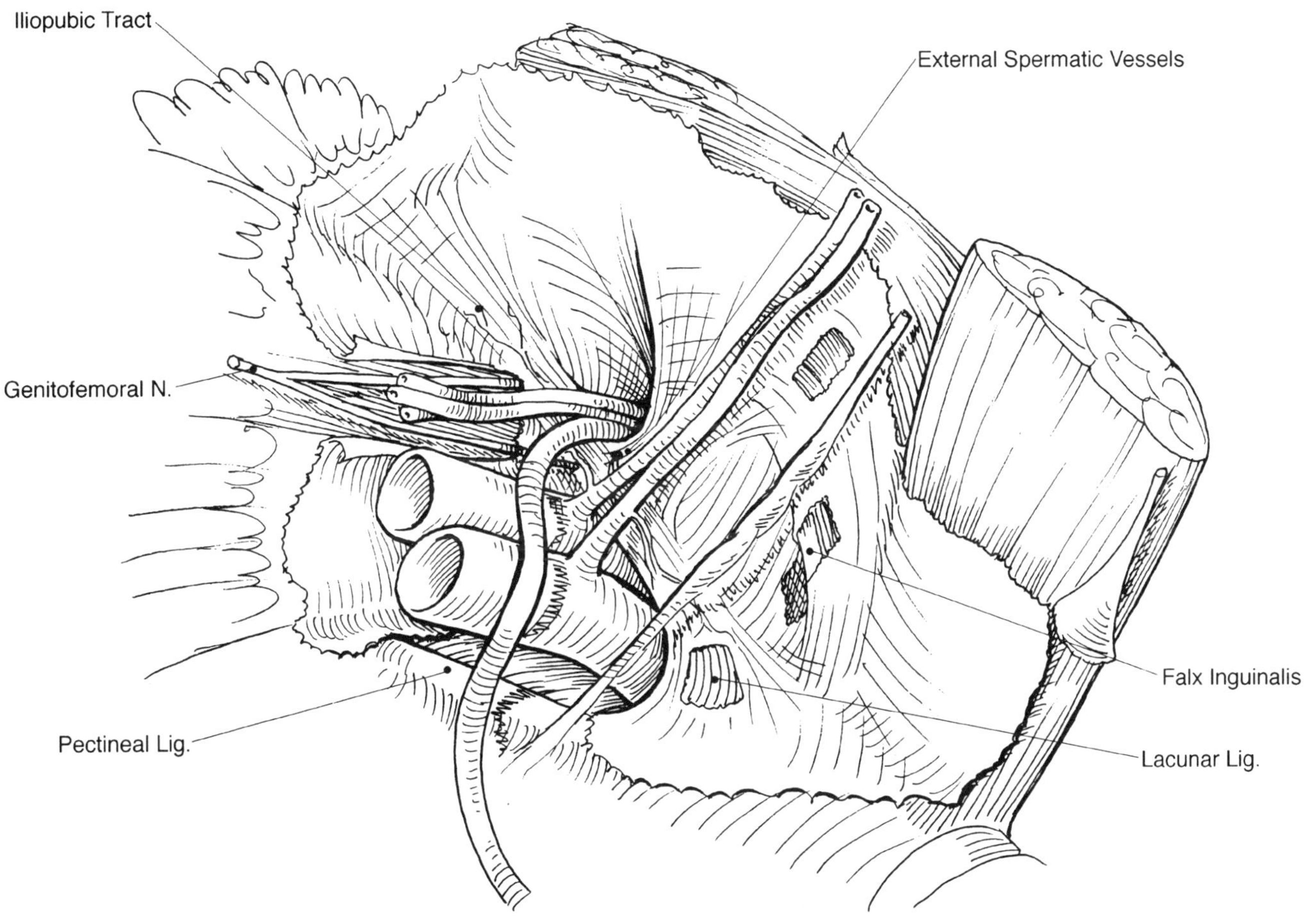

Fig. 3.21

Physiological or functional competence of inguinal structures has long been recognized as an important factor in groin hernia. The arching lower fibers of transversus abdominis and internal oblique muscles (Fig. 3.22A) are thought to flatten and narrow the direct space of Hesselbach's triangle on muscular exertion (fig. 3.22B), creating a shutter mechanism that reinforces the area against the strain of increased intraabdominal pressure. Inherent weakness or progressive disruption of this shutter mechanism predisposes to hernia formation and enlargement. Anatomic hernia repairs such as the iliopubic tract repair, which reapproximate layers in their original configuration, may theoretically preserve some of this mechanism.

Another component of a competent inguinal floor is the flexibility conferred by the iliopubic tract and its loose adherence to the shelving edge of the inguinal ligament (fig. 3.22C). This combined flexible band may act as a shock absorber and dissipate strain energy. Repairs that anchor the transversus aponeurotic arch to the rigid pecitineal ligament may thus have a slight disadvantage, although clinically there is a minimal difference in recurrence rates. The greater distance the falx must be brought down to reach pectineal ligament may add some tension to the repair despite the use of a relaxing incision.

In recent years, emphasis has been placed on tension-free hernia repair to prevent recurrence. The use of synthetic mesh placed via anterior, preperitoneal, and laparoscopic approaches has increased as a result, even for primary hernia repair.

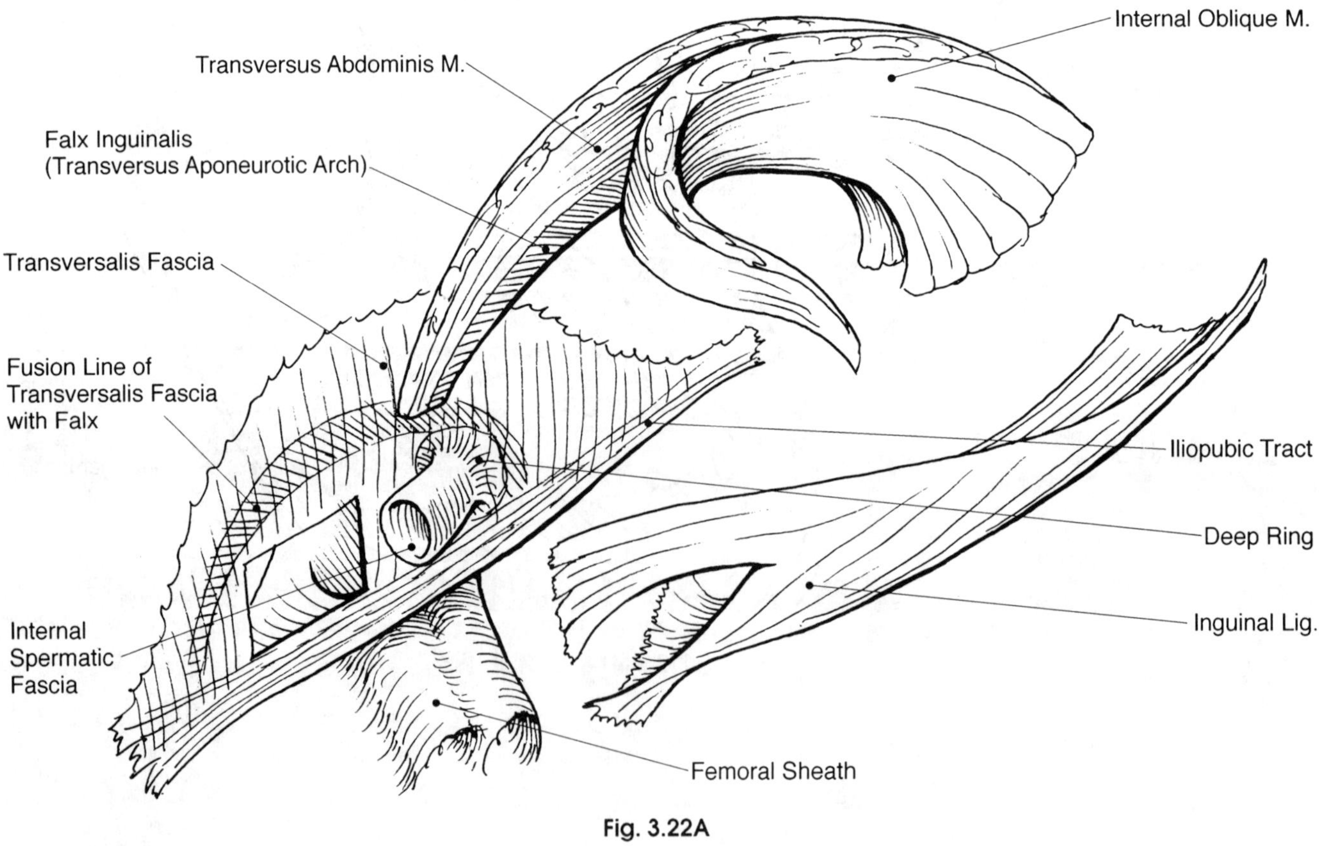

Fig. 3.22A

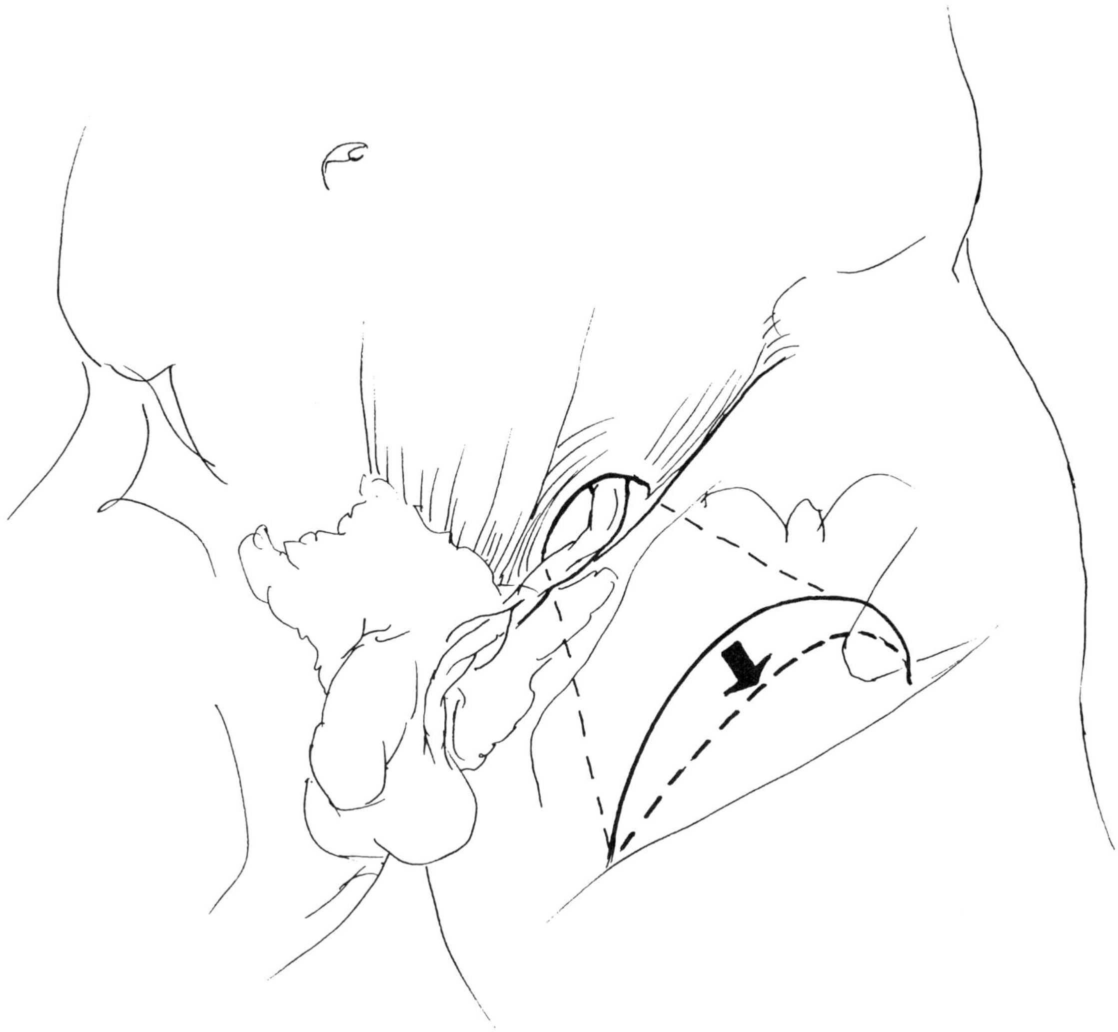

Fig. 3.22B

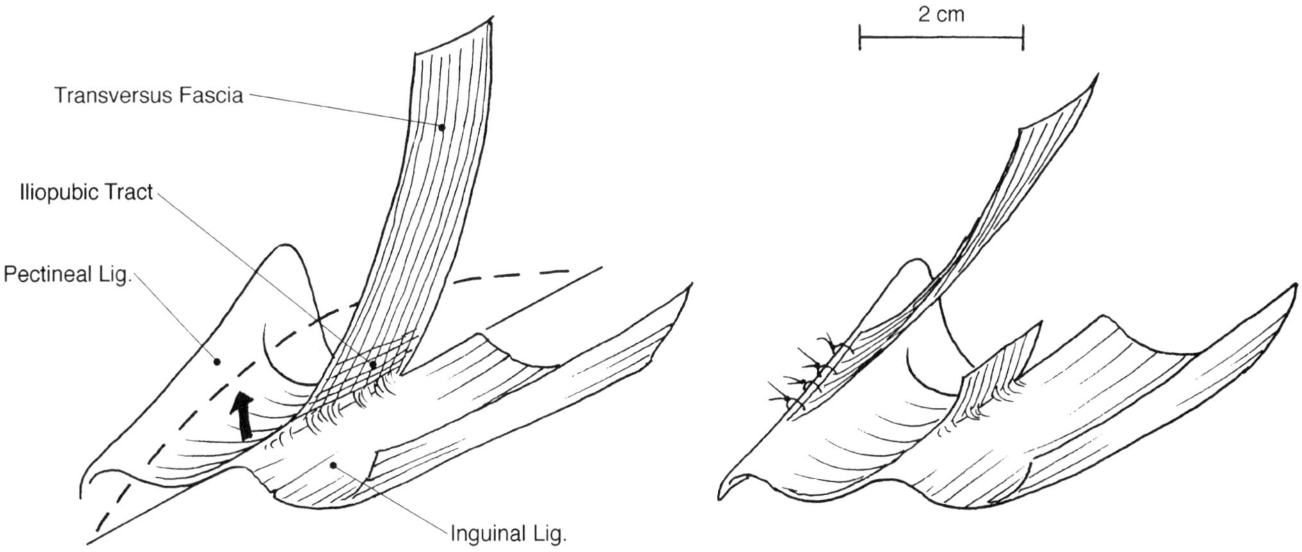

Fig. 3.22C

Classification of Hernias

The Nyhus classification of groin hernias is a useful framework for describing hernia pathology (Fig. 3.23).

Type I: Small indifect hernia without dilatation of the deep ring.

Type II: Indirect hernia with ring dilatation up to 2 cm. No impingement on the direct space.

Type III: Weakened inguinal floor

Type IIIa: Direct hernia

Type IIIb: large indirect hernia stretching the direct space

1. In the internal ring
2. In the inguinal canal
3. At the external ring
4. Scrotal

Type IIIc: Femoral hernia

Type IV: Any recurrent hernia

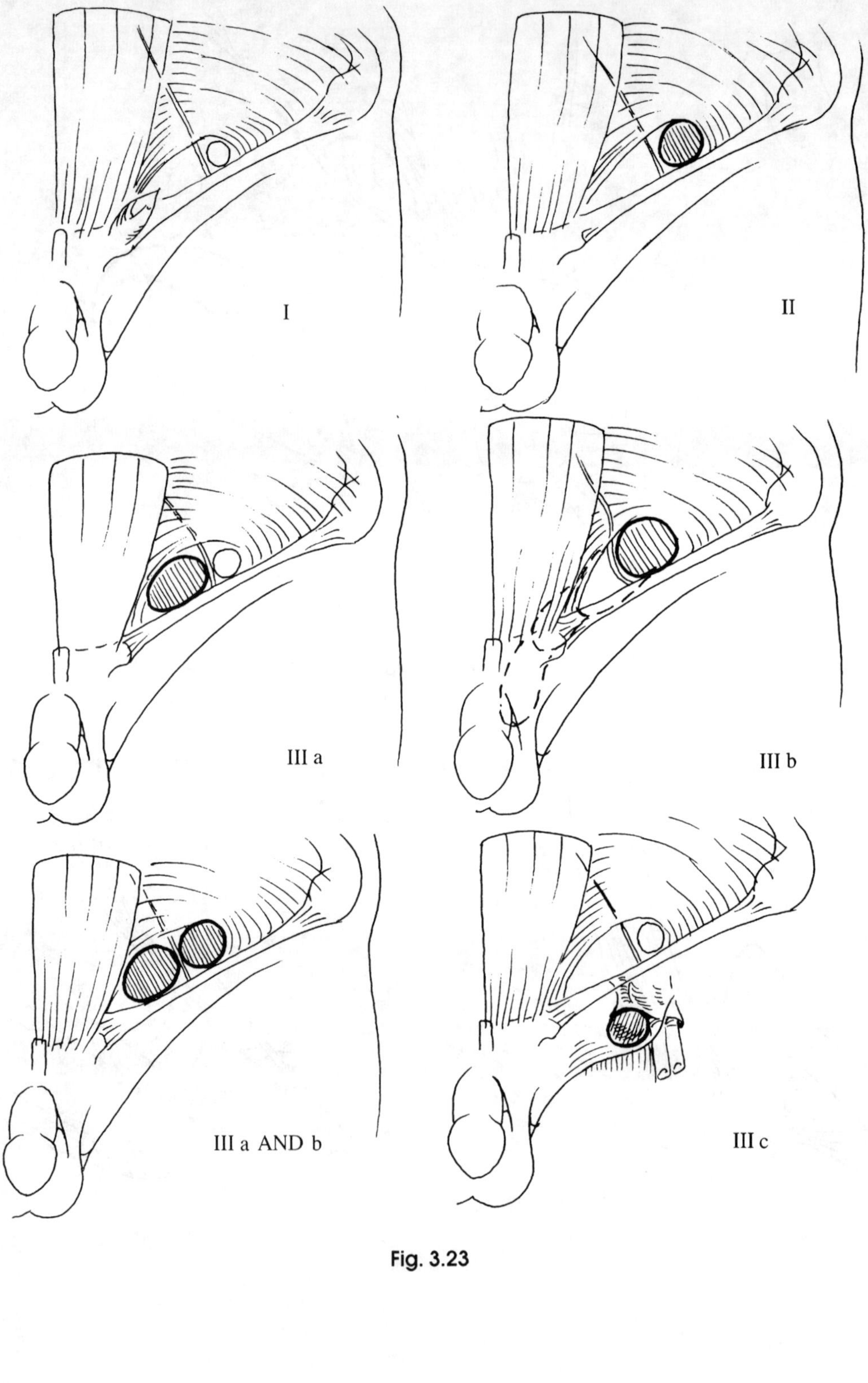

Fig. 3.23

Type I: Patent Processus Without Ring Dilatation

An indirect hernia that appears early may have caused no significant dilatation to the deep inguinal ring (Fig. 3.24). In such a pediatric or adolescent hernia, nothing more than high ligation of the sac may be necessary in an anterior approach. Some surgeons will add a few sutures between falx and iliopubic tract at the medial margin of the deep ring for additional security. Laparoscopically, a smaller patch and less dissection may be required for small hernias. Paradoxically, although the anatomic disruption of a small indirect hernia is less severe, the risk of incarceration of protruding intraabdominal structures is greater because of the narrow neck of the defect, and the urgency of repair is increased.

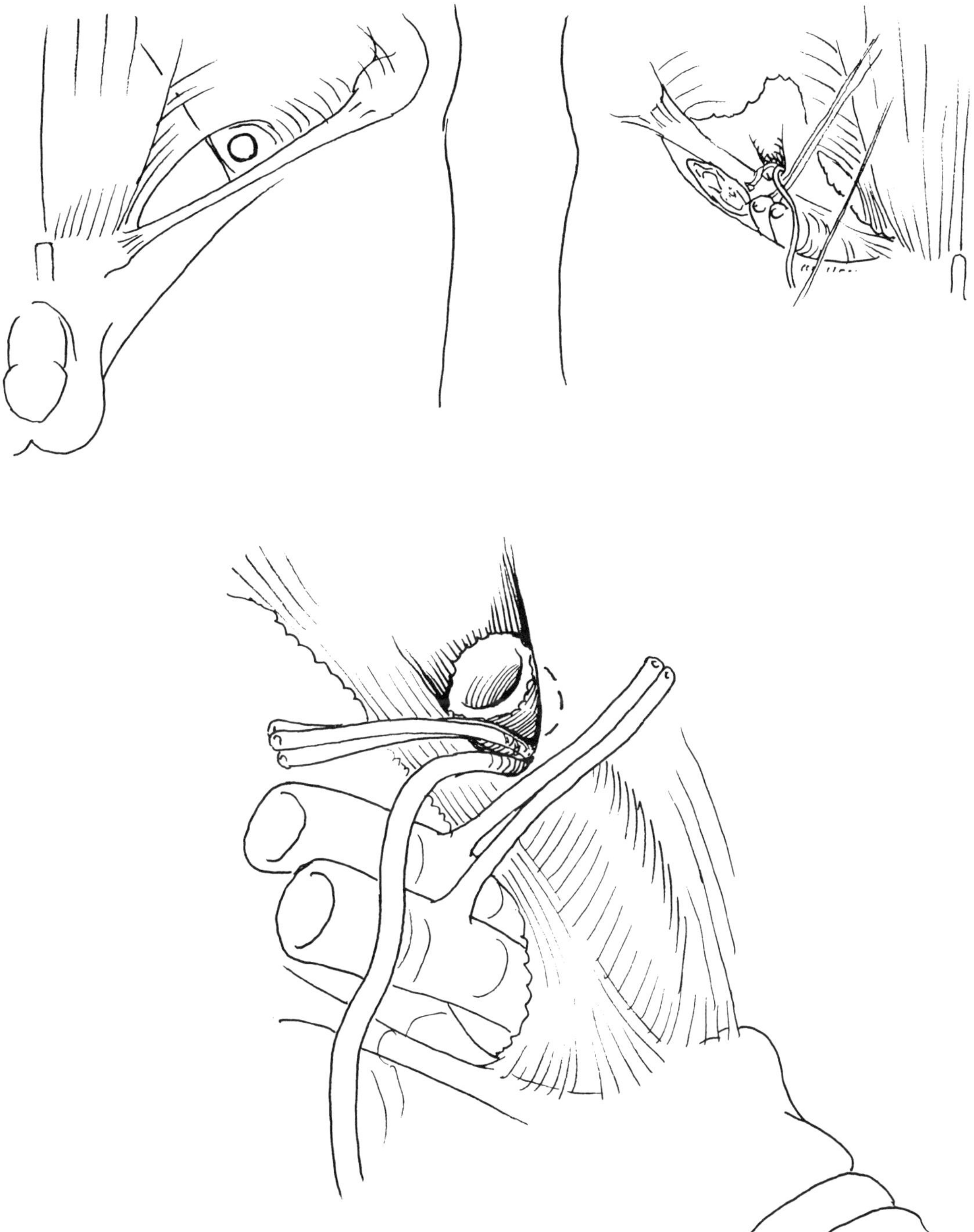

Fig. 3.24

Type II: Indirect with Minor Ring Dilatation

Small indirect hernias with ring dilatation up to 2 cm in size are most commonly seen in the population under age 40 (Fig. 3.25). The stretching of the deep ring does not cause deviation of the inferior epigastric vessels toward the direct space or weaken the transversalis fascia medial to the ring. An anterior procedure that tightens the ring is indicated, or a small laparoscopic repair may be sufficient.

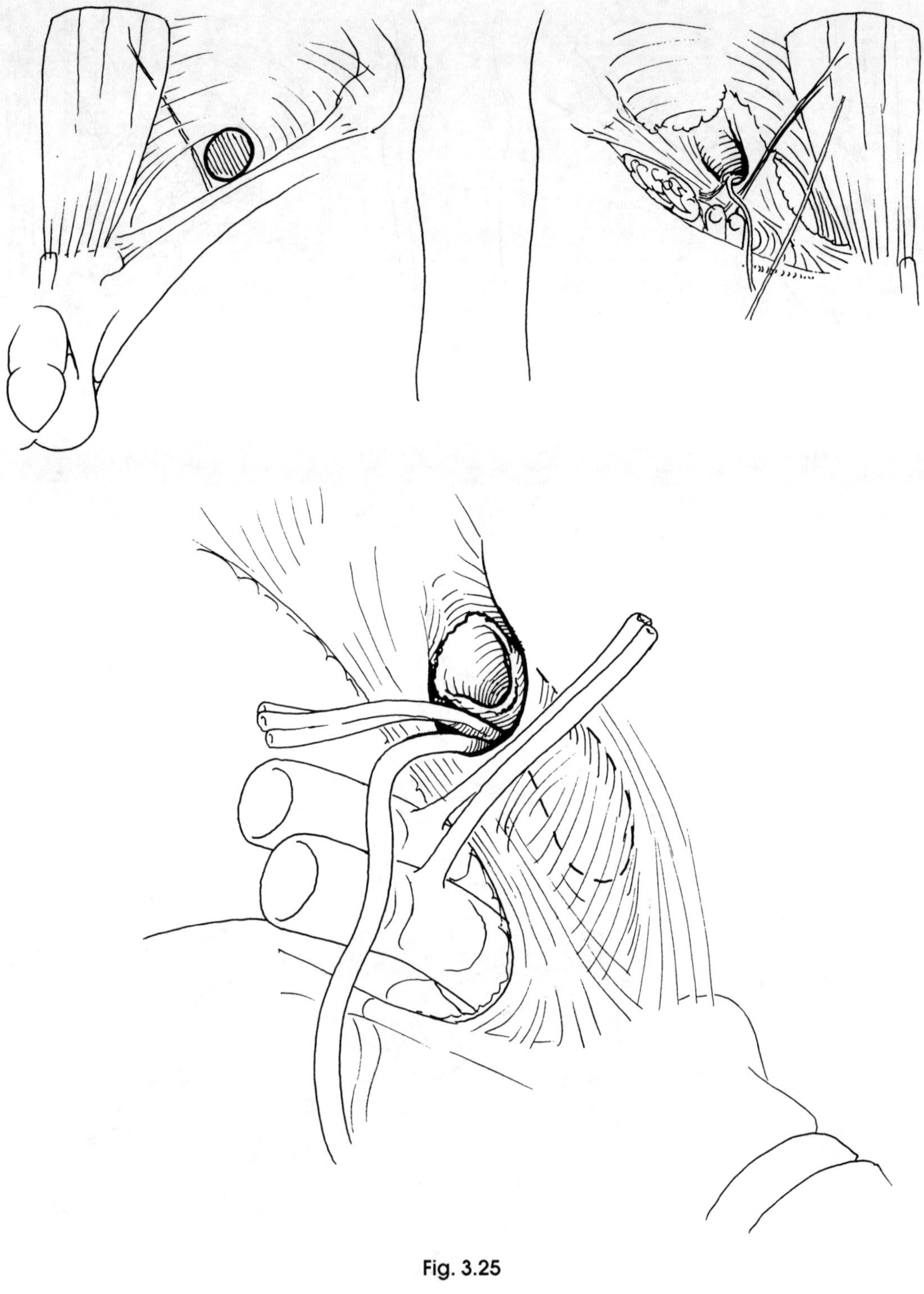

Fig. 3.25

Type IIIa: Direct Hernia

Stretching and protrusion of the transversalis fascia covering Hesselbach's triangle is a direct hernia (Fig. 3.26). Such a weakness may diffusely involve all of the direct space or may be localized to a limited defect. The broader the neck, the lower the risk of incarceration. In an anterior approach, the cremaster must always be opened and the cord inspected for an indirect hernia even if an obvious direct hernia is present. Direct hernias may occasionally extend to the scrotum and be mistaken for indirect. Repair requires reconstruction of the back wall or "floor" of the inguinal canal, with either an anterior or a laparoscopic approach.

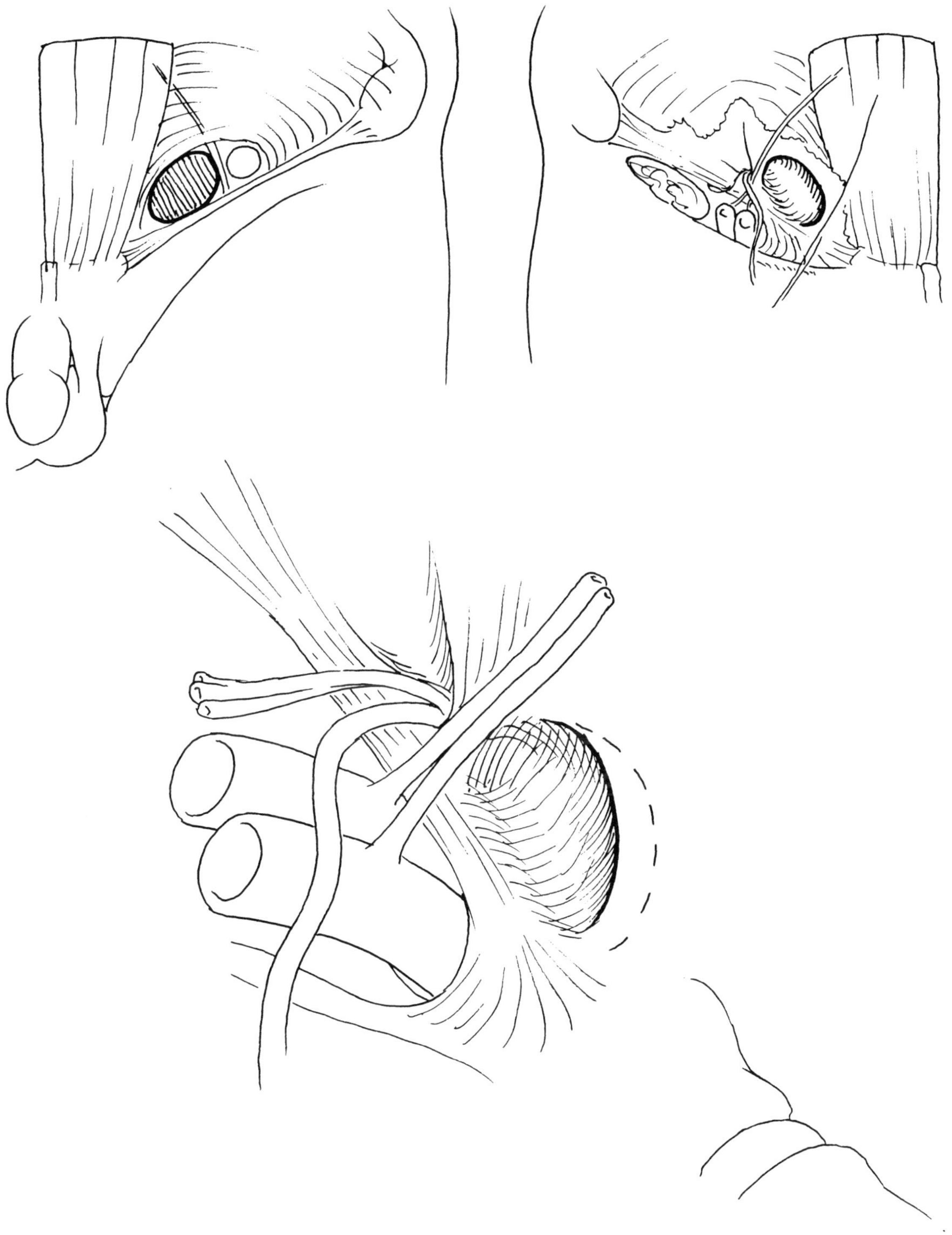

Fig. 3.26

Type IIIb: Large Indirect Hernia

When there has been significant dilatation of the deep ring, expansion takes place in the direction of least resistance, which is into the transversalis fascia of the direct space medially (Fig. 3.27). The inferior epigastric vessels are bowed medially, the area of Hesselbach's triangle is diminished and the remaining transversalis fascia may be stretched. In such cases, in addition to high ligation of the sac (anterior approach), the floor of the inguinal canal must be reconstructed to recreate a snug deep ring and repair the medial weakness. Preoperative assessment of the level (1-4) of the hernia sac allows planning for whether the sac will be dissected or divided and left in place. Manipulation of a sac that approaches the external ring can endanger the blood supply of the testis.

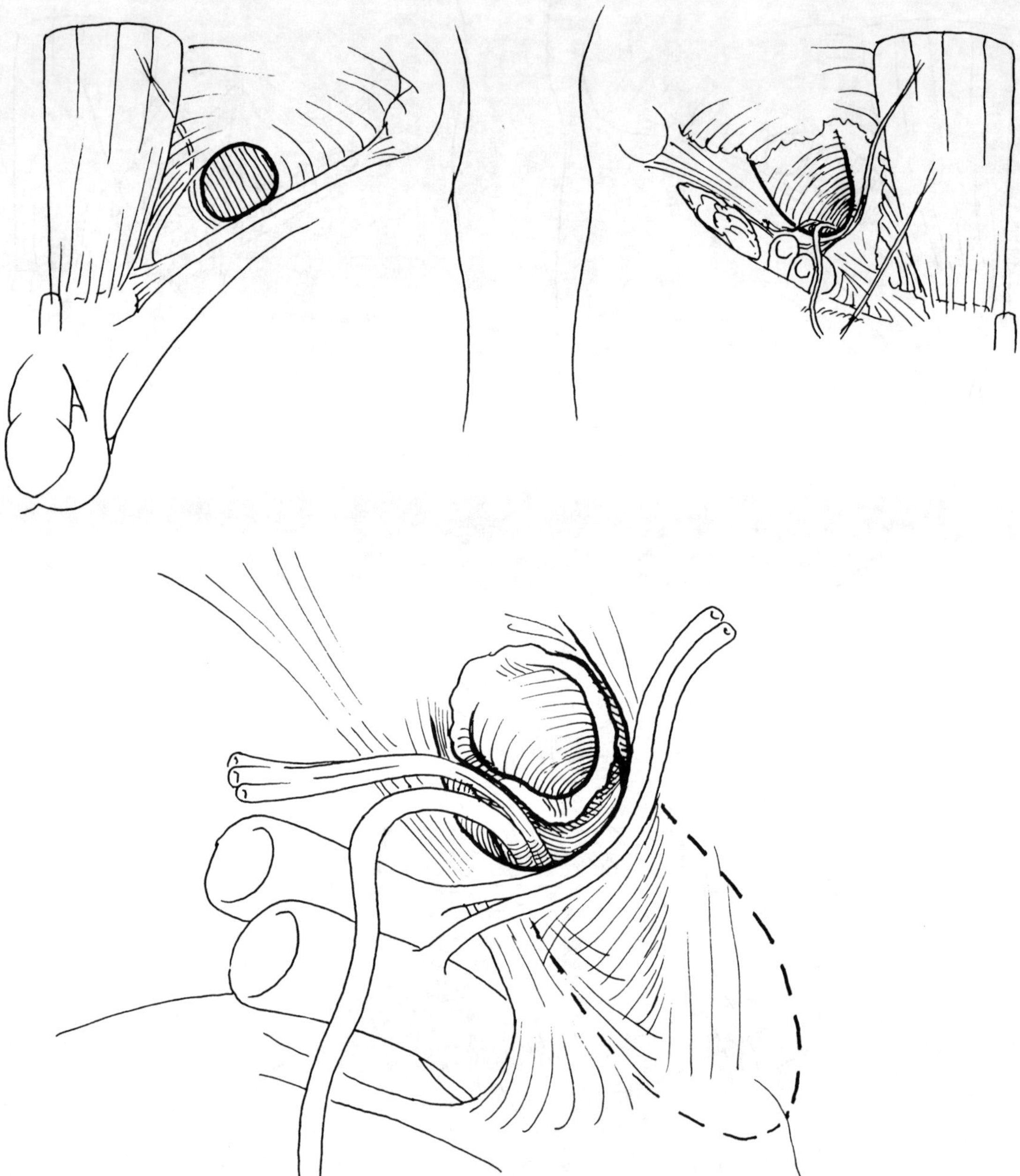

Fig. 3.27

Types IIIa, b: Combined Direct and Indirect Hernia

The combination of direct and indirect defects is fancifully referred to as a "pantaloon" hernia after the old fashioned women's garment with balloon-like legs (Fig. 3.28). The direct space is always checked in the course of repairing an indirect hernia anteriorly to determine the integrity of the transversalis floor. Examination of the inguinal floor is best done by inserting a finger into the opened sac and palpating around the epigastric vessels to the underside of the direct space. Conversely, the initial recognition of an obvious direct bulge must never deter the surgeon from opening cremaster and ruling out a concurrent indirect sac, a common cause of a "recurrent" hernia. In addition, during repair of both direct and indirect hernias, the abdominal end of the femoral canal should be palpated to rule out a hernia defect. The combined type of hernia also requires a formal floor repair. The laparoscopic view shows all floor defects at a glance.

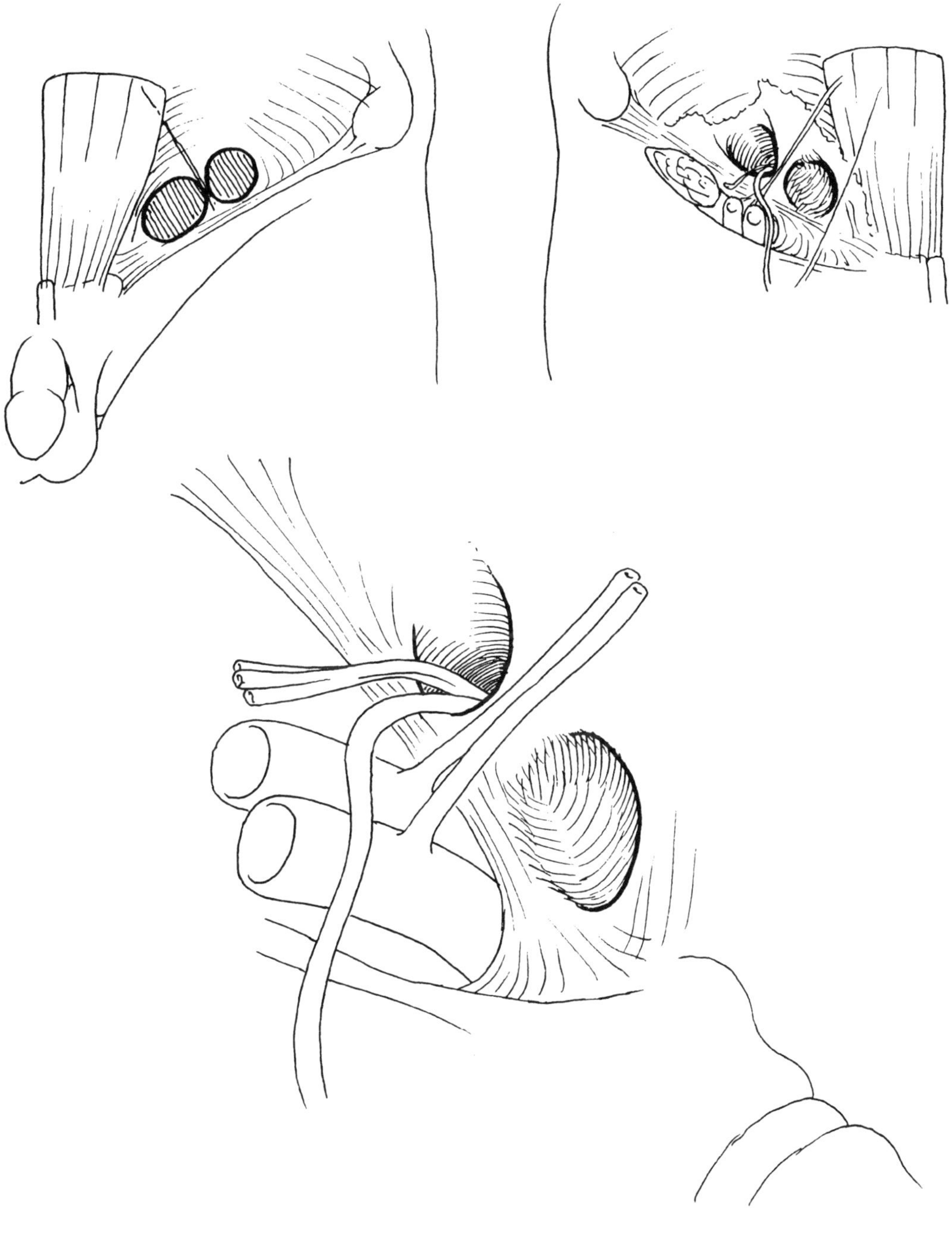

Fig. 3.28

Type IIIc: Femoral Hernia

The potential space of the femoral canal medial to the femoral vein in the femoral sheath may dilate and allow protrusion of abdominal contents (Fig. 3.29). The rigid constraints of the adjacent lacunar and inguinal ligaments and the pectineal ligament on three sides result in a tight narrow neck of a femoral hernia sac and an increased risk of incarceration. The bulge of a femoral hernia sac is deep to fascia lata but may extend upward around the inguinal ligament and be mistaken for an inguinal hernia. Repair of a femoral hernia first requires reduction of incarcerated contents and then narrowing of the femoral canal orifice. Reduction often requires surgical expansion of the neck as described below. Narrowing of the V between iliopubic tract/inguinal ligament and pectineal ligament/pectineus fascia may be accomplished from above or below the inguinal ligament. Laparoscopic repair includes a local patch over the opening of the femoral canal and a mesh sheet coverage of the entire inguinal floor.

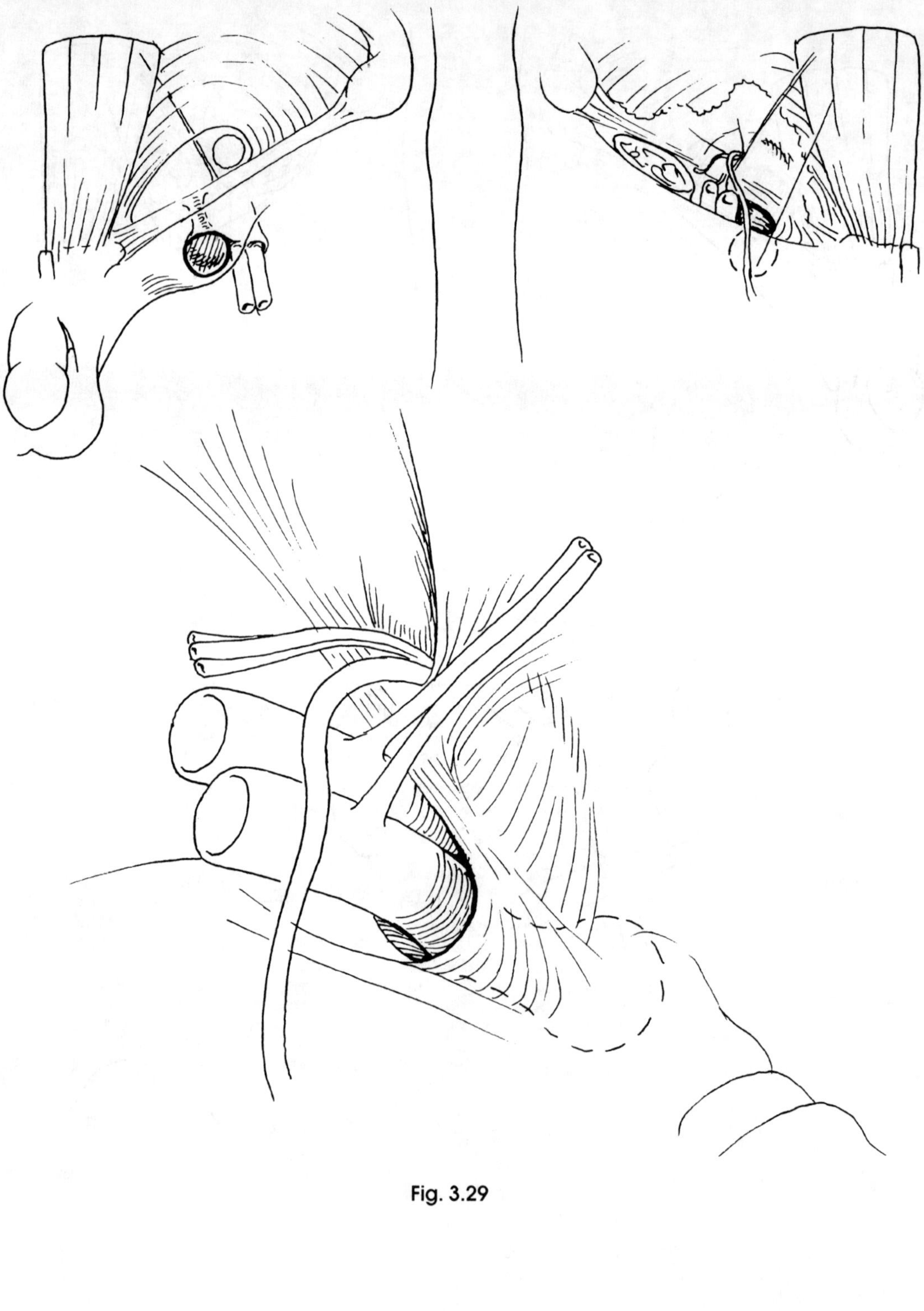

Fig. 3.29

Type IV: Recurrent Hernia

The tissue compromise incurred by prior repair and the higher risk of recurrence mitigates for the use of mesh when a recurrent hernia is approached anteriorly. The preperitoneal approach has become increasingly popular for repair of recurrent hernia because it affords access to undisturbed tissue. For the same reason, laparoscopic hernia repair is an appealing option for recurrent hernia repair. The defect is usually visible laparoscopically and easily fixed whether or not mesh was used initially. When mesh was used the first time, either open, preperitoneally or laparoscopically, the defect can be repaired with an additional application of mesh without disturbing the previous mesh.

NON-LAPAROSCOPIC GROIN HERNIA REPAIR

Introduction

When operating for groin hernia, the surgeon should always explore for both indirect and direct hernia and for femoral hernia. The presence of an obvious direct or indirect defect must not distract the operator from checking for the other. A missed indirect hernia is a common cause of "recurrent" hernia. Access to the proximal end of the femoral canal is gained through an opened indirect sac or through the opened transversalis fascia. Small indirect hernias in the pediatric and adolescent age groups often require no more than high ligation for repair. In those cases, the cremaster layer is opened but not excised. Large indirect hernias may stretch the adjacent transversalis fascia causing a secondary weakness of the direct space.

Primary direct inguinal hernias are more common in older men. Several factors predispose to this type of hernia. Inherent weakness of the transversalis may be aggravated by factors which raise intraabdominal pressure such as obstructive pulmonary disease, obstructive colon lesions, obstructive uropathy, and ascites. In addition, there may be changes in collagen metabolism with age and nutrition. Decreased available protein and altered cross linking with disease states and suboptimal nutrition degrades the strength of tissues in the course of the continuous remodelling process.

Patients should be counseled that in addition to the risk of incarceration, delay of repair incurs the risk of poorer healing with age and increased recurrence rate. Delay also results in more stretching and tissue weakening, compromising the tissue available for repair. If the surgeon determines there is a primary direct space weakness or weakness secondary to a large indirect hernia, one of the following formal repairs of the inguinal floor may be used.

Anterior Iliopubic Tract Repair

With minor variations, several named inguinal hernia repairs have in common approximation of the falx inguinalis (transversus aponeurotic arch) with the iliopubic tract and inguinal ligament (Fig. 3.30). The first effective hernia repair, performed by Bassini and presented in 1887, incorporated these structures. The Shouldice technique and the iliopubic tract repair of Nyhus and Condon are modern variants. Exposure for these repairs requires mobilization or more commonly removal of the cremaster layer to reveal the posterior inguinal wall. An iliopubic tract repair can be performed without opening the transversalis fascia of the direct space by palpating and grasping the transversus aponeurotic arch with a Babcock type clamp. With traction, the fibrous ridge stands out and can be transfixed and sutured to the iliopubic tract and adjacent inguinal ligament. The weakened transversalis fascia is thus inverted. The disadvantage of not opening the fascia is that the bite of falx is less precise. Too superficial a bite may be insufficient and too deep a bite may penetrate the bladder at the medial end of the suture line.

In the open anterior iliopubic tract repair, the transversalis fascia is opened at its reflection onto the medial side of the inguinal cord (internal spermatic fascia). Careful opening of this thin layer reveals the underlying inferior epigastric vessels. The fascia is opened toward the rectus sheath parallel to the inguinal ligament. The remaining centimeter wide lateral strip of transversalis fascia is the iliopubic tract. Properitoneal fat and peritoneum are peeled away from both flaps and the attenuated fascia of the medial flap is trimmed away. Care is taken not to damage delicate pubic branches of the inferior epigastrics on the deep surface of the iliopubic tract and the occasional (~25%) aberrant obturator artery. The most common repair technique is to sew the reflected edge of the falx to iliopubic tract as a first layer. If one does not incorporate the full width of the falx in the initial repair, there will be strong tissue left to sew to (although with increased tension) if there should be a recurrence.

The second layer sutures the full thickness of the free edge of the medial flap to the inguinal ligament. These layers may be continuous or interrupted. Placing the bites a half centimeter apart results in a firm closure, especially if the bites of the second layer are offset between those of the first row. The goal should be a secure closure with the minimal number of needle perforations. This anatomical repair, if done properly without tension on the suture line, does not require a relaxing incision. The reconstructed deep ring should just barely admit a fingertip. If the iliopubic tract is weak or if primary approximation of falx to iliopubic tract will result in tension, the anterior iliopubic repair should be abandoned in favor of a tension free mesh repair.

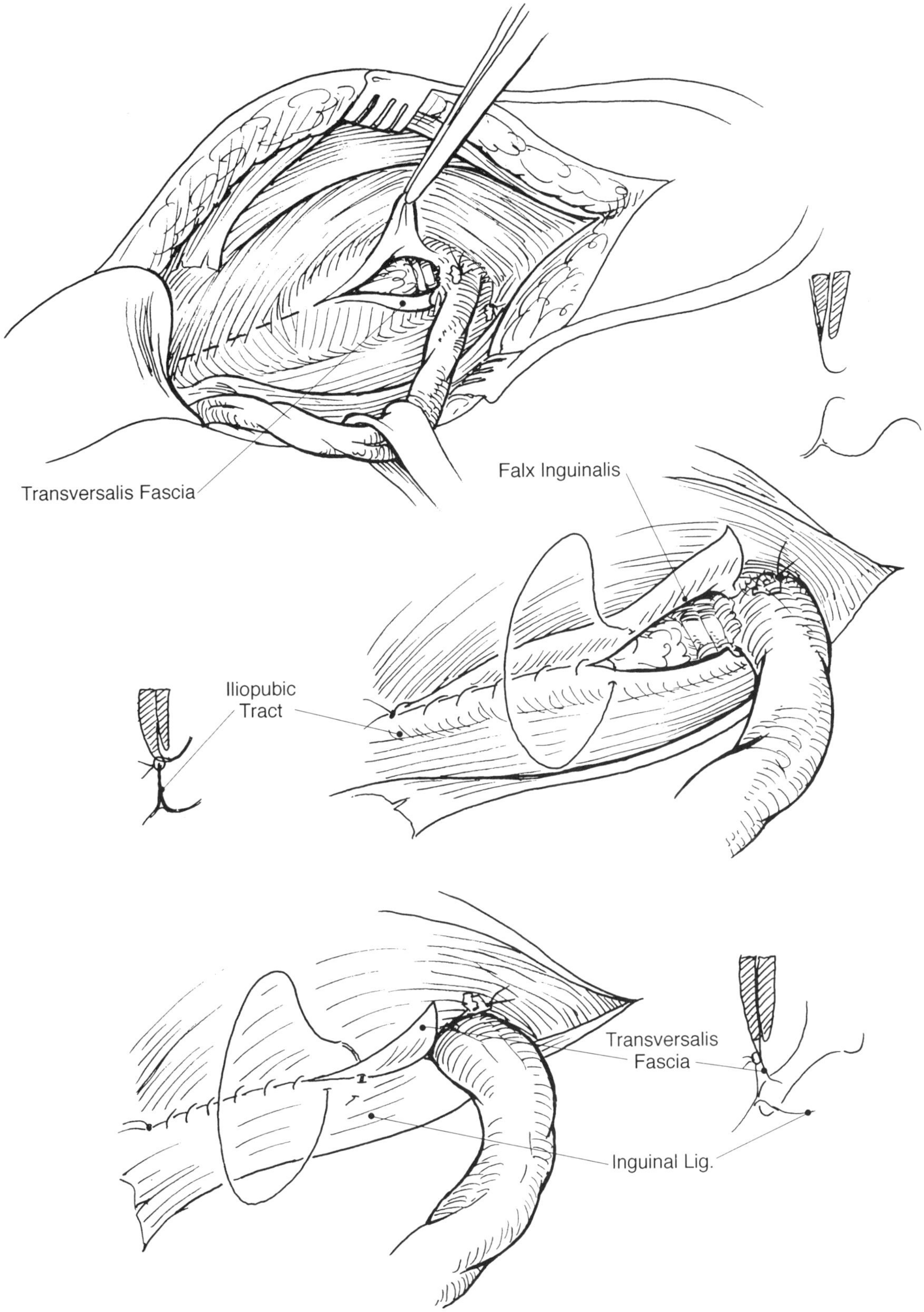
Transversalis Fascia
Falx Inguinalis
Iliopubic
Tract
Transversalis
Fascia
Inguinal Lig.

Fig. 3.30

Pectineal Ligament Repair

The pectineal ligament repair, described by Lotheissen in 1897, and popularized by McVay, approximates the falx to pectineal ligament up to the iliac vessels, then makes the transition to the more anterior iliopubic tract/inguinal ligament plane via the medial edge of the femoral sheath (Fig. 3.31). The transversalis fascia is opened as described above. The properitoneal fat and peritoneum of the lateral flap must be reflected far posterior to expose the pectineal ligament and the cephalad end of the femoral canal. Because the falx must extend farther to reach the pectineal ligament, a relaxing incision must always be made. This is a linear incision in the fused deep laminae of the anterior rectus sheath (transversus and internal oblique aponeuroses) just lateral to the medially offset fusion line of external oblique aponeurosis. The deep lamina is thus mobilized and slid laterally easing the travel of the falx. Tacking sutures may be placed from the mobilized fascial edge to rectus muscle to reduce the chance of secondary herniation at the edge of the rectus.

The falx is then sutured to pectineal ligament (periosteum of pectineal line) from the edge of the rectus sheath laterally to the external iliac vessels. A transition stitch then diverts the falx anteriorly across the medial edge of the femoral sheath (transversalis fascia). Practitioners of this repair advocate it for femoral as well as inguinal hernias. By using the transition stitch to narrow the proximal opening of the femoral canal, the femoral hernia defect is corrected. An increased incidence of femoral vein compression and laceration are associated with this step.

The remainder of the repair anterior to the iliac vessels is done using the iliopubic tract/inguinal ligament layer (McVay discounted the value of the iliopubic tract and specified the inguinal ligament for this part of the repair). The deep ring should be sized as described above.

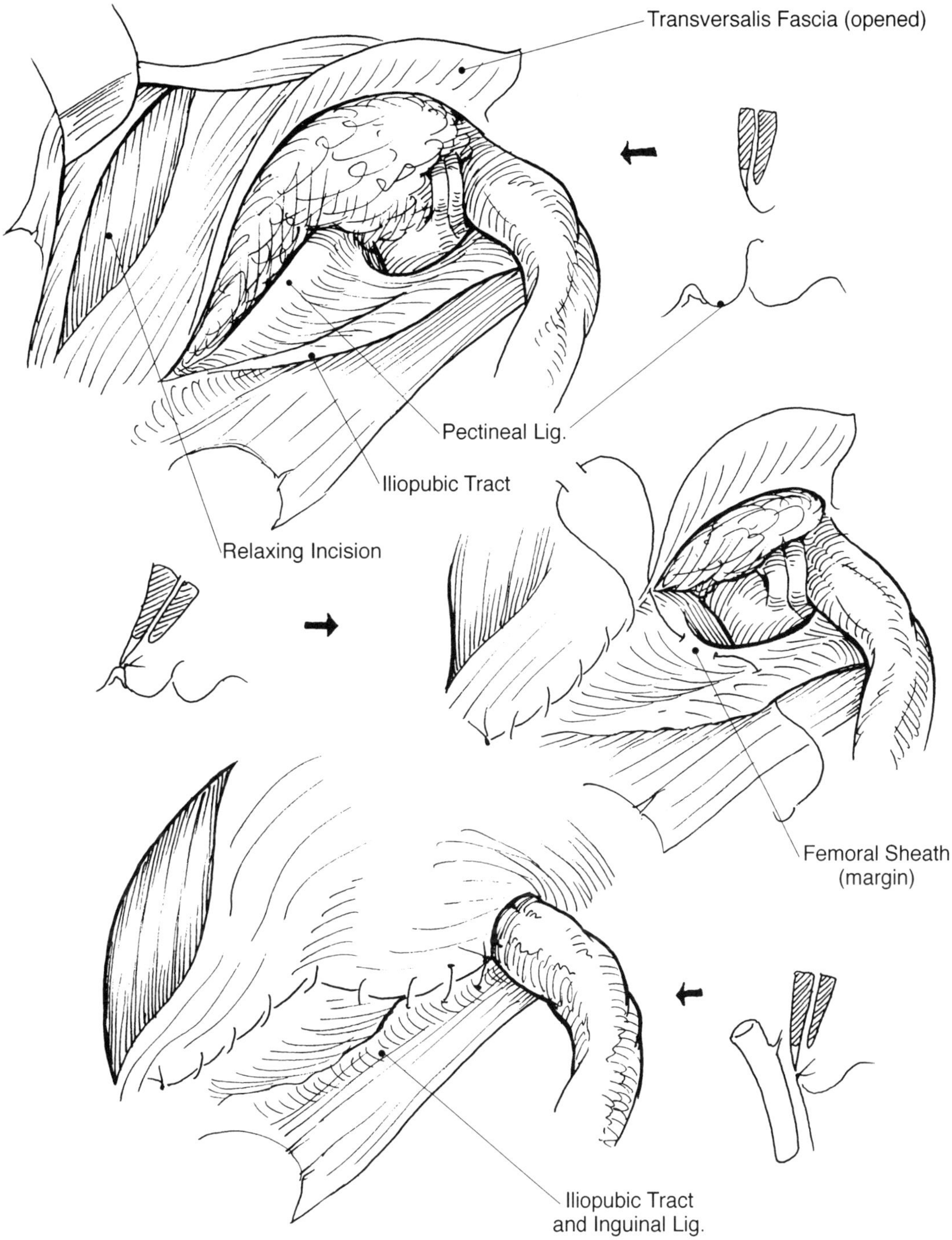

Transversalis Fascia (opened)
Pectineal Lig.
Iliopubic Tract
Relaxing Incision
Femoral Sheath
(margin)
Iliopubic Tract
and Inguinal Lig.

Fig. 3.31

Sutured Preperitoneal Repairs

Indirect, direct, and femoral hernias may all be approached using an anterior preperitoneal route first described in 1876 and most recently popularized by Nyhus (Fig. 3.32). This approach is particularly beneficial for recurrent hernias as it exposes undisturbed anatomy. An abdominal incision is made cephalad to the level of the falx, the flank muscles are divided down to the preperitoneal plane and the rectus muscle is retracted medially. The peritoneum is peeled back exposing the posterior inguinal structures. The inferior epigastric vessels may be divided to clearly delineate the full length of the falx.

A small indirect hernia sac may be carefully extracted from the inguinal canal and closed. The sac may be difficult to identify by this approach and the area over the internal spermatic vessels must be carefully dissected. This same problem arises with the total extraperitoneal laparoscopic approach where the sac is not distended with gas as in the trans-peritoneal approach. A large (approaching the external ring) indirect sac is ligated and transected and the distal end is left in situ.

For a simple indirect hernia, the deep ring may be tightened by suturing falx to iliopubic tract, preferably medial to the deep ring (Fig. 3.32A). Sutures in the iliopubic tract lateral to the deep ring (Fig. 3.32B) endanger the lateral femoral cutaneous nerve. The falx medial to the ring is normally more aponeurotic and stronger. A full length iliopubic tract repair of the floor is also easily accomplished if there is no tension across the direct space (Fig. 3.32C). If there is tension, mesh should be used as described below. The femoral canal orifice can be narrowed by suturing iliopubic tract to pectineal ligament (Fig. 3.32D).

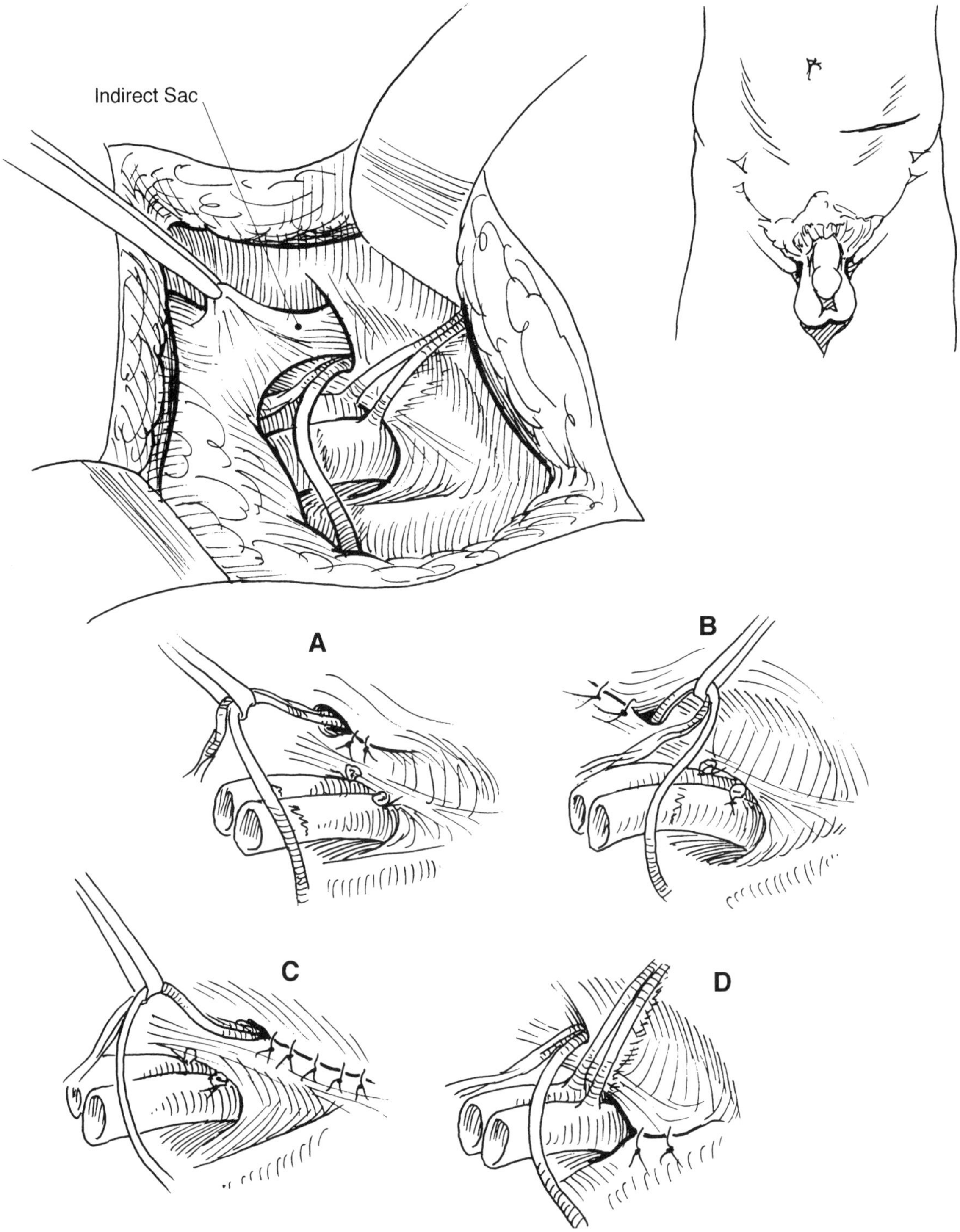

Fig. 3.32

Preperitoneal Mesh Repair

Synthetic mesh (polypropylene) may be placed via the anterior preperitoneal approach (Fig. 3.33). Mesh may be used alone after an indirect sac is dealt with, or it may supplement the repairs described above. Use of a wide sheet of mesh covering the inguinal areas bilaterally was described by Stoppa in 1968 and modified for unilateral application by Wantz. These wide sheets are held in place by intraabdominal pressure until fibrous ingrowth occurs. Recurrences typically occur at the inferolateral edges of the mesh over the deep rings.

Smaller pieces of mesh are more commonly sutured in place over the floor defects. The lower edge of the mesh is anchored to pectineal ligament. The mesh is tailored to comfortably overly the external iliac vessels with some redundancy to prevent recurrence beneath the mesh edge.

The lower medial portion of the mesh is sutured to pectineal ligament. The cephalad and lateral margins of the generous mesh patch are sutured to the deep fascia of the rectus abdominis and transversus muscle (transversalis fascia). No sutures are placed in the iliopubic tract over the vessels because of danger to the vessels themselves and to the underlying femoral branch of the genitofemoral nerve. Deep bites above and lateral to the deep ring endanger the iliohypogastric and ilioinguinal nerves, where they lie between transversus and internal oblique muscles. Nyhus leaves a long cephalad sheet of mesh that he incorporates in the abdominal wall closure.

The converging structures of the cord may be mobilized and surrounded by slitting the mesh or may be left below the lower edge of the mesh. Mobilization and the sharp edges of the mesh cutout present risks to the delicate vessels and to the genital branch of the genitofemoral nerve

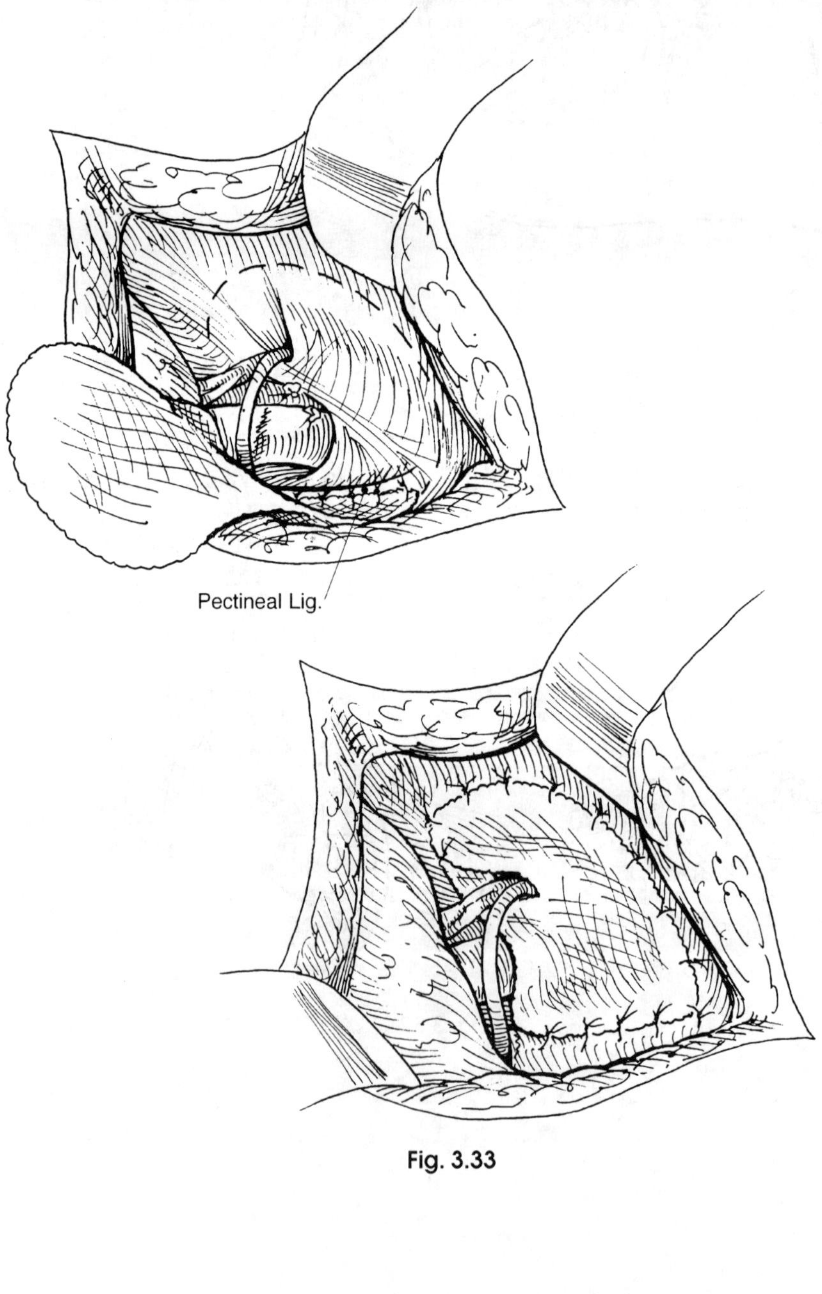

Fig. 3.33

Tension Free Anterior Mesh Repair

Anterior onlay of mesh in the inguinal canal to provide tension free reinforcement of the posterior wall and deep ring has been advocated by Lichtenstein and Gilbert (Fig. 3.34). The mesh is sutured to the deep layer of rectus sheath medially, to internal oblique above and to inguinal ligament below with tails of mesh encircling the inguinal cord at the deep ring. In addition to the freedom from tension, part of the success of this approach is due to ingrowth of tissue and incorporation of the mesh.

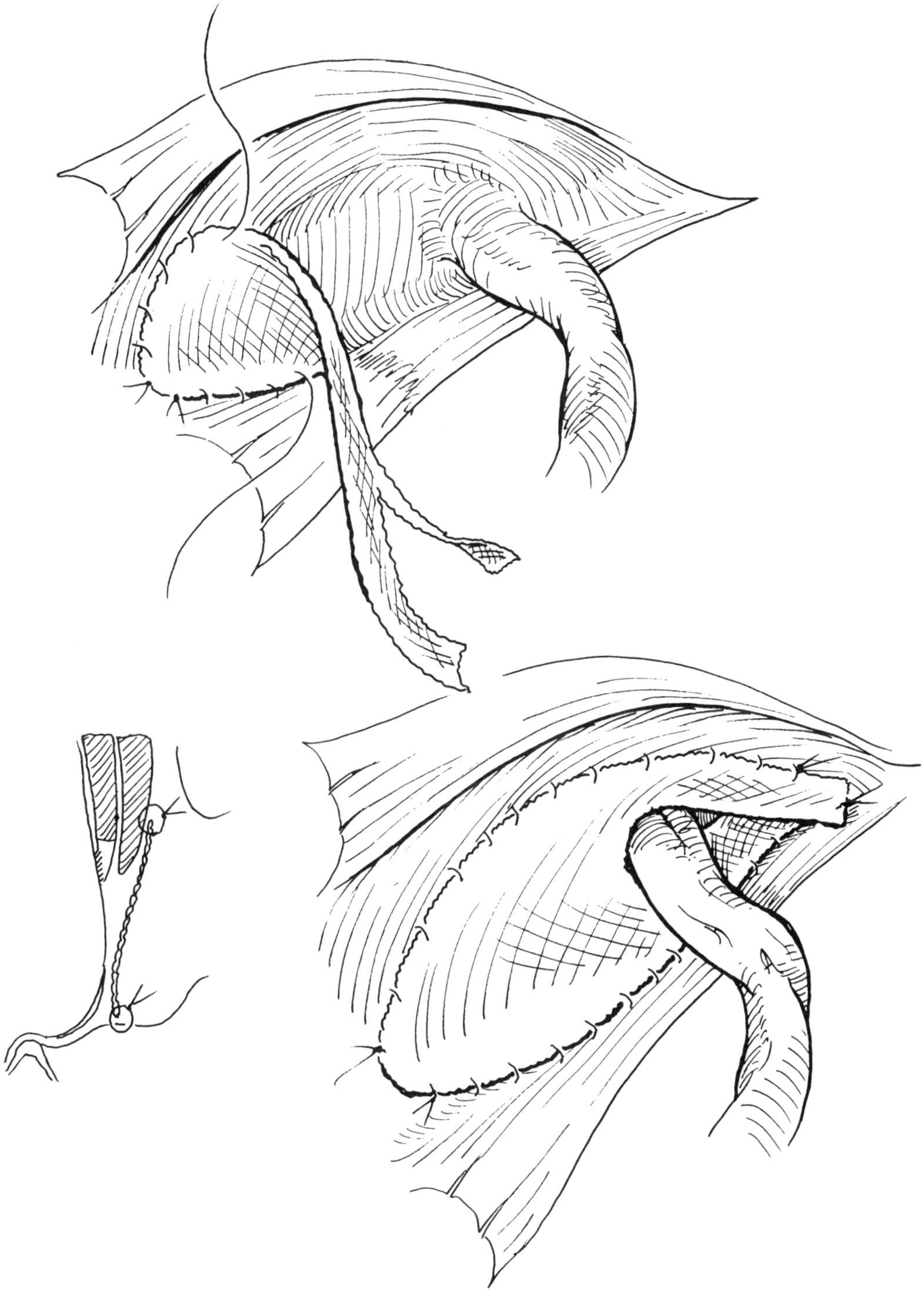

Fig. 3.34

Inferior Femoral Hernia Repair

A femoral hernia may be approached by opening the fascia lata below the inguinal ligament (Fig. 3.35). Femoral sheath is dissected off the sac and the sac opened to assess viability of contents. The disadvantage of this approach is that an abdominal counterincision must be made if bowel must be resected. If there is no evidence of bowel infarction, the hernia is reduced. This usually requires enlarging the fibro-osseus sac neck consisting of inguinal ligament anteriorly, lacunar ligament medially and pectineal ligament posteriorly. The lacunar or inguinal ligaments may be carefully divided, keeping in mind the potential proximity of an aberrant obturator artery cephalad to these structures.

The inguinal ligament and underlying iliopubic tract may then be sutured either to pectineal ligament or the more easily accessible pectineus fascia to narrow the femoral canal. Care must be taken not to injure or compress the adjacent femoral vein. The advantage of this approach is that the normal anatomy of the inguinal canal need not be disrupted as in a pectineal ligament approach and the abdominal wall need not be opened as in a preperitoneal approach.

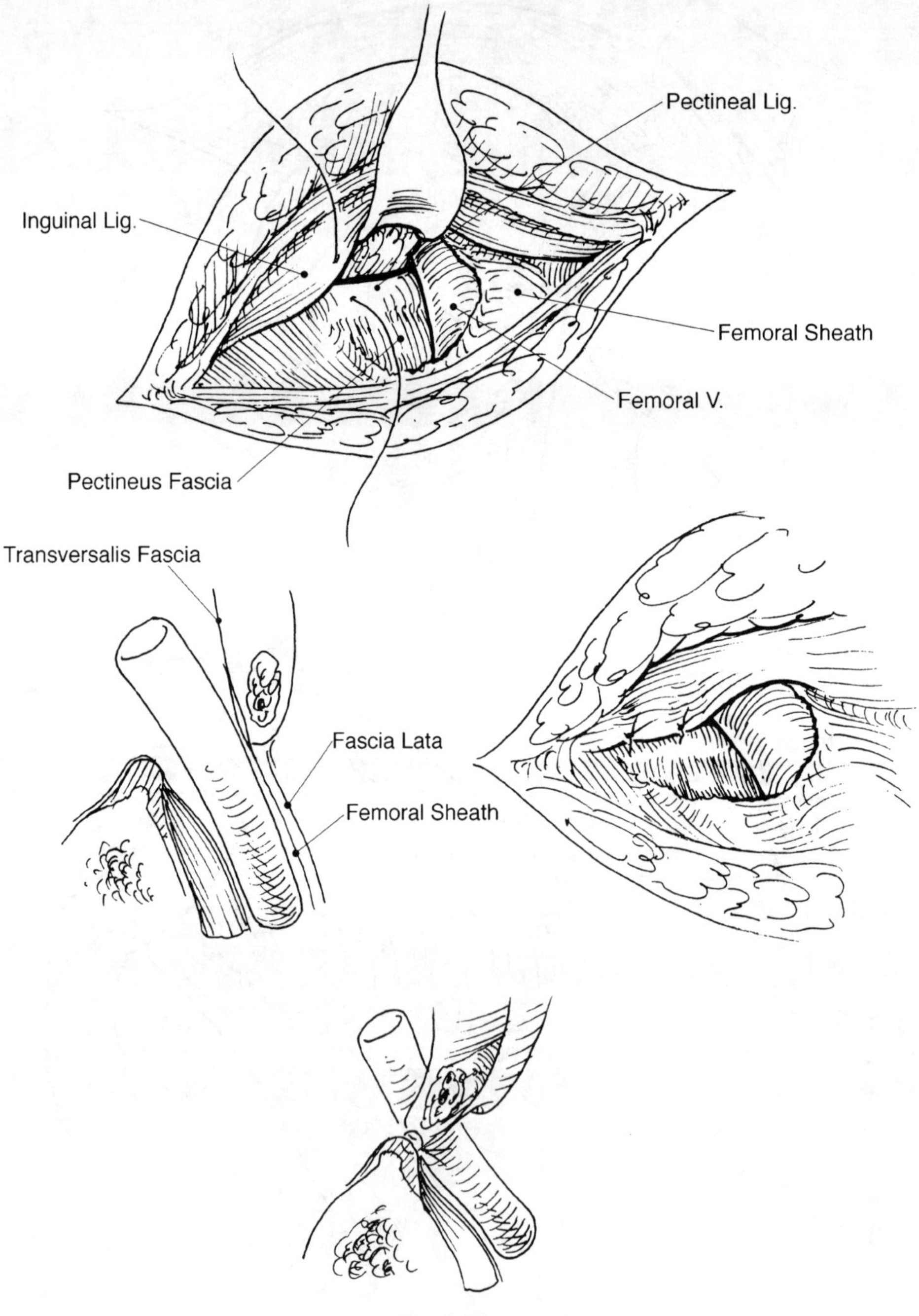

Fig. 3.35

Summary

Firm understanding of conventional approaches implies a solid grasp of groin anatomy which is the basis for laparoscopic techniques. In addition, any surgeon who operates laparoscopically must be skilled in alternatives if laparoscopic repair cannot be accomplished. The surgeon must also be prepared to deal with complications such as injury to an obturator artery or the iliac vessels.

LAPAROSCOPIC GROIN HERNIA REPAIR

Experience with laparoscopic groin herniorrhaphy is growing. Widespread acceptance will depend on several factors. Laparoscopic repair must compare favorably to the effectiveness and low morbidity of modern herniorrhaphy techniques. Patient acceptance is high for open herniorrhaphy as is physician comfort level for performing open herniorrhaphy. Laparoscopic herniorrhaphy can be more technically demanding and the learning curve is long.

Laparoscopic herniorrhaphy offers a reduction in discomfort, shorter convalescence, and quicker return to full activity. It also offers a clean approach to recurrent hernia, excellent anatomic exposure for large hernias and a low morbidity option for repair of bilateral hernias. For hernias in these categories, the early laparoscopic recurrence rates compare favorably to open repair results, but the follow-up period is still short.

The negative aspects of laparoscopic repair include the cost of the technology, the unfamiliarity with the posterior approach to groin anatomy, the difficulty of performing pressurized insufflation under local anesthesia, the current lack of standardization of techniques, the lack of long-term proof of effectiveness, and concern about the long-term risks of prosthetic material. For the transabdominal laparoscopic approach, which is most popular at present, the violation of the peritoneal cavity adds risks of morbidity, particularly visceral injury and later bowel obstruction, that are not inherent in open herniorrhaphy.

Technology can be expected to continue to improve in terms of simplicity and cost. Training and experience will bring surgeons up to speed on the posterior approach to groin anatomy and in technical skills. In experienced hands, there is no significant time difference between open and laparoscopic herniorrhaphy. The application of established hernia repair principles should yield long-term results that are comparable and await the proof of time. Some reassurance about the long-term fate of prosthetic material in the groin is known from experience with the Stoppa (25 years) and Nyhus (20 years) posterior approaches. Some concerns about infection, adhesions to exposed mesh, and erosion into organs and blood vessels remain. Patients, especially those below age 40, should be advised of these uncertainties until they are resolved. Pressurized herniorrhaphy under local anesthesia has been reported, and abdominal lifting devices are appearing for nonpressurized laparoscopy.

The learning curve for laparoscopic hernia repair is longer than for laparoscopic cholecystectomy. The first several cases can be a humbling experience and take a considerable amount of time.

Position and Port Placement

Consent is obtained for possible bilateral hernia repair because of the significant number of undetected contralateral hernias found at surgery and the benefit of saving the patient an additional procedure with minimal added risk. The patient is draped with the groin areas exposed to allow external pressure for assessment and staple placement during the procedure. With the patient supine and a Foley catheter in place, a large subumbilical port is placed after standard insufflation through the lower part of the umbilicus (Fig. 3.36A). In patients with a short umbilicus to pubis distance, the port is placed cephalad to the umbilicus. The patient is placed in steep Trendelenburg position to slide the viscera out of the pelvis. Both inguinal areas are examined. If a hernia is found only on the anticipated side, a second large port is placed at the edge of the rectus muscle above the level of the umbilicus on the side of the hernia and a 5-mm port is placed on the opposite side between the umbilical port and the anterior superior iliac spine (Fig. 3.36a). If bilateral hernias are present, two other large ports are placed at the edges of the rectus muscles parallel with the umbilical port (Fig. 3.36B). The camera is moved to the rectus port on the side to be repaired, and the surgeon stands on the side opposite the hernia. The camera operator stands on the side of the hernia. The bevel of the telescope is directed to give the surgeon the most direct view looking from the surgeon's side and upward. The surgeon operates bimanually through the two ports closest to him or her. An optional 5-mm port may be placed superomedial to the anterior superior iliac spine on the side of the hernia for assistance in a large or complicated hernia.

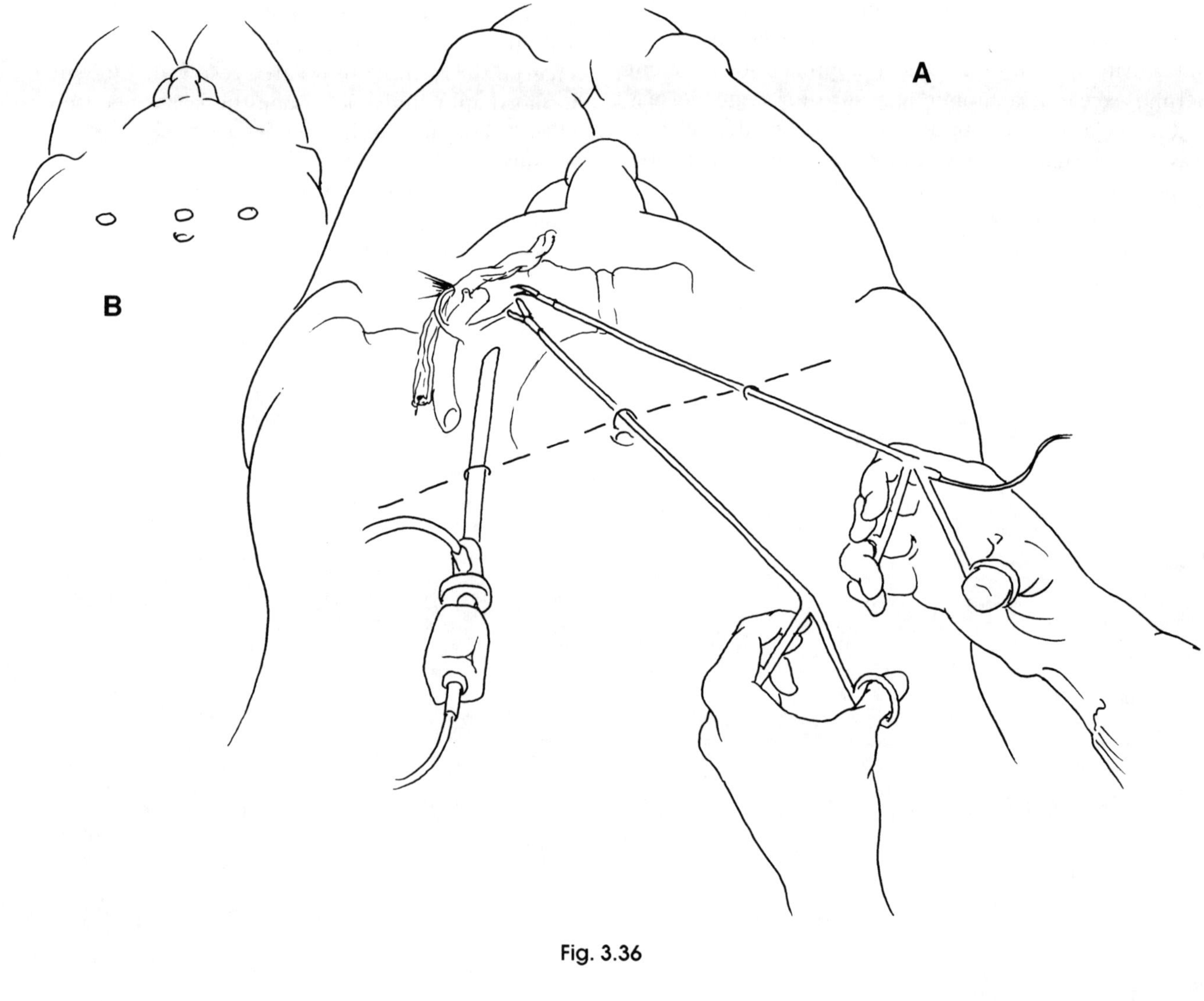

Fig. 3.36

Exposure

On inspection of both groins, a normal internal ring appears as a dimple at the junction of the internal spermatic vessels and the vas, just lateral to the inferior epigastric vessels (Fig. 3.37A). An acute angle is normally seen between the inferior epigastric vessels and the medial umbilical ligament. An indirect hernia sac is usually inflated by the intraabdominal gas and is evident on inspection (Fig. 3.37B). A large indirect hernia (Nyhus type IIIb) pushes the epigastric vessels medially into the direct space. In patients with abundant properitoneal fat, a direct defect may be difficult to identify initially (Fig. 3.37C). An important hint to the presence of a direct hernia is a widening of the angle between the inferior epigastric vessels and the medial umbilical ligament so that they are parallel to each other. External pressure with a finger through the external ring may be helpful in demonstrating the defect. A femoral hernia may be evident in most cases before dissection of the peritoneal flaps. Other times, it becomes evident as dissection of the lower flap proceeds and usually contains incarcerated properitoneal fat.

The medial umbilical ligament may have a curtain of redundant properitoneal fat and must be retracted medially for exposure. The inferior epigastric vessels, the transversalis sling of the deep ring, the external iliac vessels and overlying spermatic vessels, pectineal ligament and the vas deferens are identified through the peritoneum.

The three current options for laparoscopic hernia repair are intraperitoneal onlay mesh (IPOM), transabdominal preperitoneal (TAPP) and totally extraperitoneal (TEP). If intraperitoneal placement of soft synthetic material like Polytetraflouroethylene (PTFE) is elected for repair, no peritoneal dissection is performed. Intraperitoneal onlay is problematic at this time for two reasons. An ideal unreactive material to be left in contact with viscera is not yet available and the staples may not

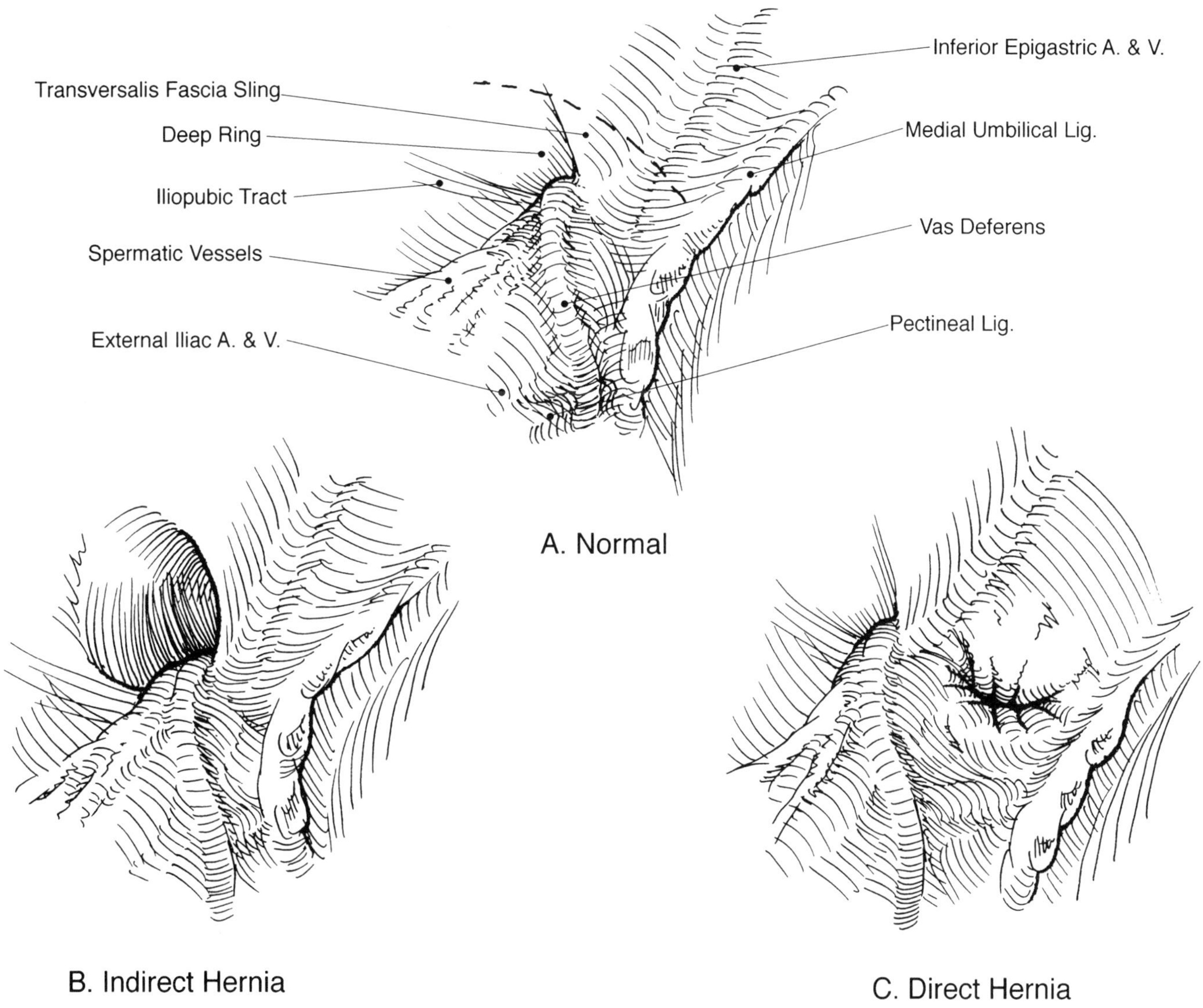

Fig. 3.37

reach the transversalis fascia because of the preperitoneal fat layer. Staples in peritoneum alone have allowed the mesh to slide into the defect causing persistence and recurrence of the hernia. These problems are avoided by placing the mesh in the preperitoneal position by a trans-abdominal or extraperitoneal route.

Trans-abdominal Dissection

A generous arching peritoneal incision touching the upper margin of the deep ring is carried from a point 2 cm lateral to the deep ring to the medial umbilical ligament (Fig. 3.38A). The incision should not extend medial to the medial umbilical ligament because of the danger of injuring bladder. Embryologically, the umbilical arteries lay on either side of the bladder (see pelvic embryology) and their remnants, the medial umbilical ligaments, are good guideposts to the margins of the bladder. The incision is carried through properitoneal fat down to transversalis fascia taking care not to injure the inferior epigastric vessels (Fig. 3.38B). After the peritoneum lateral to the ligament is open, blunt dissection easily moves the ligament and bladder medially as far as the midline.

A small indirect hernia sac may be successfully peeled out of the inguinal canal and be reflected with the lower flap. Any lipoma of the cord should be identified and excised to help prevent recurrence. The lipoma enters the deep ring from lateral to medial and lifts up the lower edge of the unfixed mesh inferiorly if it is not removed. If the defect is small enough and appropriate for a patch repair only, the medial dissection of the flaps is not as extensive as for a large defect. Attempts to remove a large sac or one that extends below the pubic tubercle may injure the cord and compromise the testicular blood supply. Large sacs should be disconnected ("ring excision") from the peritoneum at their neck and left in situ (Fig. 3.38C). The fatty preperitoneal fascia layer is opened to expose the proper plane of dissection on the transversalis fascia above the iliopubic tract. In the case of direct hernias, it is often necessary to peel peritoneum and properitoneal fat out of the defect using two instruments in a hand-over-hand manner (Fig. 3.38D). The fascial edges of a primary or recurrent direct hernia should be defined in this way. The incarcerated properitoneal fat in a femoral hernia can be dissected out as the lower flap is mobilized.

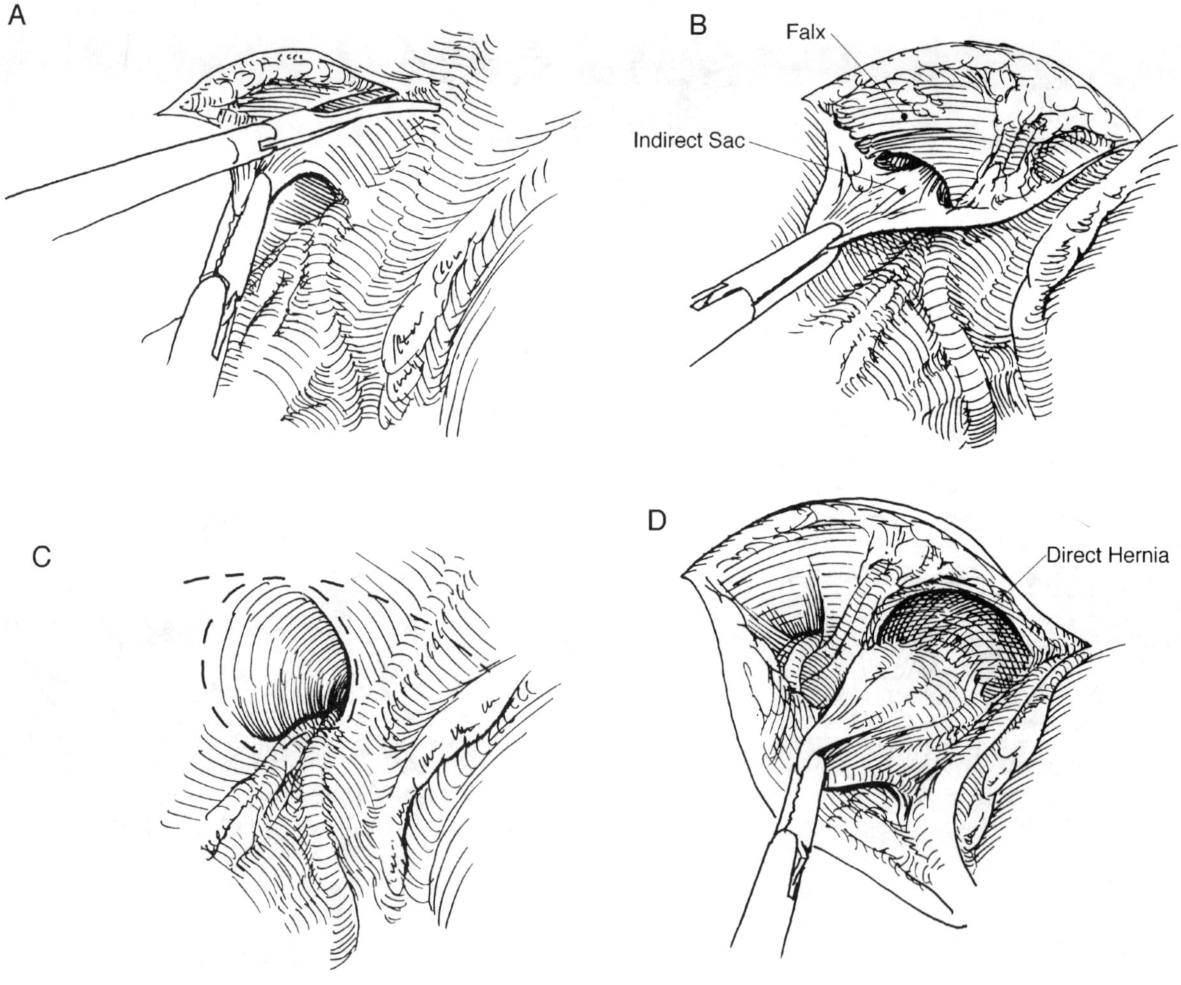

Fig. 3.38

A wide dissection of the flaps to create space for the mesh is then carried out so that the margins of the mesh lie well outside (at least 2 cm) the borders of the defect. The superior flap is lifted to expose the undersurface of the transversus muscle up to the level at which the inferior epigastric vessels penetrate the rectus muscle (Fig. 3.39A). Unlike the dissection of the upper flap, the plane of dissection of the lower flap is just beneath the peritoneum, leaving the preperitoneal fascia on the vessels and vas below (Fig. 3.39B). The peritoneum may be adherent over the junction of epigastric, iliac, internal spermatic vessels and vas, and dissection should proceed carefully. Similar care should be taken for the delicate pubic branch of the inferior epigastric vessels and the aberrant obturator artery when present. Once the lower flap is mobilized, gently pushing aside the preperitoneal fascia from medial to lateral reveals the caudal limit of dissection, the pectineal ligament from pubis to the external iliac vessels (Fig. 3.39C). Inspection of the femoral canal is then possible. The lateral limit of dissection is the transversus muscle and iliopubic tract 2 cm lateral to the deep ring. The medial limit of dissection is the back of the rectus muscle and the pubic bone below. The inferior epigastric vessels may be clipped or bipolar coagulated and divided for clear access to the inguinal floor (Fig. 3.39D).

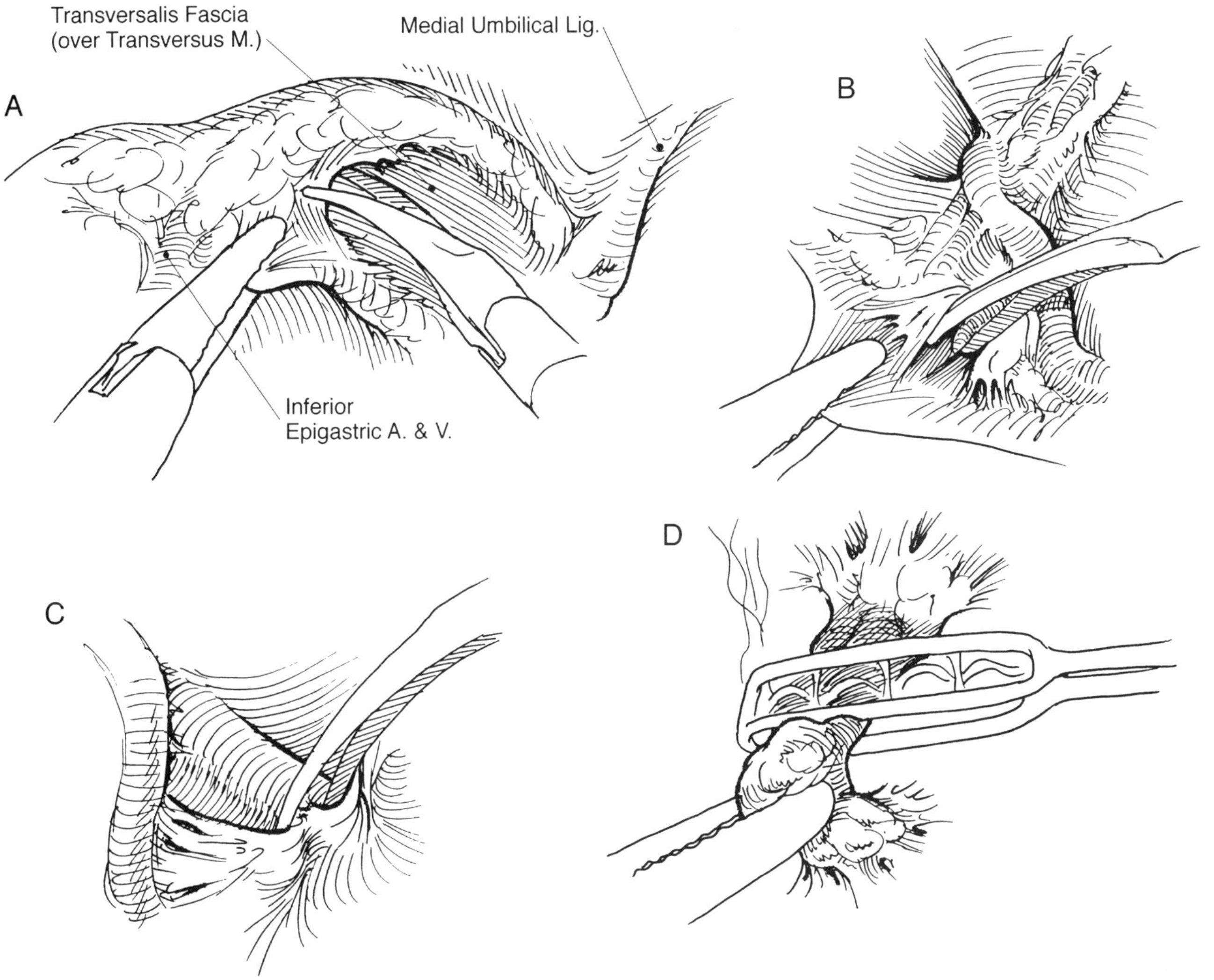

Fig. 3.39

Trans-abdominal Preperitoneal Repair

Staple or suture of a direct or indirect hernia before mesh placement is possible, but incurs the risks of nerve injury and tension and is not advocated. Simple suture closure of a hernia defect without mesh has a higher recurrence rate (2.6%, Phillips). Placement of an unsutured mesh plug in indirect defects has proven unsatisfactory due to distal migration and high recurrence. Small indirect hernias (Nyhus type I and II) may be treated without extensive dissection using a local patch or a single mesh (polypropylene) sheet, but the saving in initial dissection is at the price of the chance of a later direct recurrence and a more difficult secondary dissection. For large hernias, a double layer repair has a lower recurrence rate than single layer (1% vs. 3%) in reports to date. One method of double layer repair illustrated here, the butterfly patch (Dudai), has been used under a mesh sheet with good results.

To create the butterfly patch, a 6 × 12 cm sheet of polypropylene mesh is folded as illustrated (Fig. 3.40) and sutured at one end with a 2-0 suture of the same material. Each fold is cut individually so that adjacent strips are not exactly superimposed on one another and they will not stick together. The resulting patch has eight individual limbs and a short central hub.

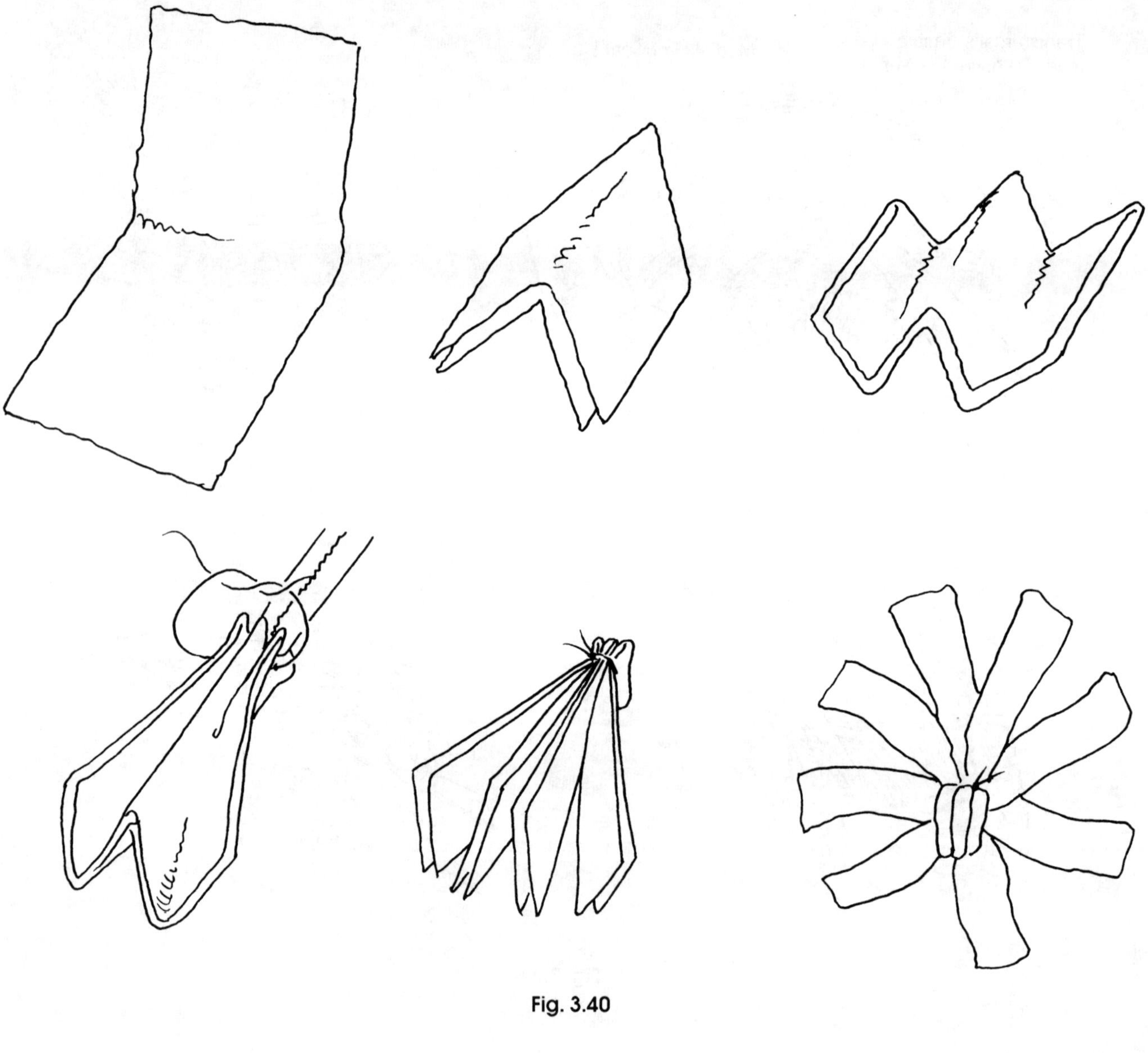

Fig. 3.40

The patch is introduced through a large port, and the hub is held in place in the indirect, direct or femoral defect (Fig. 3.41). The first arm is stapled in the 12:00 position (lateral to the intact epigastric vessels or at the site of the transected vessels), the second on the superolateral side of the defect, and the third lateral to the defect above the iliopubic tract. The fourth arm is stapled to the falx or the rectus muscle and the fifth to the mid-point of pectineal ligament (using 4.0-mm limbed staples; the longer 4.8-mm limbed staples used for the rest of the procedure hit the bone of the pectineal ridge and fail to close properly). The remaining three arms are laid over, medial and lateral to the iliac and spermatic vessels without staples.

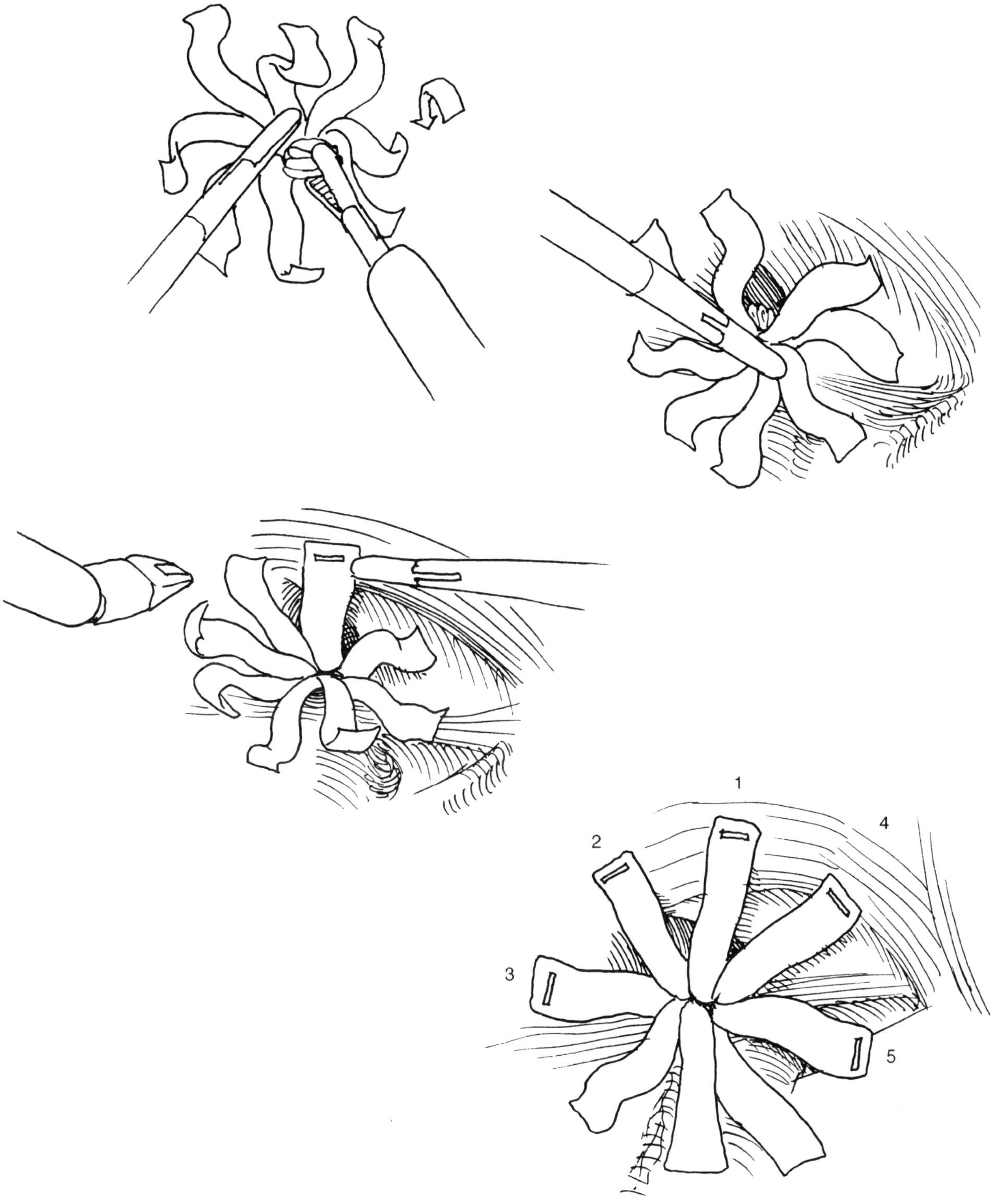

Fig. 3.41

Next, a measurement of the width of the dissected area is made with a ligature (Fig. 3.42) and a patch of mesh slightly larger than posterior inguinal wall (and overlapping the defect on all sides by at least 2 cm) is cut. The mesh is passed through the 11-mm port. The trimmed mesh can be placed into the abdomen through a large port directly or by using an introducer sheath.

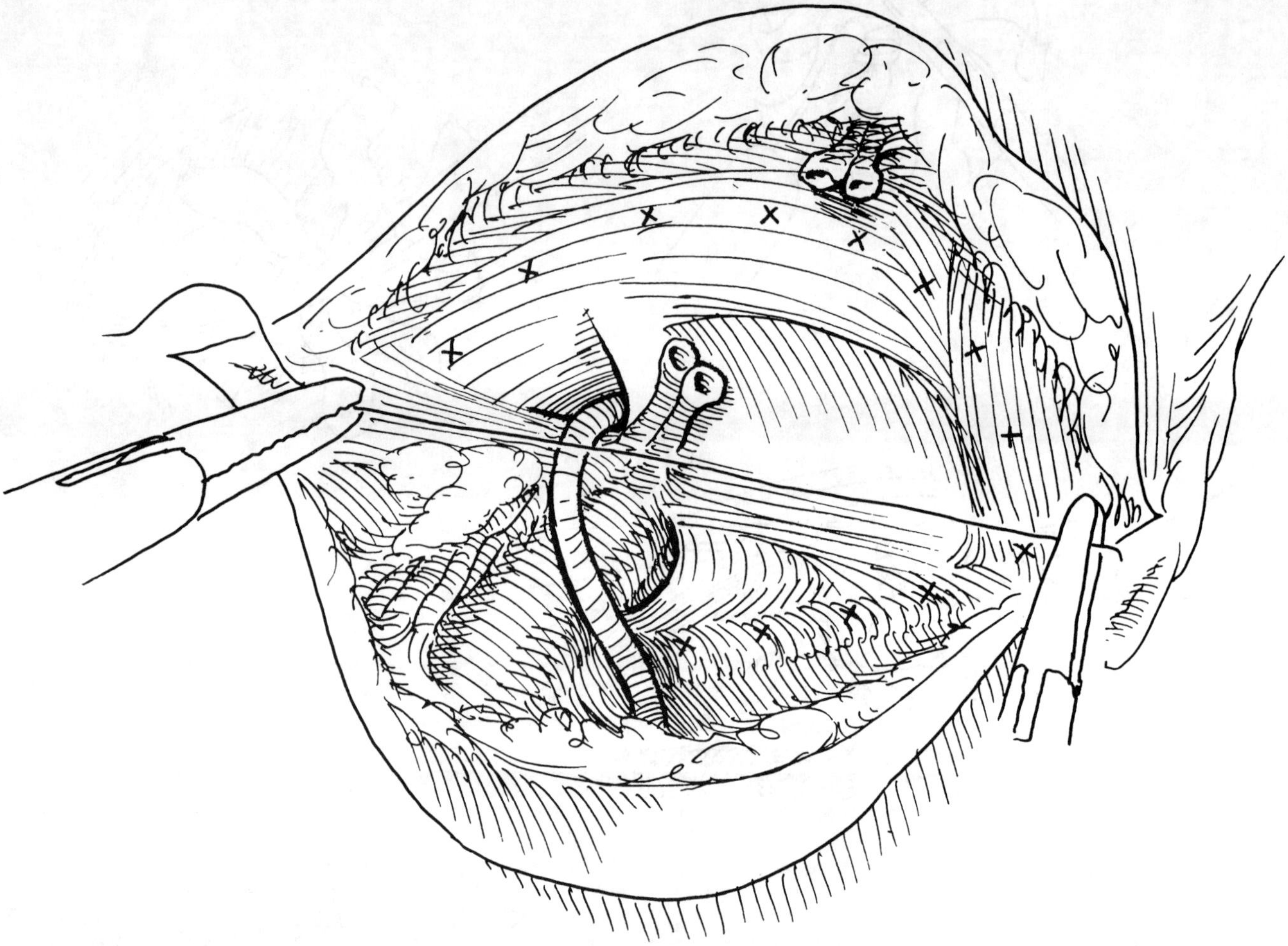

Fig. 3.42

An elegant way to introduce the mesh is to form a double scroll-like roll (Dudai) with a temporary suture fixing the lateral side. The mesh is wet so that it will adhere to the abdominal wall (Fig. 3.43A). The surgeon holds the center of the fixed roll and positions it beneath the flaps, bisecting the field, and the loose roll is spread toward the medial side (Fig. 3.43B, C).

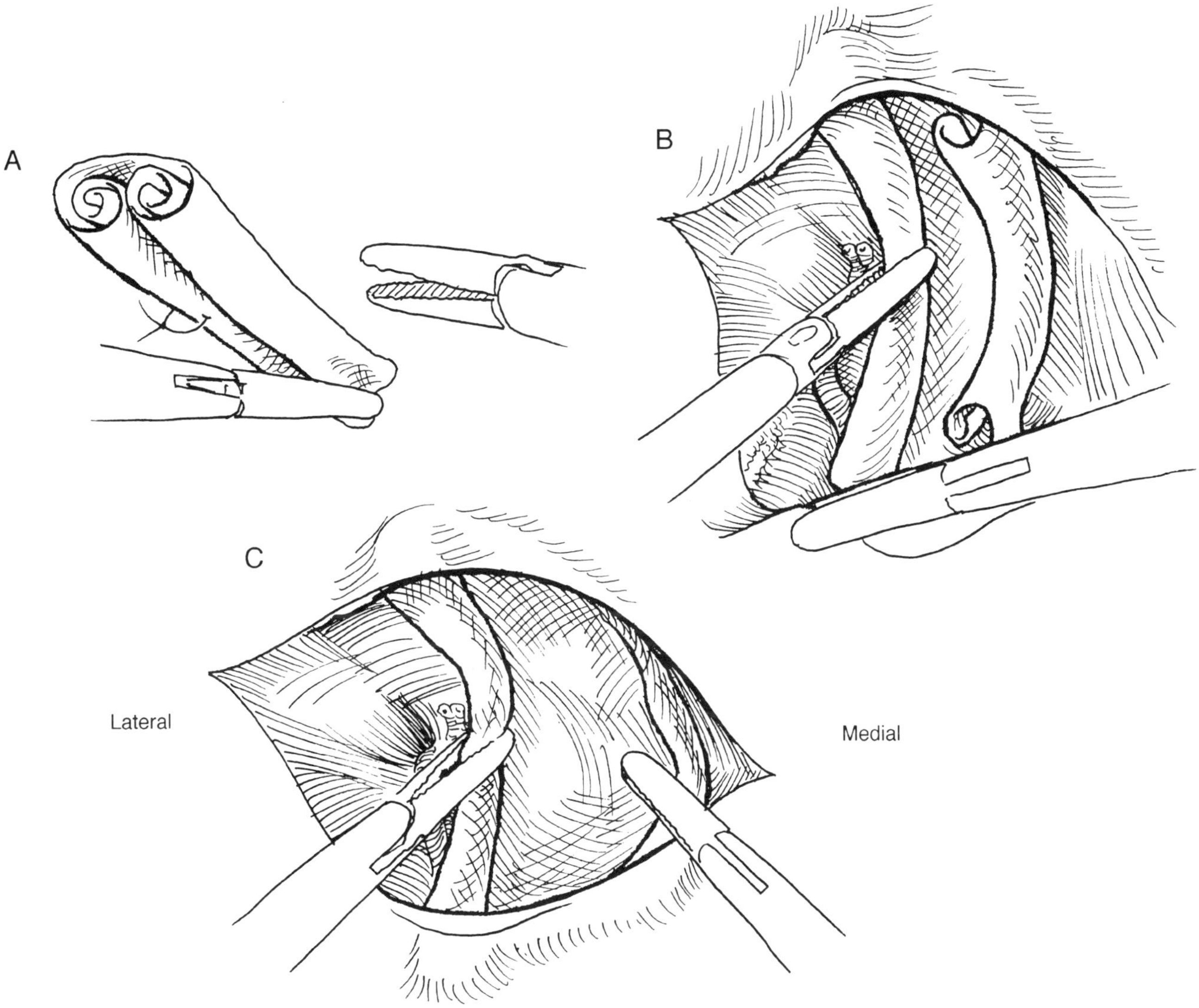

Fig. 3.43

The first (4.0 mm) staple is placed in the pectineal ligament next to the iliac vein and vas. Three additional staples are placed medially in the pectineal ligament (Fig. 3.44). The remaining borders of the mesh are stapled with 4.8-mm staples. Staples are placed in the body of the pubis and in a wide arch across transversalis fascia over the rectus and

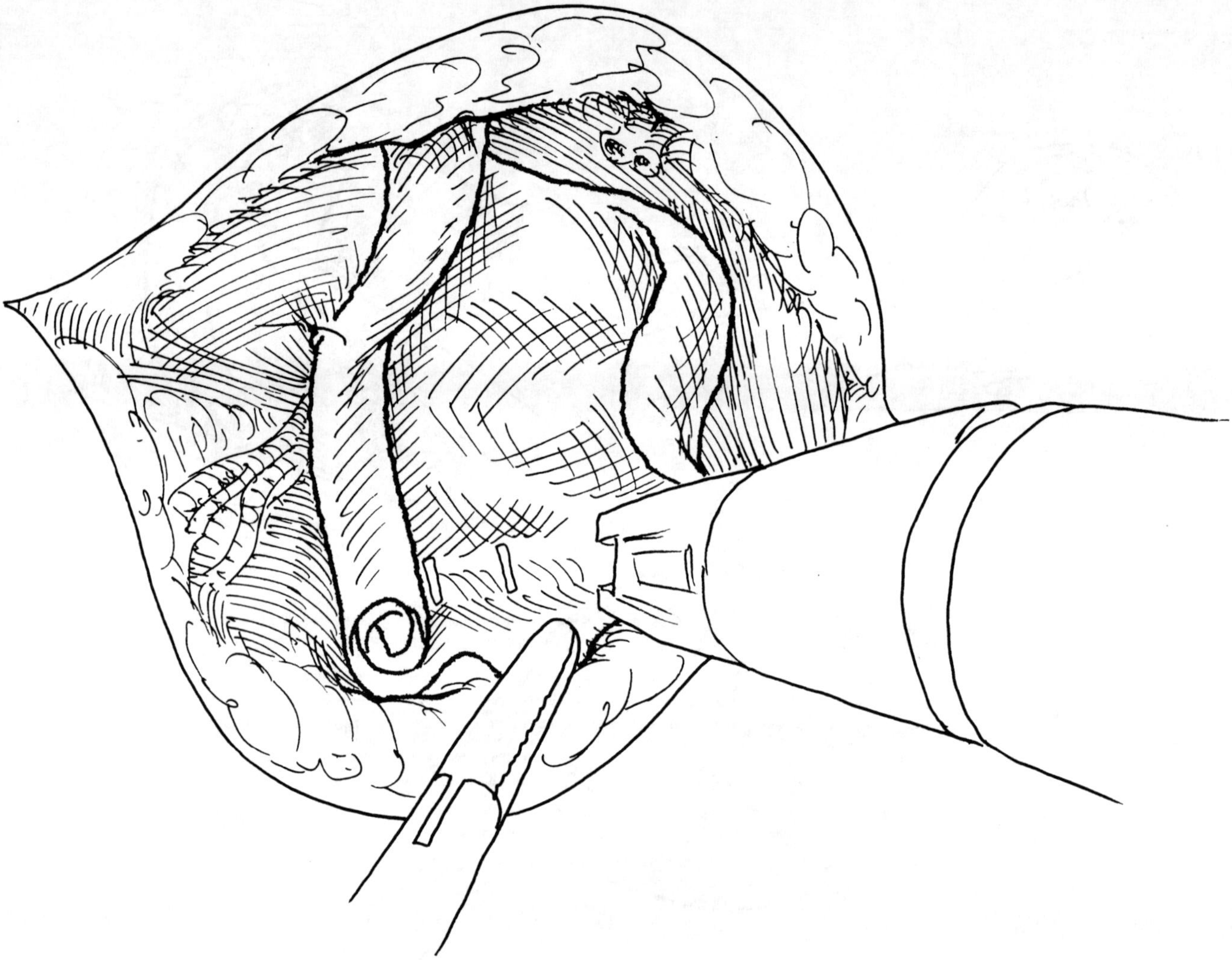

Fig. 3.44

transversus abdominis muscles (Fig. 3.45). A stapler with an articulating head is necessary to properly place the staples, especially in the steeply angled upper edges of the mesh. The most lateral staple should be placed above the iliopubic tract to avoid injuring the lateral femoral cutaneous nerve. These lateral staples should be oriented vertically to decrease chances of catching the nerve. The ilioinguinal nerve is at risk from deep staple placement toward the lateral part of the arch. If nerve entrapment occurs it may be necessary to go back later and remove the offending staple. Relief of pain has been achieved in such cases. Identifying such a staple may be difficult unless the videotape of the procedure is available for review.

It is only the lining transversalis fascia, not muscle, that has holding power and the fascia is easily encompassed by the staple. Mobilization and encirclement of the cord structures is dangerous to the cord structures and is unnecessary if a long apron of mesh is left over the vessels.

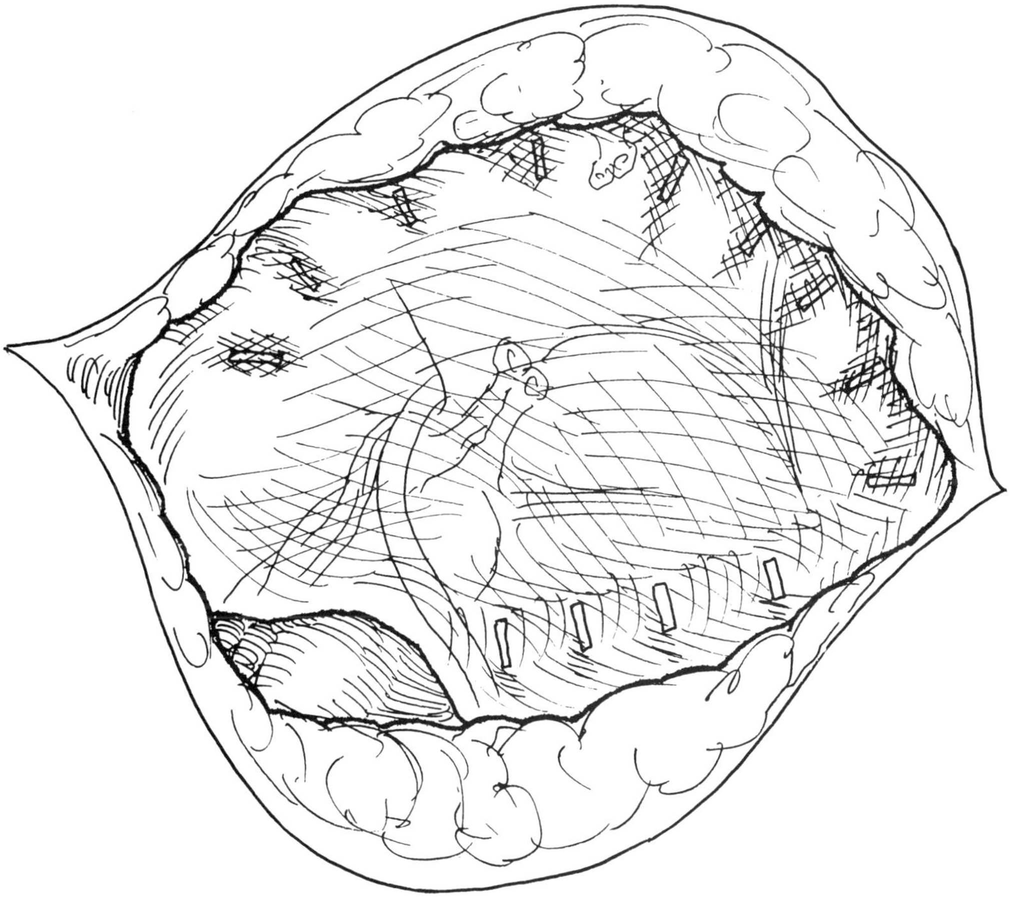

Fig. 3.45

A long-acting local anesthetic may be sprayed on the area of dissection before flap closure or injected beneath the flaps after closure. The intraabdominal pressure is reduced to 6–8 mm Hg to relax the flap edges and the edges are closed with staples (Fig. 3.46) or clips. Staples are easier to apply but leave gaps where bowel may intrude, whereas clips give complete parallel edge-to-edge closure. Several cases of intestinal obstruction due to bowel incarcerated through the peritoneal closure have been reported. The technique of clip application is illustrated (Fig. 3.47). The patient may ambulate when awake and is discharged the same evening or the next day.

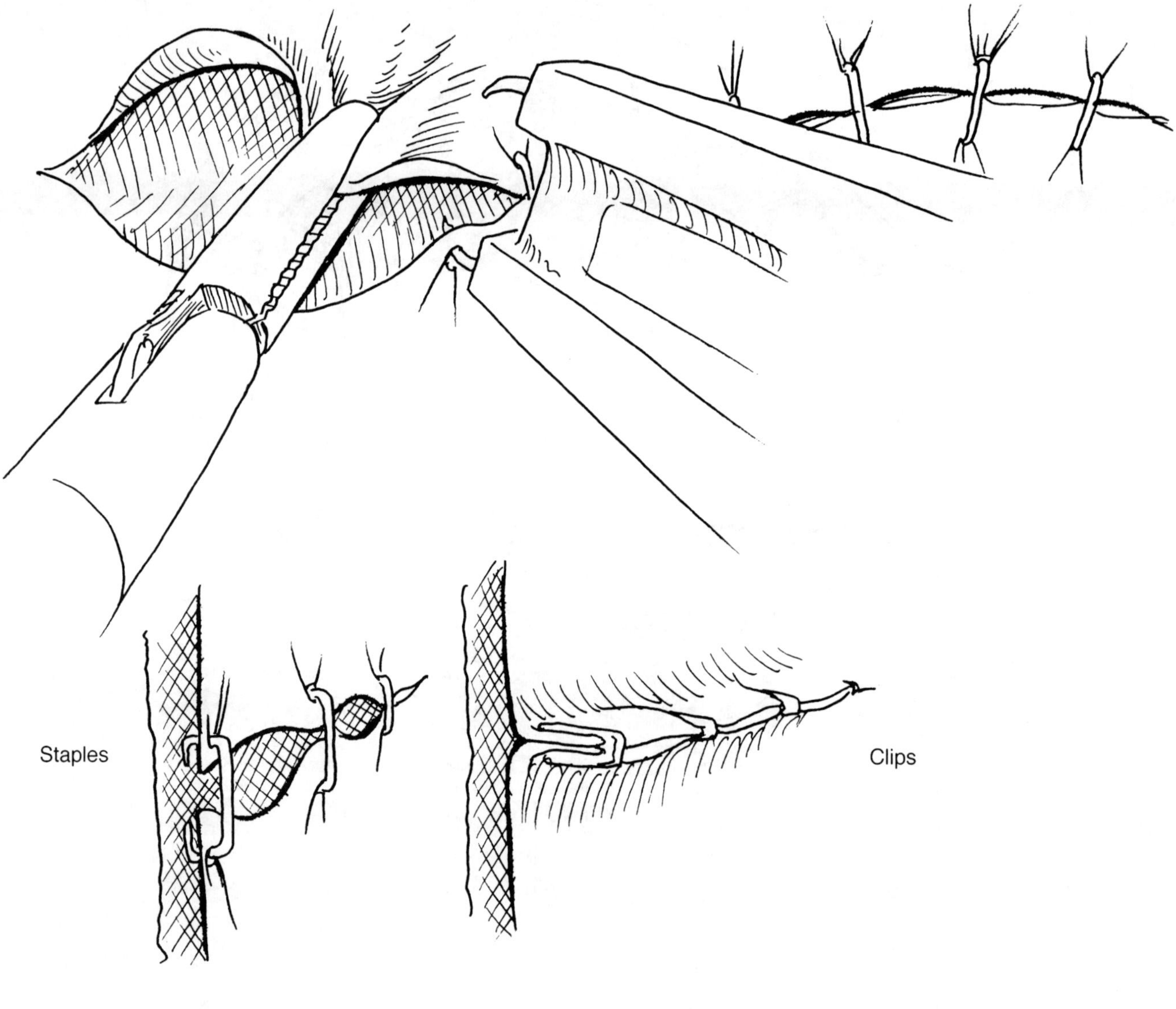

Fig. 3.46

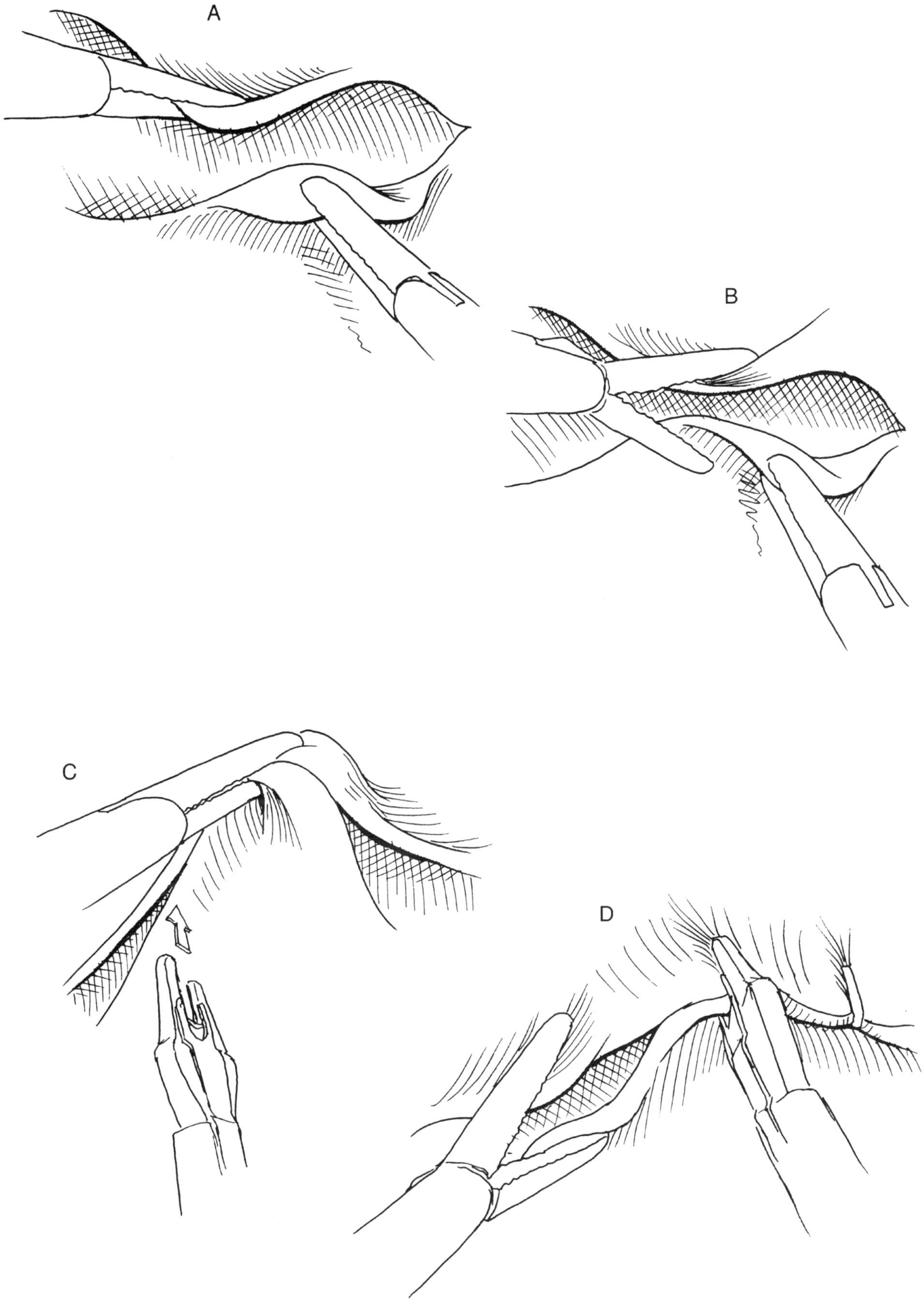

Fig. 3.47

Total Extraperitoneal Repair

For the total extraperitoneal approach, dissection of the lower abdominal preperitoneal space is begun using a balloon dilator introduced through a small subumbilical incision (Fig. 3.48). The remainder of the dissection exposing the inguinal floor is done under direct vision with ports placed as for the TAPP approach. Prior lower abdominal surgery and prostate surgery and some complicated recurrences make the dissection difficult and are contraindications. The balloon invariably reduces a direct sac. An indirect sac must be identified, separated from the cord structures and reduced or divided. This can be very difficult for a large scrotal hernia and is contraindicated in sliding hernia. Once the inguinal floor is exposed, a larger mesh than that used in the TAPP approach is introduced and placed. It is tacked in place to pectineal ligament and is observed to ensure that it lies flat as the pressure is reduced and the abdominal contents press it into place like in the Stoppa repair.

This approach has several advantages. It avoids violating the peritoneal space and the associated potential complications. It requires lower pressure and may be done with epidural or spinal anesthesia. It provides wide access to the inguinal floor although the instrument maneuvering room is more limited than in the transabdominal approach. The other disadvantages are the limitations of hernia types that can be repaired by this approach, the wide area of dissection necessary in all cases and the more difficult learning curve. Significant postoperative fluid can collect in the large space created.

Recurrence

Experience with recurrence of laparoscopic hernia repair is just beginning to accumulate. The plug and patch technique had an unacceptably high recurrence rate (9%) and has been abandoned. In the largest reported series (Phillips), short term recurrence was 0% for total expraperitoneal, 1% for trans-abdominal, and 2% for intraperitoneal onlay. The majority of recurrences appeared within the first year. Early recurrences were most commonly due to technical errors. The major factors were incomplete dissection, inadequate size of the mesh, inadequate overlap, and inadequate fixation. The first three factors all have to do with the size of the mesh relative to the defect, which is the major reason for recurrence. An undissected lipoma of the cord may widen the deep ring and also predispose to recurrence. In most cases there is more than one factor. Missed or inadequately treated indirect hernias accounted for 29% of

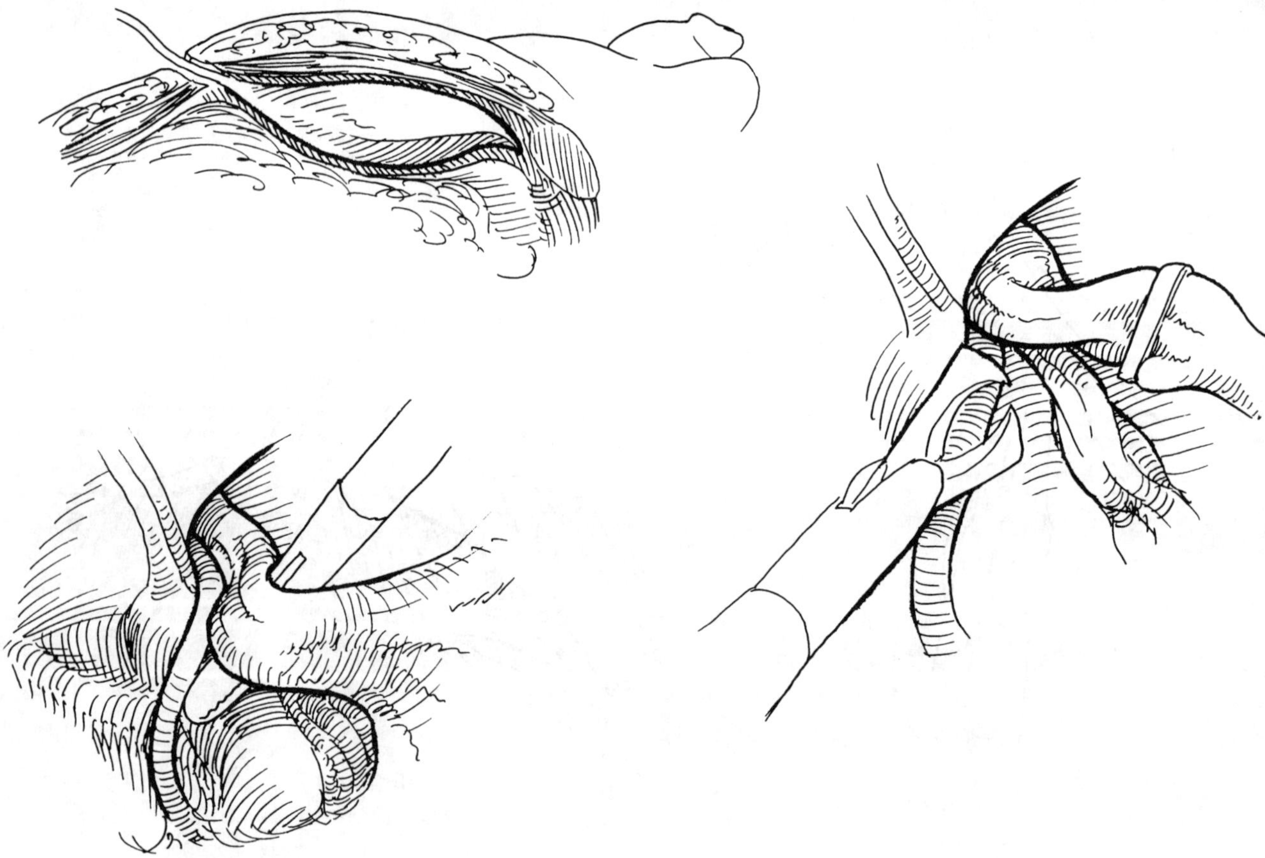

Fig. 3.48

recurrences in one series. Direct recurrences were more common and a femoral component was less common. Other factors include displacement, twisting and folding of the mesh, tension, and intrinsic floor weakness. Recurrence rates will reflect the learning curve and type of repair in individual series, and only when cumulative data are available will valid comparisons be possible. In most cases laparoscopic repair of recurrent laparoscopic hernia is easier than open repair. Most of the time, the recurrence is at the edge of the mesh and can be easily identified. The original mesh should not be disturbed, and the dissection should be done only in the area of recurrence. An additional patch of mesh should be placed to cover the defect and to overlap the original mesh.

Chapter 3: The Inguinal Region

EMBRYOLOGY

Skandalakis JE, Gray SW. Embryology For Surgeons, Philadelphia: Williams & Wilkins, 1994: 577-582.

ANATOMY

Condon RE. The anatomy of the inguinal region and its relation to groin hernia. In: Nyhus LM and Condon RE (eds.). Hernia. Philadelphia: J.B. Lippincott, 1989: 18-64.

Condon RE, Carilli S. The biology and anatomy of inguinofemoral hernia. Sem Laparosc Surg 1994; 1: 75-85.

Gilroy AM, Marks Jr. SC, Lei Q, et al. Anatomical characteristics of the iliopubic tract: implications for repair of inguinal hernias. Clin Anat 1992;5:255-263.

Quinn TH, et al. Dissection of the anterior abdominal wall and the deep inguinal region from a laparoscopic perspective. Clin Anat 1995; 8: 245-251.

Skandalakis JE, et al. Embryologic and anatomic basis of inguinal herniorrhaphy. Surg Clin North Am 1993; 73: 799-836.

Spaw AT, Ennis BW, Spaw LP. Laparoscopic hernia repair. The anatomic basis. J. Laparoendoscopic Surg 1991;1: 269-277.

OPEN HERNIORRHAPHY

Condon RE. Iliopubic tract repair of inguinal hernia: the anterior (inguinal canal) approach. In: Nyhus LM, Baker RJ (eds.). Mastery of Surgery, Boston: Little Brown 1984:1274-1282.

Fischer E, Wantz GE. Traditional preperitoneal approach to inguinal hernias. Sem Laparosc Surg 1994; 1: 86-97.

Gilbert AI. Sutureless repair of inguinal hernia. Am J Surg 1992; 163: 331-335.

Glassow F. The Shouldice repair. In: Nyhus LM, Baker RJ (eds.). Mastery of Surgery. Boston: Little Brown 1984: 1268-1282.

Lichtenstein IL, Schulman AG, Amid PK, et al. The tension-free hernioplasty. Am J Surg 1989; 157: 188-193.

McVay CB. Cooper's ligament repair of groin hernia. In: Nyhus LM, Baker RJ (eds.). Mastery of Surgery. Boston: Little Brown 1984: 1239-1249.

Nyhus LM. Iliopubic tract repair of inguinal and femoral hernia: the posterior (preperitoneal) approach. In: Nyhus LM, Baker RJ (eds.). Mastery of Surgery. Boston: Little Brown, 1984: 1283-1289.

Nyhus LM, Pollack R, Bombeck CT, et al. The preperitoneal approach and prosthetic buttress repair for recurrent hernia. Ann Surg 1988; 208: 733-737.

Ponka JL. The Ponka approach to repair of groin hernias. In: Nyhus LM, Baker RJ (eds.). Mastery of Surgery. Boston: Little Brown, 1984: 1250-1267.

Wantz GE. The technique of giant prosthetic reinforcement of the visceral sac performed through an anterior groin incision. Surg Gyn Obstet 1993; 176: 497-500.

LAPAROSCOPIC HERNIORRHAPHY

Arregui ME, Navarrete J, Davis CJ, et al. Laparoscopic inguinal herniorrhaphy. Surg Clin North Am 1993; 73: 513-527.

Bendavid R. Expectations of hernia surgery (inguinal and femoral). In: Paterson-Brown S, Garden J, editors. Principles and practice of surgical laparoscopy. London: WB Saunders Co. Ltd., 1994: 389-426.

Broin EO. Meralgia paresthetica following laparoscopic inguinal hernia repair. Surg Endosc 1995; 9: 76-78.

Brooks DC. A prospective comparison of laparoscopic and tension-free open herniorrhaphy. Arch Surg 1994; 129: 361-366.

Dion Y-M, Morin J. Laparoscopic inguinal herniorrhaphy. Can J Surg 1992; 35: 209-212.

Dion Y-M. Laparoscopic inguinal herniorrhaphy: an individualized approach. Surg Laparosc Endosc 1993; 3: 451-455.

Dudai M. Laparoscopic hernia repair of large and small hernias using the Dudai butterfly with or without mesh, according to Nyhus hernia type. In: Nyhus LM, Condon RE. Hernia, 4th ed. Philadelphia: J.B. Lippincott Co, 1995: 263-267.

Felix EL. Laparoscopic repair of recurrent hernias. Surg Endosc 1995; 9: 135-139.

Filipi CJ, et al. Laparoscopic herniorrhaphy. Surg Clin North Am 1992;72: 1109-1124.

Ger R, Monroe K, Duvivier R, et al. Management of indirect inguinal hernias by laparoscopic closure of the neck of the sac. Am J Surg 1990; 159: 370-373.

Katkhouda N, Mouiel J. Laparoscopic hernia repair. In: Paterson-Brown S, Garden J, editors. Principles and Practice of Surgical Laparoscopy. London: WB Saunders Co. Ltd., 1994: 415-424.

MacFayden Jr. BV, Mathis CR. Inguinal herniorrhaphy: complications and recurrences. Sem Laparosc Surg 1994; 1: 128-140.

McKernan B. Prosthetic inguinal hernia repair using a laparoscopic extraperitoneal approach. Sem Laparosc Surg 1994; 1: 116-122.

Newman III L, et al. Is laparoscopic herniorrhaphy an effective alternative to open hernia repair? J Laparoendosc Surg 1993; 3: 121-128.

Nguyen NX, et al. Laparoscopic intraperitoneal onlay mesh inguinal hernia repair. Sem Laparosc Surg 1994; 1: 106-115.

Pendurthi TK. Laparoscopic bilateral inguinal hernia repair under local anesthesia. Surg Endosc 1995; 9: 197-199.

Phillips EH, et al. Incidence of complications following laparoscopic hernioplasty. Surg Endosc 1995; 9: 16-21.

Phillips EH, et al. Reasons for early recurrence following laparoscopic herniorrhaphy. Surg Endosc 1995; 9: 140-145.

Schultz LS, et al. Transabdominal preperitoneal approach. Sem Laparosc Surg 1994; 1: 98-105.

Zucker KA (ed.), Bailey RW, Reddick EJ (assoc. eds.). Surgical Laparoscopy Update. Quality Medical Publishing Inc. St. Louis, 1993: 377-393.

4

The Stomach

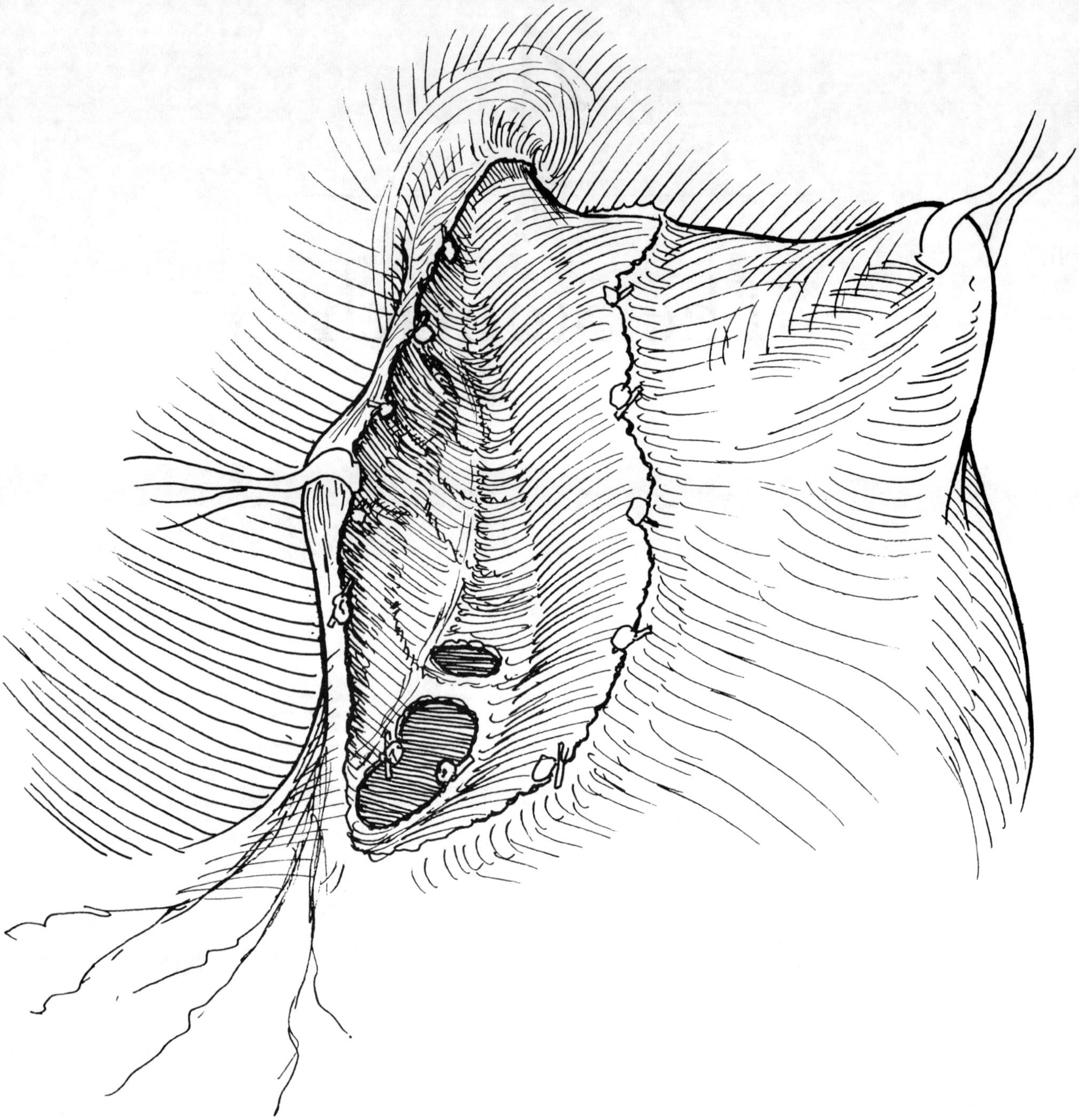

4

The Stomach

INTRODUCTION

Advances in medical management of gastroesophageal reflux disease and peptic ulcer disease have shifted treatment away from invasive surgical procedures and the associated morbidity. The advent of minimal access surgery has again made surgical options attractive alternatives for patients refractory to medical management and patients who are dependent on medication. Safe and effective laparoscopic surgery in the hard to reach area of the esophageal hiatus requires a solid three-dimensional understanding of the regional anatomy. The embryology of the foregut and diaphragm provides important insights and is a good starting point.

EMBRYOLOGY

As the cephalad and caudad portions of embryonic entoderm fold into tubular form, they are enclosed by a double layer of splanchnic mesoderm (Fig. 4.1). This median partition of primitive mesentery is divided into dorsal and ventral portions by the gut tube. The liver, biliary tree, and ventral pancreatic bud develop in the ventral part of the foregut mesentery. The portion of ventral mesentery between the gut and liver will become the gastrohepatic or lesser omentum. The ventral mesentery caudal to the bile duct regresses, leaving the free edge as the hepatoduodenal ligament. With regression of the ventral mesentery caudal to the umbilical vein, the remnant between the liver and the body wall is called the falciform ligament.

During the fifth week of gestation, the gastric portion of the gut tube begins to dilate and flatten from side to side. The esophageal segment of gut between the tra-

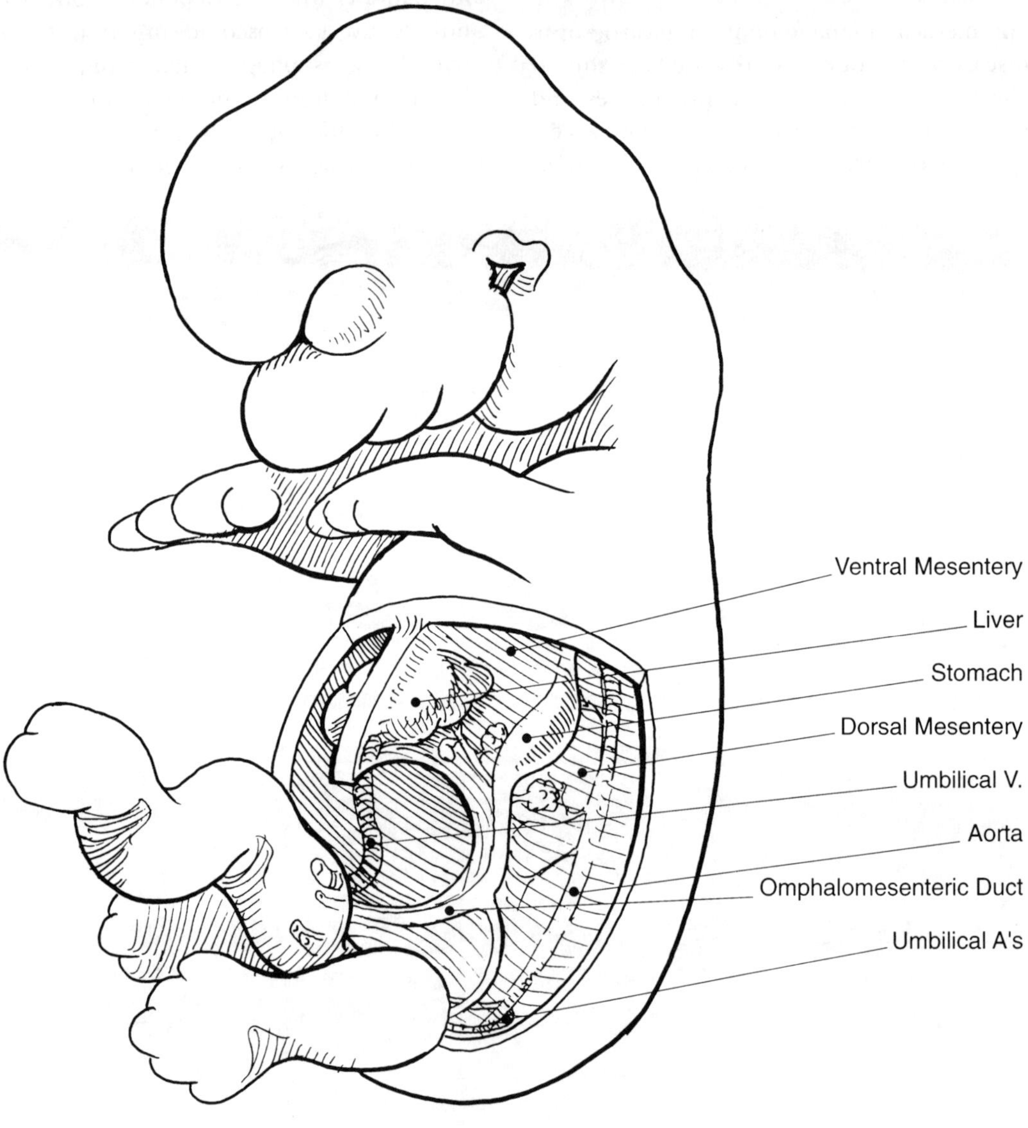

Fig. 4.1

cheal diverticulum and stomach progressively elongates to reach a mature proportion by the seventh week. The dorsal border of the stomach grows more rapidly than the ventral border, forming the greater curve. This border moves axially to the left (thought to do so by differential growth rather than by rotation). At the same time, the dorsal mesogastrium balloons to the left, forming the beginnings of the omental bursa and greater omentum (Fig. 4.2). The spleen develops in the left side of the dorsal mesogastrium in parallel with the stomach dilatation and shift and moves to the left with the expanding omental bursa. The inlet of the omental bursa is bounded ventrally by the hepatoduodenal ligament and dorsally by the inferior vena cava and body wall.

The proximal sac of the omental bursa adheres posteriorly and laterally to parietal peritoneum. The fused pancreatic buds in the posterior wall of the sac come to lie diagonally across aorta and left kidney. The tail of the pancreas lies close to the splenic hilum and the splenic vessels run along its cephalad border. The upper pole of the spleen is separated from the esophagogastric junction by a very short span of dorsal mesogastrium. As the omental sac and dorsal border of the spleen attach to the dorsal parietal peritoneum, the esophagosplenic segment of dorsal mesentery also fuses, fixing the fundus of the stomach posteriorly. The distal omental sac drapes over the rotating colon and the two layers of sac fuse forming the greater omentum lying across the transverse colon (Chapter 6).

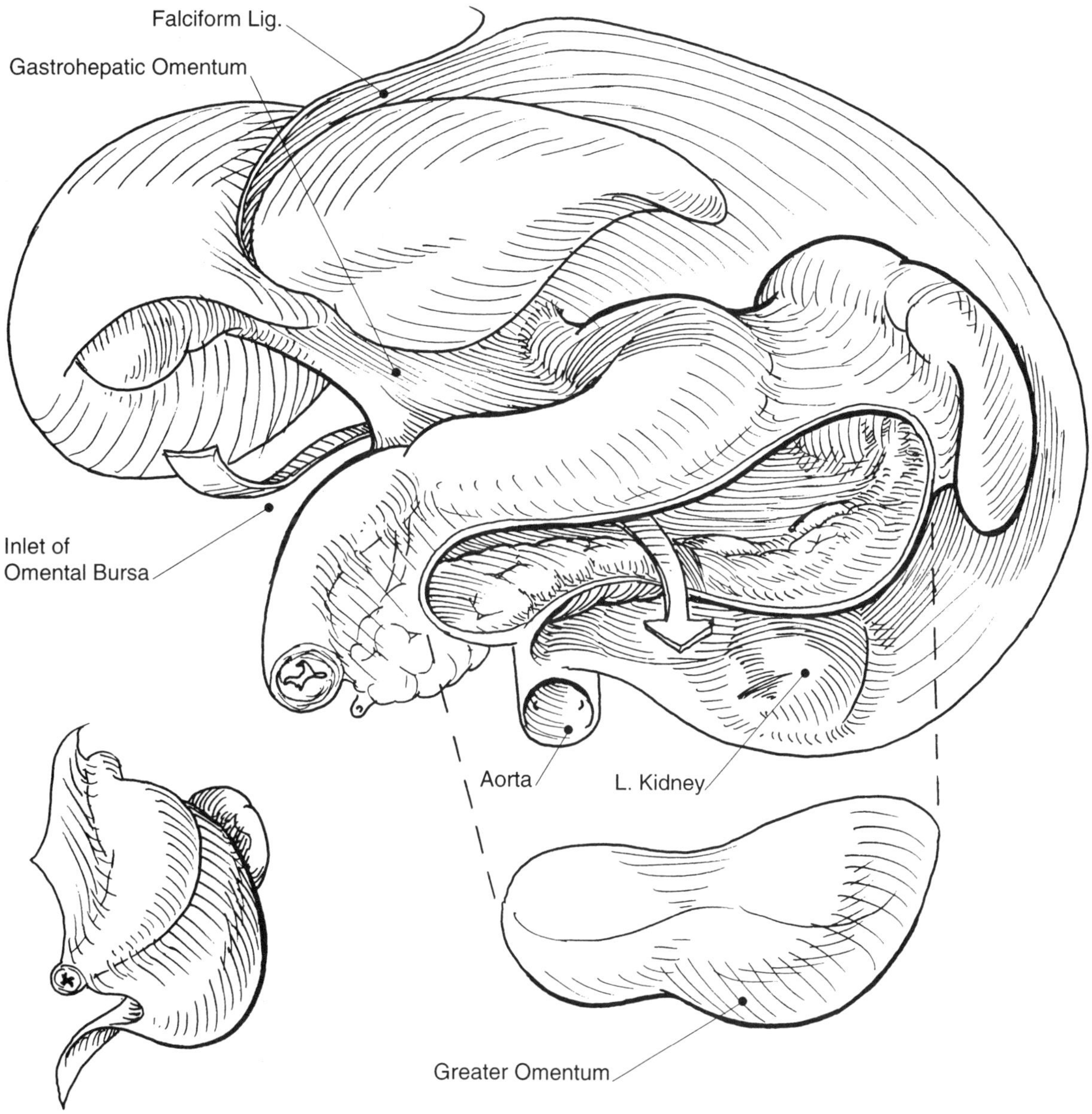

Fig. 4.2

While these changes are taking place from week four to week eight in the foregut and its mesenteries, the diaphragm is developing between the future chest and abdominal cavities. The first component of the diaphragm is the transverse septum, the area of mesenchyme between the growing pericardial cavity above and the open midgut below (Fig. 4.3). By nature of its origin, the septum is continuous with the area that will become mediastinum around the closing central midgut. Dorsolaterally, the communication between the pleural and peritoneal cavities is bridged by membranes which join the transverse septum and the mediastinum. Later expansion of the pleural cavities shifts an inner layer of muscle from the body wall onto the diaphragm, dorsal groups forming the crura and lateral groups forming the peripheral skirts of diaphragmatic muscle. Failure of these muscle groups to meet posteriorly results in the Bochdalek type of diaphragmatic hernia. Incomplete anterior muscular ingrowth may result in the parasternal hernia of Morgagni or eventration (absence of the muscular component leaving only a membranous diaphragm). A congenitally wide esophageal hiatus may result from delayed elongation of the esophagus, with the hiatus forming around the proximal gastric dilatation. The development of the liver in the caudal part of the septum transversarum, leaves the thin cranial part associated with the diaphragm.

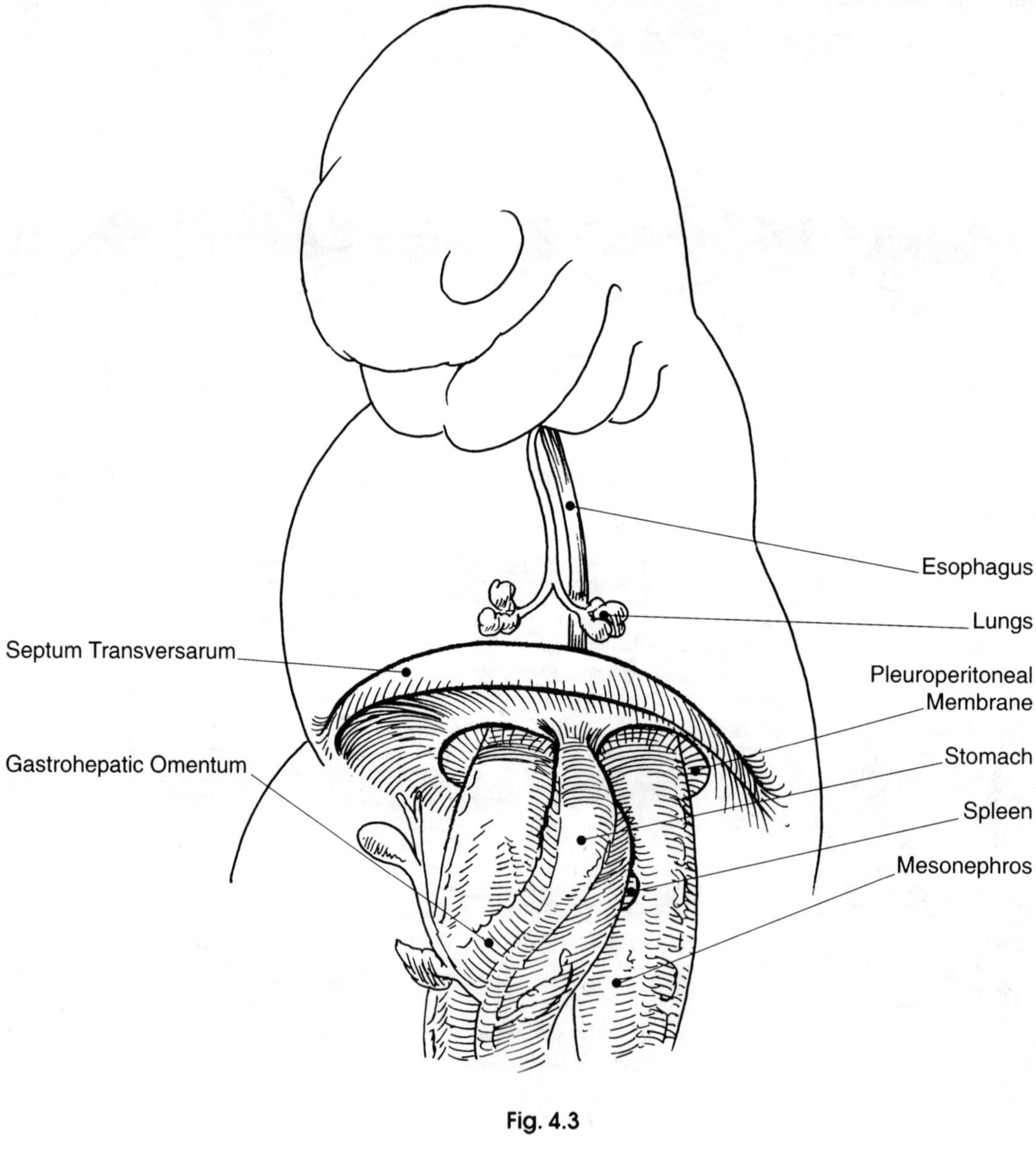

Fig. 4.3

ANATOMY

Reflections

The peritoneal reflections around the esophagogastric junction are a direct result of the fusions of the proximal omental bursa with the dorsal parietal peritoneum to the left of the midline (Fig. 4.4). The caudal reflection of peritoneum onto the esophagogastric junction contains the left gastric artery and the left gastric (coronary) vein. To the left of the esophagus, there is a short gastrophrenic segment of unfused dorsal mesogastrium. A posterior gastric artery from the splenic artery to the fundus of the stomach may sometimes be found in this membrane. The continuation of this fold becomes the gastrosplenic ligament containing the gastrosplenic (short gastric) vessels. The fused portion of proximal dorsal mesogastrium forms the posterior wall of the omental bursa and covers a small portion of diaphragm and the left adrenal gland (cross hatched area). To the right of the anterior esophagophrenic reflection, the remnant of ventral mesogastrium between stomach and liver is represented by the gastrohepatic (lesser) omentum. This membrane extends between the lesser curve of the stomach and the hilum of the liver (Chapter 2). The support for the structures tethered by these reflections is provided by areolar connections between the esophagus and the diaphragm, the true esophagophrenic membrane.

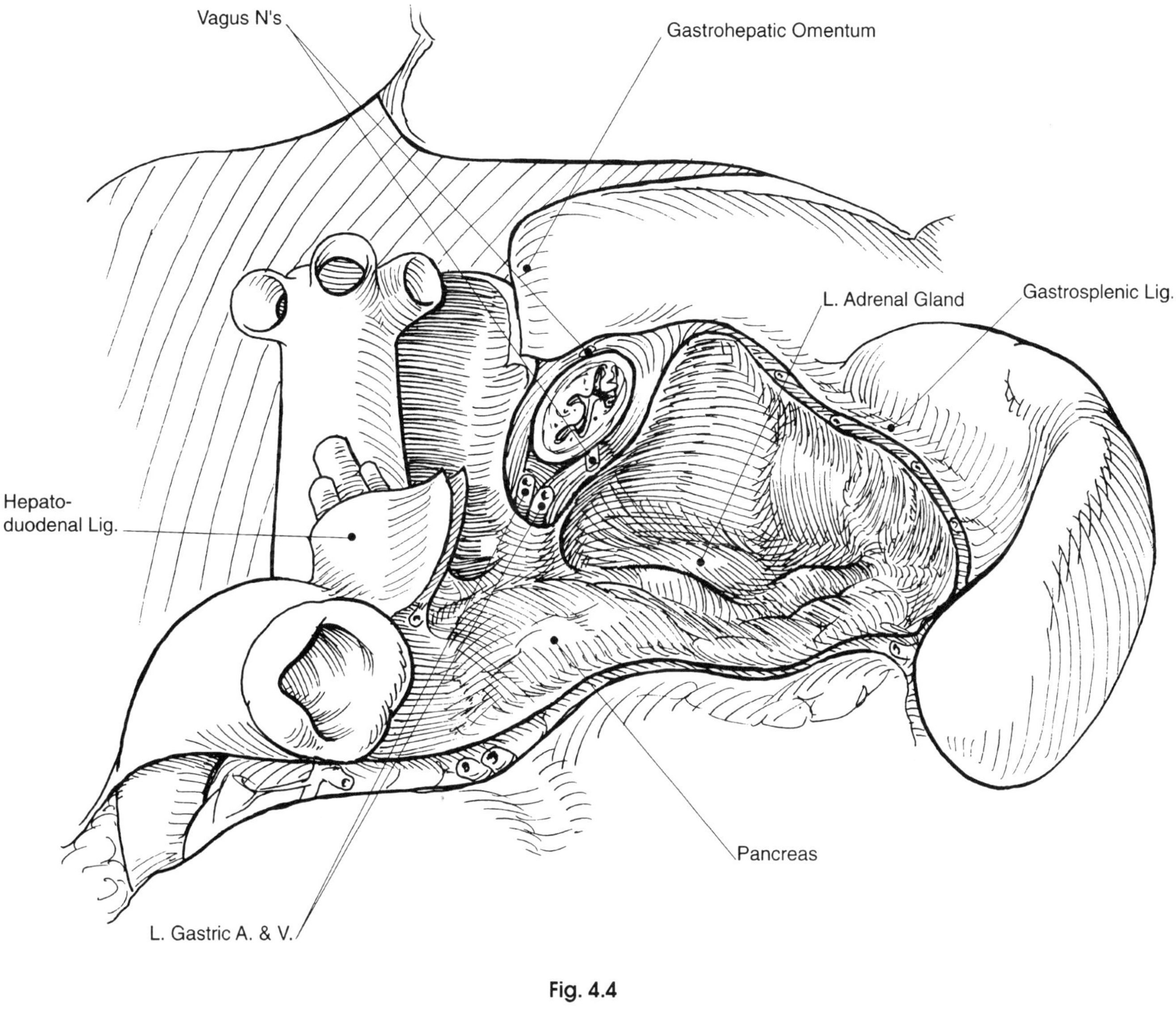

Fig. 4.4

Diaphragm

The mature diaphragm consists of paired muscular domes capped by a dense tri-lobed membrane (Fig. 4.5A). The diaphragmatic domes are divided posteriorly by the ridge of the vertebral column and the overlying aorta. The esophageal hiatus lies almost directly anterior to the aorta and behind the pericardial attachment to the central lobe of the membranous diaphragm. To the right of the esophageal hiatus, the inferior vena cava pierces the central lobe to enter the base of the right atrium of the heart.

The diaphragmatic attachments are visible from the caudal perspective (Fig. 4.5B). The rims of the domes attach to the costal cartilages around the inferior thoracic aperture. Posteriorly, the muscle fibers arise from lateral and medial fibrous lumbocostal arches spanning the quadratus lumborum and psoas muscles respectively. The "roots" of the diaphragm centrally, the crura, consist of muscular bundles arising from the lateral bodies of the first three lumbar vertebrae on the right and first two on the left.

The right and left muscular crura fan out toward the respective domes and mingle centrally over the aorta forming the aortic hiatus. The esophageal hiatus is surrounded by crural fibers derived primarily from the right side in about two thirds of individuals. The most frequent variation is a contribution to the right side of the hiatus from

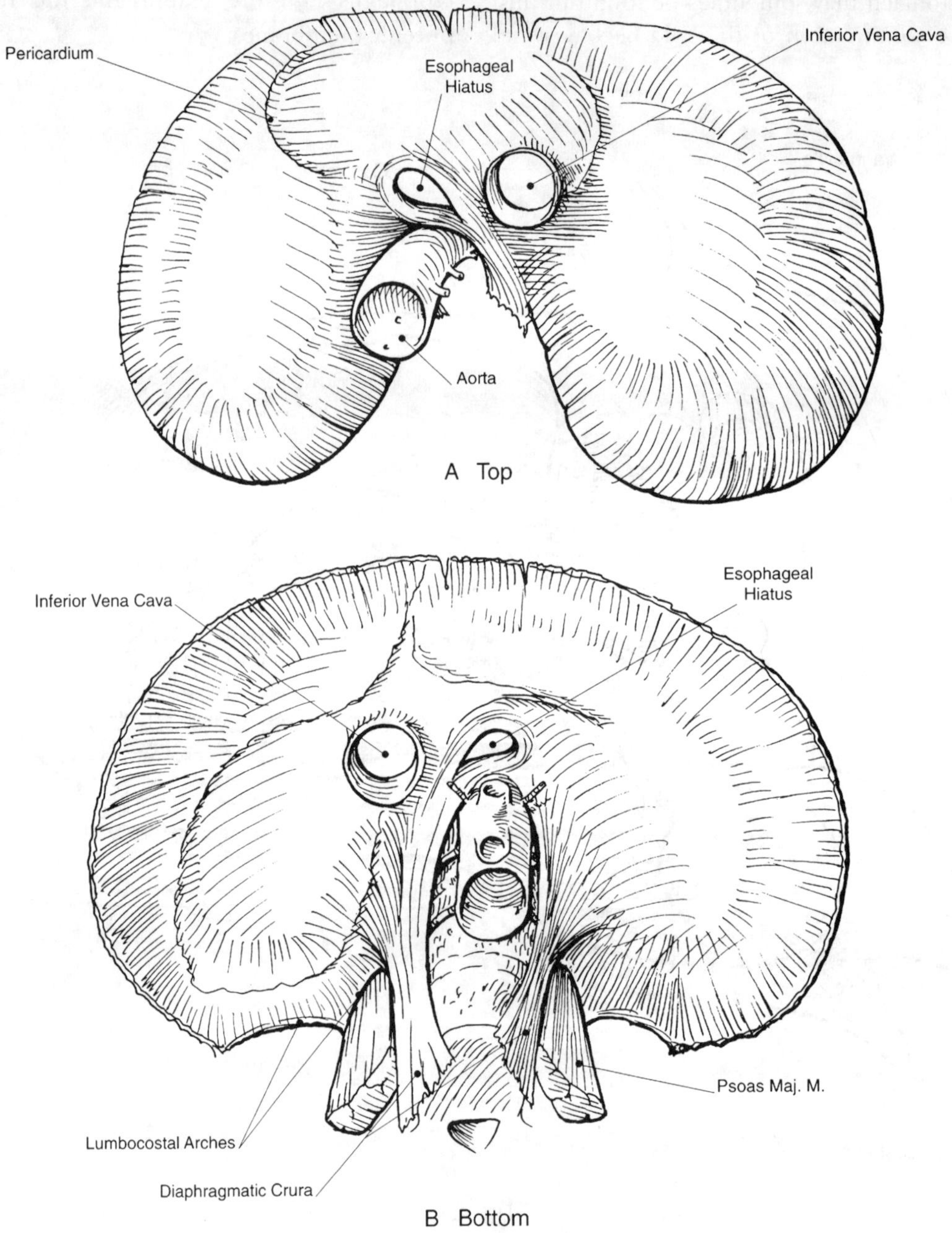

Fig. 4.5 A & B

the left crus. The esophagus is attached to the diaphragm by fibroelastic connective tissue continuous with the endothoracic and endoabdominal connective tissues and sandwiched between pleura above and peritoneum below. The combined connection is called the phrenoesophageal ligament. When the peritoneum is opened from below, the enclosed connective tissue is found to be soft, areolar, and easily separated by blunt dissection.

Seen from an anterior perspective, the diaphragm presents two domes, the right higher than the left, and a lower central cardiac plateau (Fig. 4.5C). The vena caval hiatus at the level of T9 is most cephalad of the three normal openings, the esophageal hiatus lies at the level of T10 and the aortic hiatus lies at the level of T12. The aortic hiatus is actually a muscular bridge between the right and left crura anterior to the aorta with a fibrous band (median arcuate ligament) spanning the inverted V of the arch. The central blood supply to the diaphragm seen from below (Fig. 4.5D) consists of variable inferior phrenic arteries, which may arise symmetrically from the beginning of the abdominal aorta below the hiatus or from a single trunk. They also commonly arise from a variety of neighboring vessels including the celiac trunk. The venous drainage from the left half of the diaphragm may pass anterior to the esophageal hiatus on its way to the inferior vena cava and may be injured in opening the esophagophrenic peritoneal reflection.

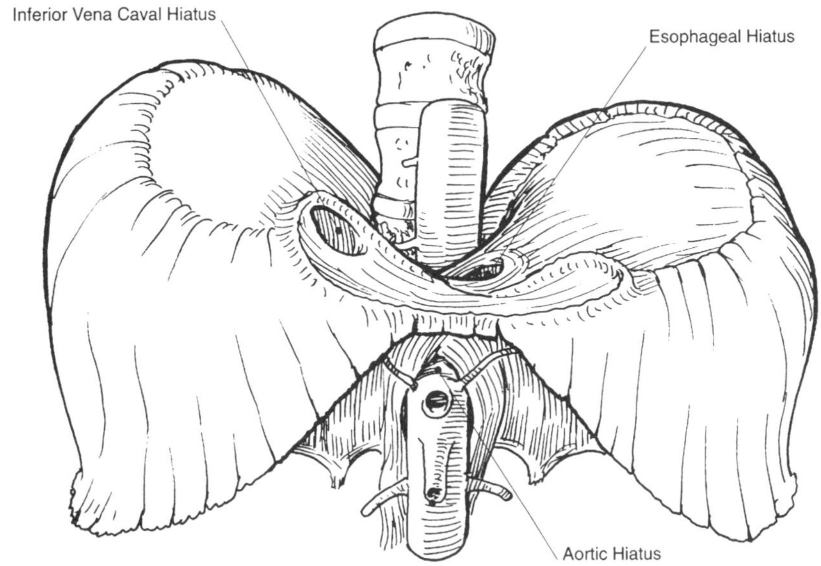

C Anterior

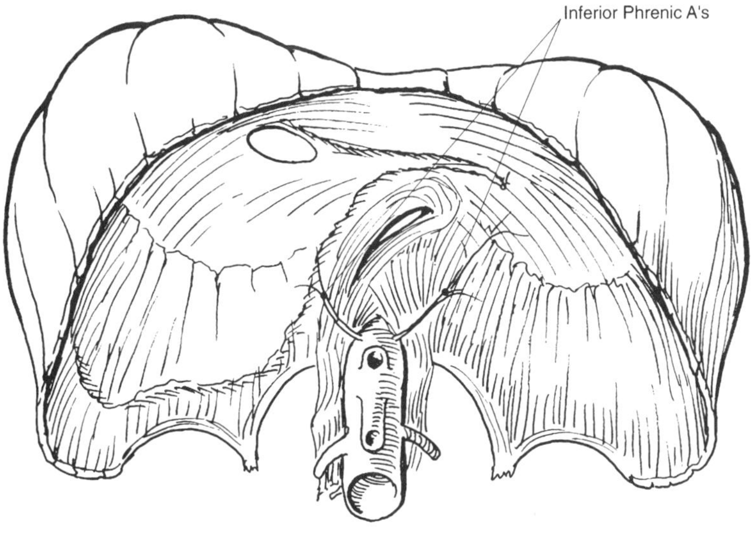

D Inferior

Fig. 4.5 C & D

Viewed posteriorly (Fig. 4.6), the distance between the esophageal and aortic hiatus can be seen. Small superior phrenic branches supply the cephalad surface of the diaphragm. The azygous and hemiazygous veins flank the aorta and the thoracic duct rises to the right of the aorta from the cisterna chyli. The lower mediastinum directly behind the limbs of the right crus is in close contact with the left pleura, posing the risk of pneumothorax when mobilizing the esophagus. Manipulation far down between the limbs of the right crus could potentially injure the underlying thoracic duct. Through this supporting structure, the esophagus passes from the thorax into the abdomen.

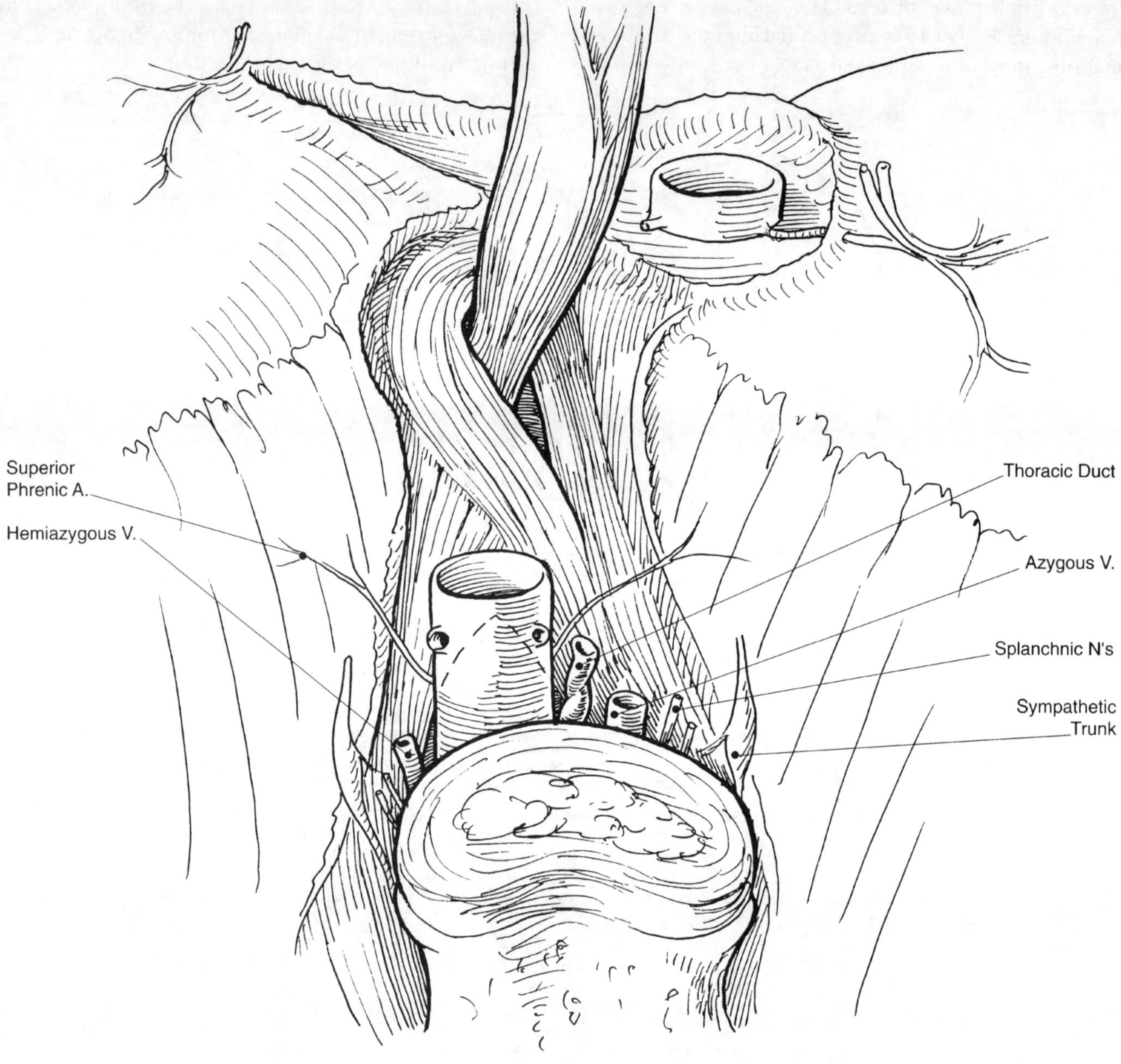

Fig. 4.6

Esophagus

To reach the esophageal hiatus, the esophagus descends through the posterior mediastinum to the right of the aortic arch and finally anterior to the descending thoracic aorta at the diaphragm (Fig. 4.7). It is bounded anteriorly by the trachea and then by the left atrium.

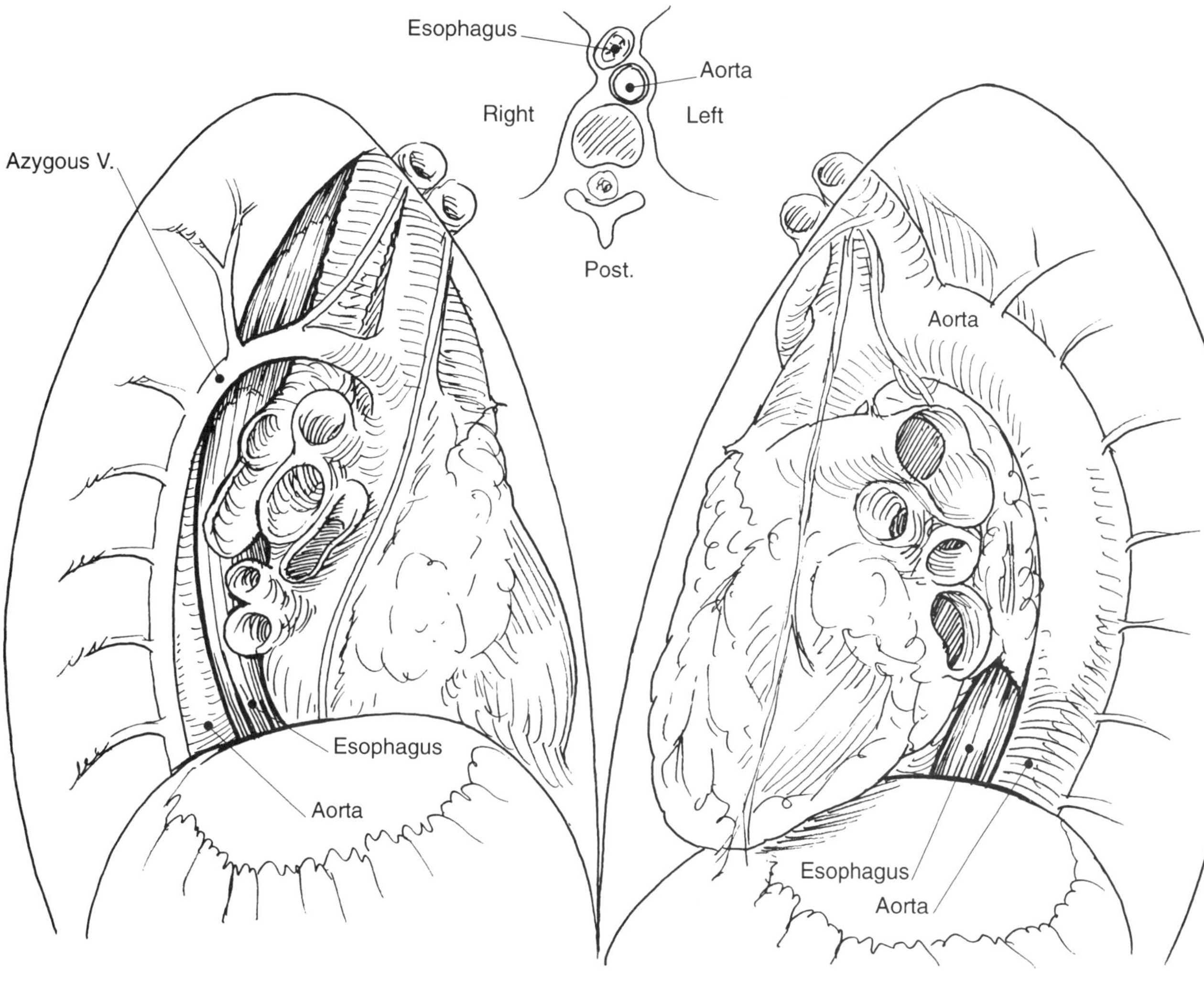

Fig. 4.7

The blood supply of the lower esophagus comes from the bronchial arteries, small aortic branches, and ascending branches of the inferior phrenic and left gastric arteries (Fig. 4.8). Venous drainage flows into the azygous and hemiazygous above the diaphragm and into the portal vein via the left and right gastric veins below the diaphragm. The venous plexus around the esophagogastric junction connects the portal with the systemic circulation and becomes dilated in the presence of portal hypertension.

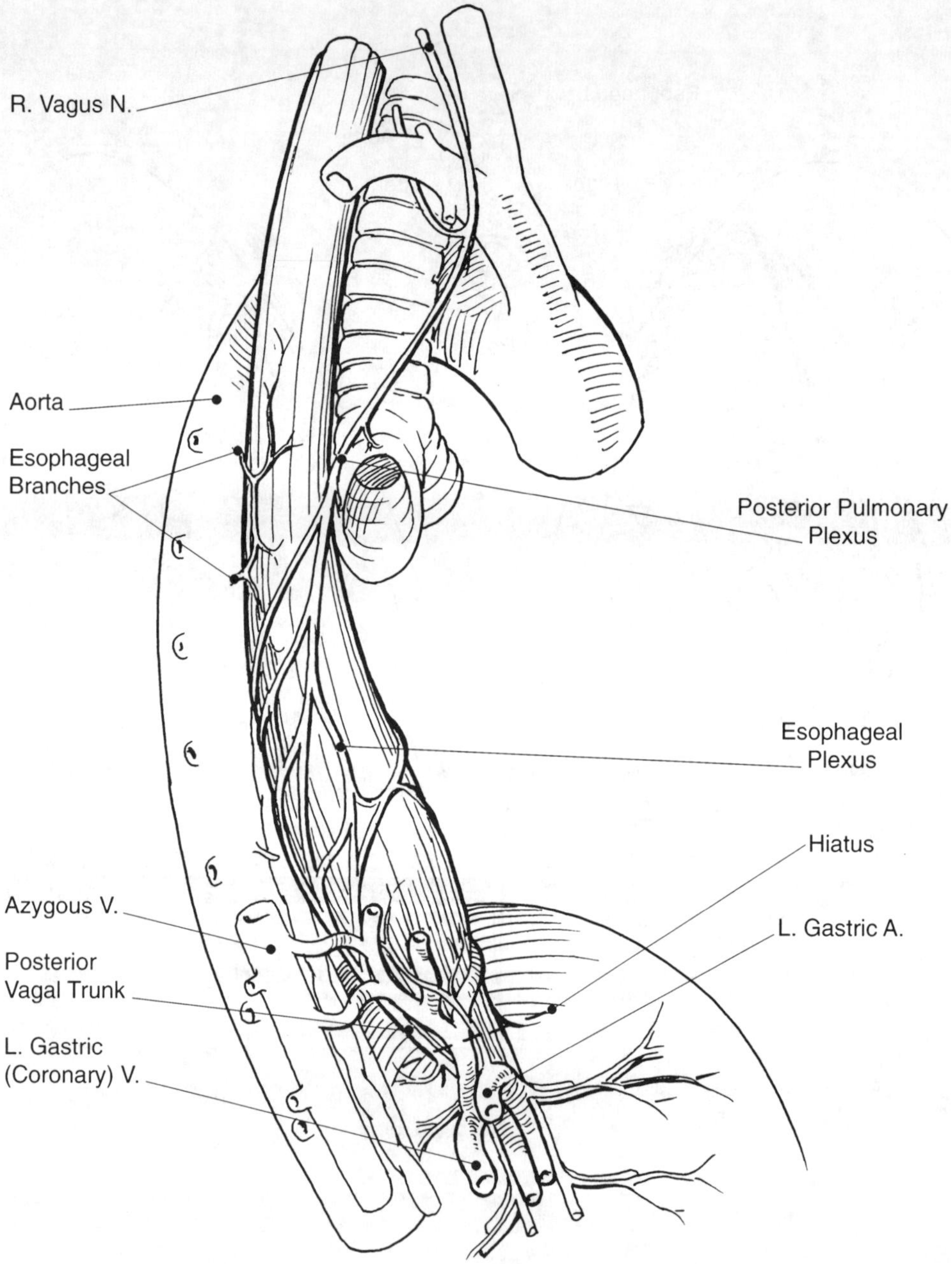

Fig. 4.8

The right and left vagus nerves divide into multiple branches behind the right and left mainstem bronchi forming posterior pulmonary plexuses. Continuing branches spread on the surface of the esophagus to form the esophageal plexus. After interconnecting, most of the esophageal plexus branches reconstitute above the esophageal hiatus forming an anterior trunk containing predominantly left sided fibers and a posterior trunk containing mostly fibers from the right vagus. The small branches that were not included in the fusion presumably reach the stomach by alternate routes that are not completely mapped at this time.

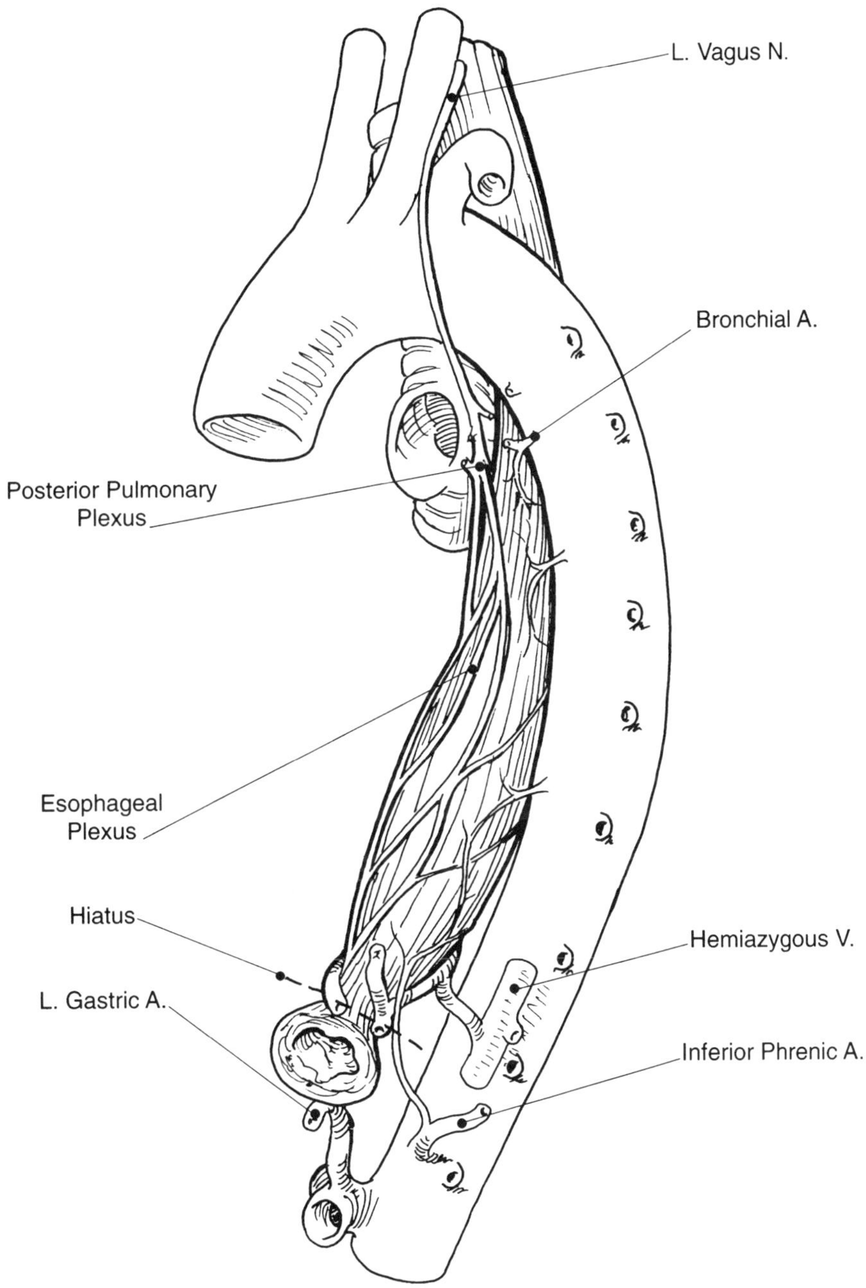

Fig. 4.8

From a caudal perspective (Fig. 4.9), the intra-abdominal esophagus occupies a central location in the body, lying immediately anterior to the aorta.

Because of the long rise of the crura from their lumbar origins, the esophagogastric junction is separated from the terminal intrathoracic aorta behind it by a

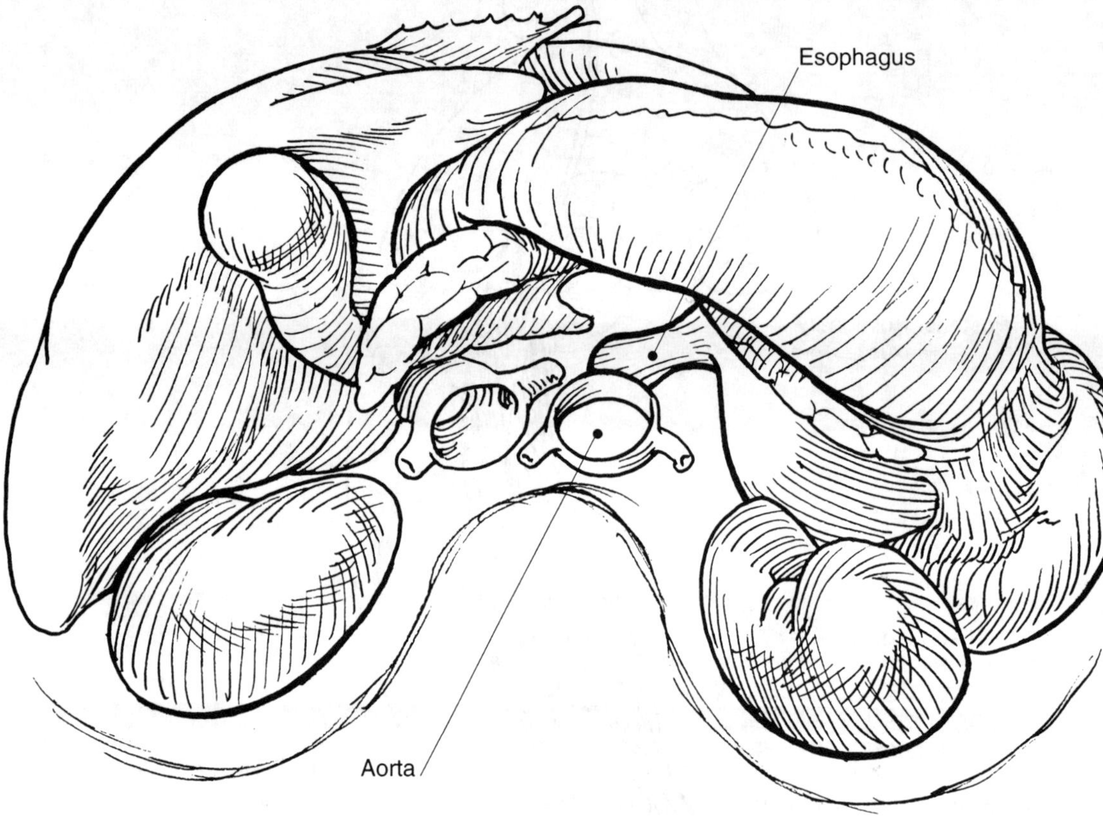

Fig. 4.9

sheet of crural fibers (Fig. 4.10). Dissection of the limbs of the right crus opens the lower posterior mediastinum. If the thin layer of mediastinal pleura on either side of the esophagus and aorta is violated a pneumothorax may result and compromise ventilation.

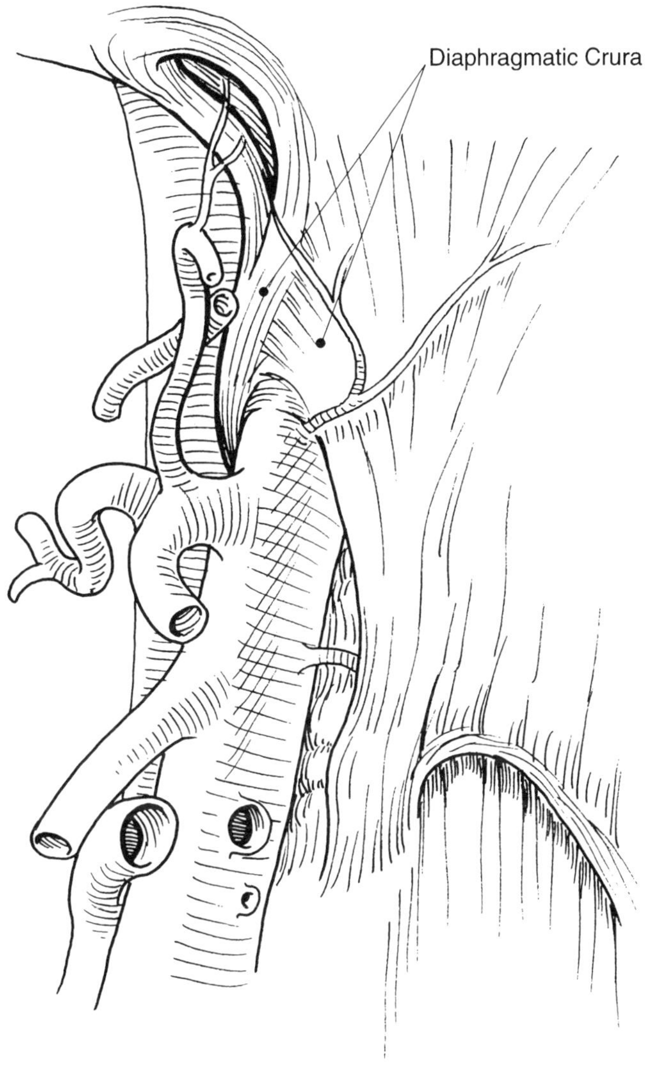

Fig. 4.10

Intra-abdominal Vagus Nerves

At the esophageal hiatus two major vagal trunks (Fig. 4.11) are most commonly found (88%). The anterior vagus gives off a hepatic branch which runs in the gastrohepatic omentum to the hilus of the liver. The posterior vagus gives off a celiac branch which runs along the left gastric artery to the celiac plexus at the base of the celiac trunk. Fibers not included in the vagal trunks may reach the stomach through the gastrophrenic ligament,

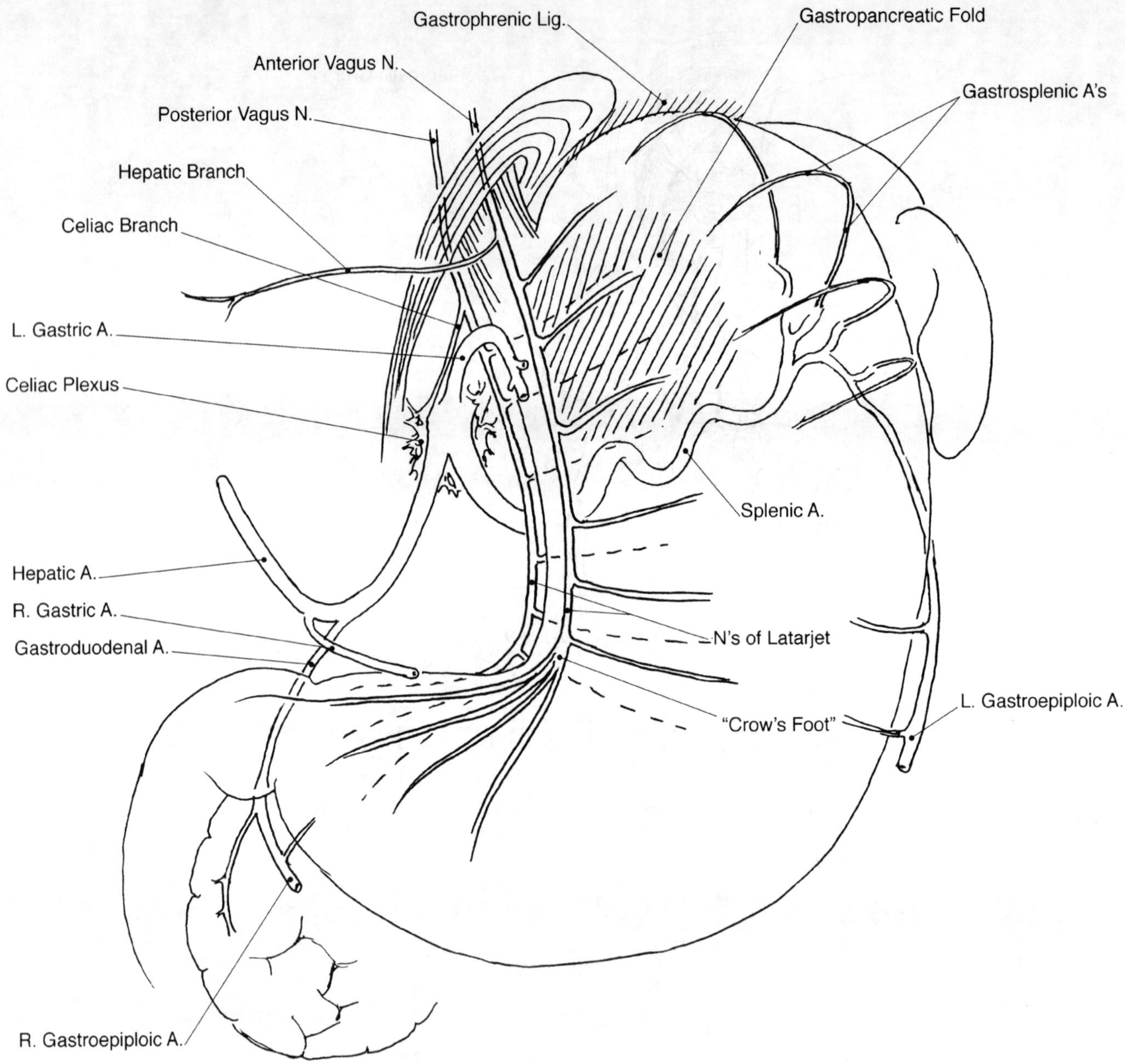

Fig. 4.11

gastropancreatic fold and along vascular pathways via the celiac trunk. When multiple nerve branches are found, they are either early bifurcation into hepatic and celiac divisions and tributaries (Fig. 4.12A, B or late fusion of esophageal plexus strands (Fig. 4.12C). The trunks are most often (80%) to the right of midline and

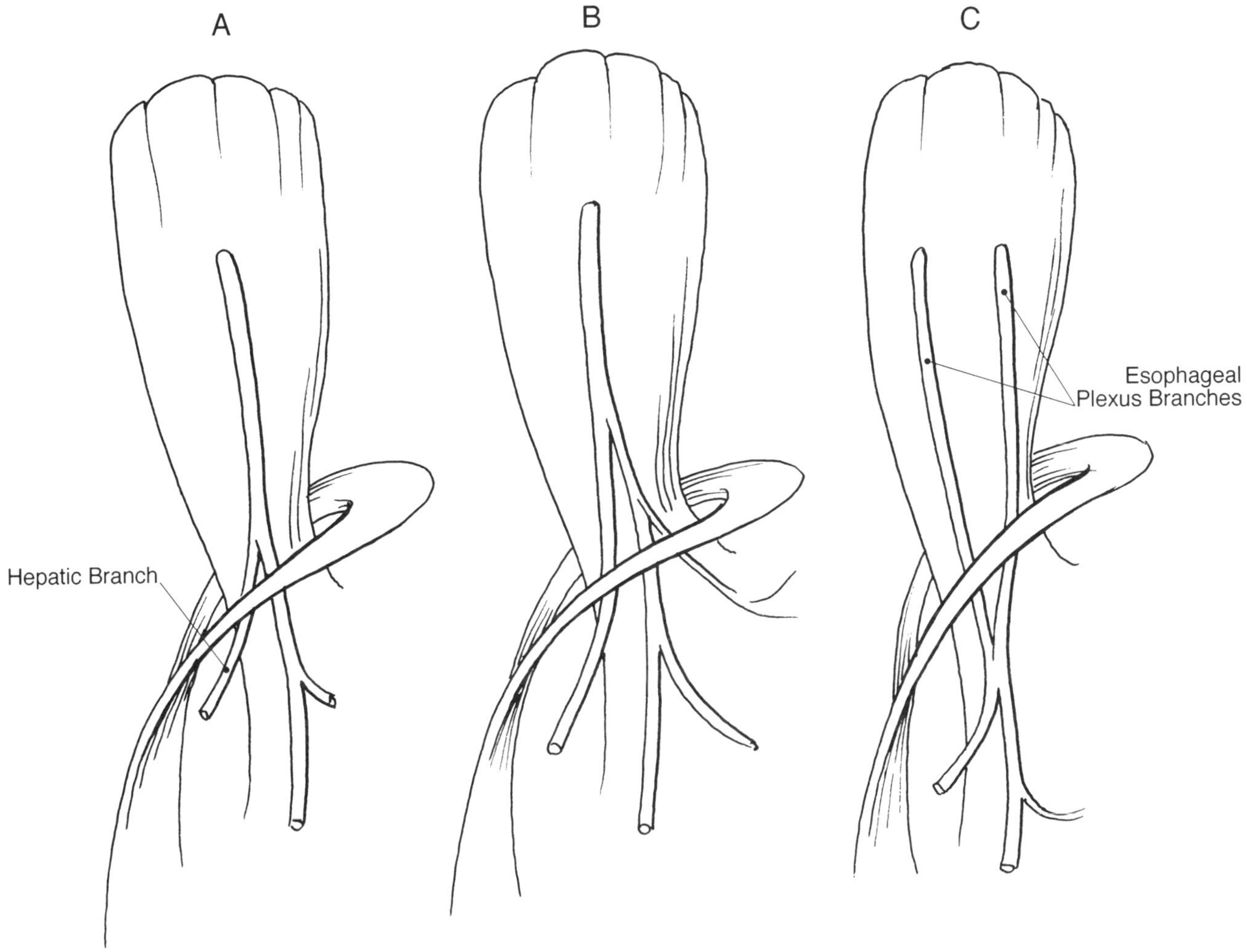

Fig. 4.12

the posterior trunk is more widely separated from the esophagus than the anterior trunk (Fig. 4.13).

The anterior vagal trunk is most commonly (96%) a single nerve (of Latarjet) on the anterior lesser curva-

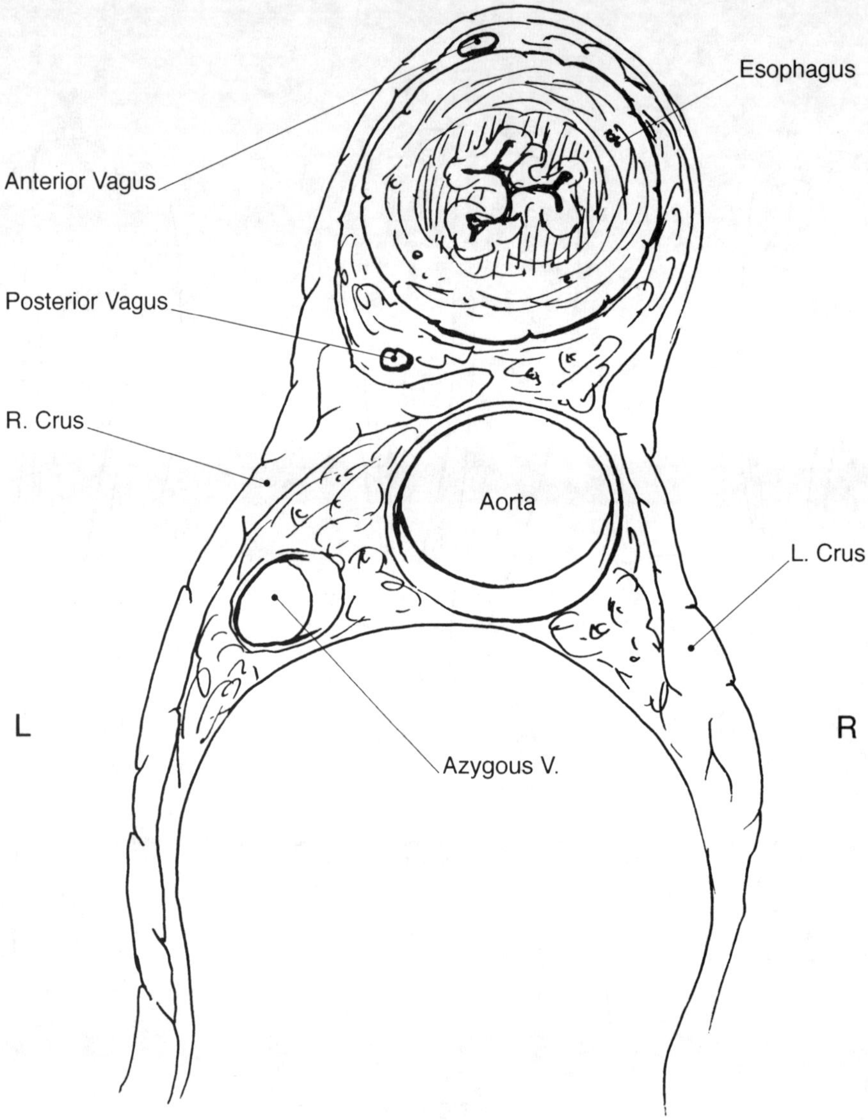

Fig. 4.13

ture of the stomach (Fig. 4.14A). The hepatic branch may be multiple and commonly gives rise to a pyloric twig. In the absence of a dominant anterior trunk (Fig. 4.14B), the gastric branches arise from the hepatic division. The number of gastric branches vary between 2 and 12 with an average of 6. The anterior trunk terminates in pyloric branches, which have an inhibitory effect on the tonic contraction of the pyloric sphincter and allow gastric emptying.

The celiac branch of the posterior vagus nerve is usually single and runs with or near the left gastric artery to reach the celiac plexus around the celiac trunk (Fig. 4.14C). A dominant posterior nerve is also the common (82%) pattern, with gastric branches arising from the celiac (Fig. 4.14D) in the minority of individuals. The posterior vagal branches do not reach the pylorus but terminate in branches to the antral musculature (posterior "crow's foot" area).

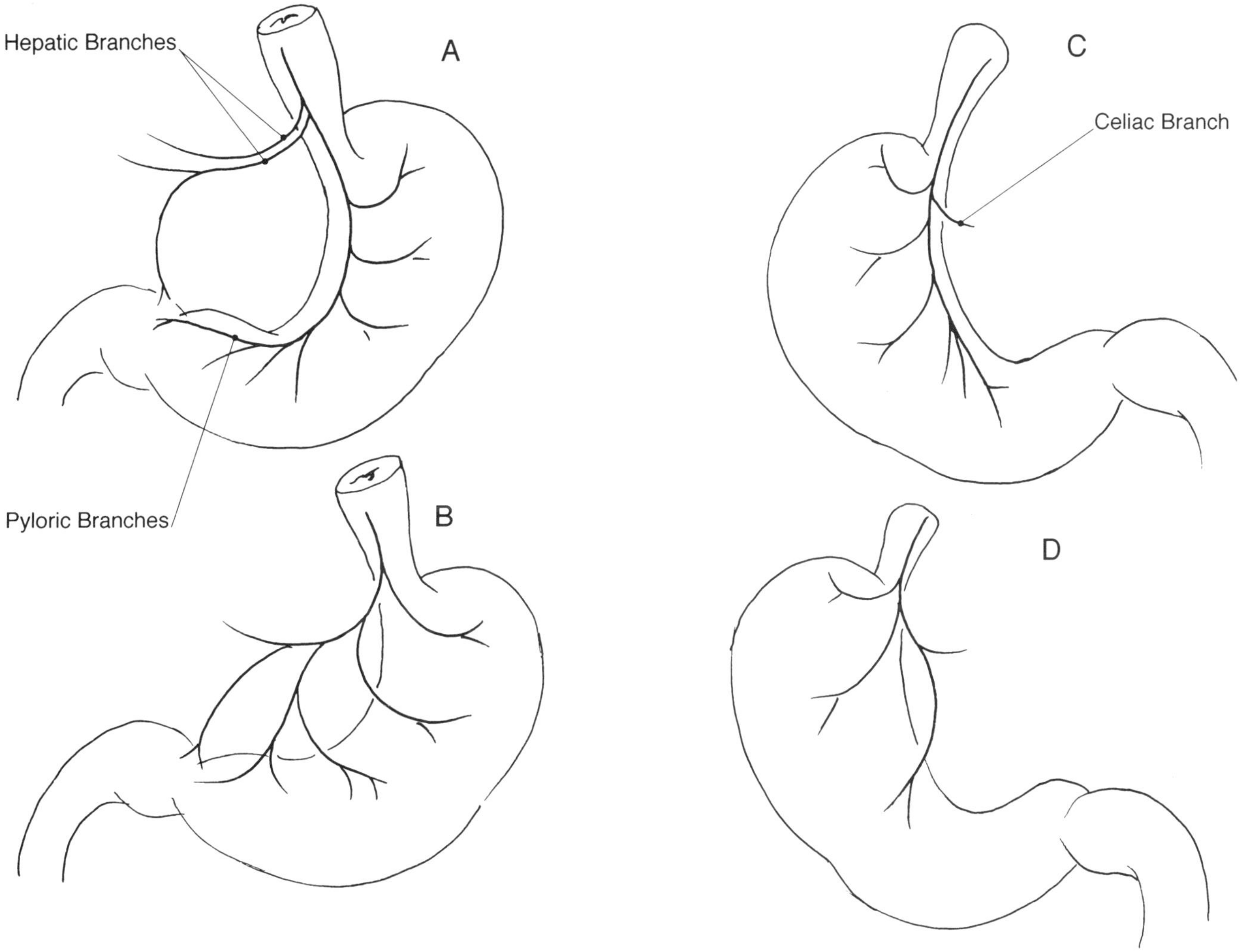

Fig. 4.14

Intra-abdominal Esophagogastric Vessels

The left gastric artery most often (86%) arises from the celiac trunk between the aorta and the bifurcation into hepatic and splenic arteries (Fig. 4.15A). A small percent of individuals have a gastrosplenic trunk (Fig. 4.15B) or an independent aortic origin of the left gastric artery (Fig. 4.15C). Other origins (celiaco-mesenteric trunk, hepatic) are rare.

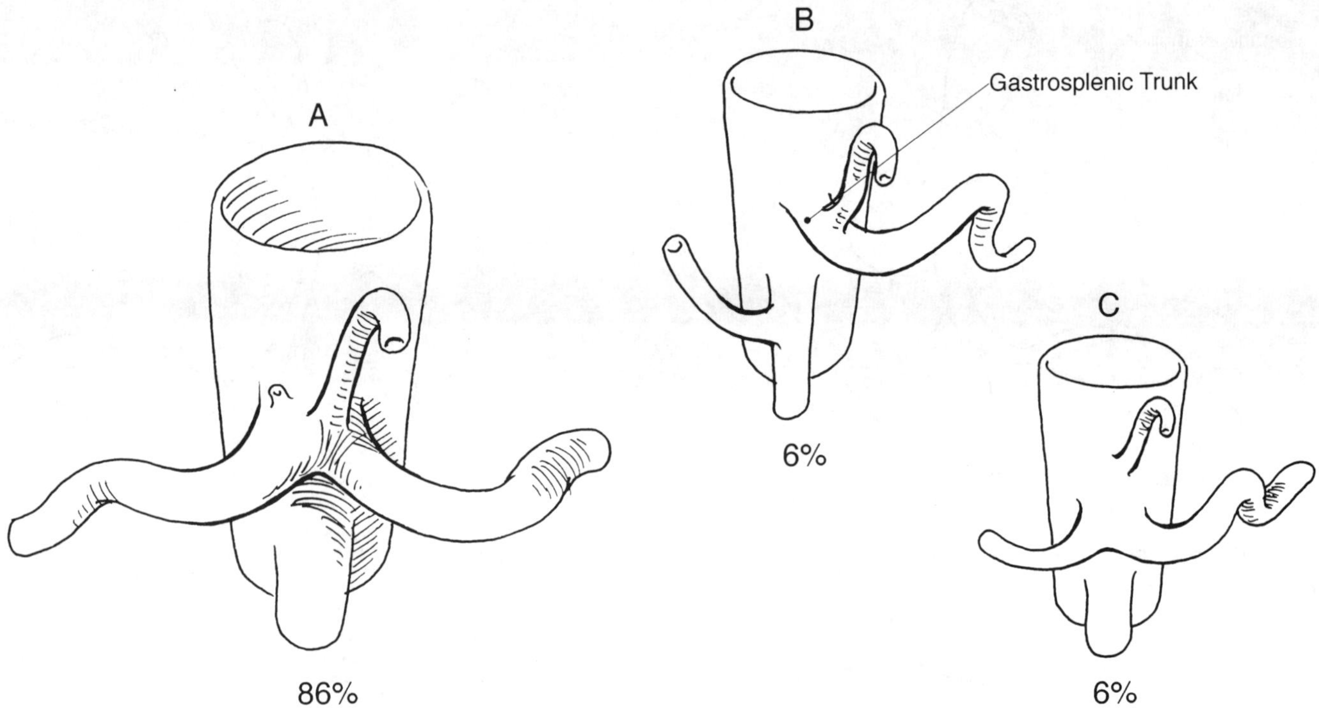

Fig. 4.15

The left gastric artery rises vertically beneath the posterior peritoneum of the lesser sac (Fig. 4.16) to reach the proximal lesser curve of the stomach. There it turns to run between the nerves of Latarjet. An ascending esophageal branch arises from the arch of the left gastric artery and may be joined by branches from the inferior phrenic arteries. The inferior phrenics themselves may arise from the celiac trunk. The available space behind the proximal stomach is limited by the origin of the left gastric artery and the tethering effect of the posterior vagus and its celiac branch. The posterior position of the posterior vagus and the separation from the esophageal wall makes for a wider passage behind the esophagus when the nerve is left posterior as opposed to including it with the esophagus (inset).

A significant number of individuals (30%) have an aberrant left hepatic artery which invariably arises from the left gastric artery (Fig. 4.17). The aberrant left hepatic runs within the proximal gastrohepatic omentum and may be injured when this structure is opened.

The cardia of the stomach receives a branch of the splenic artery in about a third of individuals. This posterior gastric artery lies beneath the fusion fascia in the high posterior wall of the lesser sac. This vessel may be injured when the portion of cardia between the esophagus and the gastrosplenic vessels is mobilized.

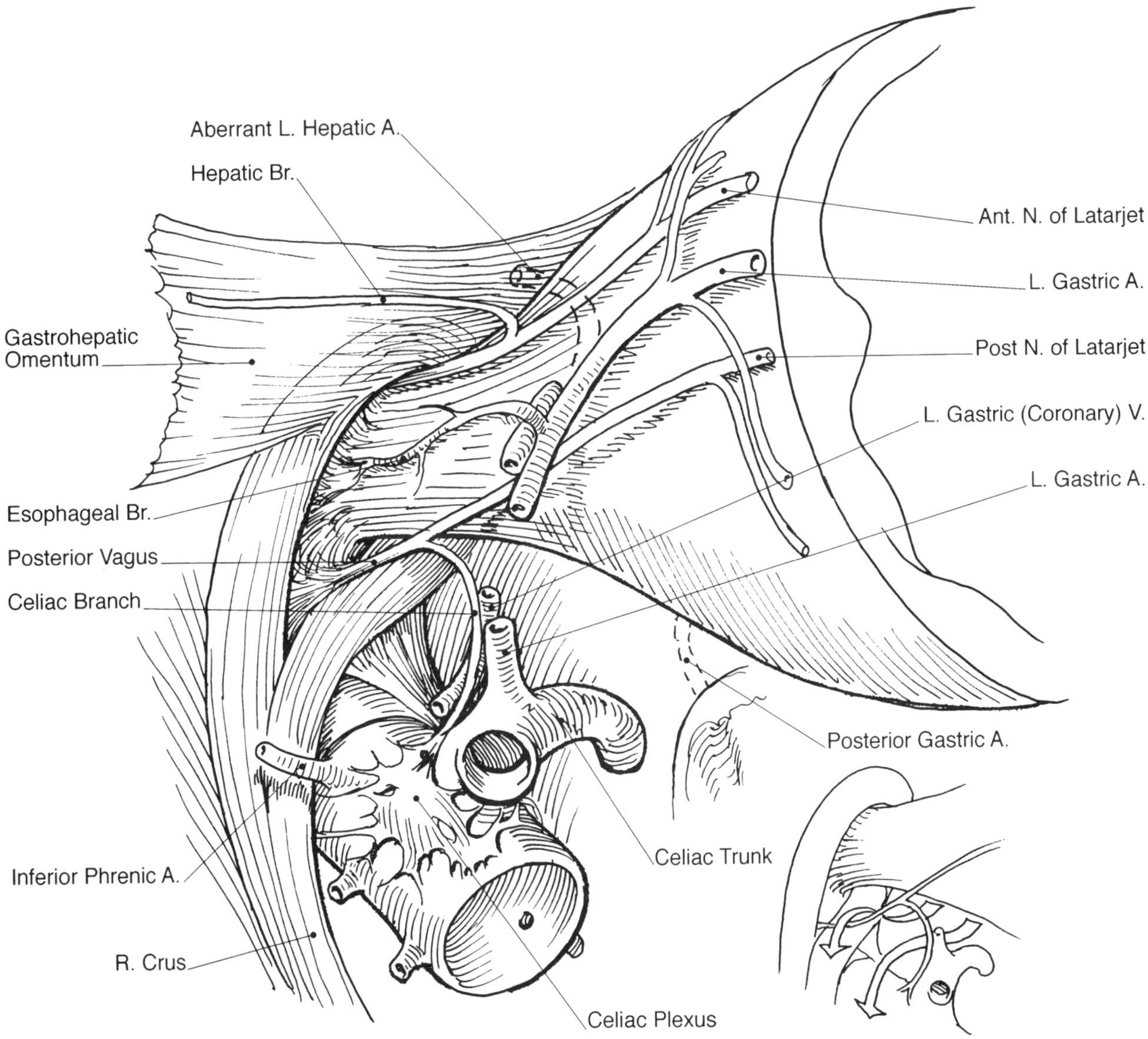

Fig. 4.16

The esophageal plexus of veins drains into the left gastric vein and across the cardia to the short gastric veins (Fig. 4.18). The left gastric vein crosses the retroperitoneum of the lesser sac to join the beginning of the portal vein. The right gastric vein from the distal lesser curve drains into the portal vein close to the entry of the left gastric forming a lesser curve circuit. The inferior phrenic vein may cross from left to right near the anterior lip of the esophageal hiatus.

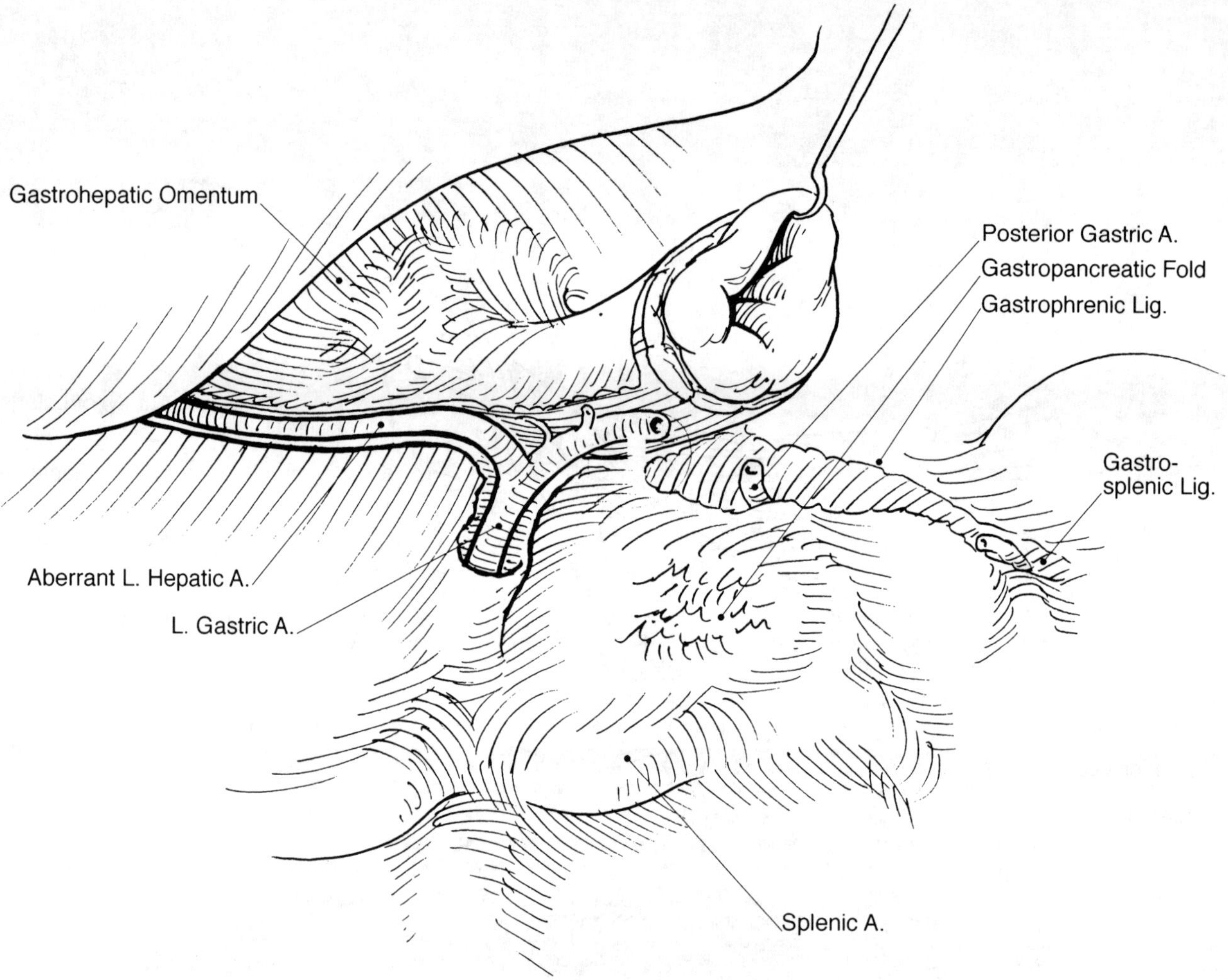

Fig. 4.17

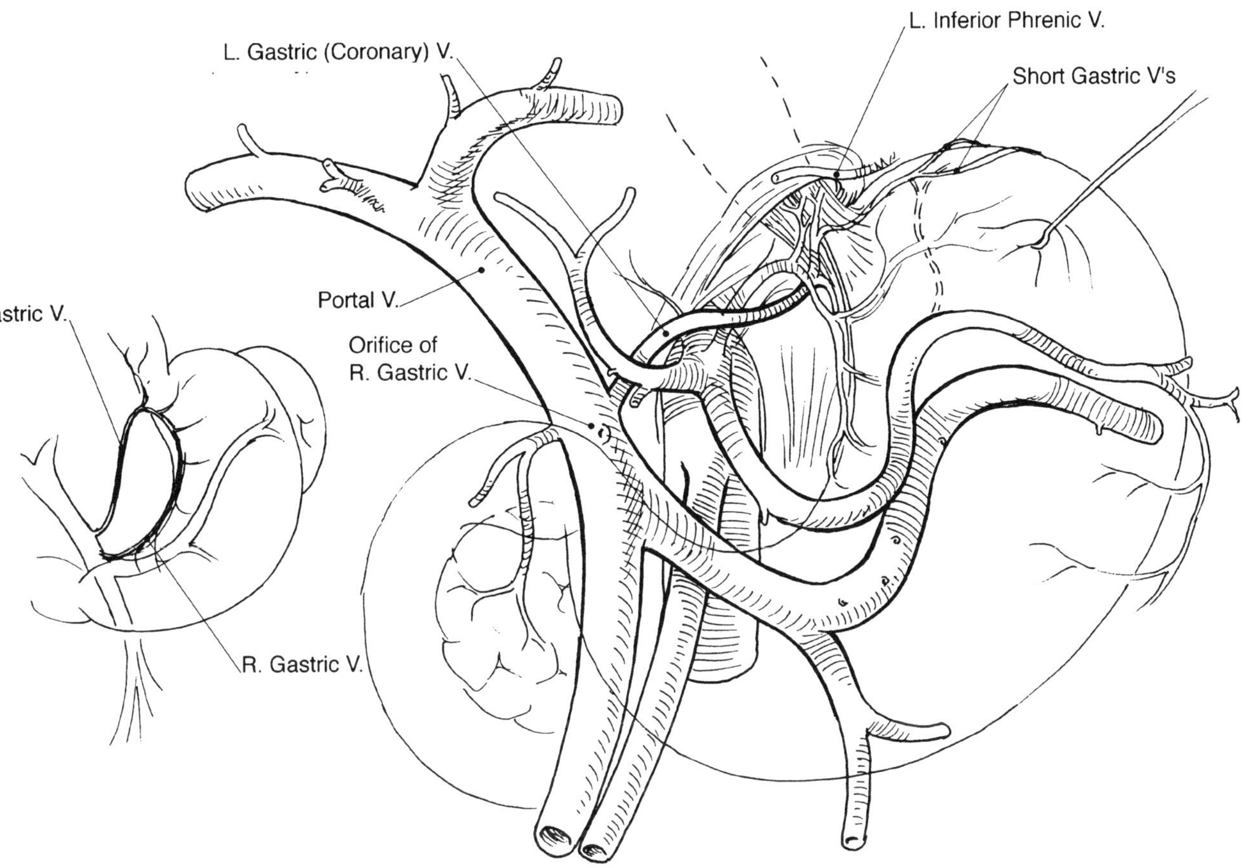
L. Gastric (Coronary) V.
L. Inferior Phrenic V.
Short Gastric V's
Portal V.
L. Gastric V.
Orifice of
R. Gastric V.
R. Gastric V.

Fig. 4.18

ANTIREFLUX SURGERY

Indications

The symptoms of mild gastroesophageal reflux disease are managed medically with antacids, weight loss, elevation of the head of the bed, cessation of smoking, avoidance of drugs that decrease lower esophageal sphincter pressure and modification of dietary habits (avoid large and late meals). More severe reflux disease may require H_2 blockers and more intensive medical management. A small subset of patients who do not respond to medical therapy or are dependent on medication because of relapsing symptoms benefit from a surgical antireflux procedure. Success depends as much on patient selection as on the technique.

Exposure of the lower esophagus to acid reflux from the stomach is mediated by three things. The competence of the lower esophageal sphincter (mediated by resting tone, the valve created by the intact esophagogastric angle, and fixation at the hiatus where it is subject to abdominal pressure) normally resists acid reflux while appropriate physiological relaxation allows passage of food. Esophageal peristalsis, the second factor, normally strips acid reflux back into the stomach, minimizing contact time with the esophageal mucosa. The third factor, normal function (emptying and acid production) of the stomach determines the potential for acid reflux and the gastric pressure behind it. Over half of patients with increased esophageal acid exposure have a defective lower esophageal sphincter mechanism. About a third of patients have delayed gastric emptying or aerophagia forcing acid up into the esophagus past a normal lower esophageal sphincter. Gastric emptying is evaluated along with reflux during barium radiographic study. Only a small percent of patients have abnormally high acid production.

Only the patients with reflux associated with a proven lower esophageal dysfunction are candidates for antireflux surgery. Patients with esophageal motility problems do not have the propulsive power to overcome the pressure of a fundoplication superimposed on a normal lower esophageal sphincter and develop symptoms of esophageal obstruction. Primary esophageal motility problems should be differentiated from secondary motility impairment from the reflux itself. For patients with an abnormal lower esophageal sphincter and motility problems, a partial fundoplication has been advocated. Those patients with gastric emptying problems are prone to the gas bloat syndrome with a fundoplication and need the primary pathology (usually pyloric outlet obstruction from peptic ulcer disease) taken care of. The small subset (5%) of patients with both an incompetent lower esophageal sphincter and hyperacidity are candidates for a fundoplication combined with a highly selective vagotomy.

Failure to control reflux over long periods can lead to esophagitis, stricture, ulceration, bleeding, and Barrett's esophagus. The latter, extension of the squamo-columnar junction more than 2 cm above the esophagogastric junction, is associated with ulceration, stricture, and a dramatically increased risk of cancer. Young patients with significant reflux are more prone to develop complications and surgical correction of reflux should be considered earlier.

Those who will benefit from surgery are patients who do not respond to an adequate (8–12 wk) course of intensive acid suppression, who have severe (above the 95th percentile) increased esophageal acid exposure on 24-hour esophageal pH monitoring (pH less than 4 for more than 4 1/2 hr, episodes longer than 19.8 min at a time), who have a defective (<6 mm Hg) lower esophageal sphincter mechanism by manometry, and have adequate esophageal motor function. Patients who are medication dependent, who have severe lifestyle and dietary restrictions, and patients whose symptoms are primarily respiratory (asthma and pneumonia from aspiration) are also good candidates for surgery. These patients will benefit from having surgery early, before complications occur.

In addition to patients with general systemic contraindications to laparoscopic surgery (COPD, severe bleeding disorders, portal hypertension etc.) patients who have had prior upper abdominal surgery or who have a shortened esophagus are poor candidates for an abdominal laparoscopic approach. A hiatus hernia that does not reduce with the patient in the upright position during barium swallow may indicate a shortened esophagus. In clinical practice, an adequate length of esophagus can almost always be mobilized for fundoplication. In cases of true short esophagus, the hiatus can be sutured around the rim of the wrap with no compromise in results, or a gastroplasty may be performed to increase esophageal length.

Paraesophageal hiatus hernia is a clear indication for surgical treatment. In addition to reflux associated problems, patients with paraesophageal hiatus hernia are subject to a high risk of life threatening complications like incarceration, torsion, strangulation and perforation. The surgical dissection is much more difficult and dangerous with a higher risk of esophageal perforation. Surgery for paraesophageal hiatus hernia should only be performed by experienced (30 or more routine reflux procedures) laparoscopic surgeons. An antireflux procedure should be added to all cases to prevent postoperative reflux. The hernia sac should be resected and a gastropexy preformed to help prevent recurrence. The gastropexy consists of suturing the greater curvature to the posterior rectus sheath.

The objectives of fundoplication are to restore the competence of the lower esophageal sphincter (increased pressure and increased length of the high pressure zone, keeping two centimeters of lower esophagus in the abdomen without tension, and recreation of the esophagogastric angle) while allowing free antegrade passage of food. The latter is accomplished by keeping the wrap loose or "floppy" and short (2 cm). In the uncomplicated patient meeting these criteria, these goals are reliably achieved (80–90% effectiveness, minimal morbidity) with laparoscopic Nissen fundoplication.

Position and Setup

For work at the esophagogastric junction, the patient is placed in the spread leg position with the thighs slightly flexed at the hips and the knees slightly bent to achieve a semisitting position when the table is tilted in reverse Trendelenburg (Fig. 4.19). The camera operator stands to the patient's right, the assistant to the left and

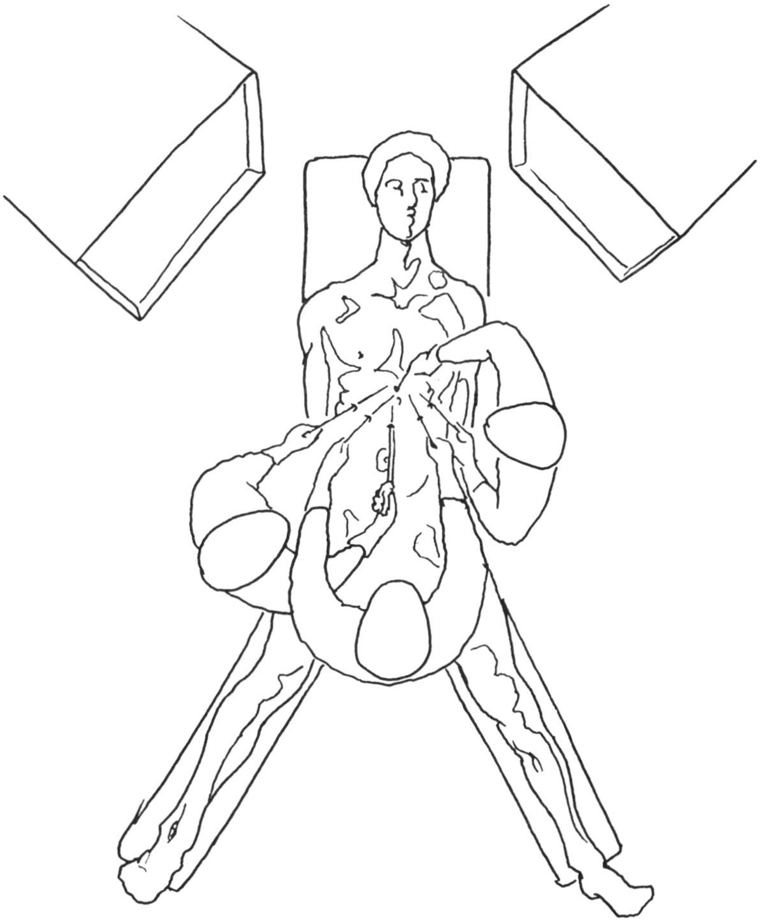

Fig. 4.19

the surgeon between the legs. Gastric and bladder decompression is followed by standard establishment of pneumoperitoneum.

After insufflation, the 10- or 11-mm camera port is placed midway between xiphoid and umbilicus to allow adequate reach to the deep central location of the esophagogastric junction (Fig. 4.20). A 30-degree telescope angled downward offers optimal visualization. The patient is placed in 30–40 degrees of reverse Trendelenburg position. Four to five additional ports are placed. The critical positions are a right sided port for liver retraction, a subxiphoid port (an alternate port for the surgeon's left hand), a left-sided port for gastric and esophageal retraction and two para-rectus ports for dissecting and suturing.

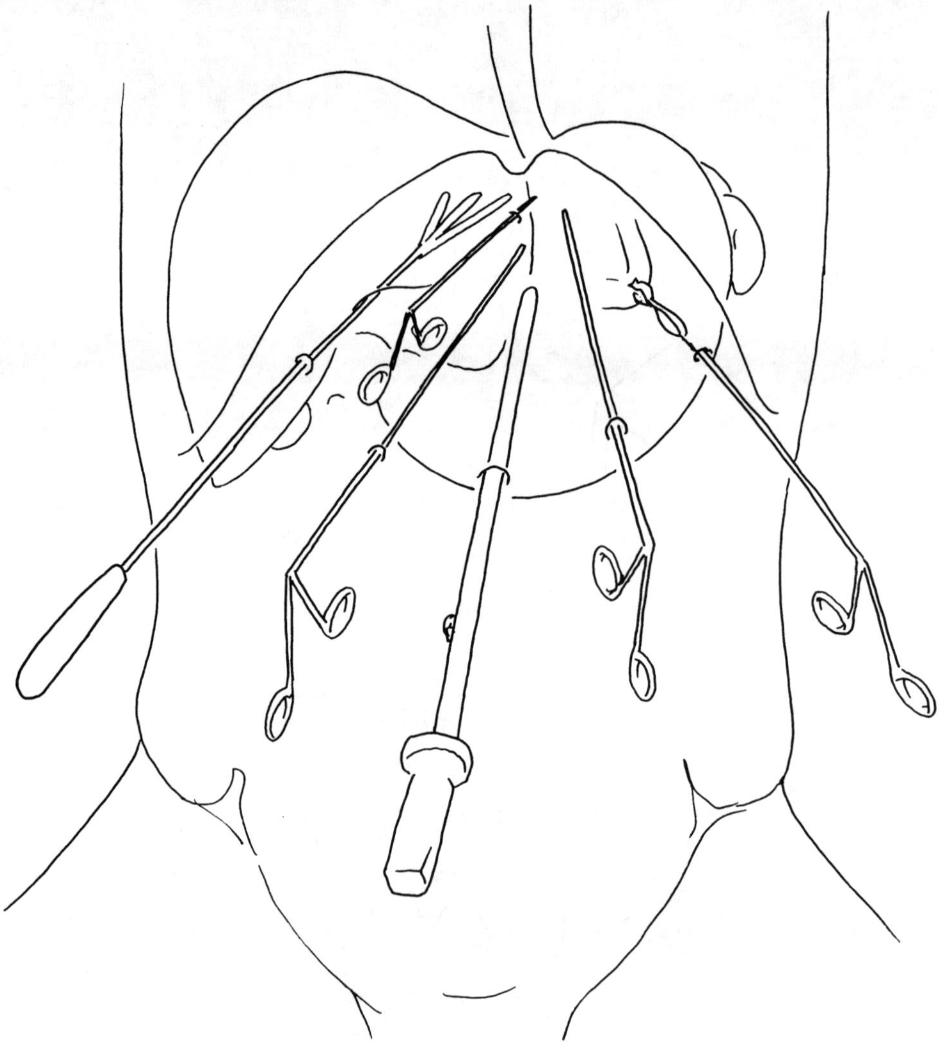

Fig. 4.20

Fundoplication

With the stomach decompressed by nasogastric tube (18 Fr) and the left lobe of the liver elevated with a retractor or a grasper attached to the undersurface of the diaphragm (Fig. 4.21), the gastrohepatic omentum is opened above the hepatic branch of the anterior vagus nerve, taking care to avoid the aberrant left hepatic artery found in about one tenth of individuals. The esophagus is identified at the right limb of the right crus and the space between the crus and the proximal lesser curve is dissected down to the left gastric artery. Alternately, the dissection can begin at the gastrophrenic ligament to the left of the esophagus and proceed to the right, preparing the way for the retro-esophageal window. When dividing the gastrophrenic ligament, the surgeon should keep in mind the occasional posterior gastric artery from the splenic artery running behind the posterior peritoneum of the lesser sac. The peritoneal incision is extended across the anterior surface of the esophagus. The left inferior phrenic vein is often found beneath the peritoneum just anterior to the esophageal hiatus and should be avoided.

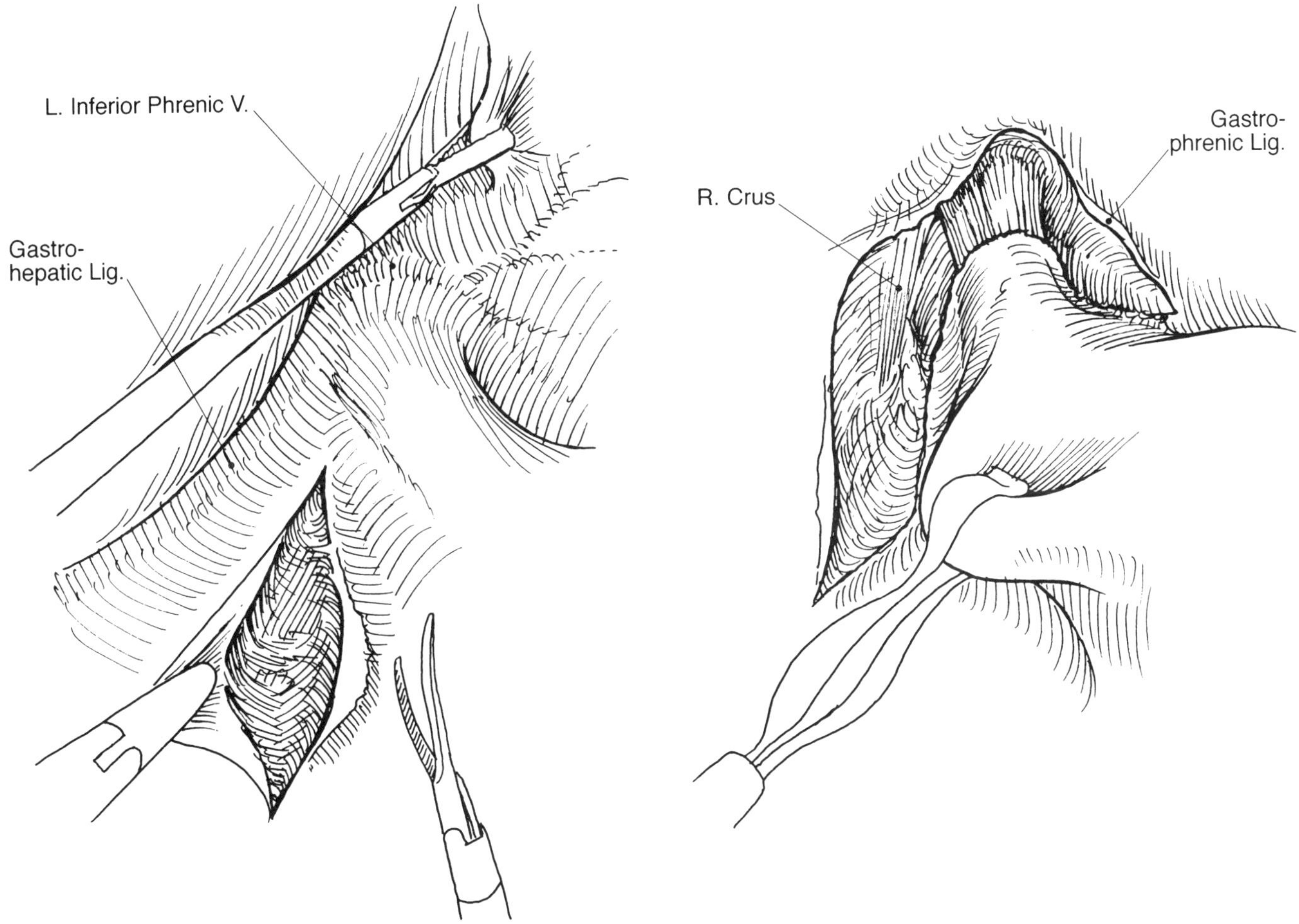

Fig. 4.21

The areolar connections of the esophagus to the hiatus (esophagophrenic ligament) are divided and a 4- to 5-cm length of esophagus is mobilized from both sides creating a posterior window (Fig. 4.22). Care should be taken not to open the left pleura during dissection. A Penrose drain is passed through the window and used to retract the esophagus. The anterior vagus nerve is left on the esophagus. The posterior vagus nerve is easily identified and left in the areolar tissue separated from the posterior esophagus and is placed posterior to the crural repair and the wrap.

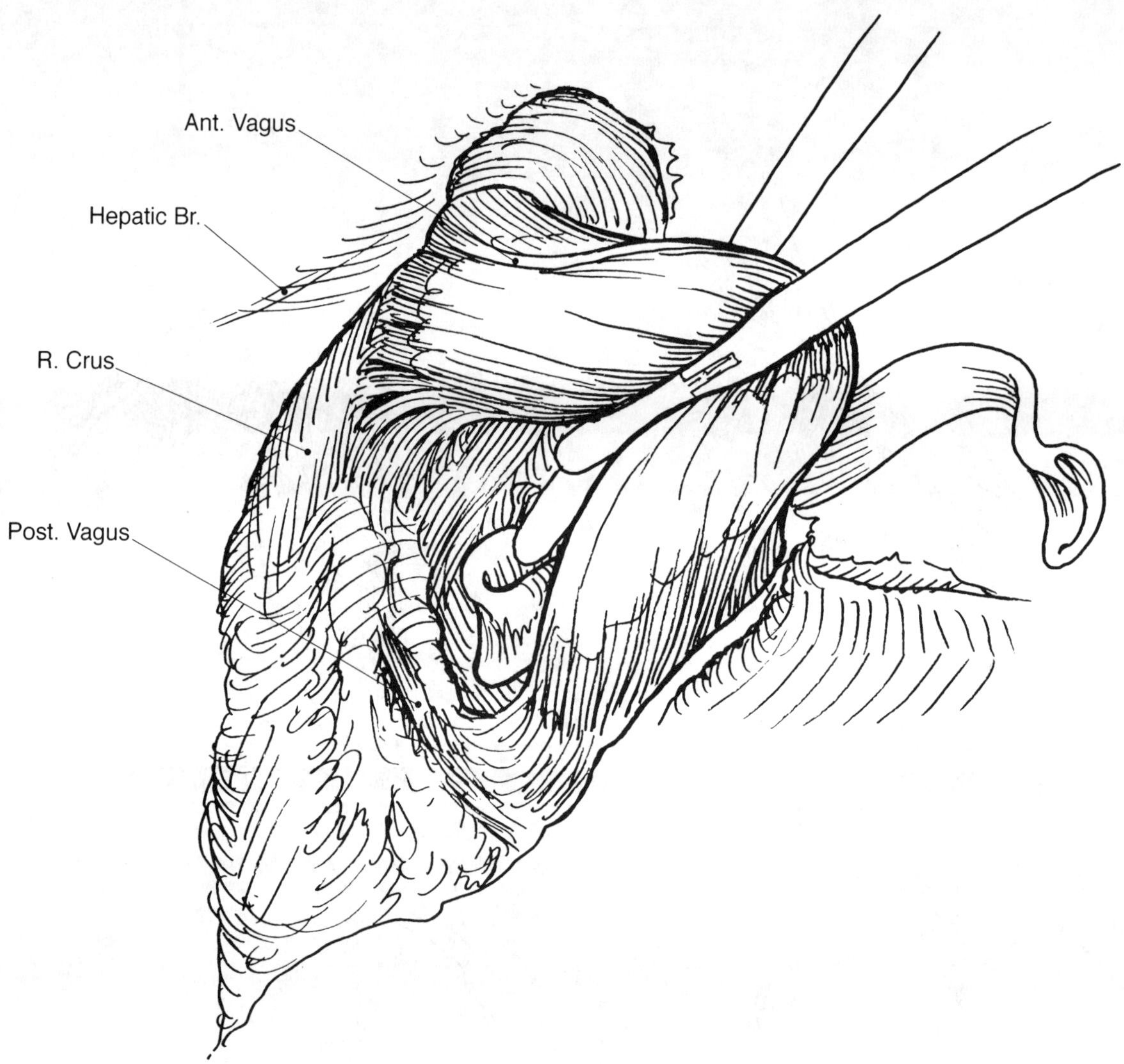

Fig. 4.22

Division of the short gastric vessels should be done routinely to ensure a loose wrap. The dissection is safer and easier when done from distal to proximal. The surgeon retracts the fundus down and to the right while the assistant gently elevates the spleen side of the gastrosplenic ligament (Fig. 4.23). The gastrosplenic ligament is opened into the lesser sac about 15 cm from the esophagogastric junction and the short gastric vessels are clipped and divided (the ultrasonic scalpel is efficient for this purpose) in order. Division of the short highest gastrosplenic vessel opens the lesser curve up to the previously divided gastrophrenic ligament.

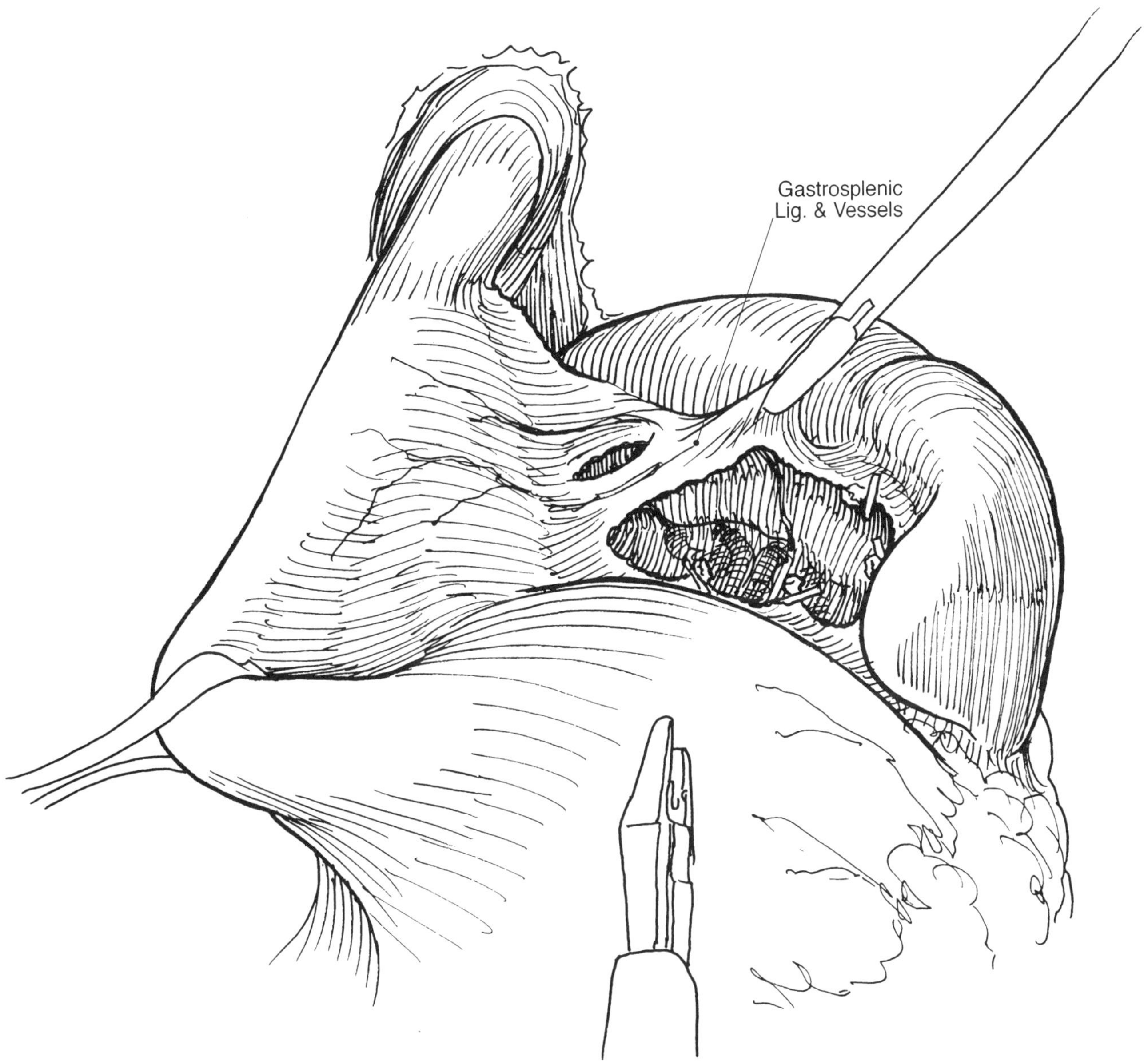

Fig. 4.23

The mobilized fundus is passed behind the esophagus by grasping it through the window from the right side and released to check that it stays in place without tension (Fig. 4.24). Several trial passes may be necessary.

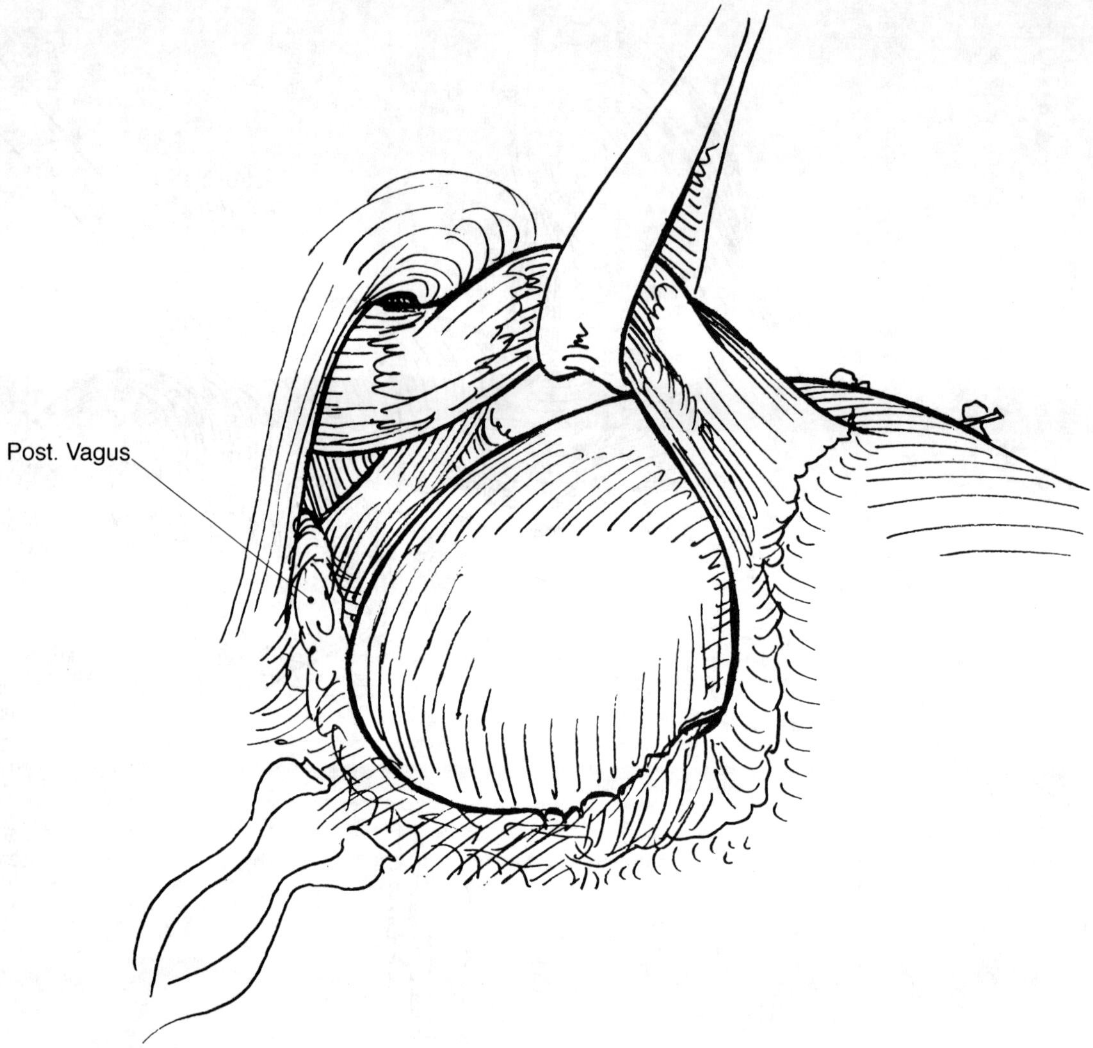

Fig. 4.24

A large Maloney dilator is placed in the esophagus either with or in place of the nasogastric tube. If the 18-French NG tube is left in place, a 40-French dilator is used. If the NG is removed, a 60-French dilator is used. The advantage of leaving the NG tube is that it eliminates the risk of perforation incurred by repassing it after the wrap is done. The esophagus is elevated, and the crura are approximated to a loose comfortable fit around the dilator using 2-0 non-absorbable sutures (Fig. 4.25).

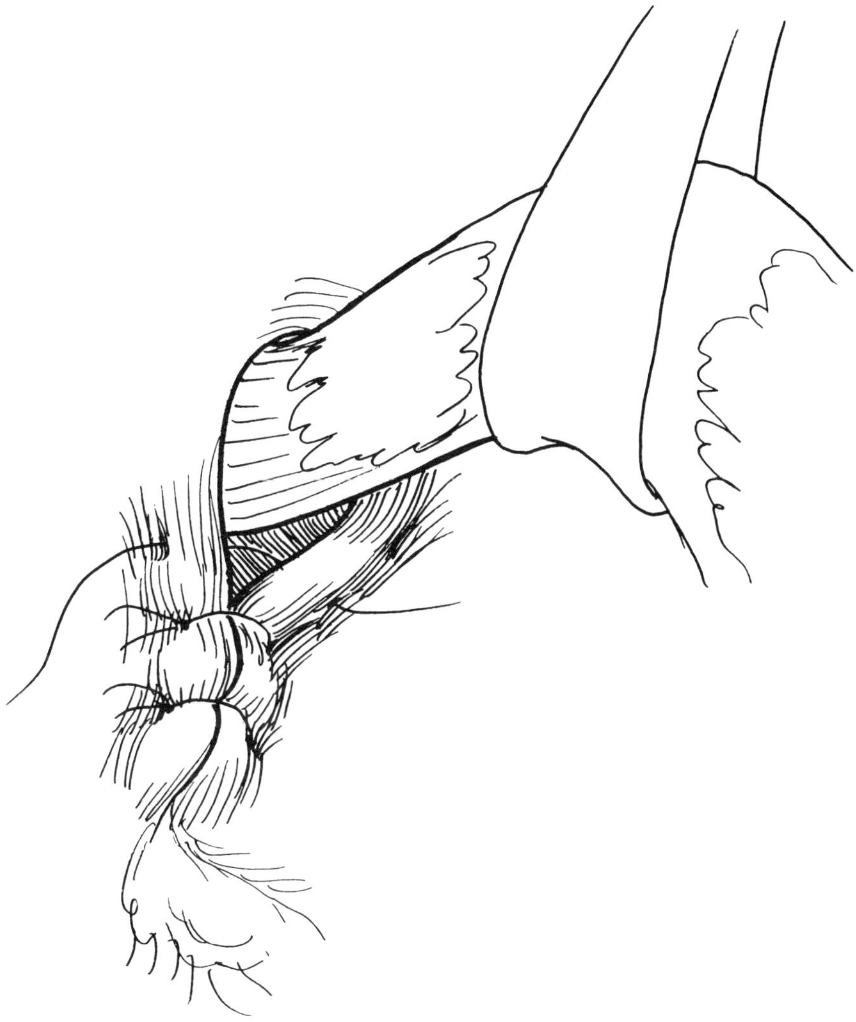

Fig. 4.25

The fundus is again passed behind the esophagus and the first non-absorbable plication suture is placed through the fundus and esophagus at the esophagogastric junction and tied with an extracorporeal knot for control (Fig. 4.26). The bites in both fundus and esophagus must be deep enough to include the strong collagen-containing submucosa. The second stitch is placed two centimeters distal to the first. A third stitch taking only the fundus is placed between the first two. An additional stitch may be placed to recreate the gastroesophageal angle (of His). With the dilator in place, the wrap should be loose enough to comfortably admit the tip of a dissector. At the conclusion of the procedure, the dilator is removed and the 18-Fr nasogastric tube is left to prevent gastric dilatation and wrap disruption in the immediate postoperative period.

A gastrografin swallow is performed with the nasogastric tube in place the morning after surgery to check for leaks, obstruction, displacement, or disruption. If the study is normal, the nasogastric tube is removed and the patient is started on clear fluids. More than a third of patients have significant early edema and patients should be started initially on liquids and advised to chew their food well and avoid swallowing large chunks during the immediate post operative period..

PEPTIC ULCER DISEASE

Indications

The effectiveness of medical management of peptic ulcer disease with H_2 blockers, proton pump inhibitors, and treatment of H. pylori infection has left only patients with complications and intractability in the surgical domain. While early laparoscopic closure of perforated duodenal ulcer is practical and effective, hemorrhage and pyloric stricture do not easily lend themselves to laparoscopic treatment. Patients with intractable or medication-dependent disease on the other hand may be significantly benefitted with minimal morbidity by some form of laparoscopic highly selective vagotomy.

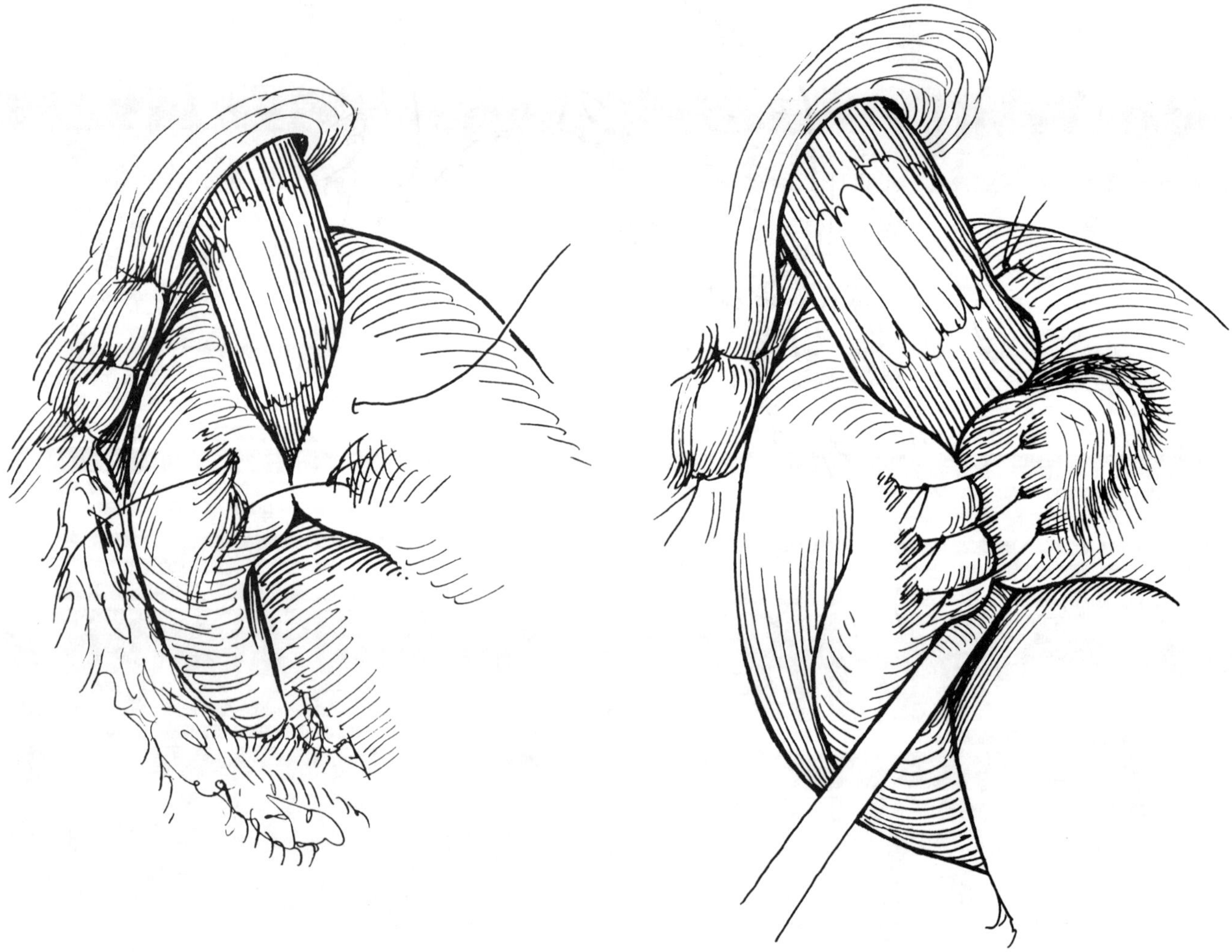

Fig. 4.26

Physiology

The objective of highly selective vagotomy has been to interrupt stimulatory preganglionic vagal fibers to the acid secreting parietal cell mass of the proximal stomach while preserving the innervation of the antrum and pylorus and of the biliary system and small bowel. The antral fibers stimulate muscular contraction and antral emptying and the pyloric fibers are inhibitory, causing relaxation at the end of the antral peristaltic wave. This strategy eliminated the need for a drainage procedure seen in some patients with truncal vagotomy. Further studies showed that pyloric inhibitory fibers are found mainly in the anterior gastric nerve (of Latarjet). The benefit of this knowledge to the laparoscopic approach is that the simpler truncal vagotomy can be substituted for the difficult to reach posterior vagal nerve without compromising pyloric innervation.

Additional advancement of our understanding of vagal innervation came with the demonstration by Donahue of other fibers circuitously reaching the greater curvature of the stomach. Congo red demonstration of persistent greater curvature secretion after highly selective vagotomy led to neuroanatomic demonstration of fibers to this area in the rat and ferret and presumably in man. The exact routes of these fibers is not yet clear, but some presumably travel with celiac trunk branches (splenic and gastroduodenal arteries) to the short gastric arteries and gastroepiploic arch. Others may lie outside named vascular pathways as in the gastropnacreatic fold. Supplementary denervation of some of these fibers is called extended highly selective vagotomy. Concerns about the adequacy of the residual gastric blood supply led Donahue to divide the right and left gastroepiploic pedicles but to leave the short gastrics (Fig. 4.27). Because the short gastrics carry vagal fibers

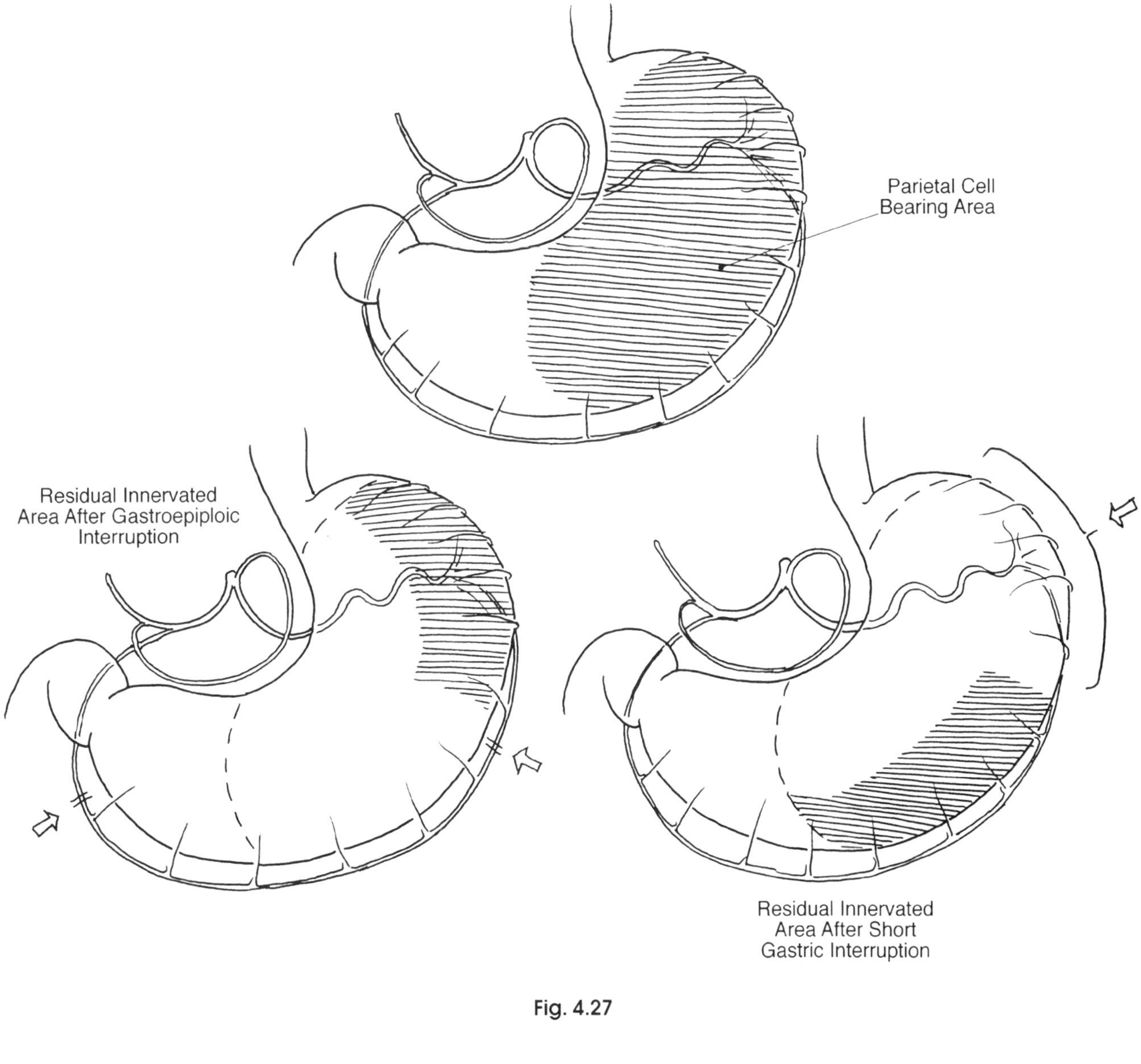

Fig. 4.27

that supply the large area of parietal cell bearing body and fundus of the stomach and only the left half of the gastroepiploic arch supplies parietal cell areas, Dudai has suggested the reverse approach, dividing the short gastrics and leaving the gastroepiploic arch intact. Division of either set of vessels can easily be accomplished laparoscopically.

Surgical Options

The full range of surgical options used in open surgery has been applied laparoscopically (Fig. 4.28). These include bilateral truncal, posterior truncal with anterior seromyotomy or anterior highly selective, bilateral highly selective, and extended highly selective vagotomy.

Bilateral truncal vagotomy with pyloric stretch, drainage procedure, or antrectomy can be accomplished laparoscopically, but has proven disadvantages and has the highest morbidity. Some have reported a low incidence of delayed gastric emptying after laparoscopic truncal vagotomy and those patients respond to postoperative endoscopic pyloric balloon dilatation. However, most laparoscopic surgeons reserve truncal vagotomy via a transthoracic route for patients without evidence of gastric outlet obstruction who are high surgical risks and patients with recurrent ulcer after prior vagotomy

A second option is posterior truncal and anterior highly selective vagotomy. This approach was adopted early by laparoscopic surgeons because of the simplicity compared with a posterior highly selective vagotomy. Theoretically, the absence of posterior vagal fibers reaching the pylorus should avoid delayed gastric emptying although some has been reported. Because vagal fibers to the small bowel via the celiac branch of the posterior vagus are interrupted there is a high incidence of diarrhea with this procedure. The ulcer recurrence rate is also higher than extended highly selective vagotomy, perhaps because the extent of esophageal clearing of vagal fibers is not as complete.

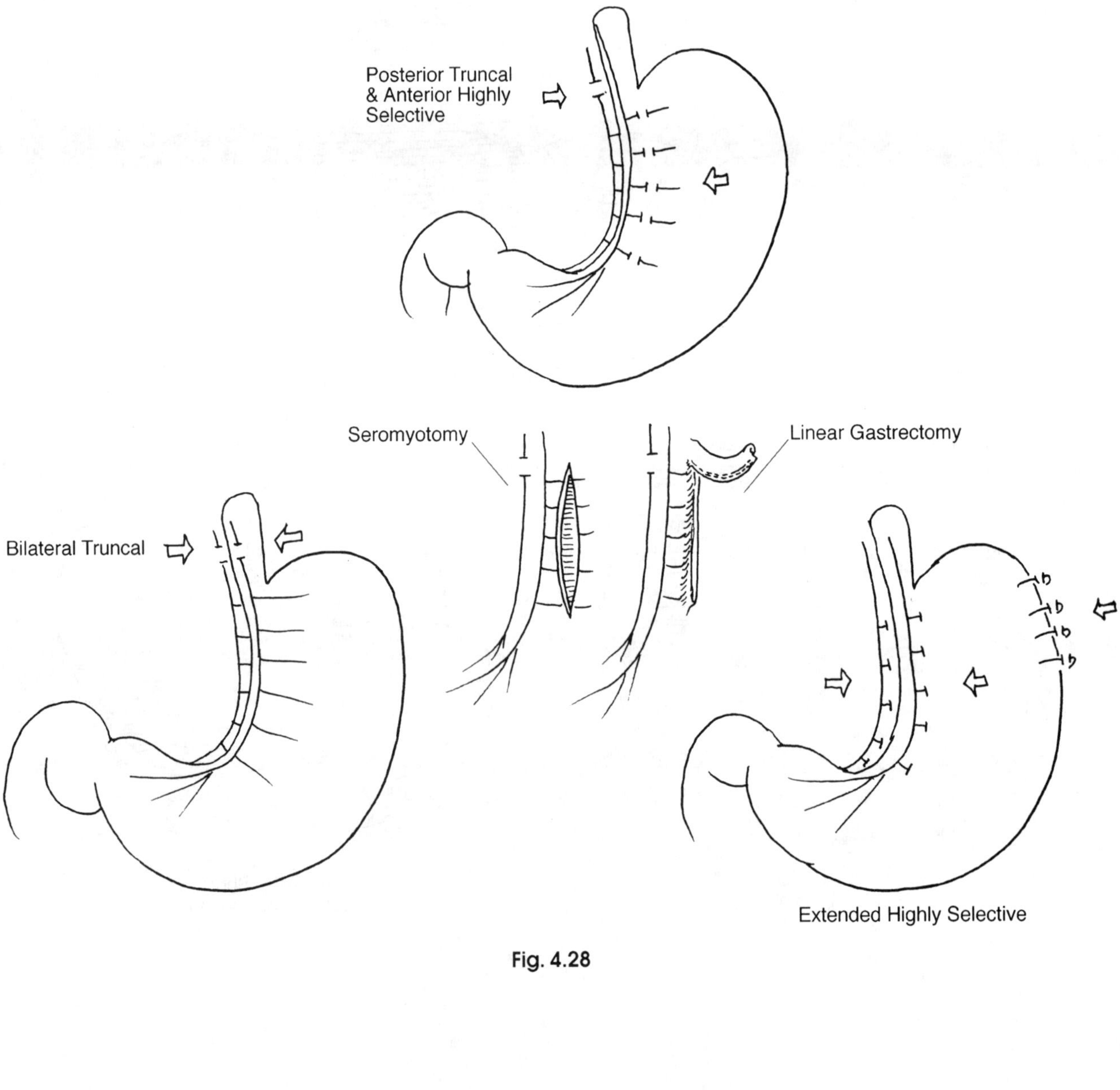

Fig. 4.28

Time saving alternatives to anterior highly selective vagotomy have been tried. These include anterior seromyotomy and anterior linear gastrectomy. In the former approach, the gastric branches of the anterior vagus are interrupted by making a linear incision down to submucosa with cautery. The second approach uses multiple applications of the linear stapler to accomplish the same end. The danger of perforation and leak attend these approaches.

The most rigorous, technically demanding (and time consuming) abdominal approach is extended anterior and posterior highly selective vagotomy which preserves posterior celiac and antral branches. Because there is complete separation of the left gastric artery from the lesser curve with this procedure, there is greater devascularization than with a posterior truncal vagotomy, although the feared necrosis of the lesser curve is very rare (0.2%). Preservation of posterior pyloric fibers may be unnecessary for relaxation, but preservation of all rather than half of the antral motor fibers may be significant for antral motility and gastric emptying. With experience, the procedure can be done efficiently and provides benefits of low side effects and effective ulcer control. Adding interruption of alternate vagal fibers (extended highly selective vagotomy) shows promise of reducing recurrence rates even further. For purposes of anatomic demonstration, the extended highly selective vagotomy is described.

Laparoscopic Extended Highly Selective Vagotomy

Position and trochar placement are similar to that used in laparoscopic antireflux surgery but ports are placed slightly lower on the abdomen to accomplish the more caudal parts of the operation (Fig. 4.29). The surgeon, standing between the legs, operates through the two lateral rectus ports with the camera in the central

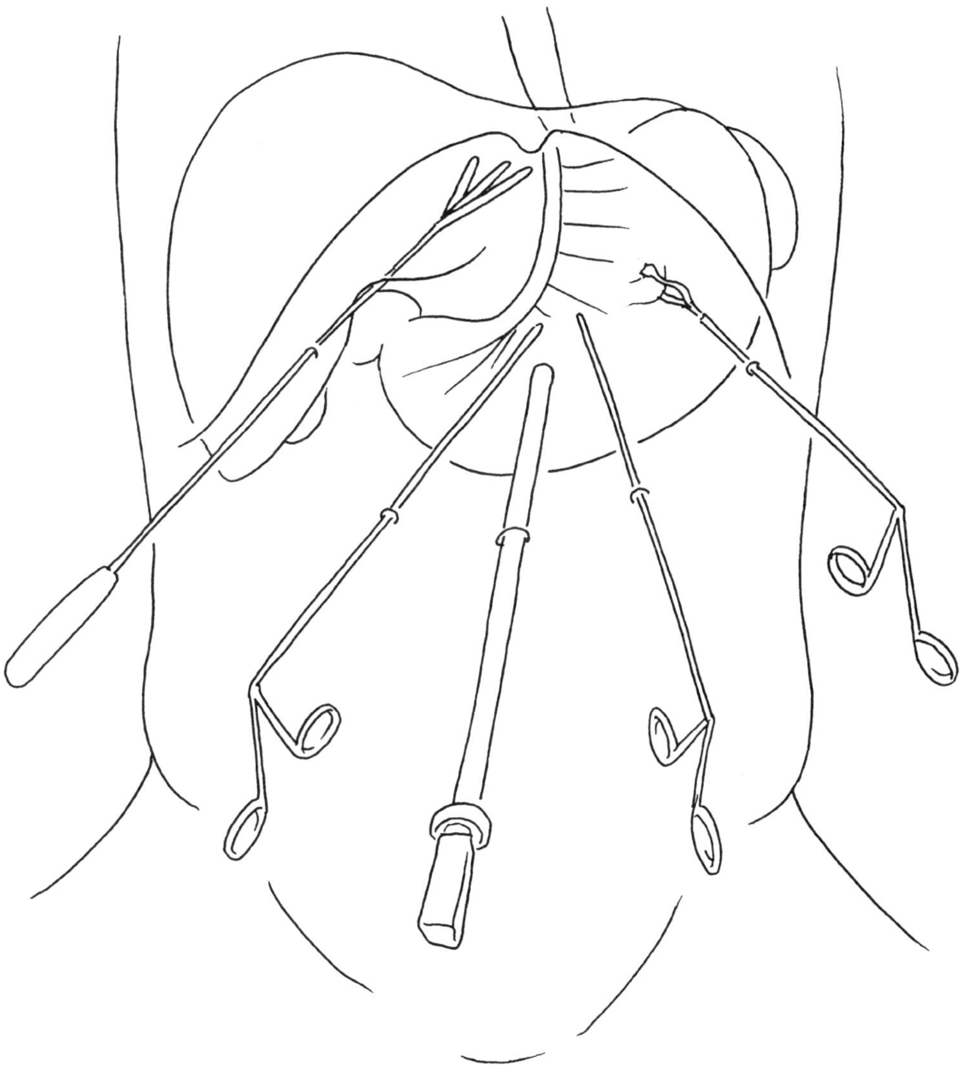

Fig. 4.29

position through the umbilical port. The assistant on the left works through an anterior axillary line port while the assistant on the right retracts through a mid-clavicular line port.

The nerve anatomy is identified (Fig. 4.30). The parietal branches if the anterior vagus come off at a right angle, and the lowest branch to be divided is distinguished from the first branch of the antral "crows foot"

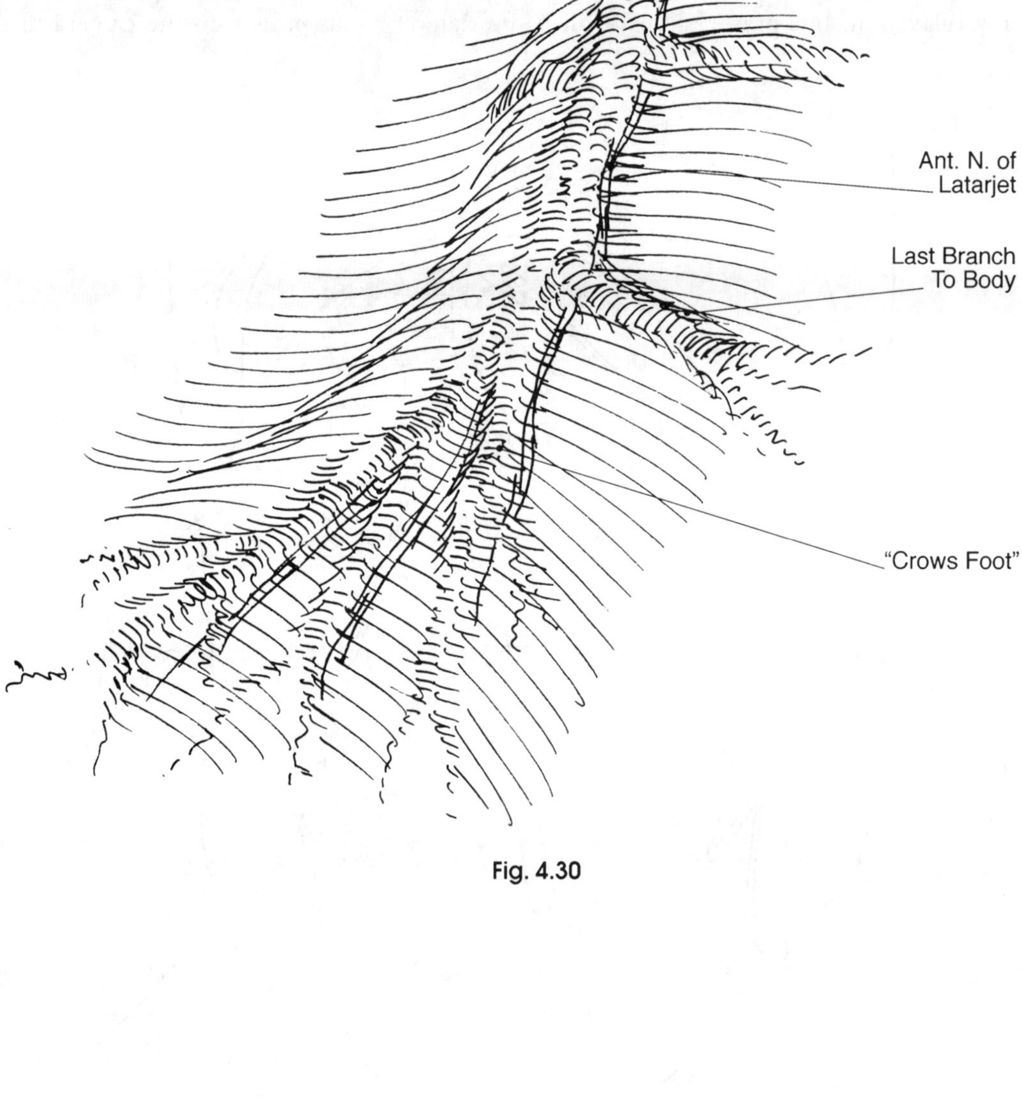

Fig. 4.30

by the acute angle of the latter relative to the vagus (actually a linear continuation of the line of the upper lesser curve). The peritoneum is opened alongside each neurovascular bundle with grasper and scissors, the bundle is isolated, clipped, and divided (Fig. 4.31). The process is repeated up to the gastroesophageal angle and the gastrophrenic ligament is divided to the left of the esophagus.

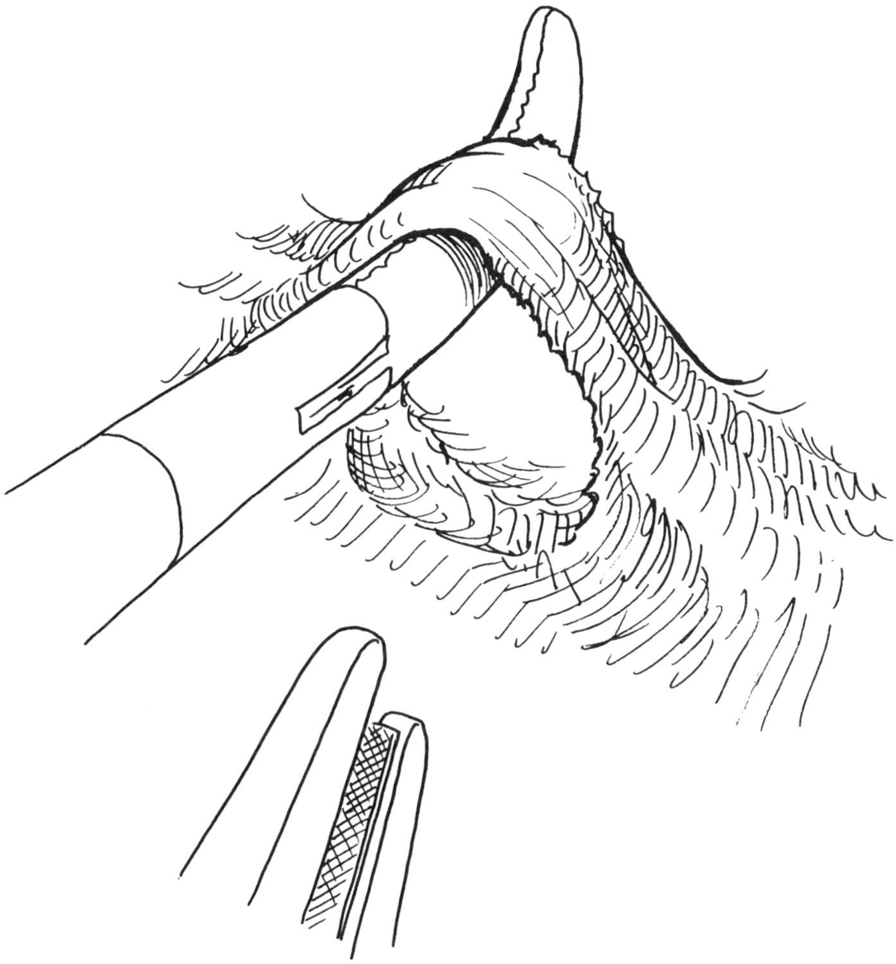

Fig. 4.31

The lesser sac is then entered near the crow's foot by following close to the lesser curve posteriorly (Fig. 4.32). The posterior branches are divided in a similar manner working up to the esophagus.

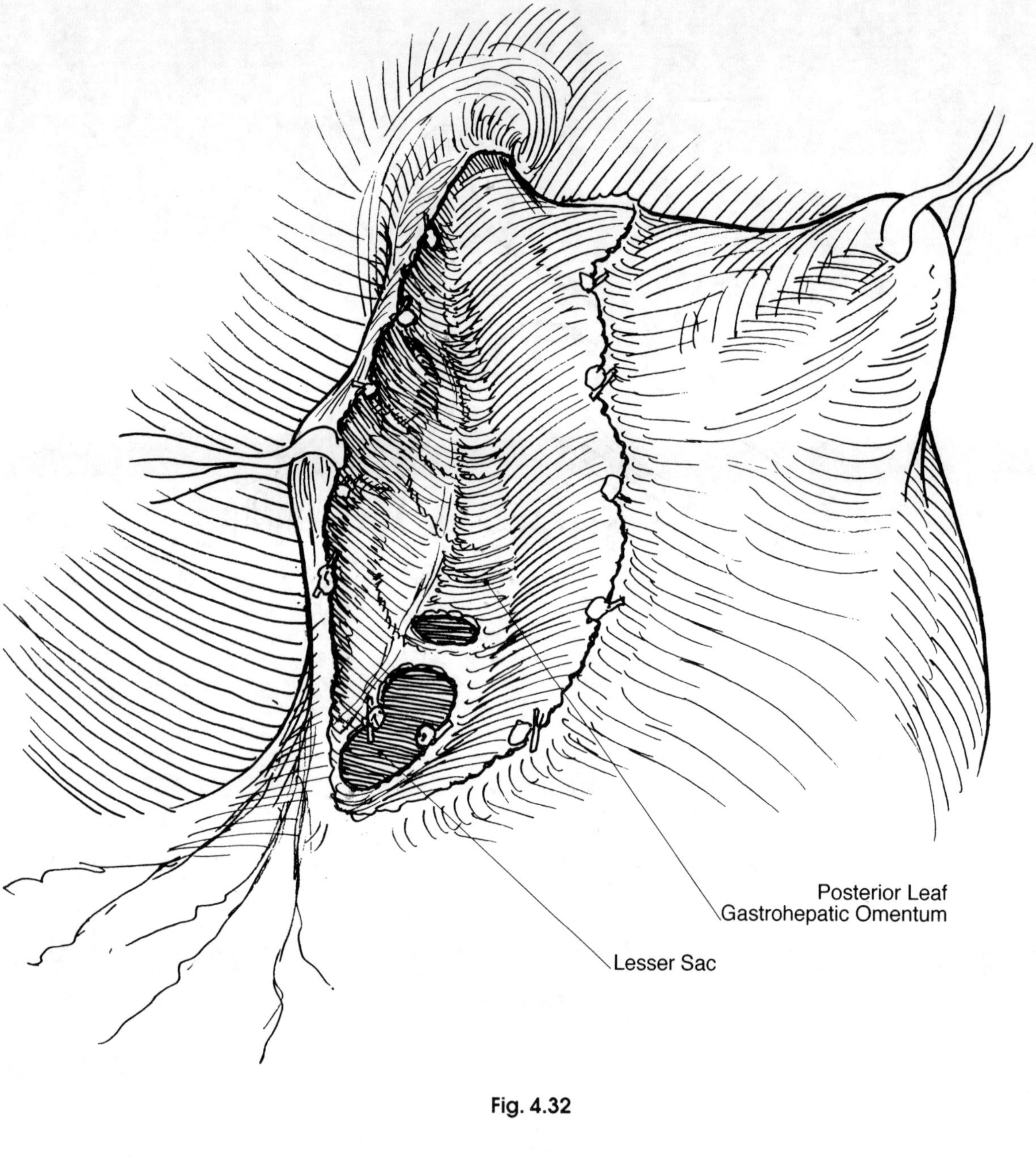

Fig. 4.32

The esophagus is exposed by further mobilizing the gastrohepatic omentum containing the vagal nerve trunks (Fig. 4.33). No effort is made to visualize the trunks to avoid neuropraxia. The esophagophrenic ligament is divided circumferentially, clearing the esophagus of all additional vagal fibers for a distance of 6–7cm.

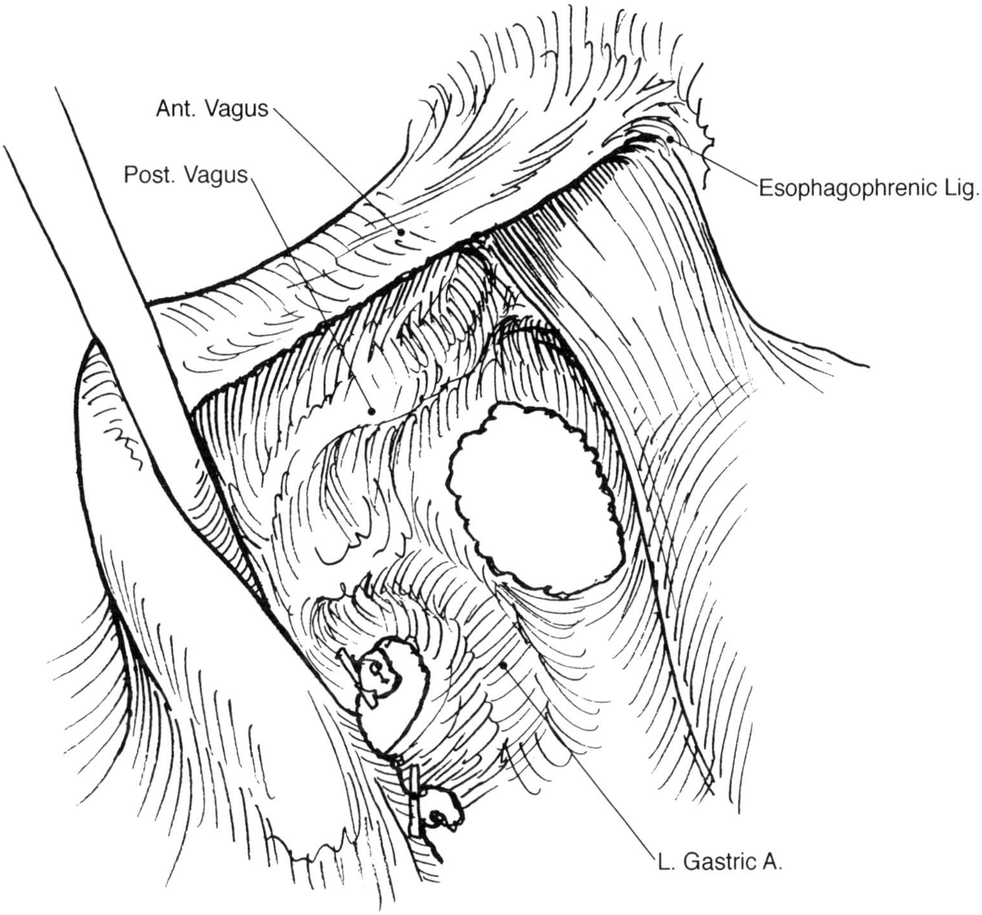

Fig. 4.33

The crura of the esophageal hiatus are dissected posterior to the esophagus and all areolar fibers are divided up into the lower mediastinum to interrupt small independent parasympathetic fibers (Fig. 4.34). The posterior vagus and occasionally the anterior trunk may be exposed at this point.

With the stomach elevated to the left, all attachments of the posterior gastric wall to the diaphragm and pan-

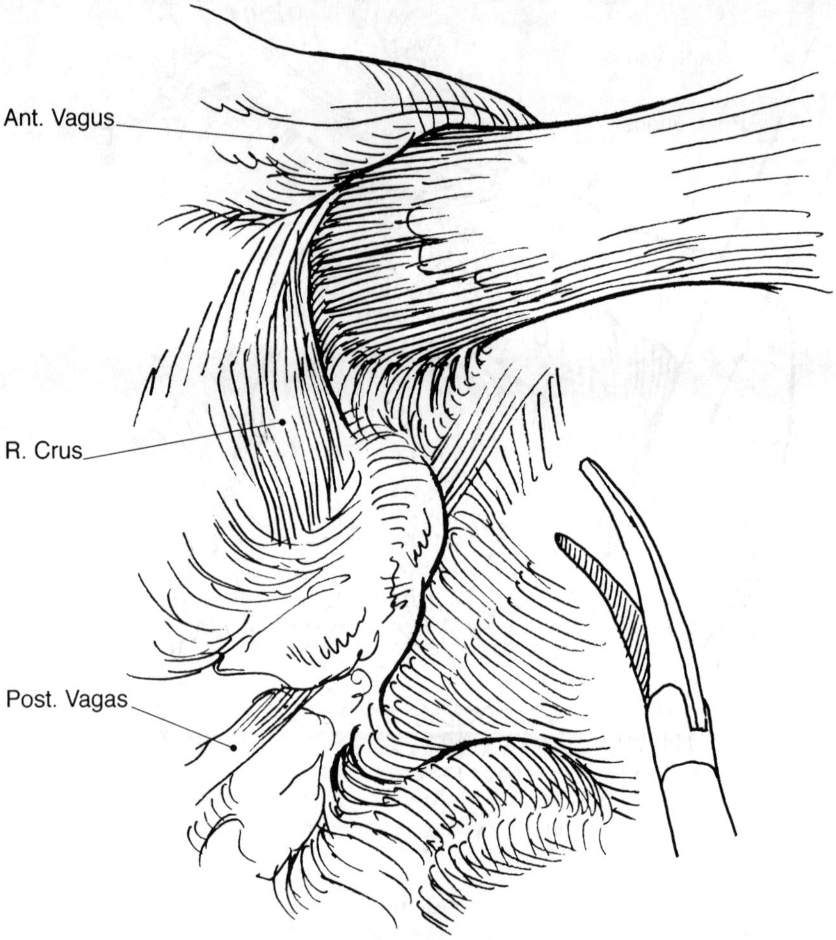

Fig. 4.34

creas (gastropancreatic fold) that might contain parasympathetic fibers are divided (Fig. 4.35). The occasional posterior gastric artery is easily visualized with this exposure. With this exposure, the greater curve can be

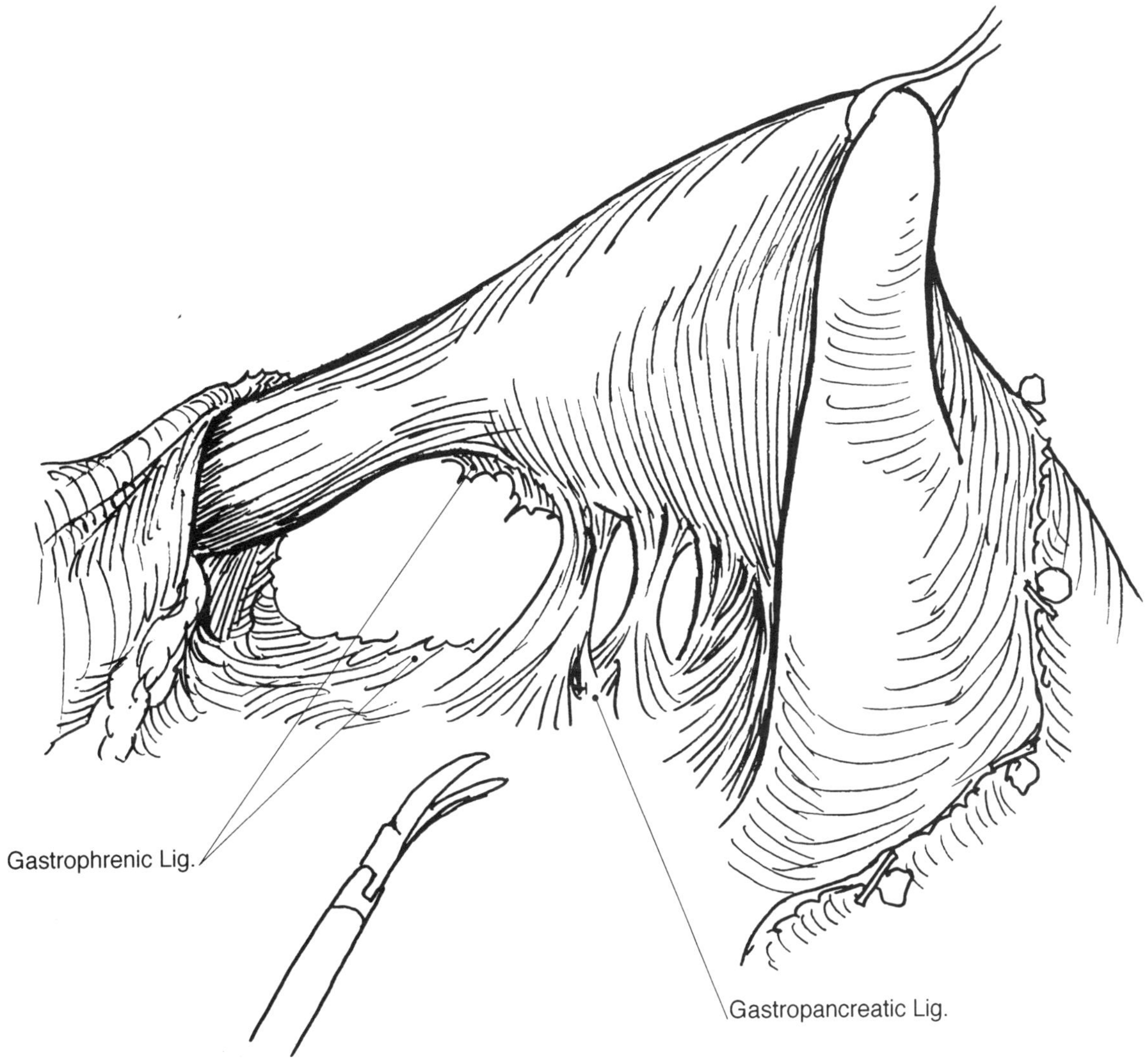

Fig. 4.35

pulled to the right beneath the lesser curve (Fig. 4.36), and the short gastric vessels can be divided posteriorly (Dudai). Because the gastrohepatic ligament is wide open, this approach is safe and time saving and is a short-

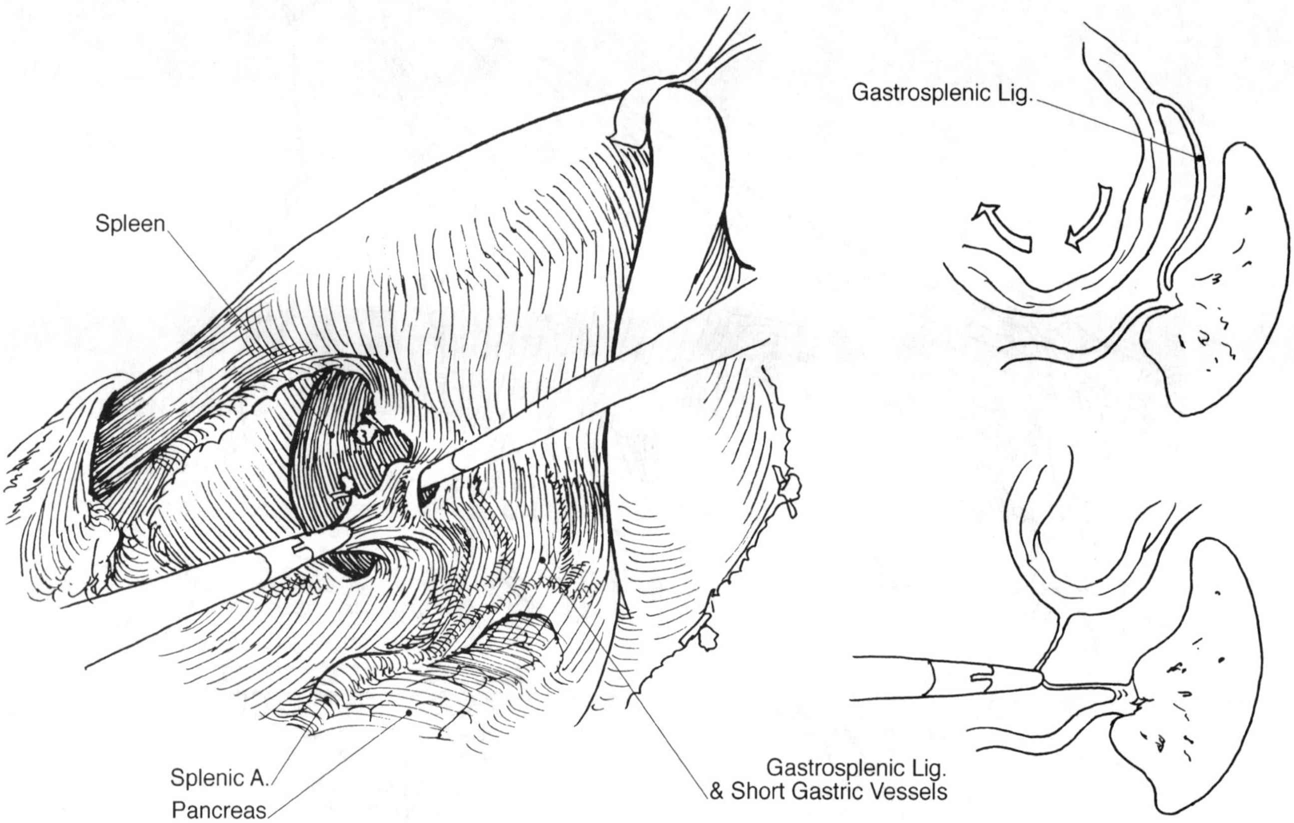

Fig. 4.36

er more direct route than the anterior approach.

Finally, intermediate fibers between the vagal trunks at the incisura are cleared to complete the procedure (Fig. 4.37).

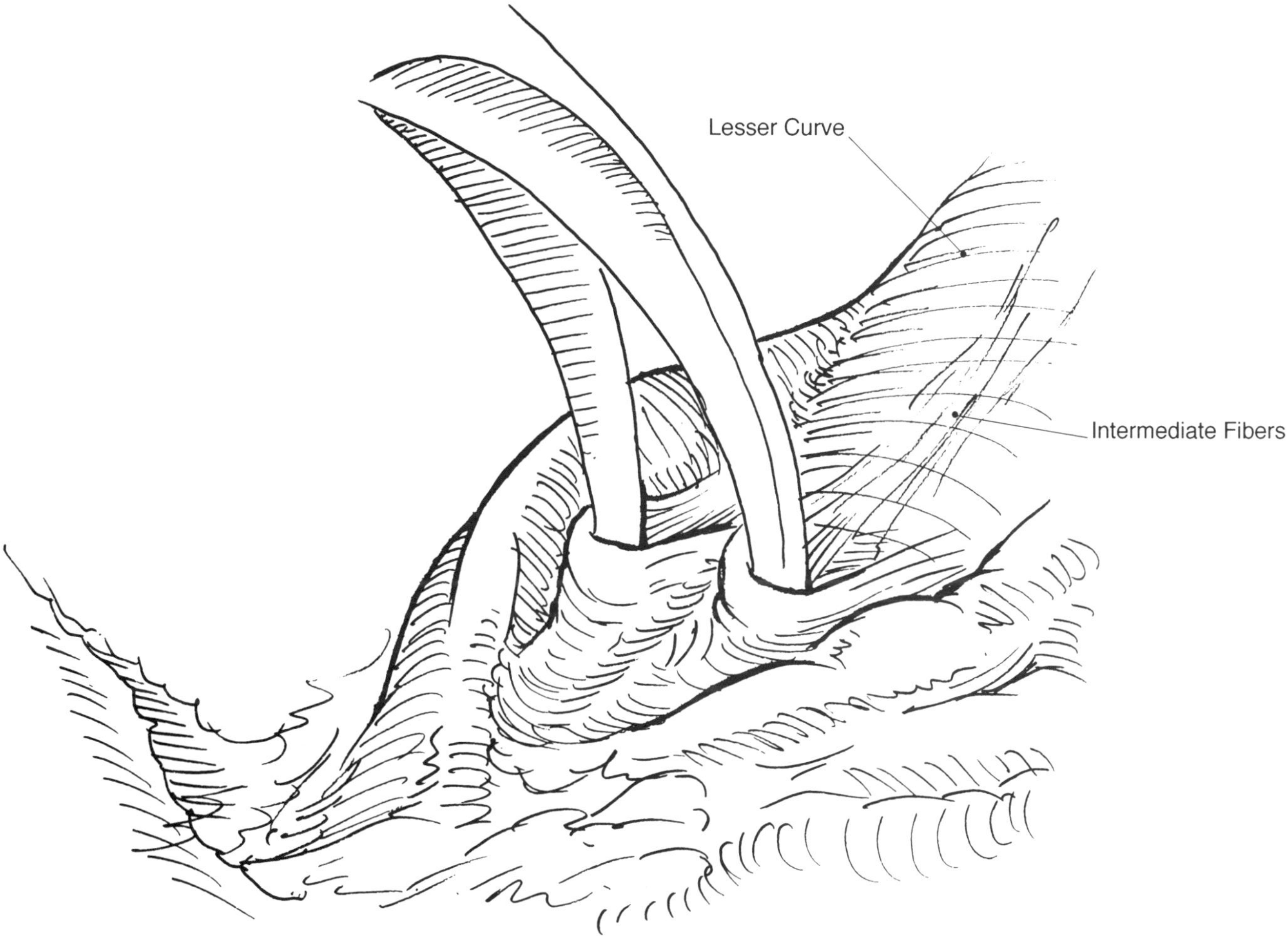

Fig. 4.37

Chapter 4: The Stomach

EMBRYOLOGY

O'Rahilly R, Muller F. Human Embryology and Teratology. New York: Wiley Liss, 1992: 139-159, 173.

Skandalakis JE, Gray SW. Embryology for Surgeons. Philadelphia: WB Saunders, 1972: 63-66, 101-104.

ANATOMY

Bergman RA, Thompson SA, Afifi AK, et. al. Compendium of Human Anatomic Variation. Baltimore, 1988: 76, 77, 166.

Cuschieri A, Hennessy TPJ. Anatomy and physiology of the esophagus. In: Hennessy TPJ, Cuschieri A. Surgery of the Esophagus, 2nd ed. Butterworth Hinemann, 1982: 1-16.

Derbyshire SA. Distribution of the vagus nerve to the human pyloric antrum and possible surgical implications. Clin Anat 1990; 3: 25-31.

Gray H, Clemente CD, Ed. Anatomy of the Human Body, 30th American Ed. Phila: Lea & Febiger, 1985: 1446, 1447, 1463-1472

Naik KS, et al. Distribution of antral G cells in relation to the parietal cells of the stomach and anatomical boundaries. Clin Anat 1990; 3: 17-24.

Skandalakis LJ, et al. The vagus nerve and its vagaries. Surg Clin North Am 1993; 73: 769-773.

Thomas DM, et al. The anatomic basis for gastric mobilization in total esophagectomy. Br J Surg 1979; 66: 203-233.

VanDamme J, PJ. Behavioral anatomy of the abdominal arteries. Surg Clin North Am 1993;73:699-725.

Wastell C, Nyhus LM, Donahue PE. Surgery of the Esophagus, Stomach and Small Intestine, 5th ed, Boston: Little, Brown and Company, 1995:32-37, 45-54, 388-415.

ANTIREFLUX SURGERY

Collard JM, et al. Laparoscopic antireflux surgery, what is real progress. Ann Surg 1994; 220: 146-154.

Cuschieri A, Hennessy TPJ. Hiatal hernia and reflux esophagitis. in Hennessy TPJ, Cuschieri A. Surgery of the Oesophagus, 2nd ed, Butterworth Hinemann, 1982: 194-208.

Dudai M, et al. Laparoscopic repair of various types of hiatus hernia (abstract). International Symposium on New Trends in Endoscopic surgery, Tel Aviv, Israel 1995.

Dudai M, et al. Laparoscopic reapir of paraesophageal hiatus hernia type II and III (abstract), International Symposium on Vagotomy and Hiatus Hernia, Bordeaux, France 1994.

Hinder RA, Philipi CJ. The technique of laparoscopic Nissen fundoplication. Surg Lap Endosc 1992; 2: 265-272.

Hinder RA, et al. Laparoscopic Nissen fundoplication is an effective treatment for gastroesophageal reflux disease. Ann Surg 1994; 220: 472-483.

Hinder RA, Filipi CJ. The laparoscopic management of gastroesophageal reflux disease. In: Cameron JL (ed). Adv Surg, St. Louis: Mosby, 1995:41-58.

Jamieson GG, Duranceau A. What is a Nissen fundoplication? Surg Gyn Obstet 1984; 159: 591-593.

Jamieson GG. Laparoscopic Nissen fundoplication. Ann Surg 1994; 220: 137-145.

Katkhouda N. Laparoscopic treatment of gastroesophageal reflux disease-defining a gold standard, (editorial). Surg Endosc 1995; 9: 765-767.

Paterson-Brown S, Garden J (eds.). Principles and Practice of Surgical Laparoscopy. London: WB Saunders Co. Ltd., 1994: 246-261.

Peters JH, Demeester TR. Minimally Invasive Surgery of the Foregut, St. Louis: Quality Medical Publishers, 1994: 38-70, 119-176, 188-196.

Zucker KA. Surgical Laparoscopy Update. St. Louis: Quality Medical Publishing, 1993: 217-239.

PEPTIC ULCER DISEASE

Dudai M, et al. Transthoraacoscopic truncal vagotomy for recurrent ulcer (abstract). SAGES, Orlando 1995.

Dudai M, et al. Laparoscopic highly selective vagotomy (abstract). EAES, Luxenburg 1995.

Dudai M, et al. Laparoscopic vagotomy in 57 cases with four year follow up (abstract). ACS, New Orleans 1995.

Laws HL, McKernan JB. Endoscopic management of peptic ulcer disease. Ann Surg 1993; 217: 584-556.

McKernan JB, et al. Laparoscopic repair of duodenal ulcer and gastroesophageal reflux. Surg Clin North Am 1992; 72: 1153-1167.

Mouiel J, Katkhouda N. Laparoscopic posterior truncal vagotomy and anterior seromyotomy: In: Paterson-Brown S, Garden J, Eds., Principles and Practice of Surgical Laparoscopy. London: WB Saunders Co. Ltd.: 314-327.

Peters JH, Demeester TR. Minimally Invasive Surgery of the Foregut, St. Louis: Quality Medical Publishers, 1994: 199-235.

Swanstrom L, Wayne R. Spectrum of gastrointestinal symptoms after laparoscopic fundoplication. Am J Surg 1994; 167: 538-541.

Wastell C, Nyhus LM, Donahue PE. Surgery of the Esophagus Stomach and Small Intestines, 5th ed, Boston: Little Brown & Company, 1995:505-519, 754-769.

Zucker KA. Surgical Laparoscopy Update. St. Louis: Quality Medical Publishing, 1993:241-286.

5

The Spleen

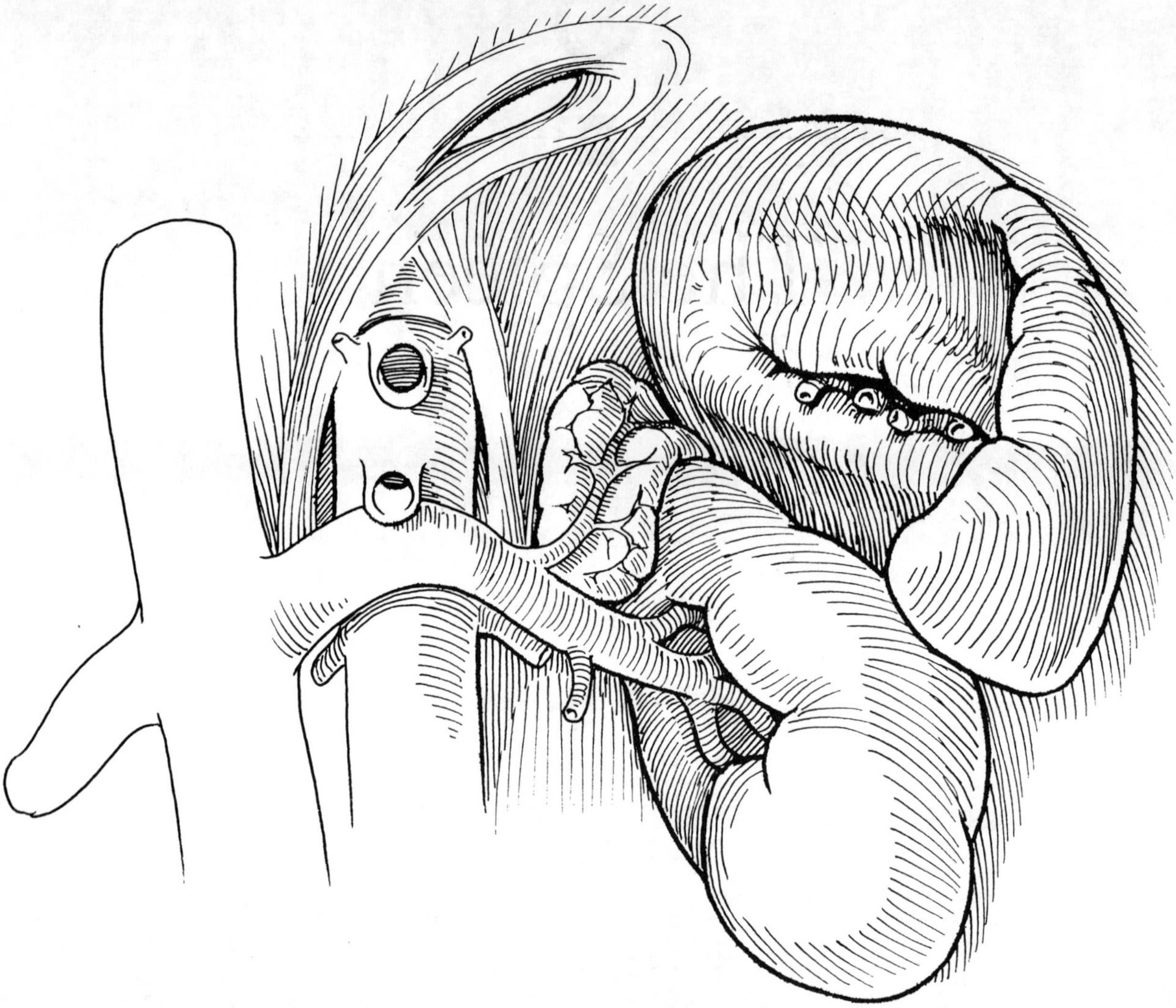

5

The Spleen

EMBRYOLOGY

The spleen develops in the dorsal mesogastrium, the portion of the mesentery between the aorta posteriorly and the developing stomach (Chapter 4). Islands of mesenchymal cells coalesce on the left side of this membrane and become vascularized during the eighth or ninth weeks. The vessels that acquire responsibility for supplying these islands are the multiple unpaired midline vessels running between the aorta and the dorsal, greater curve side of the stomach (Fig. 5.1). One of these vessels becomes dominant and survives as the splenic artery. By visualizing the spleen as a secondarily acquired way station in the course of the splenic artery, one can understand the relationship of the gastrosplenic (short gastric) vessels to the splenic artery.

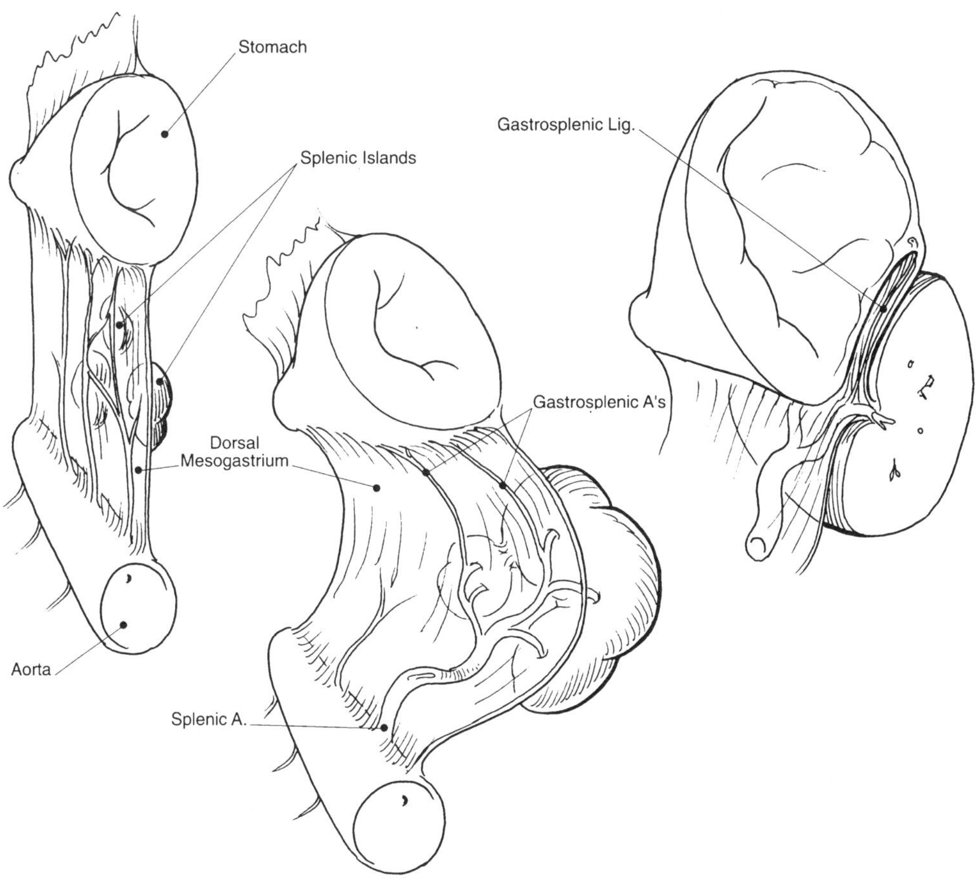

Fig. 5.1

The independent vascularized mesenchymal aggregates are two to four in number, each with its own blood supply (Fig. 5.2). When these unite, they result in a spleen that is segmented and has limited (15%) communication between its segmental vessels.

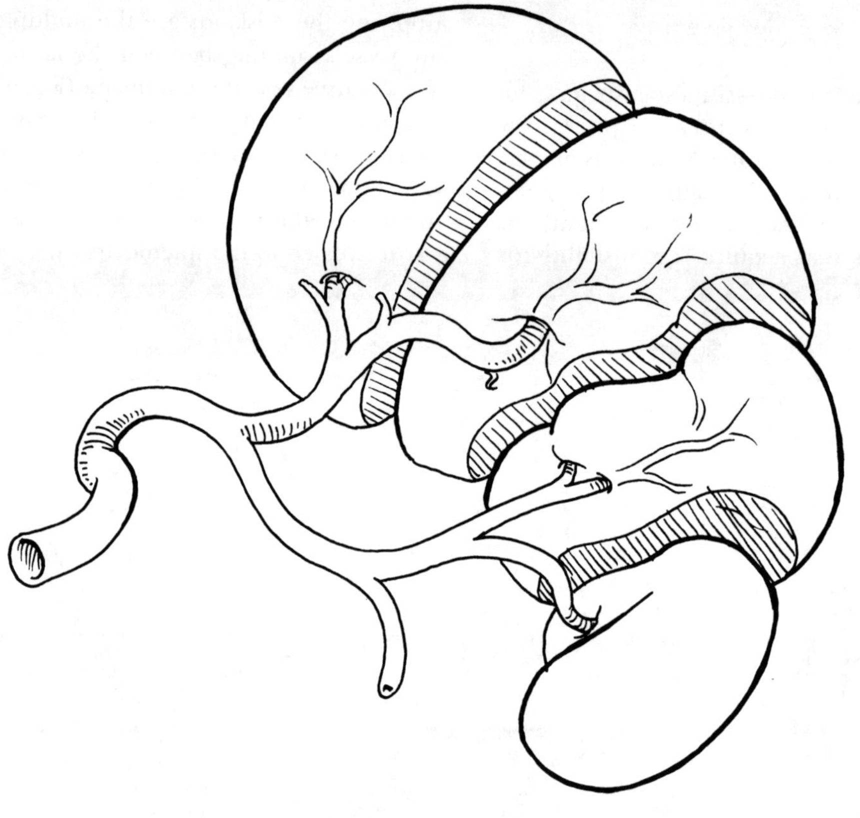

Fig. 5.2

The ballooning of the dorsal mesogastrium to form the greater omentum carries the spleen to the left (Fig. 5.3). At the same time that the spleen is forming, the dorsal pancreatic bud is also growing into the dorsal mesogastrium parallel to the course of the future splenic vessels. This dorsal pancreatic precursor approaches the splenic islands and forms the tail of the pancreas. The future splenic vessels run along its upper border.

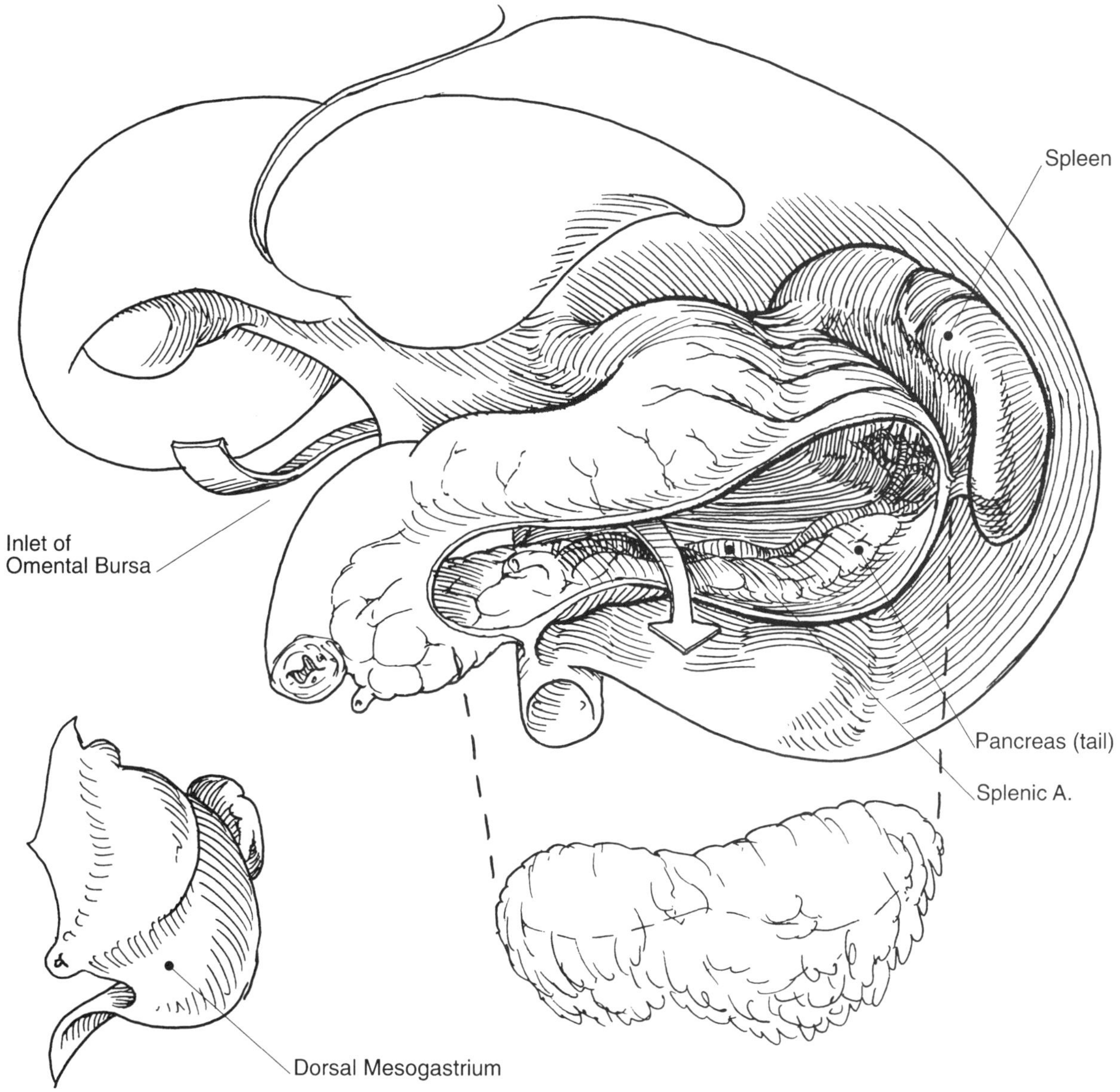

Fig. 5.3

The part of dorsal mesogastrium between spleen and aorta becomes apposed to the dorsal parietal peritoneum and fuses with that layer (Fig. 5.4). It covers the posteromedial part of the left hemidiaphragm, the left adrenal gland, and the upper part of the left kidney. The pancreas drapes across the middle of the left kidney, lying on what will become renal (Gerota's) fascia. The resulting fusion fascia forms the posterior wall of the omental bursa (lesser sac). When the spleen and tail of the pancreas are mobilized surgically, the original dorsal mesentery is recreated.

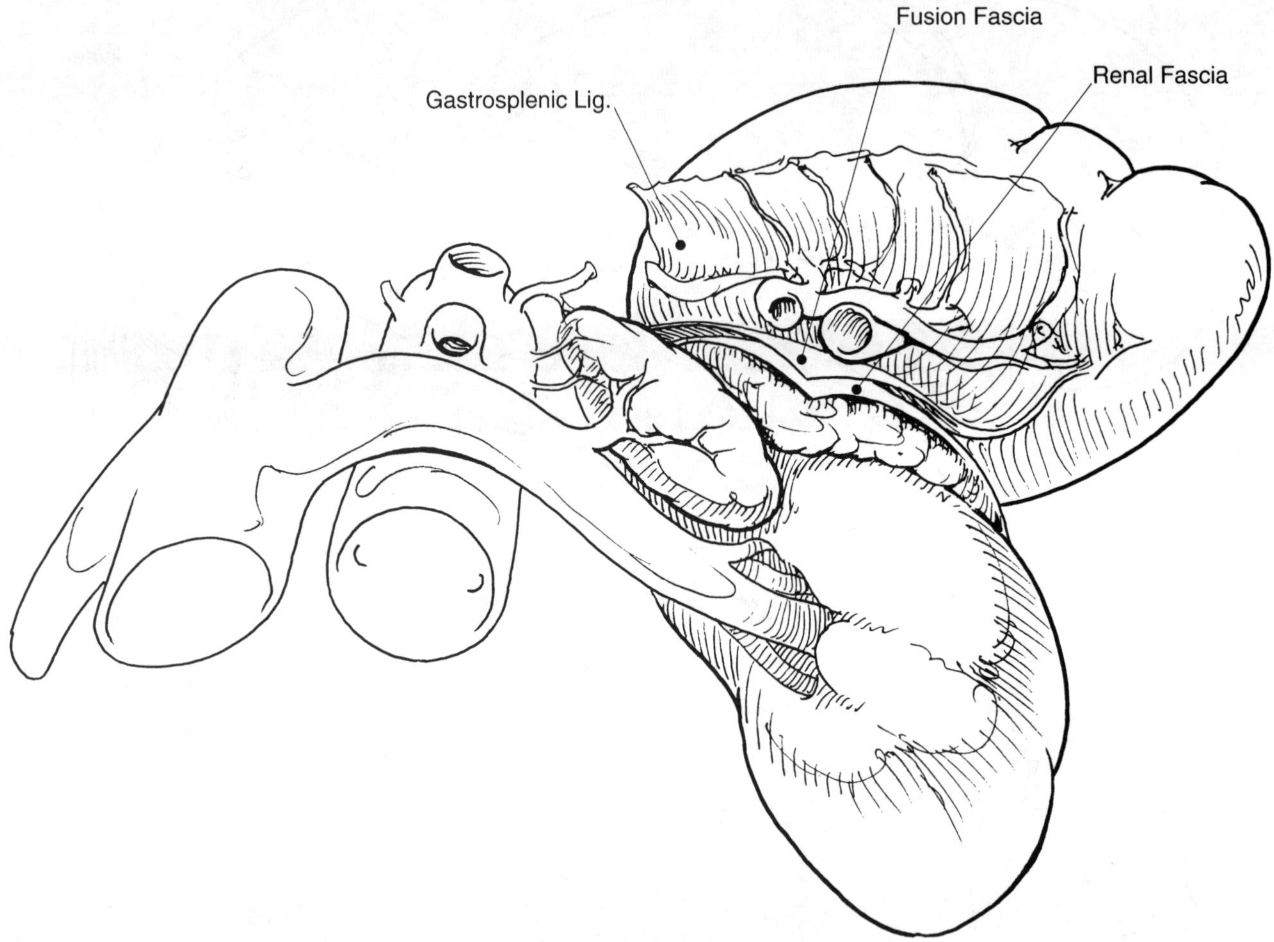

Fig. 5.4

ANATOMY

Relationships

The spleen is located high posterolaterally beneath the left hemidiaphragm (Fig. 5.5). Its long axis is oriented along the course of the 10th rib and its lower pole is

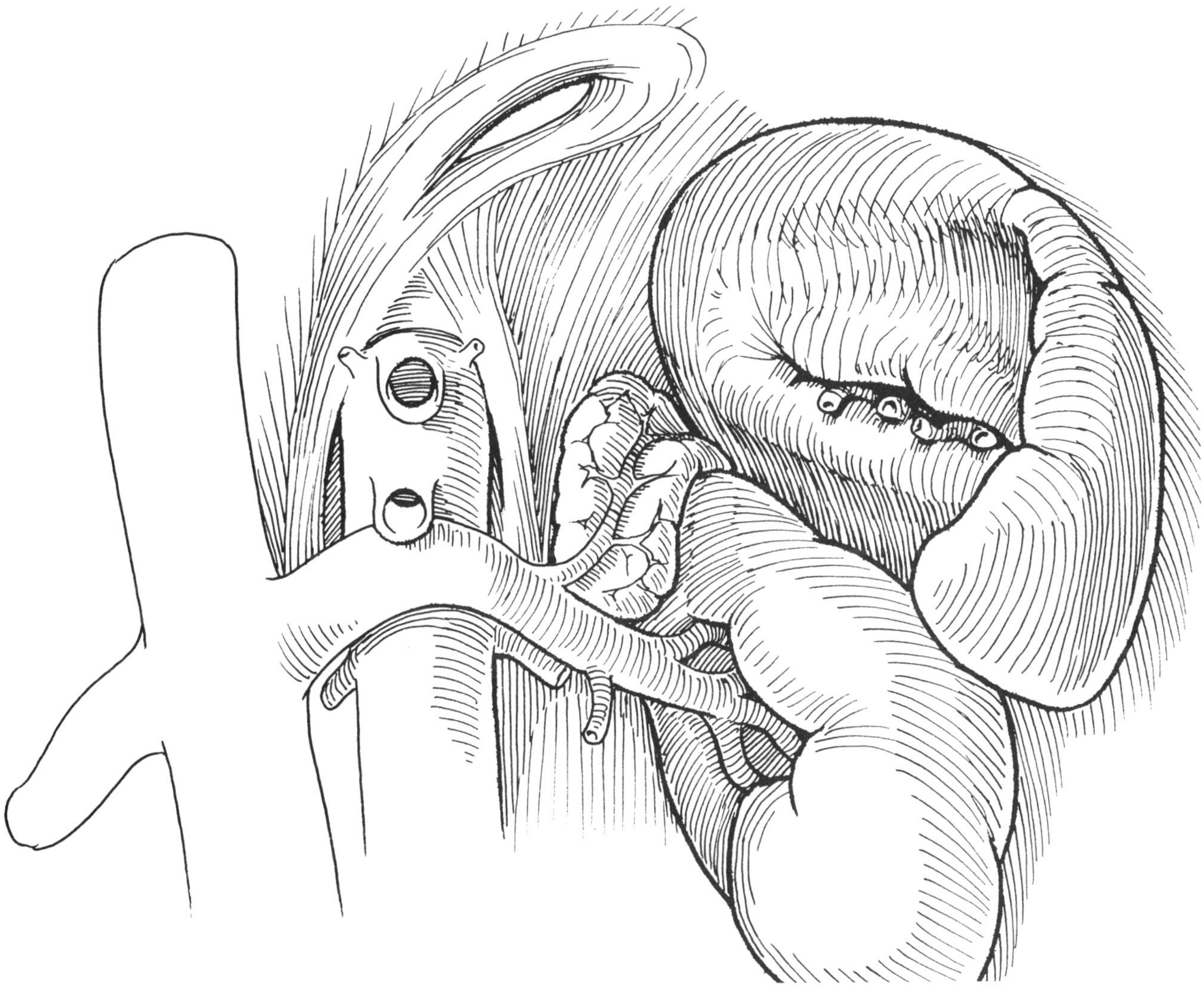

Fig. 5.5

normally not close enough to the costal margin to palpate (Fig. 5.6). The outer surface of the spleen is in contact with the diaphragm and the pleural reflection on the thoracic side of the diaphragm overlies the upper third of the spleen. The anterior two thirds of the hilar side of the spleen indents the posterior wall of the fun-

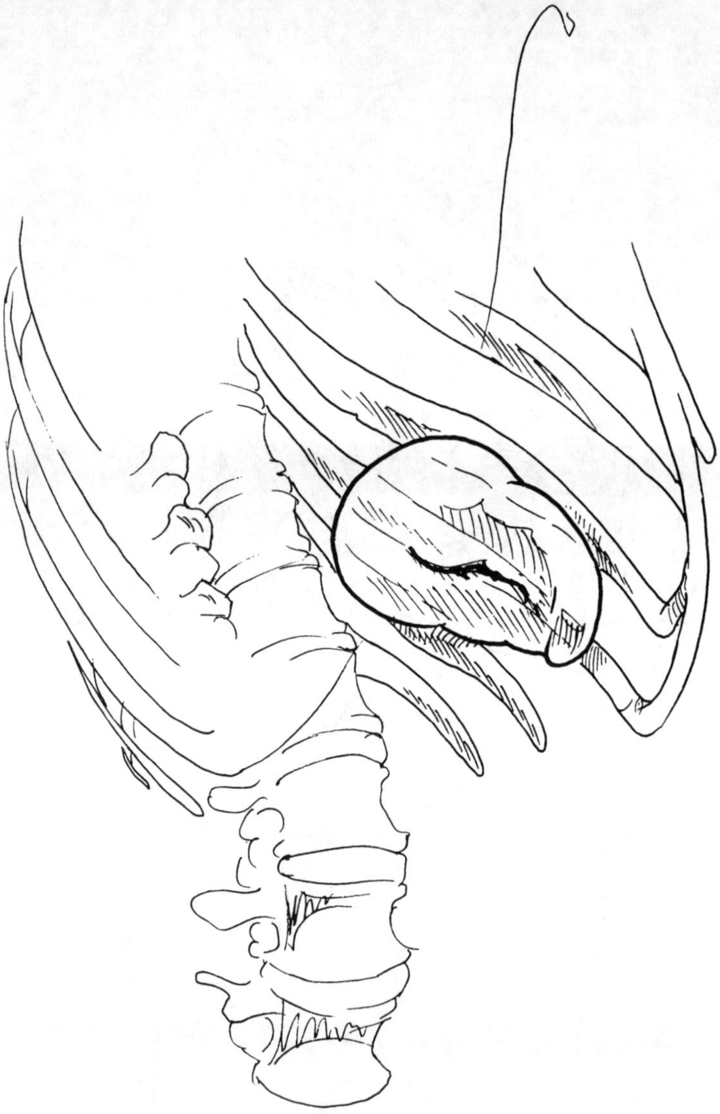

Fig. 5.6

dus and upper body of the stomach (Fig. 5.7). The posterior third of the spleen's inner surface is indented by the underlying left kidney.

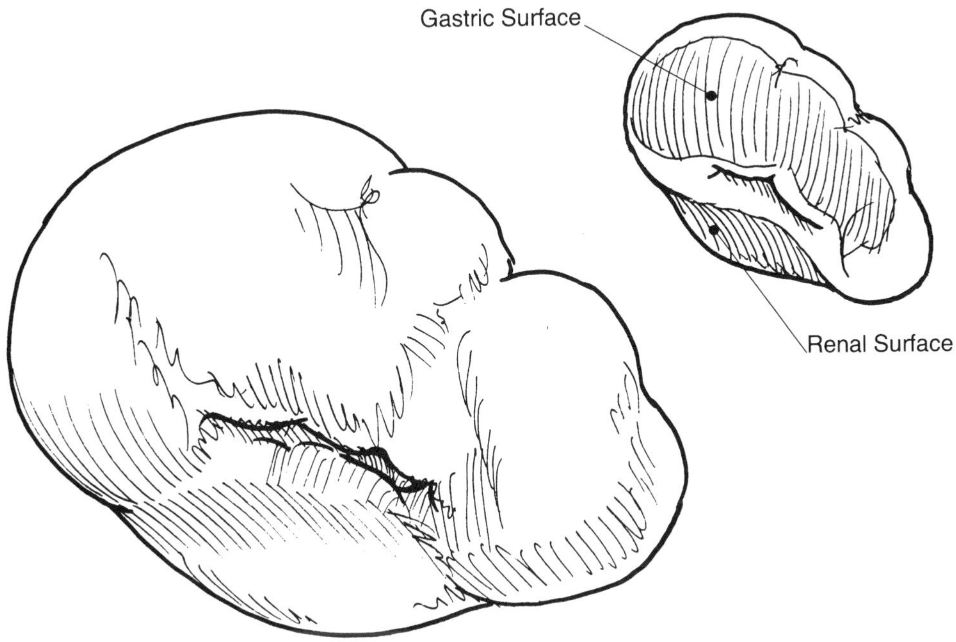

Fig. 5.7

The interface between the spleen and kidney merits special attention because the separation of this plane is critical in mobilizing the spleen. The perirenal fat and the renal fascia intervenes between the kidney and spleen (Fig. 5.8). The renal indentation of the spleen is applied to the renal fascia. Many descriptions of splenic anatomy state that the main splenic vessels are contained in the splenorenal ligament. The attachment between spleen and renal fascia actually begins just inside the lip of the posterior splenic border at the lateral peritoneal reflection. This broad-based attachment contains few if any vessels due to the fact that it is an embryological fusion plane. The hilum of the spleen lies at the medial end of this fusion plane. The tissue between the splenic vessels and the renal fascia could still be considered part of the splenorenal ligament, but more properly this plane should be thought of as the splenopancreatic continuation of the original dorsal mesentery.

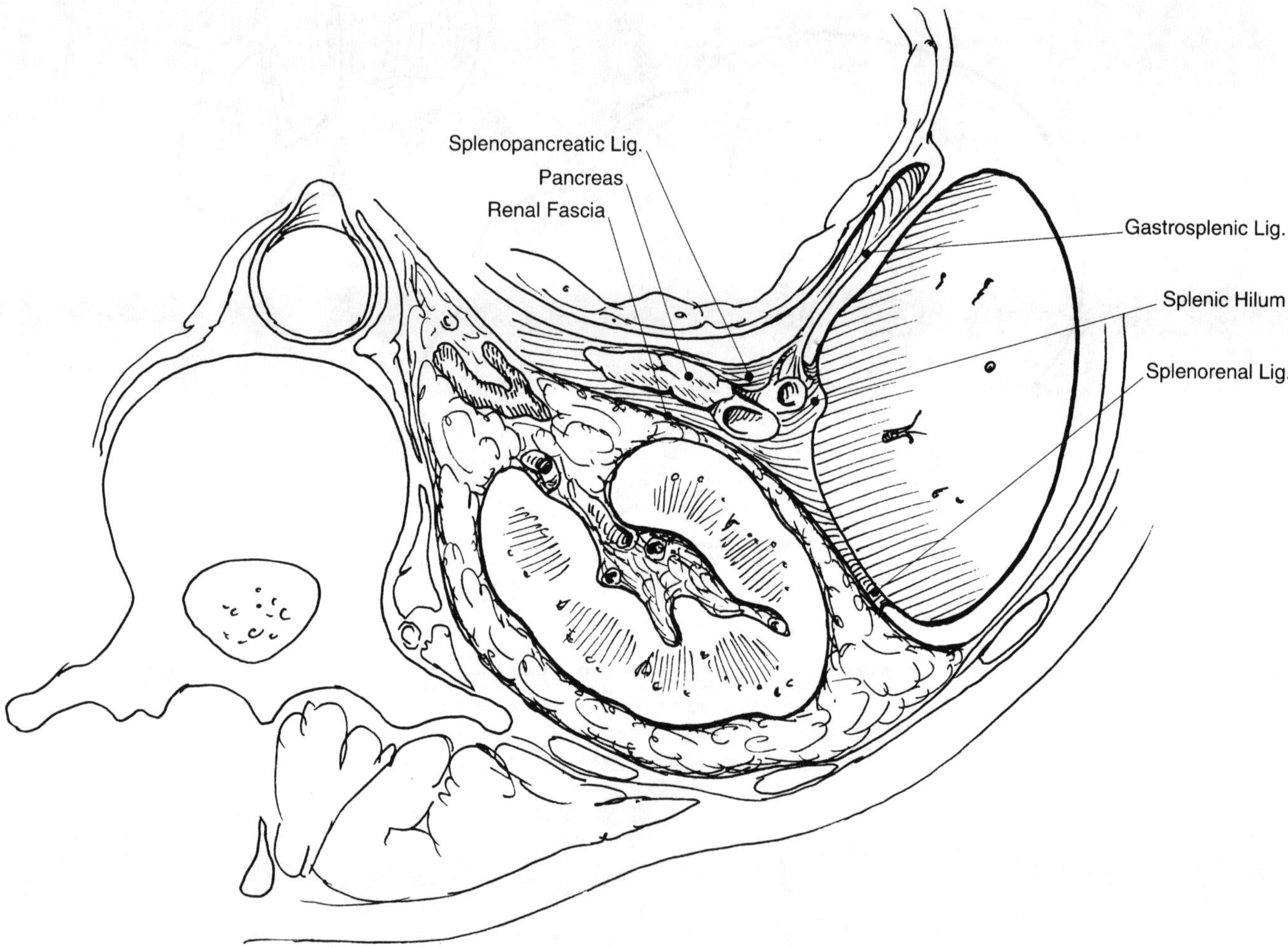

Fig. 5.8

In a sectional view (Fig. 5.9), the lower pole of the spleen diverges from the lower pole of the left kidney. The upper pole of the spleen is lateral to the left adrenal gland. The gastrosplenic ligament running from the hilum of the spleen to the greater curve of the stomach lies flattened between the gastric surface of the spleen and the posterior stomach wall. This ligament is broader at its caudal end, resulting in easier surgical access to the

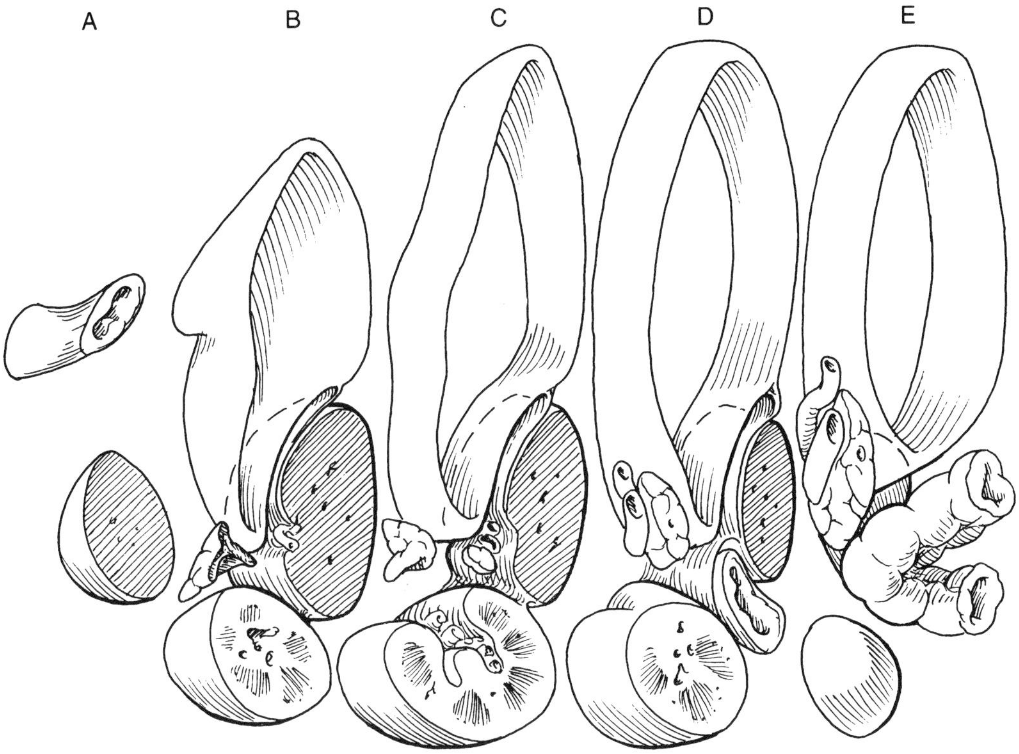

Fig. 5.9

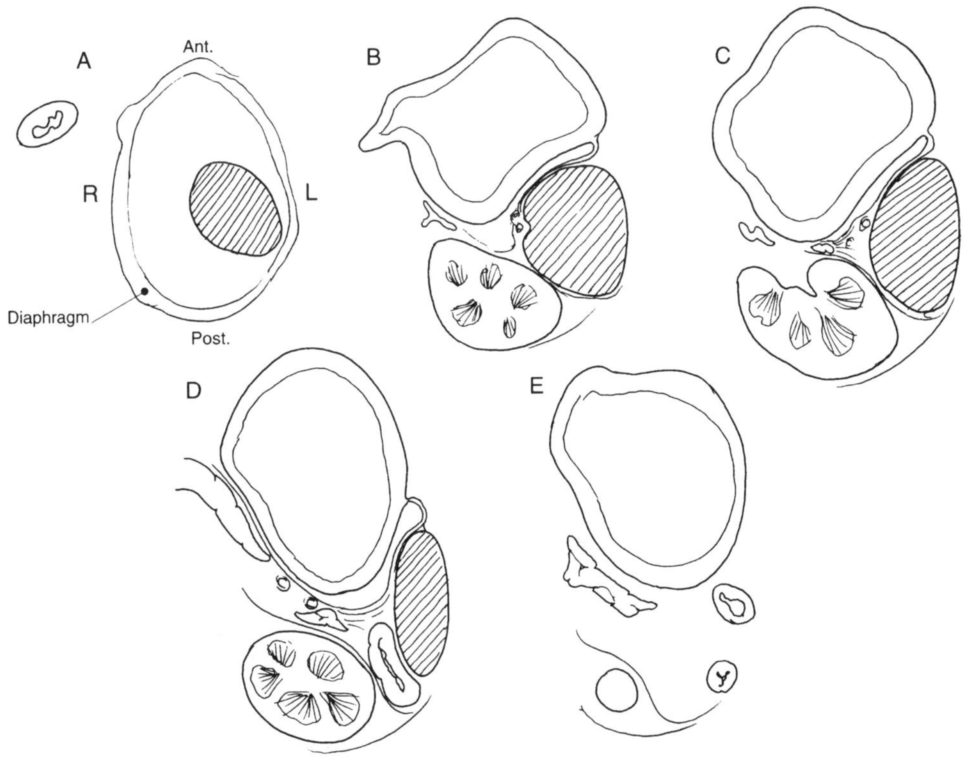

Fig. 5.9 key

short gastric vessels near the lower pole of the spleen than to the highest short gastrics at the upper pole. Between the divergent lower poles of the spleen and kidney is found the highly variable splenic flexure of the colon.

The tail of the pancreas is most often (92%) found toward the caudal end of the hilum (Fig. 5.10). It is found in close contact (70%) with (<1 cm) or touching (30%) the spleen in most cases.

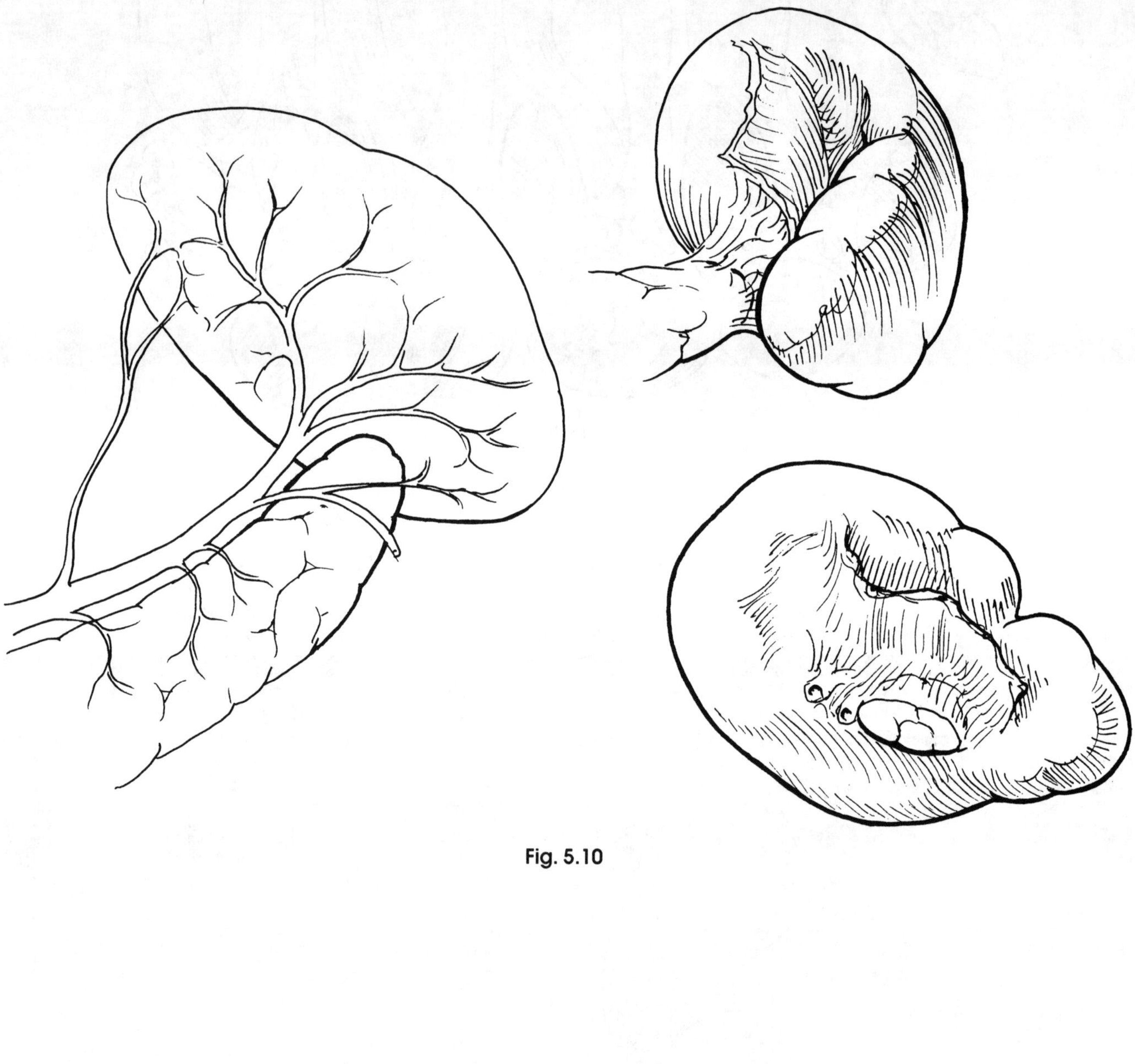

Fig. 5.10

Splenic Flexure

The splenic flexure of the colon is normally higher and more posterior than the hepatic flexure (Fig. 5.11). As can be seen from CT scan reconstructions, it varies in

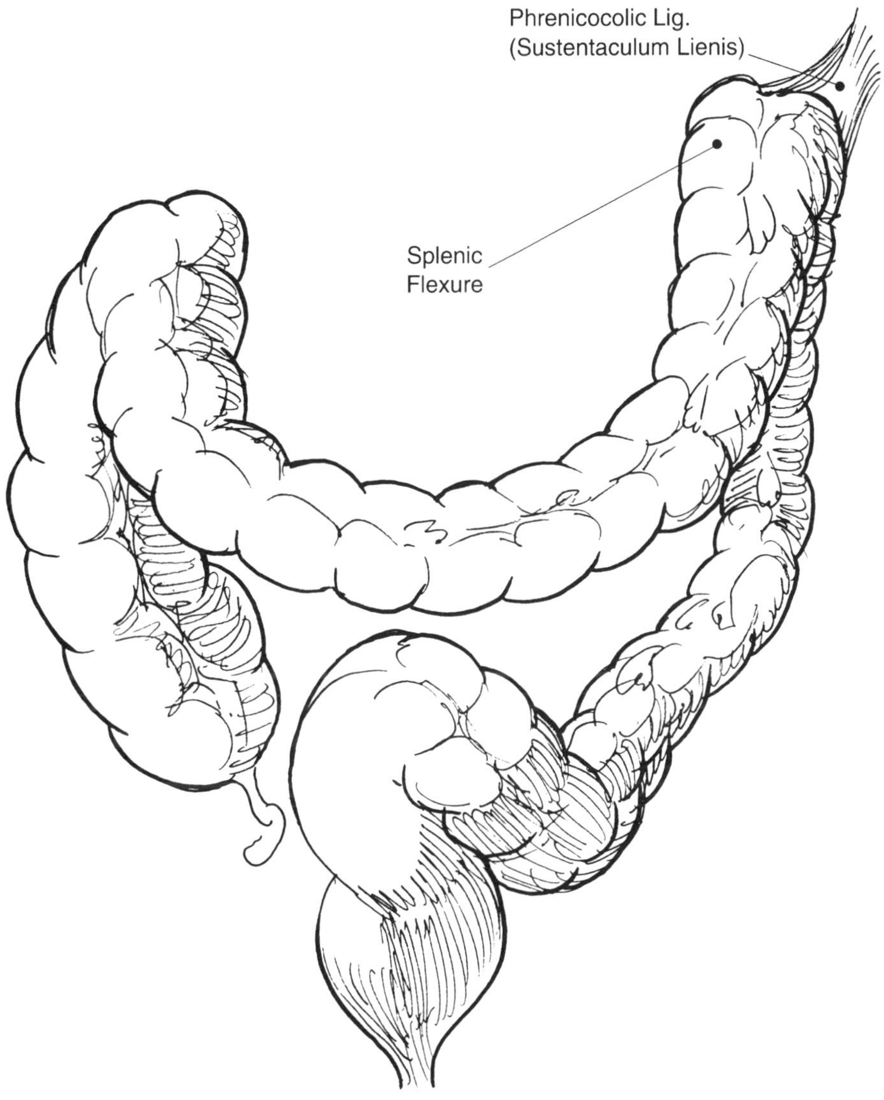

Fig. 5.11

position from individual to individual (Fig. 5.12 A-G). It may reside between the lower poles of the spleen and left kidney or it may rise between the anterior splenic border and stomach up to the dome of the diaphragm. The higher the splenic flexure rises, the more it interferes with mobilization of the spleen. In most cases the flexure is attached to the diaphragm laterally. This phrenicocolic ligament is beneath the lower pole of the spleen and separate from it. It is often described as supporting the spleen and is called the sustentaculum lienis.

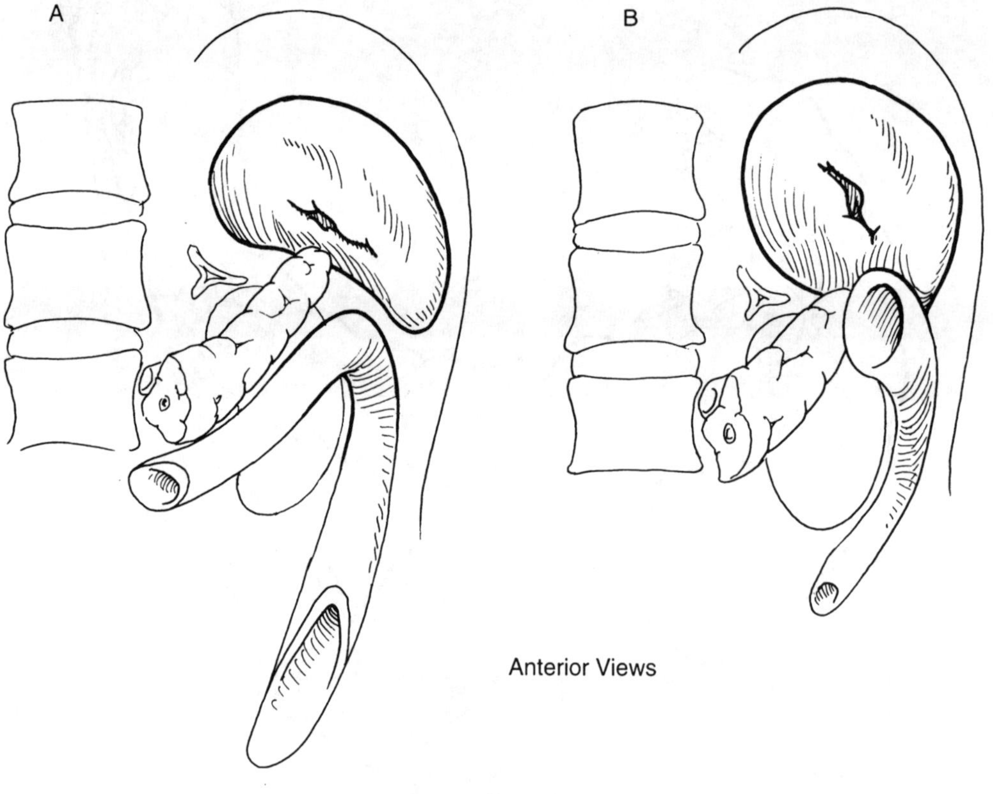

Fig. 5.12 A & B

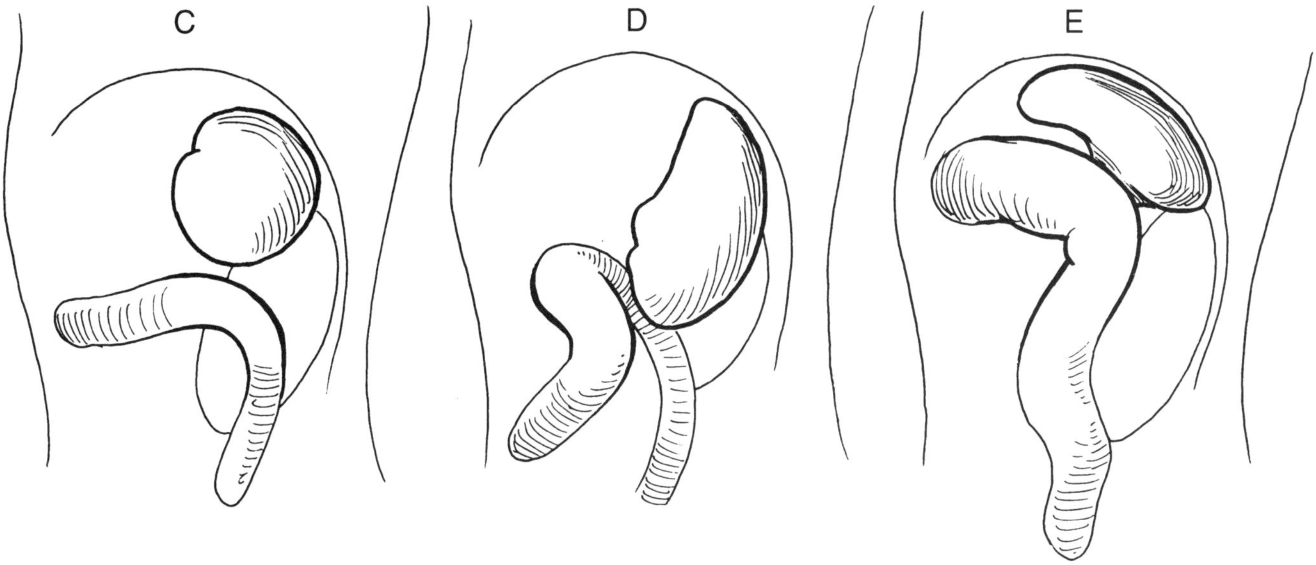

L. Lateral Views

Fig. 5.12 C, D & E

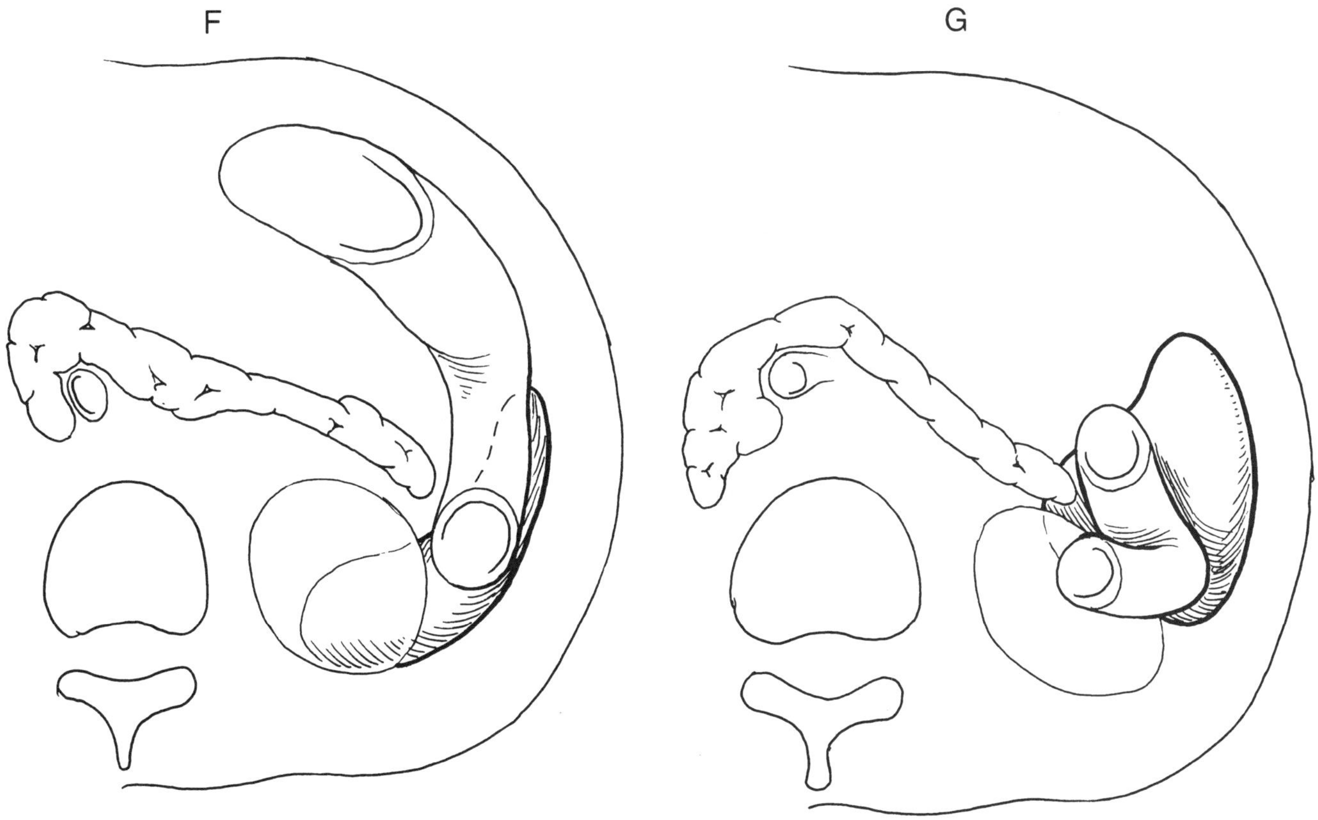

Inferior Views

Fig. 5.12 F & G

Ligaments

Descriptions of the splenic ligaments are often unnecessarily confusing. This confusion can be resolved by conceptualizing the ligaments in their embryological context (Fig. 5.1). Following the embryological dorsal mesentery from the greater curve of the stomach, one first encounters the gastrosplenic ligament (Fig. 5.13). The gastrosplenic ligament is longer inferiorly and shorter near the cardia of the stomach forming a trapezoid. The continuation of this layer along the greater curve of the stomach below the spleen is the gastrocolic portion of the greater omentum containing the left gastroepiploic vessels.

Continuing posteromedially from the splenic hilum across the back wall of the lesser sac, the peritoneum covering the pancreas and splenic vessels was originally the right side of the dorsal mesogastrium. The fusion fascia of the left side of the dorsal mesogastrium and the posterior parietal peritoneum lies between the pancreas and the renal fascia. The lateral border of the fusion lies just inside the posterior margin of the spleen is called the splenorenal ligament (Fig. 5.8). The upper part of the fusion boundary (peritoneal reflection) extends above the kidney and attaches the spleen to the diaphragm. There it is called the splenophrenic ligament and is the last connection of the spleen divided in laparoscopic splenectomy.

There is usually a secondary adherence between the lower pole of the spleen and the splenic flexure of the colon called the splenocolic ligament. The final "ligament" in the area is the connection between the tail of the pancreas and the left transverse colon which is the

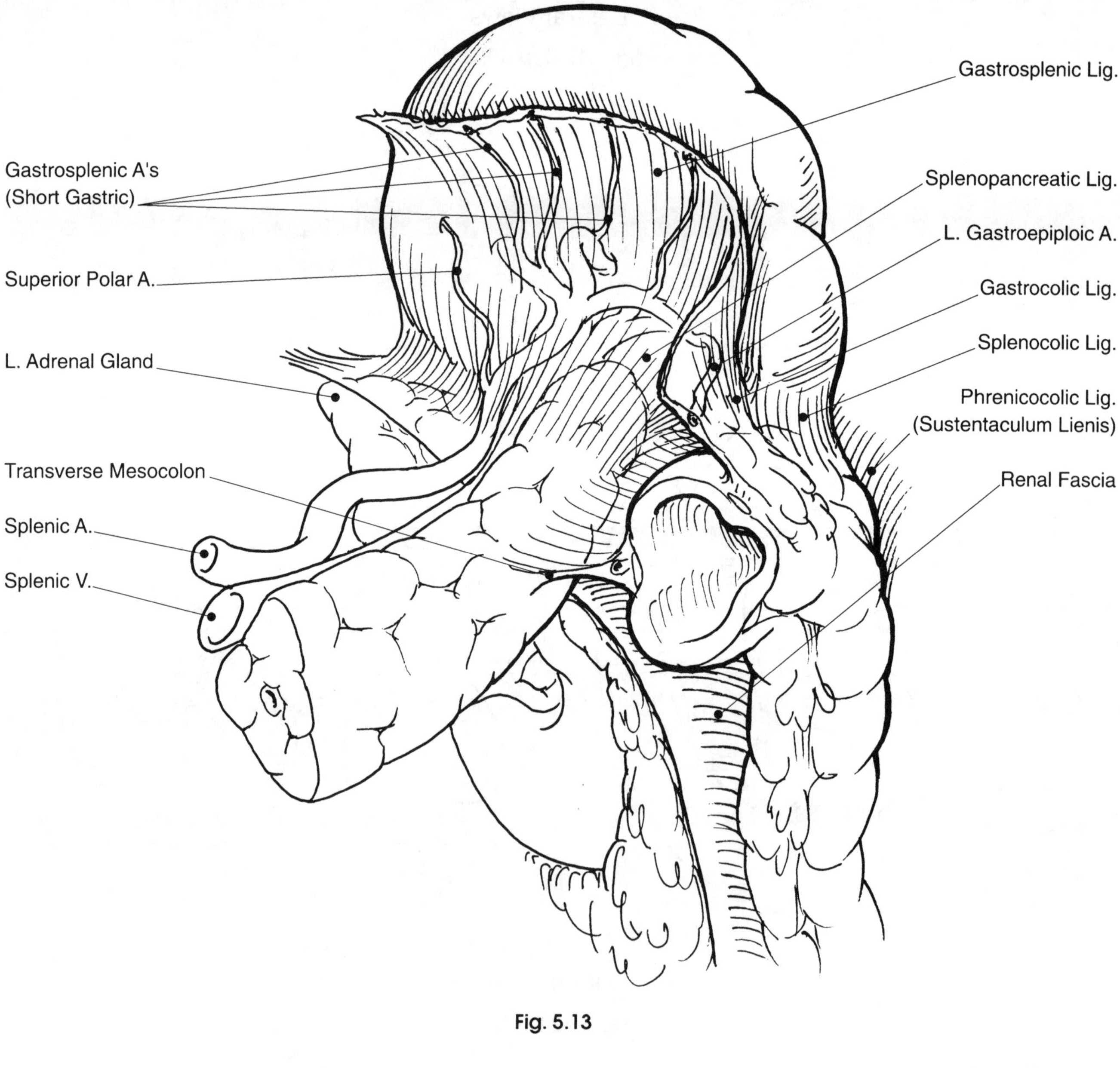

Fig. 5.13

left extremity of the transverse mesocolon. The phrenicocolic ligament mentioned above is in contact with the lower pole of the spleen but is not attached.

Accessory Spleens

Accessory splenic tissue may be found with an incidence of 10 to 20%. There are usually no more than one or two but rarely accessory spleens may be more numerous (Fig. 5.14A). They are small, measuring 1 to 3 cm. As would be expected, most are found in areas derived from the dorsal mesogastrium. They are most often found in the splenic hilum, splenic pedicle, anterior border of the spleen and greater omentum (Fig. 5.14B). They become clinically important in hematological disorders.

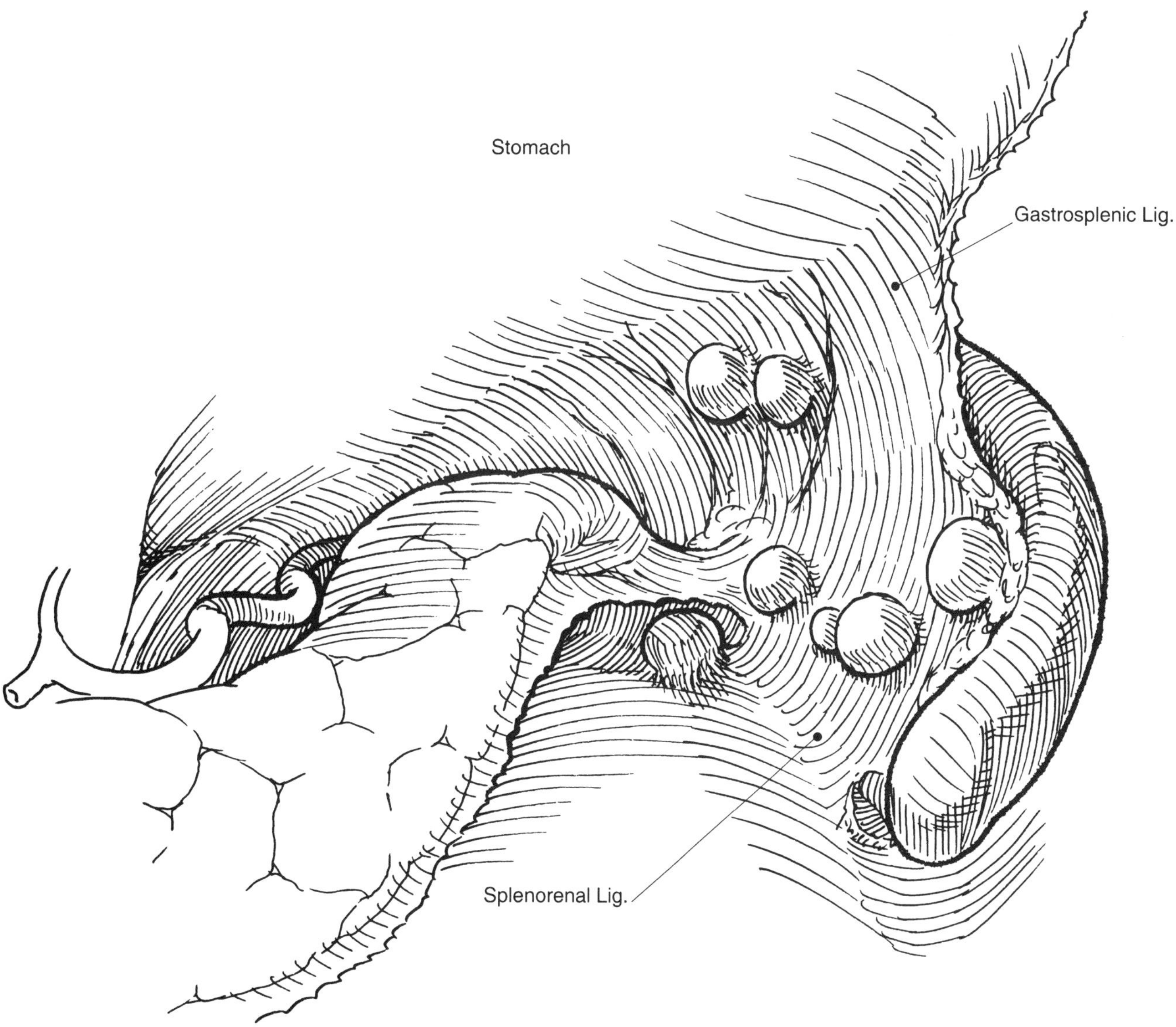

Fig. 5.14A

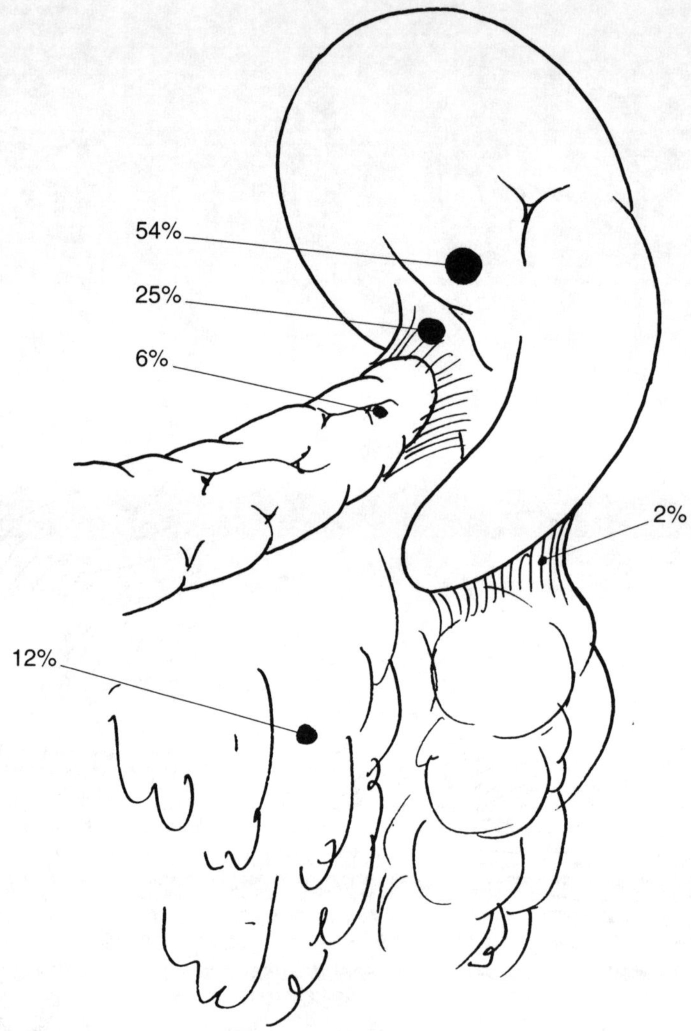

Fig. 5.14B

Splenic Vessels

The splenic artery is highly variable in its tortuosity, its pancreatic branches and its terminal branching pattern. The origin of the splenic artery is usually (~90%) from a three-branched celiac trunk (Chapter 4). The artery follows a serpentine course cephalad to the pancreatic body and tail deep to the posterior peritoneum of the lesser sac (Fig. 5.15). The splenic artery provides the major blood supply to the body and tail of the pancreas through four to five branches, two of which are usually dominant. In 60% of individuals a major branch, the dorsal pancreatic, arises from the proximal splenic artery or celiac trunk. At the distal third of the pancreas, a more constant branch, the great pancreatic artery (pancreatica magna) enters the gland. Significant anastomoses between vessels of the body and tail of the pancreas are found only 60% of the time. For this reason, the great pancreatic artery should be preserved when ligating or embolizing the splenic artery before splenectomy to avoid devascularization of the pancreatic tail. About a third of individuals have a posterior gastric artery arising from the distal splenic artery (Chapter 4).

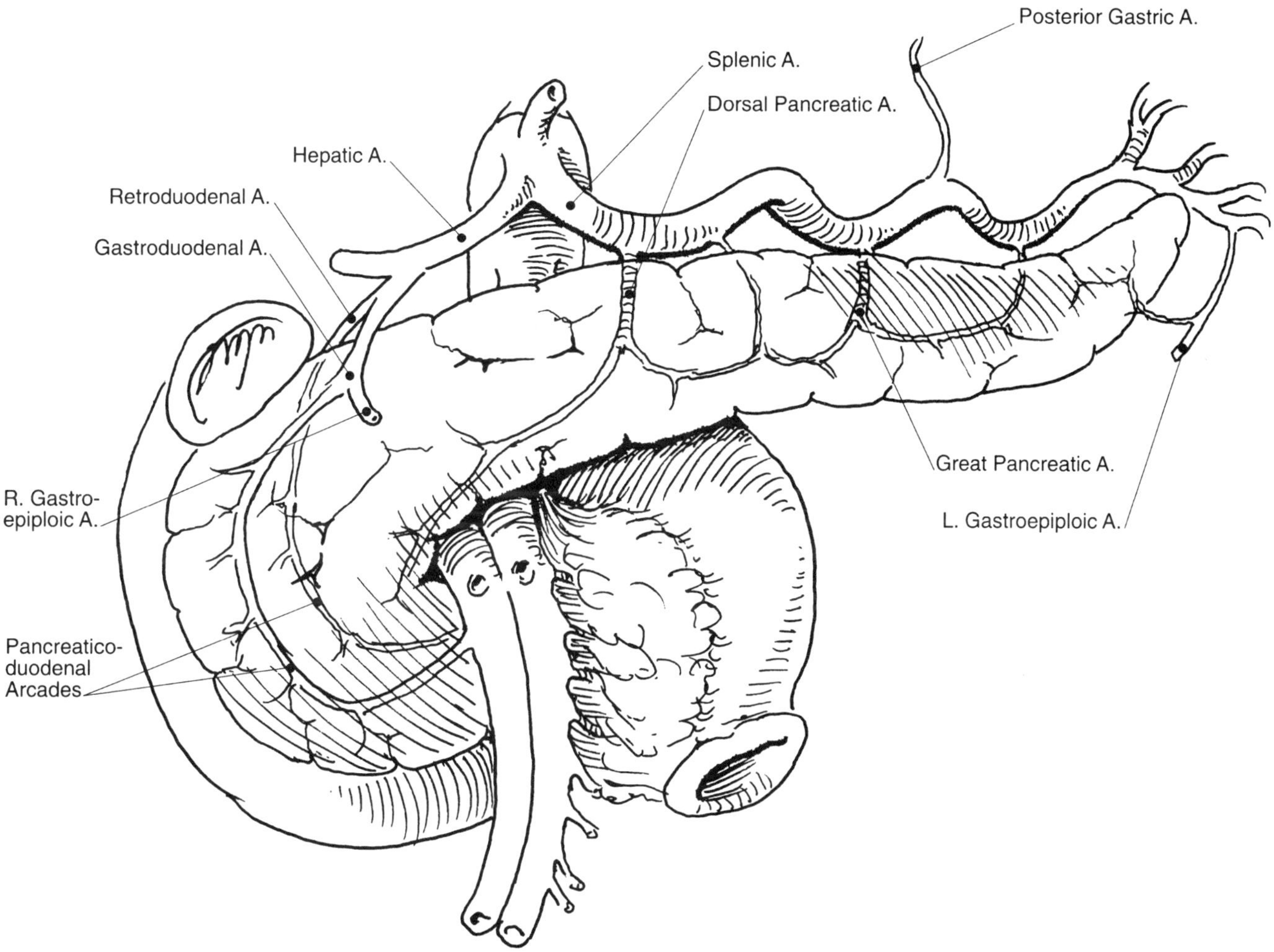

Fig. 5.15

The splenic artery is accessible in the lesser sac through the gastrohepatic omentum or, more convenient laparoscopically, through the gastrocolic omentum (Fig. 5.16). There it can be clipped before mobilizing the spleen, allowing splenic decompression for easier, safer manipulation.

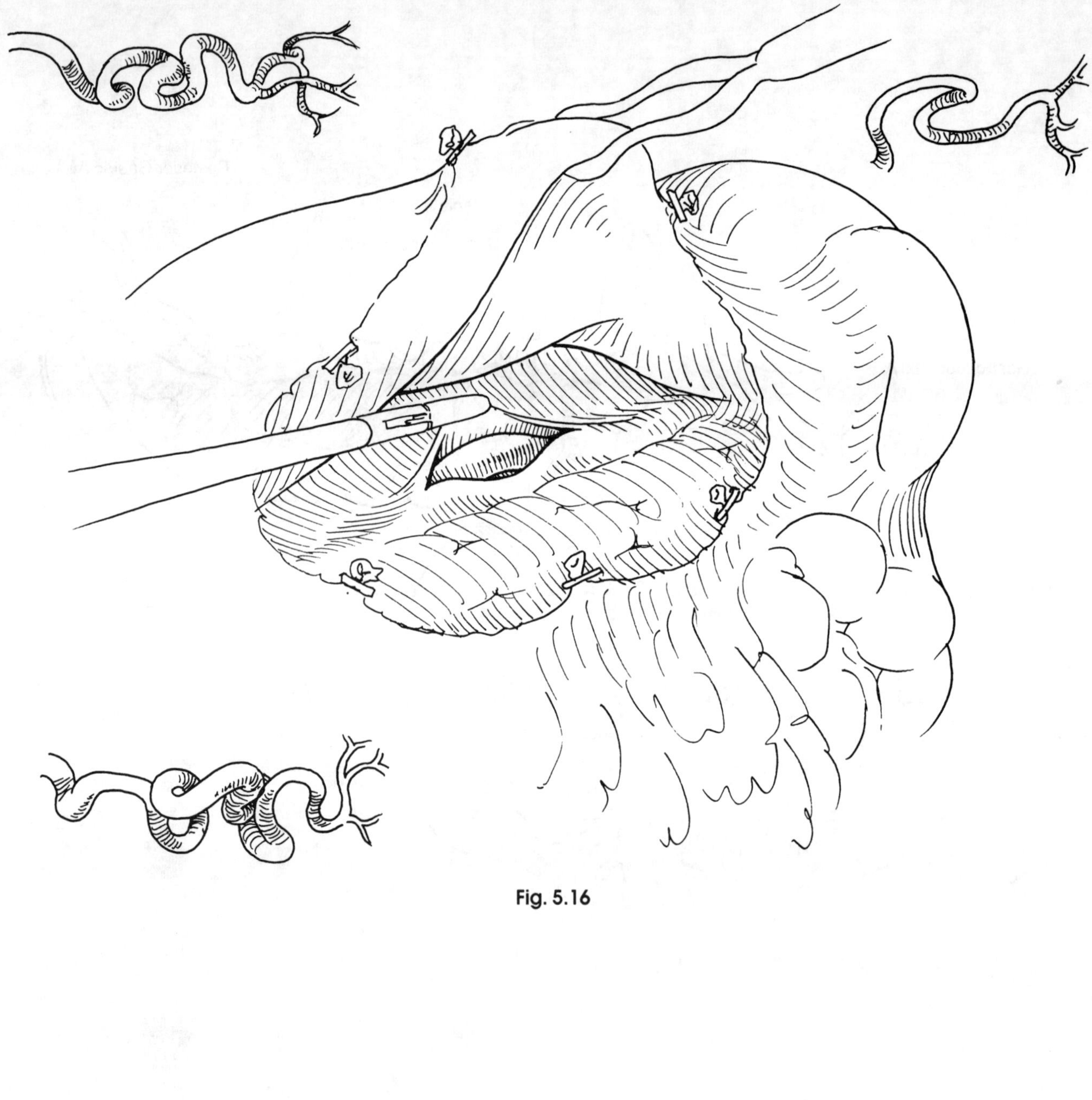

Fig. 5.16

As it approaches the splenic hilum, the splenic artery usually (~70–80%) divides into two main branches, less commonly into three (Fig. 5.17). The variable branching patterns are categorized in the literature according to the distance from the hilum of the primary branching: early branching giving a distributed pattern of vessels across a wide area of the hilar surface and a late branching (magistral pattern) giving a more compact cluster of vessels at the hilus. The distributed pattern is the more common, seen in about two thirds of individuals and the wider spread of vessels results in easier surgical access. The notching of the anterior splenic border reflects the segmental nature of the spleen.

One or more polar vessels occur in two thirds of indi-

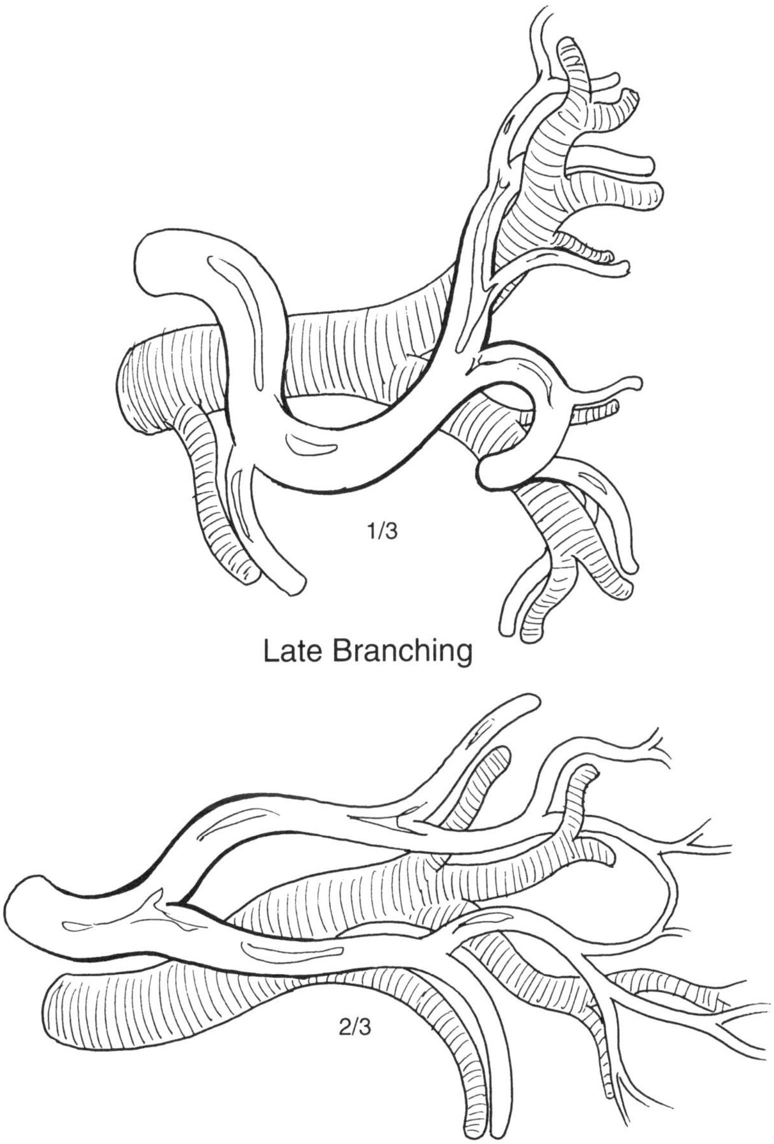

Early Branching

Fig. 5.17

viduals. One third of individuals have a superior polar vessel and about half have an inferior polar vessel. The superior polar artery arises from the distal splenic trunk and the inferior polar commonly arises from the left gastroepiploic artery (Fig. 5.18).

The gastrosplenic (short gastric) vessels extend from

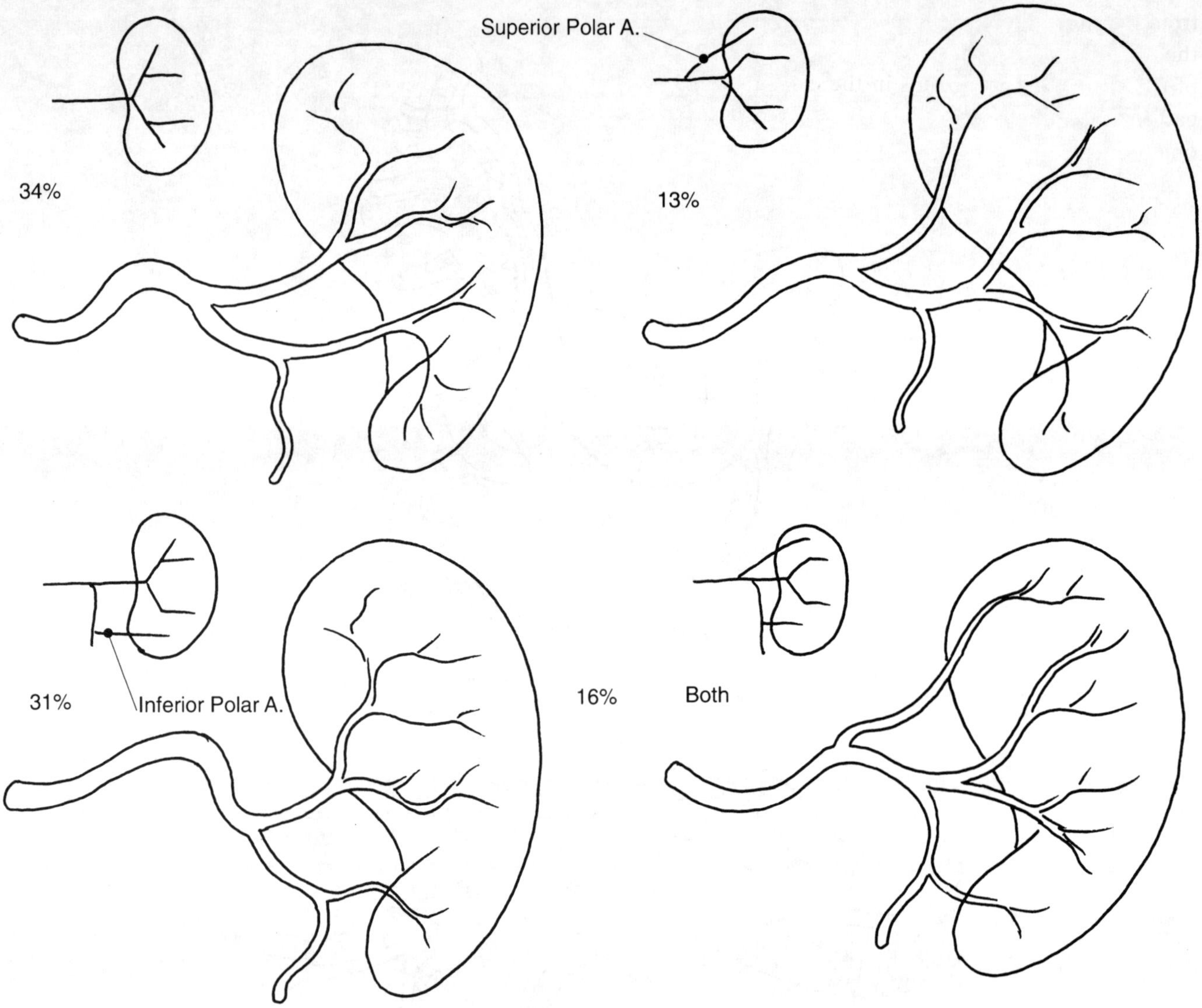

Fig. 5.18

hilar branches of the splenic artery across the gastric surface of the spleen in the gastrosplenic ligament to reach the greater curve of the stomach (Fig. 5.19). The gastrosplenic ligament is widest near the lower pole of the spleen and narrowest near the upper pole. There are usually six or fewer short gastric arteries. The highest short gastric artery is found in the short portion of the gastrosplenic ligament far posterior at the cardia of the stomach.

The left gastroepiploic artery usually (72%) arises from the splenic trunk before the primary branching. In the remainder, it arises from an inferior terminal branch of the splenic artery. It runs in the continuation of the gastrosplenic ligament as it becomes the gastrocolic omentum.

LAPAROSCOPIC SPLENECTOMY

Patient Preparation

To safely gain the benefits of reduced morbidity afforded by laparoscopy for patients requiring splenectomy, a combination of careful patient selection, meticulous technique and clear anatomic understanding must be applied. Because of the limited access afforded by the location of the spleen, only patients with a normal (~11 cm pole to pole length) or moderately enlarged (11–20 cm) spleen (eg. ITP, Hodgkin's staging) are currently considered reasonable laparoscopic candidates. Splenic size is assessed with pre-operative ultrasound. Because the upper pole is difficult to assess by ultrasound in larger spleens, CT scan can be used to resolve doubts. The

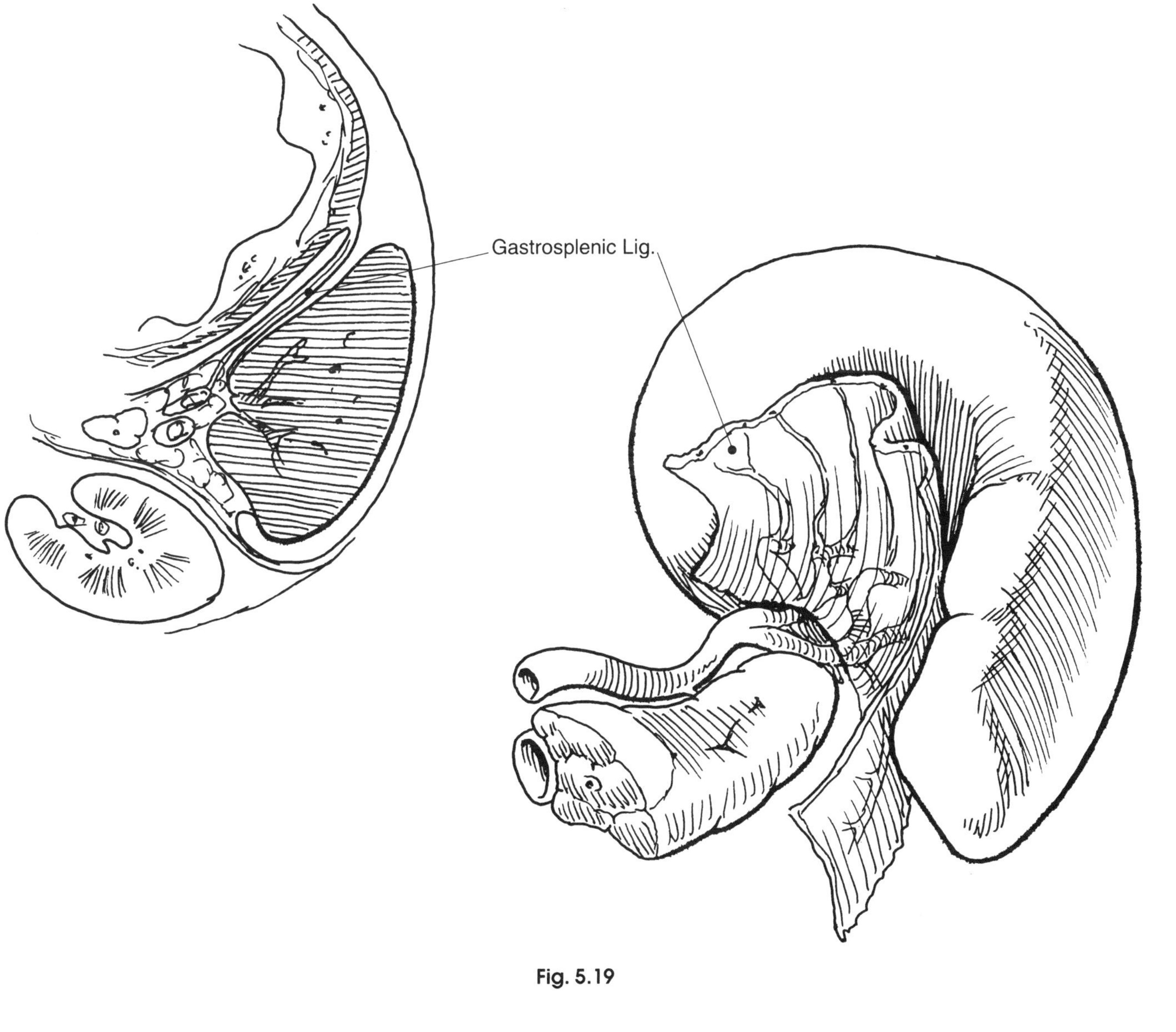

Fig. 5.19

bulk of a massively enlarged spleen filling the left upper quadrant poses prohibitive technical and safety problems. Preoperative embolization or distal clipping of the splenic artery in the lesser sac was advocated by some in the early experience with laparoscopic splenectomy to decrease blood loss and the risk of uncontrolled hemorrhage. Embolization is done with microcoils and is aimed at infarcting 80% of the splenic parenchyma (Poulin) while taking care to preserve the pancreatica magna artery. The angiographic information on the vascular pattern is also helpful in operative planning. Embolization does cause some pain, so the procedure is done the morning of surgery. Early enthusiasm for embolization has decreased, perhaps as a result of increased experience with the technique.

Position and Ports

The supine position used in the earlier experience with laparoscopic splenectomy has given way to a right lateral decubitus position similar to that used for a left lateral thoracotomy (Fig.5.20). Exploration for accessory spleens is easier supine and some surgeons start supine when operating for hematologic disease and then rotate

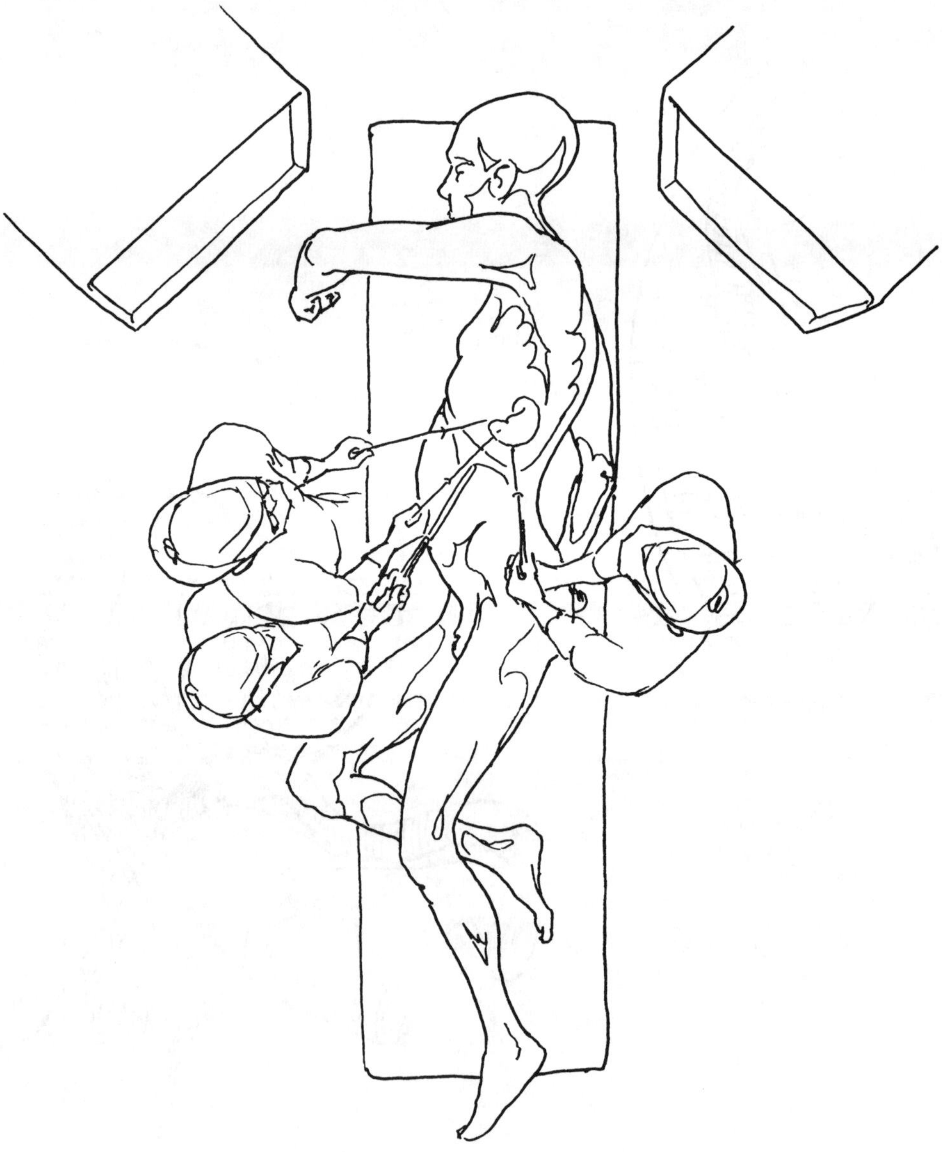

Fig. 5.20

the patient. The kidney rest is raised or the table is broken slightly to open the flank space between the ribs and the iliac crest, reverse Trendelenburg is added and the patient is rotated slightly to the anterior side. The insufflation and first camera port are placed at the umbilicus. A 30 or 45 degree telescope is used. An additional four ports are placed in an arc around the anterolateral rib cage margin (Fig. 5.21). The fourth, posterior axillary

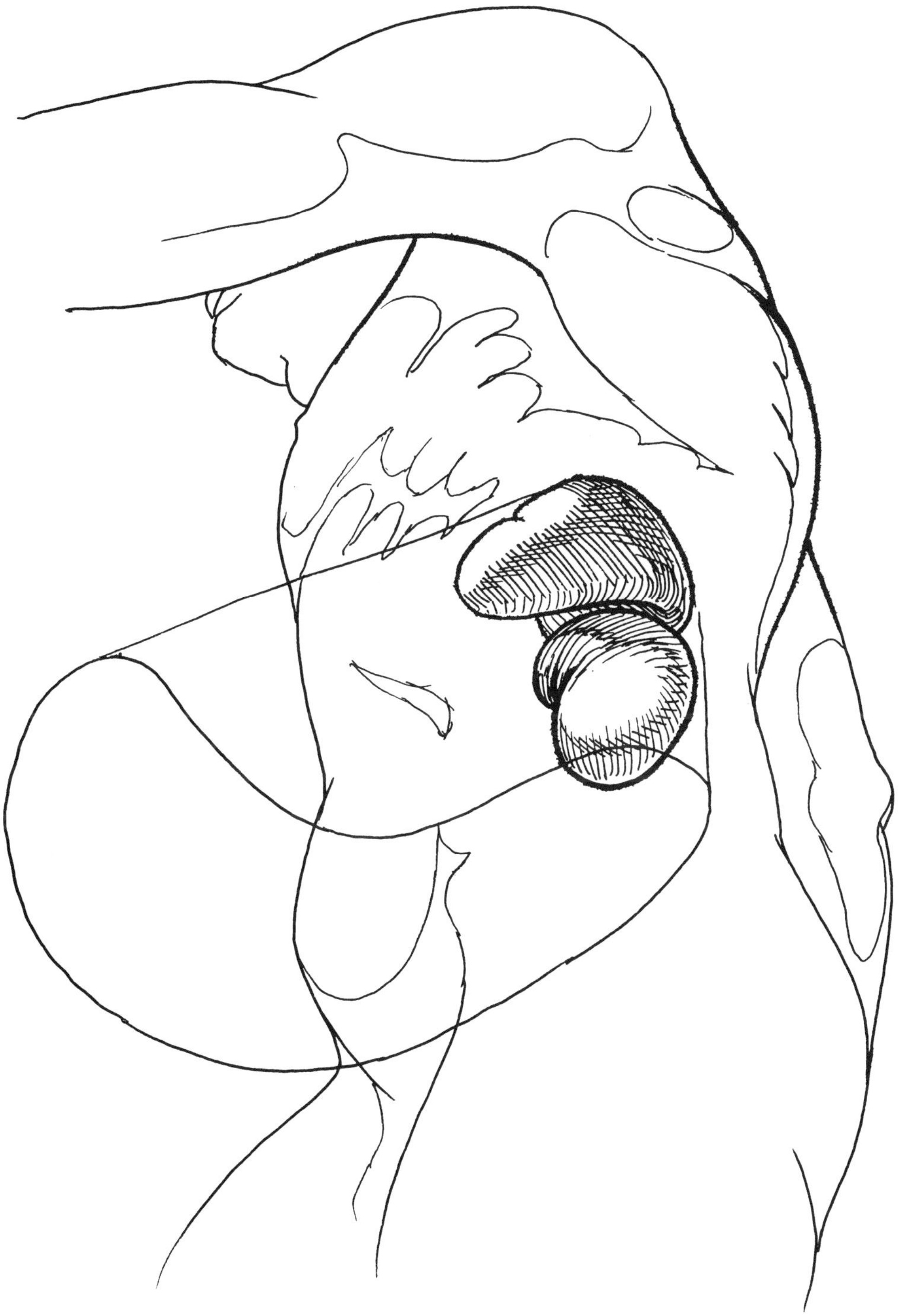

Fig. 5.21

line port is placed after the splenic flexure of the colon has been mobilized. In this position the abdominal organs drop away from the spleen and leave the spleen suspended from its renal and diaphragmatic attachments (Fig. 5.22).

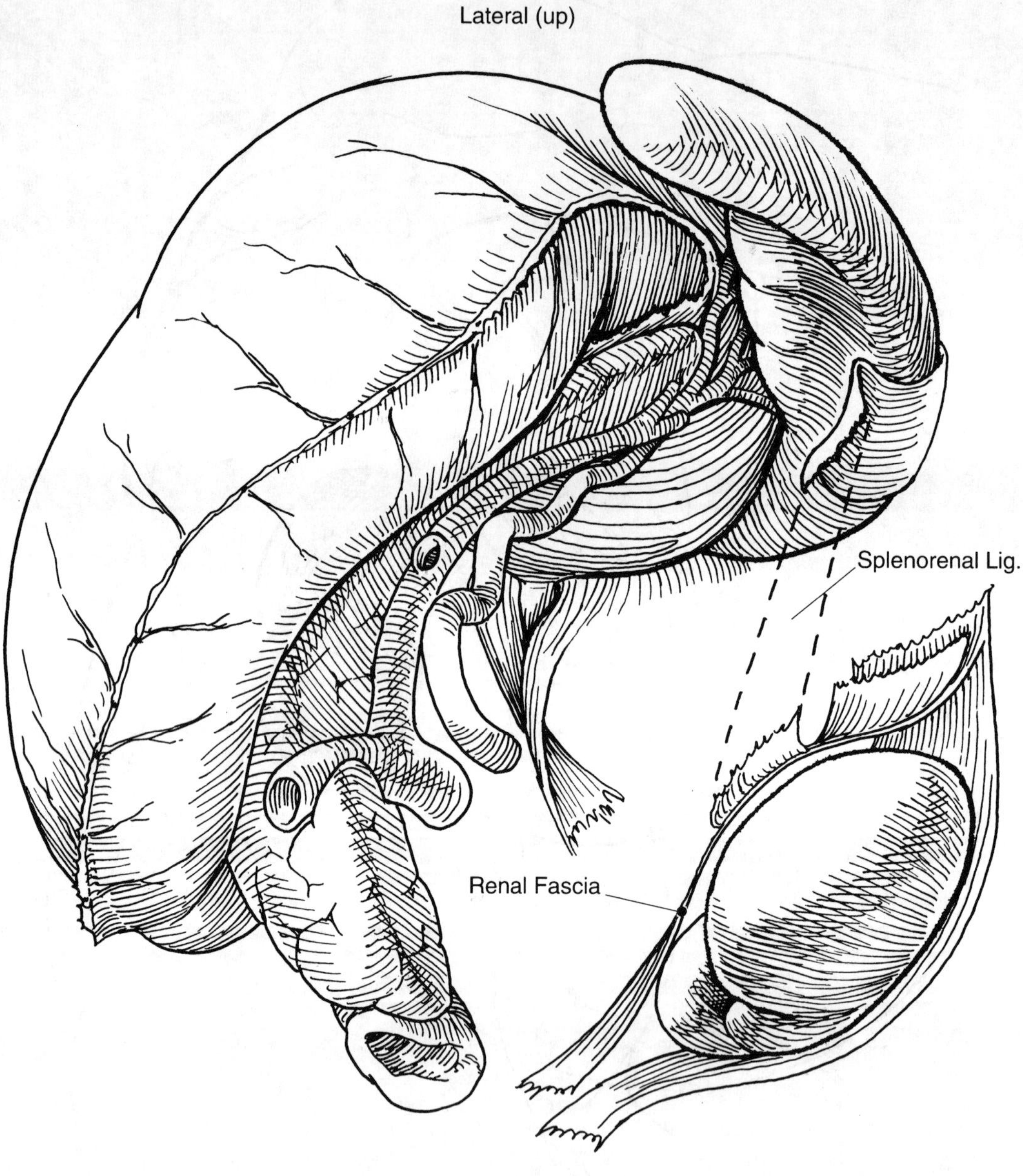

Fig. 5.22

Mobilization

Dissection is begun at the peritoneal reflection of the proximal descending colon, working up toward the splenic flexure (Fig. 5.23). The phrenicocolic ligament at the splenic flexure, the so called suspensory ligament (sustentaculum lienis) of the spleen, is divided up to the splenorenal ligament. The splenocolic attachments and

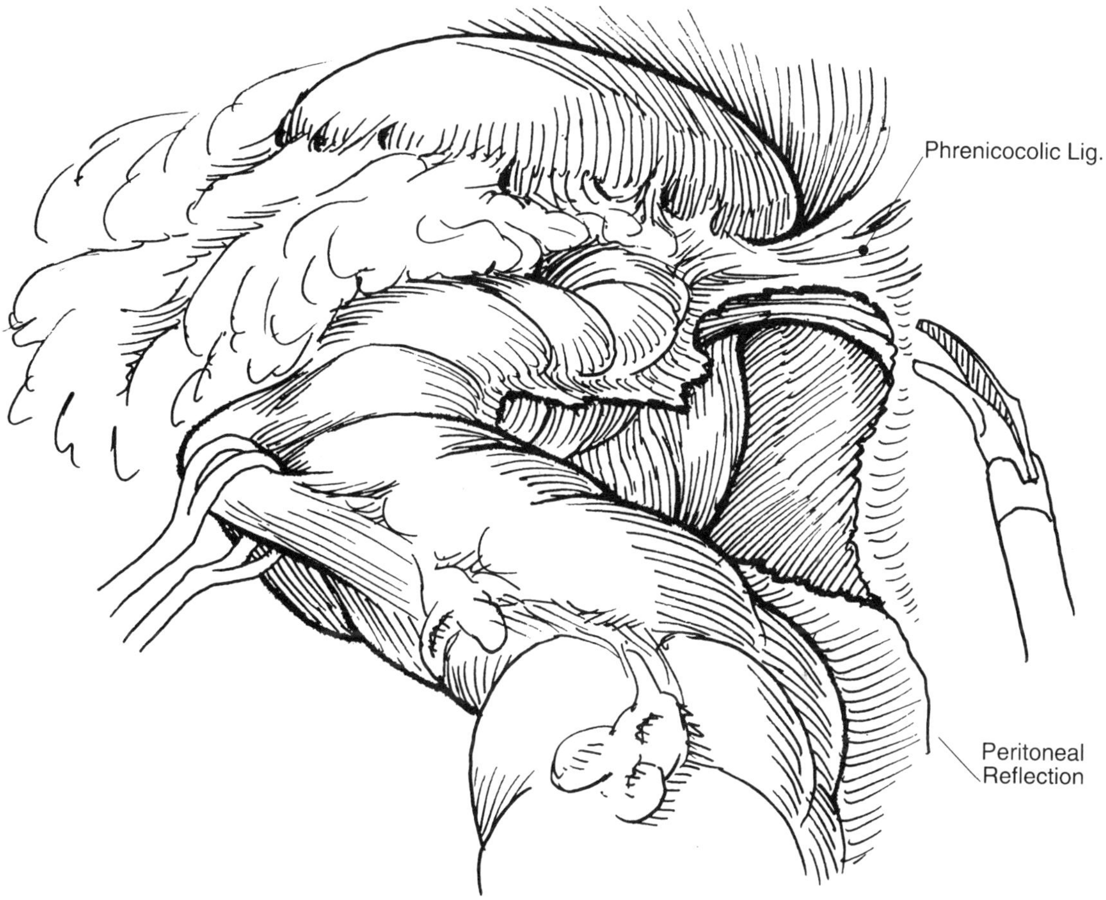

Fig. 5.23

the lower part of the splenorenal ligament are then divided with cautery scissors, freeing the lower pole of the spleen (Fig. 5.24). The lower pole of the spleen is elevated with a blunt instrument exposing the lower pole vessels in the splenic hilum.

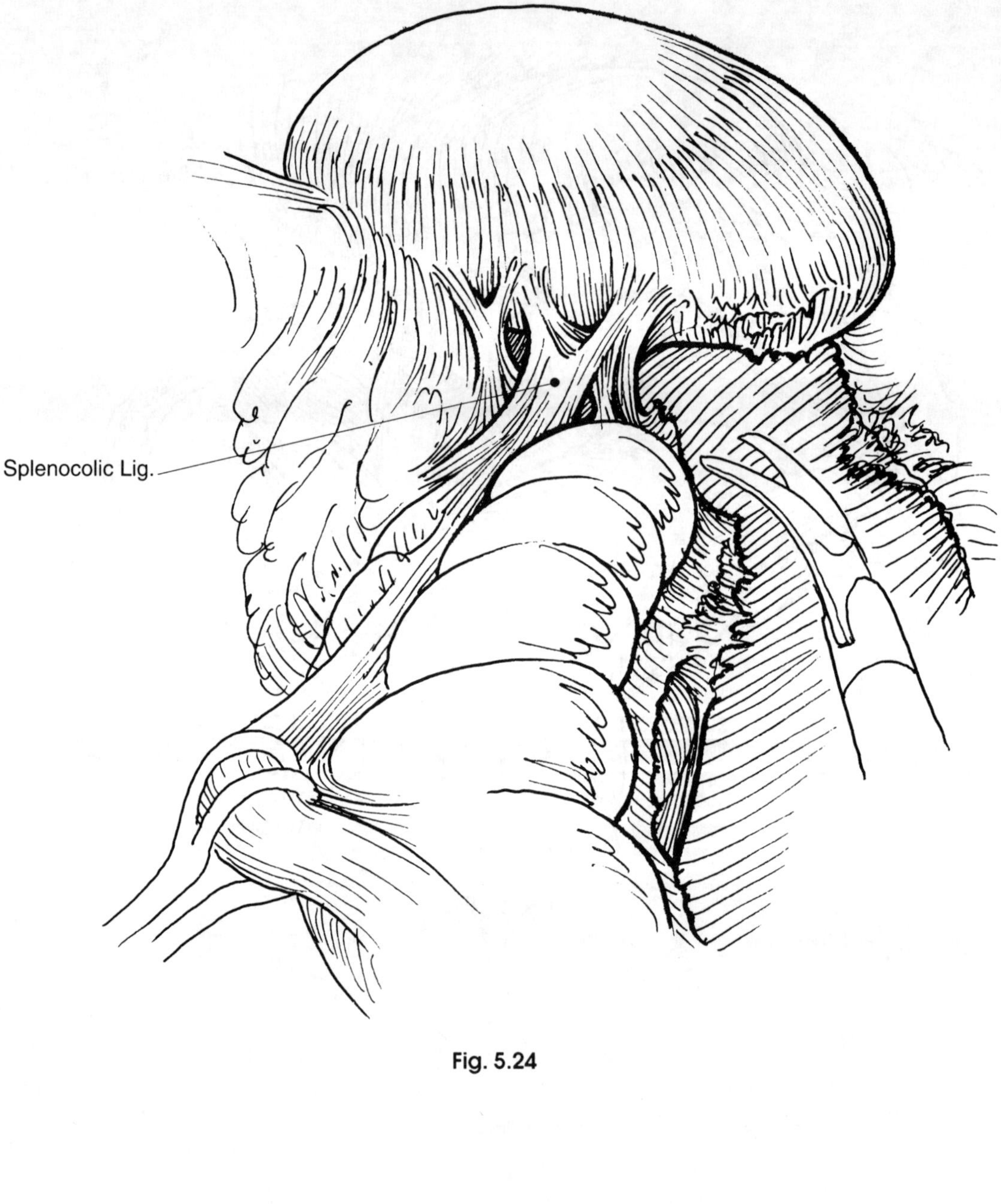

Fig. 5.24

The lower splenic hilar vessels are carefully dissected individually and clipped close to the hilus with large (10mm) clips, two proximal, one distal (Fig. 5.25). Alternately, the hilar vessels can be divided in groups with the linear stapler using a vascular cartridge. Two or three applications are used. As the hilar vessels are divided, the tail of the pancreas falls away from the spleen, leaving the spleen attached by the splenophrenic ligament posteriorly and by the gastrosplenic ligament anteriorly. The gastrosplenic ligament is next divided, secur-

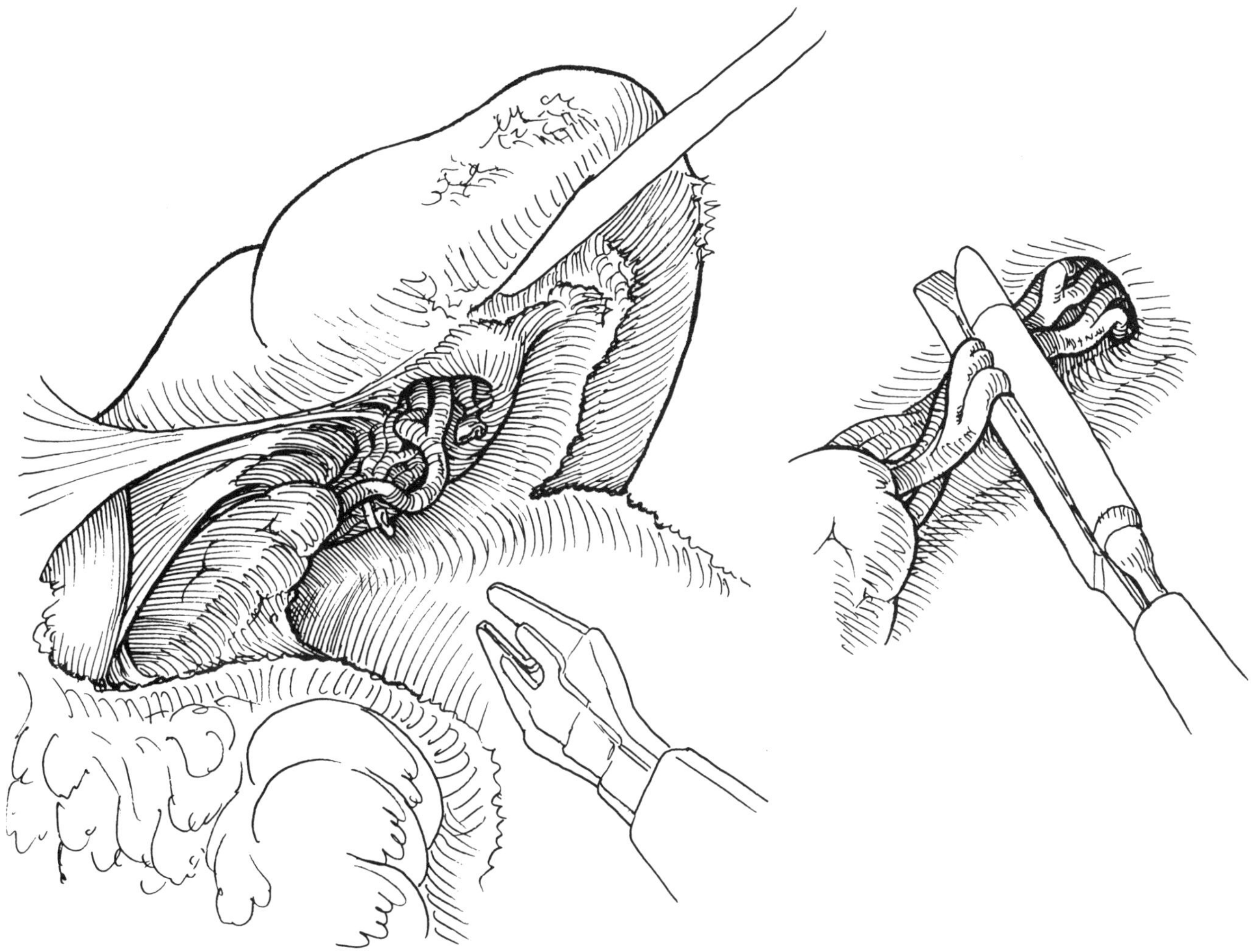

Fig. 5.25

ing the short gastric vessels in turn. The spleen can then be elevated and the last attachment at the splenophrenic ligament is divided with cautery scissors (Fig. 5.26).

The spleen is placed in a sturdy plastic bag and mechanically fragmented and aspirated from the sac.

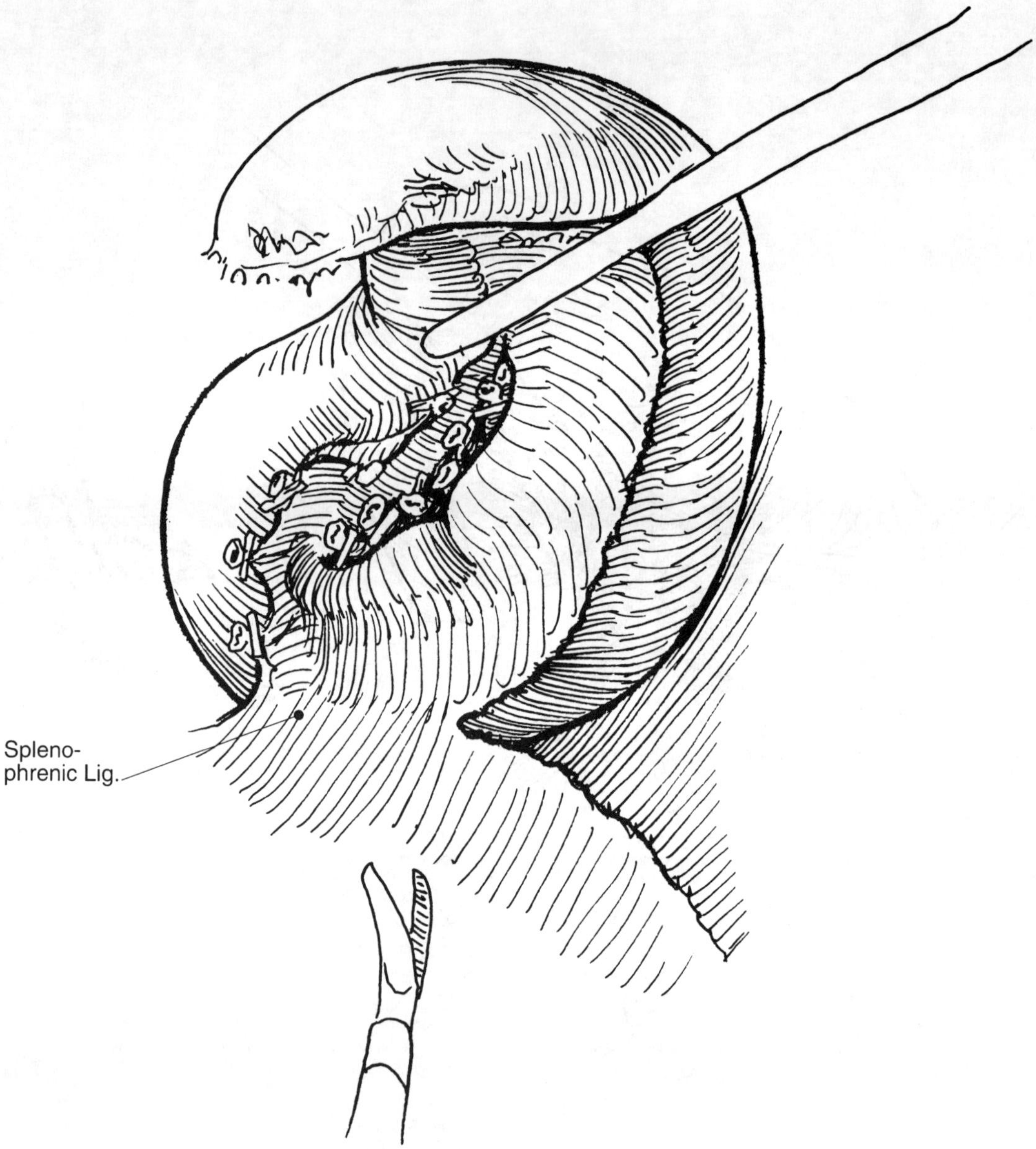

Fig. 5.26

Chapter 5: The Spleen

EMBRYOLOGY

Skandalakis JE, Gray SW. Embryology for Surgeons, Philadelphia: Williams & Wilkins, 1994:334–365.

ANATOMY

Bergman RA, Thompson SA, Afifi AK, et. al. Compendium of Human Anatomic Variation. Urban & Schwarzenberg. Baltimore-Munich. 1988:167–169.

Cuschieri A. Anatomy according to the laparoscope: left upper quadrant, eosophagus, stomach and spleen. (abstract), SAGES, 1995;??:??–??.

Fiedor P, et al. Variability of the arterial system of the human pancreas. Clin Anat 1993;6:213–216.

Gray H, Goss CM eds. Anatomy of the Human Body. Philadelphia, Lea & Febiger. 1959:1287.

Marwan F, et al. Multiple accessory spleens: case report and literature review. Clin Anat 1993;6:232–239.

Poulin EC, Thibault C. The anatomic basis for laparoscopic splenectomy. J.C.C. 1993;36:484–488.

Skandalakis PN, Colborn GL, Skandalakis LJ, et. al. The surgical anatomy of the spleen. Surg Clin North Am 1993;73:747–767.

Sylvester PA. et al. Tortuosity of the human splenic artery. Clin Anat 1995;8:214–218.

Treutner KH, Klosterhalfen B, Winkeltau G, et. al. Vascular anatomy of the spleen: the basis for organ preserving surgery. Clin Anat 1993;6:1–8.

SURGERY

Caroll BJ, Phillips EH, Semel CJ, et al. Laparoscopic splenectomy. Surg Endosc 1992;6:183–184.

Cushieri A, Shimi S, Banting S, et al. Technical aspects of laparoscopic splenectomy: hilar segmental devascularization and instrumentation. J R Coll Sur Edinb 1992; 37:414–416.

Delaitre B, Maignien B, Icard Ph. Laparoscopic splenectomy-the "hanged spleen" technique. Surg Endosc 1995;9: 528–529.

Flowers JL. Laparoscopic Splenectomy. In: Zucker K ed. et al. Surgical Laparoscopy Update. St. Louis, Quality Medical Publishing, Inc. 1993:357–371.

Poulin EC, et al. Laparoscopic splenectomy. Surg Endosc 1995;9:172–177.

Seufert RM, et al. Surgery of the Spleen, New York: Thieme, Inc., 1986:1-6,83–102.

Thibault C, Mamazza J, LeTourneau R, et al. Laparoscopic splenectomy: operative technique and preliminary report. Surg Laparosc Endosc 1992;2:248–253.

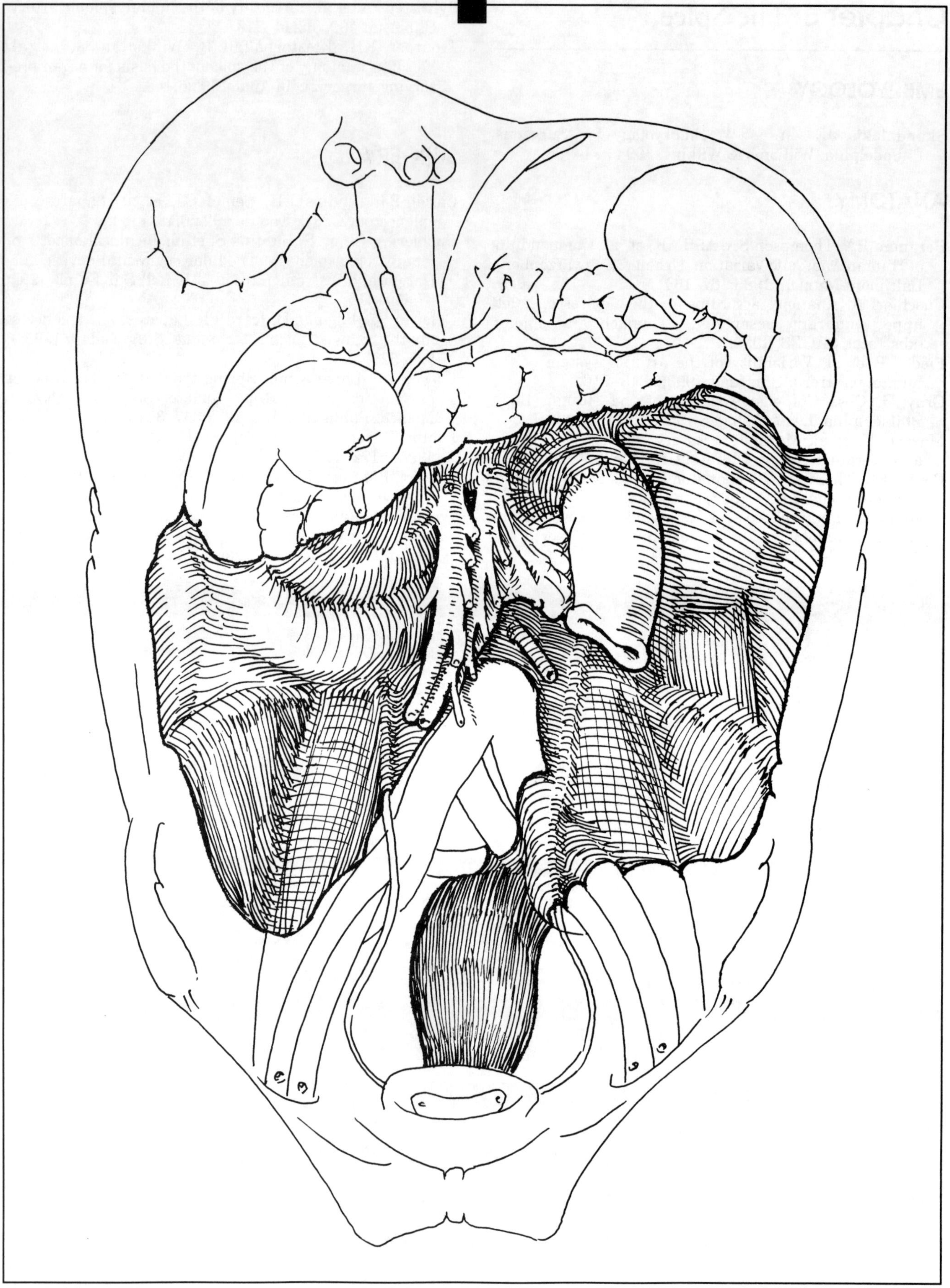

6

The Colon

EMBRYOLOGY

By the beginning of gestational week three, the embryonic gut consists of enclosed foregut and hindgut regions bracketing the midgut which is open to the yolk sac. The foregut will evolve into pharynx, esophagus and stomach, the midgut will become small bowel and proximal colon and the hindgut will become distal colon and rectum. One of the midline vitelline arteries to the yolk sac will become dominant and the others will regress leaving the midgut territory supplied by the superior mesenteric artery. The superior mesenteric artery acts as the axis around which the midgut rotates in a counterclockwise direction.

Elongation and rotation of the midgut takes place in three stages beginning at the end of week five. The connection between the midgut and the yolk sac has narrowed to a thin stalk at this time and acts as a lead point as the midgut bows ventrally toward the umbilicus (Fig. 6.1A). The future cecum is marked by a dilatation of the bowel just caudal to the yolk stalk. The midgut grows into the base of the umbilicus forming a "herniation" which will contain several loops of bowel (Fig. 6.1B). During this first stage, the herniated bowel undergoes a ninety degree counterclockwise rotation (Fig. 6.1C).

At the beginning of the first stage, the prearterial (relative to the superior mesenteric artery) portion of herniated midgut lies cranial to the postarterial segment. The prearterial side elongates faster than the postarterial side forming several loops (Fig. 6.1D). At about the eighth week, the apex of the cecum lags behind the growth of the rest of the cecum, forming the appendix. Initially in a central position at the taeneal convergence, the appendix is finally displaced medially in most individuals by differential haustral growth. While this growth is occurring, counterclockwise rotation leaves the elongated prearterial gut to the right of the cecal region, setting the stage for the return of the gut to the abdominal cavity.

The second stage of midgut development is the return of the gut to the abdominal cavity and a further 180° counterclockwise rotation. By a mechanism that is not clearly understood, the herniated gut abruptly returns to the abdominal cavity during the tenth week (Fig. 6.1E). The elongated prearterial loops reenter first, pushing the intraabdominal colon to the left. The cecal region returns last while continuing to rotate counterclockwise, leaving the colon anterior to the superior mesenteric artery (Fig. 6.1F). Due to the large size of the liver at this time, the proximal colon is displaced caudally in the abdominal cavity. Most anomalies of colon anatomy occur during this stage.

The third stage of midgut development is the completion of rotation and fixation of the colon to the abdominal wall. The final positioning proceeds from the twelfth week until some time after birth. During this period, the cecum remains in the position it attained at the end of stage two while the colon continues to elongate (Fig. 6.1G).

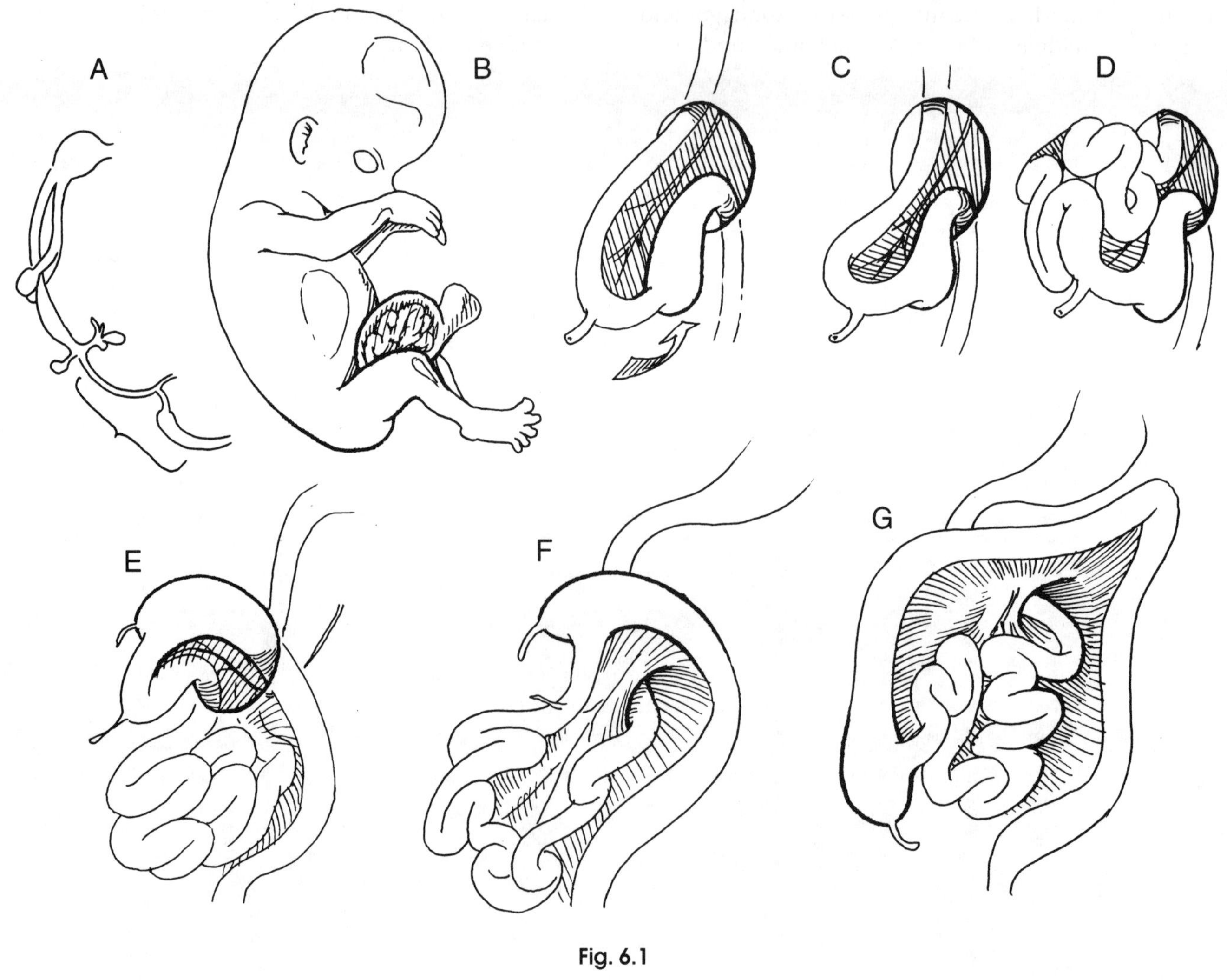

Fig. 6.1

As the colonic arc expands to form hepatic and splenic flexures, the mesenteries of the ascending and descending portions become apposed to the posterior parietal peritoneum. The lateral faces of the colon mesentery fuse with the peritoneum, leaving a line of attachment along the colon wall (Fig. 6.2A). Upward traction on the adult right or left colon creates a fold of parietal peritoneum, the so called "white line" (of Toldt), which identifies the edge of the fusion plane (Fig. 6.2B). Also during this final stage, the relationship between the greater omentum and the colon is developing.

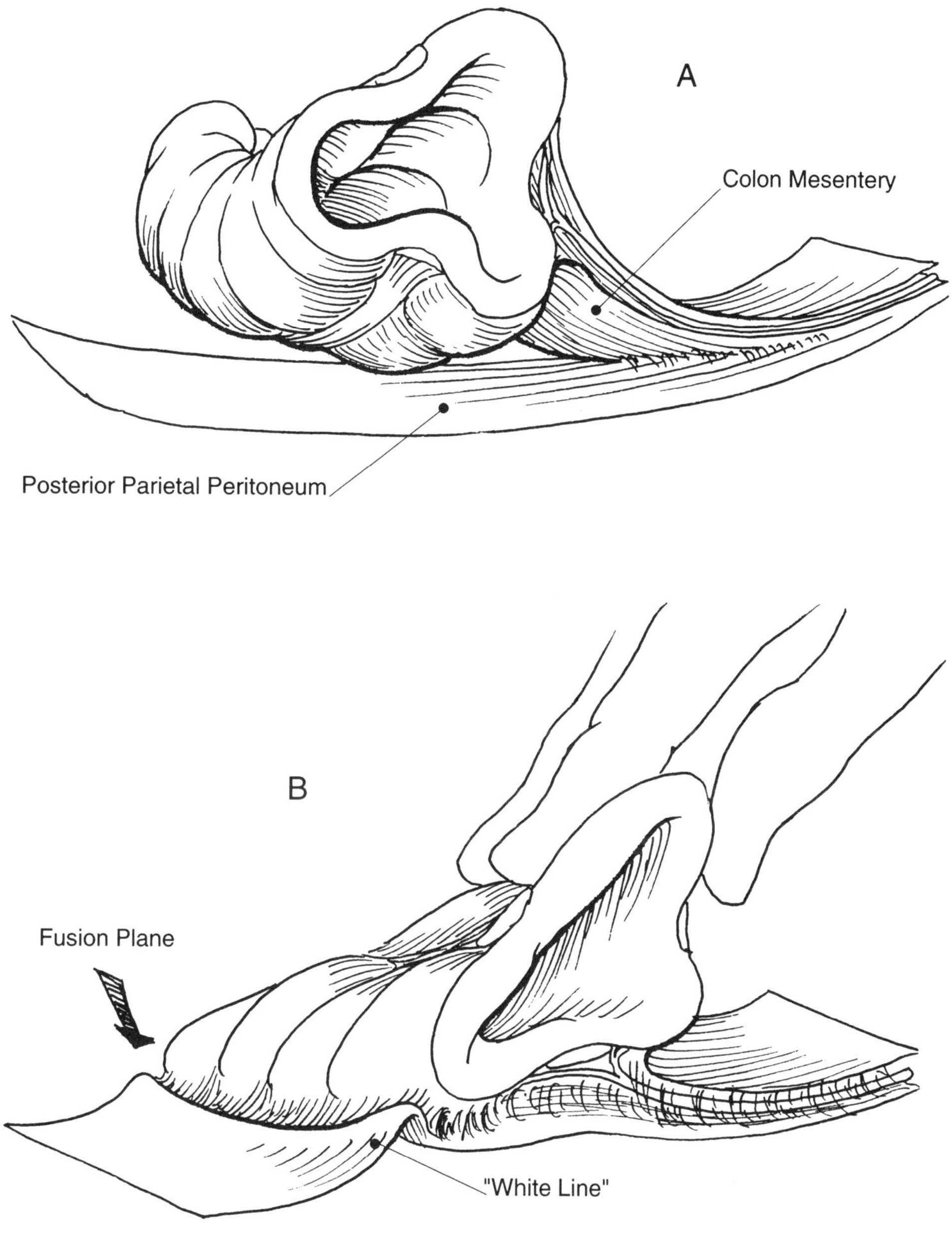

Fig. 6.2

During development of the omental bursa (Chapter 5), the bulging of the dorsal mesogastrium to the left evolves into the greater omentum. The elongating apron of greater omentum drapes over the transverse portion of the colon and fuses to itself from distal to proximal, obliterating the caudal portion of the omental bursa up to the level of the transverse colon (Fig. 6.3A). In addition, the posterior double layer of greater omentum attaches to the colon and more proximally with the cephalad surface of the transverse mesocolon. Depending on the degree of fusion within the omentum, the anterior omental layers are often partially fused with the transverse mesocolon, particularly toward the right side. Failure to recognize this fusion can lead to devascularization of the transverse colon when surgically opening the gastrocolic omentum (Fig. 6.3B).

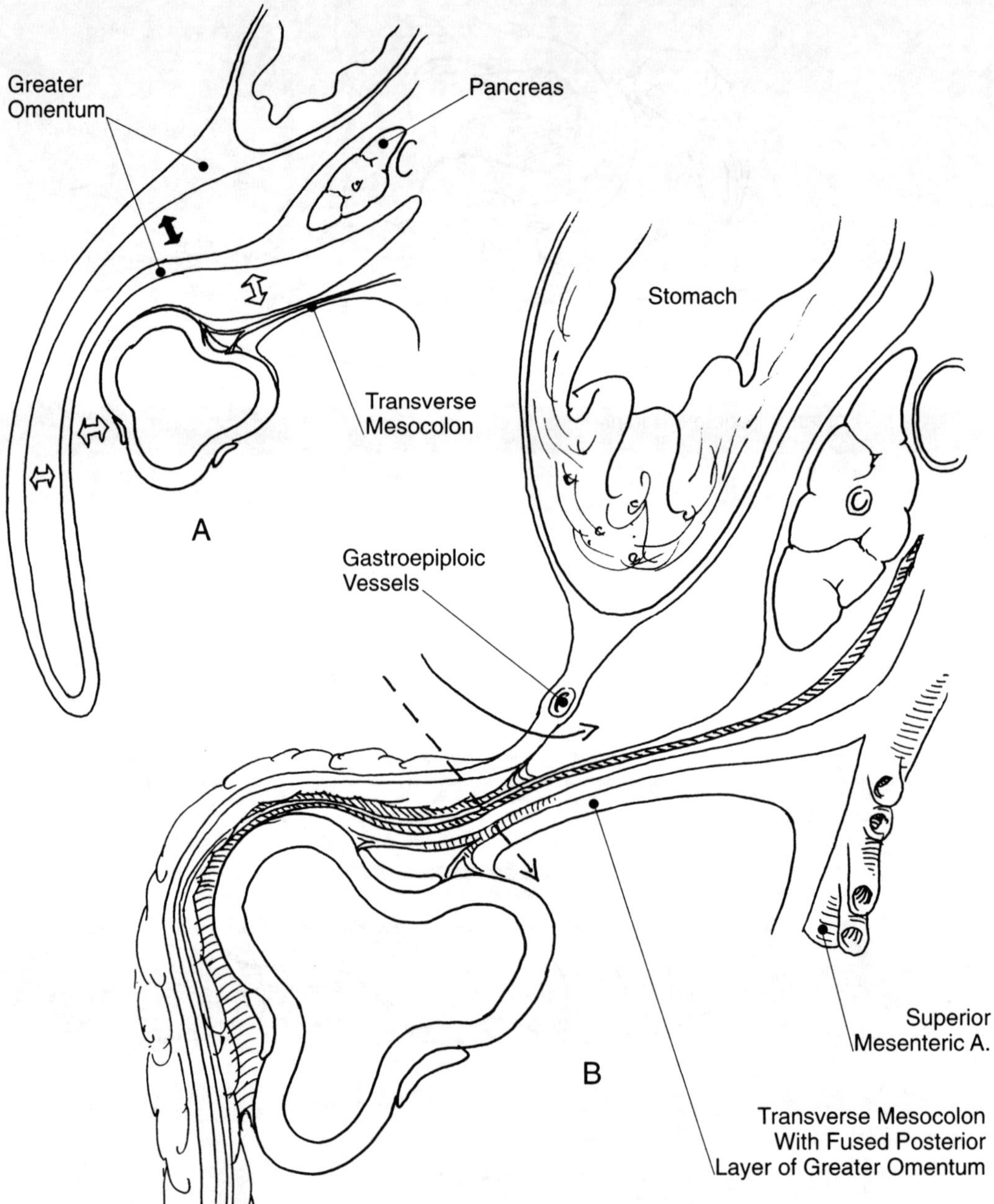

Fig. 6.3

The attachment of omentum to colon covers the surface of colon wall including one of the non-mesenteric taeniae which is designated the omental taenia (Fig. 6.4A). Separating the omentum from the colon in this plane to enter the lesser sac ultimately divides what was formerly the posterior layers of the greater omentum, an avascular layer (Fig. 6.4B). Most anatomic variation of the colon relates to rotation and fixation of the gut.

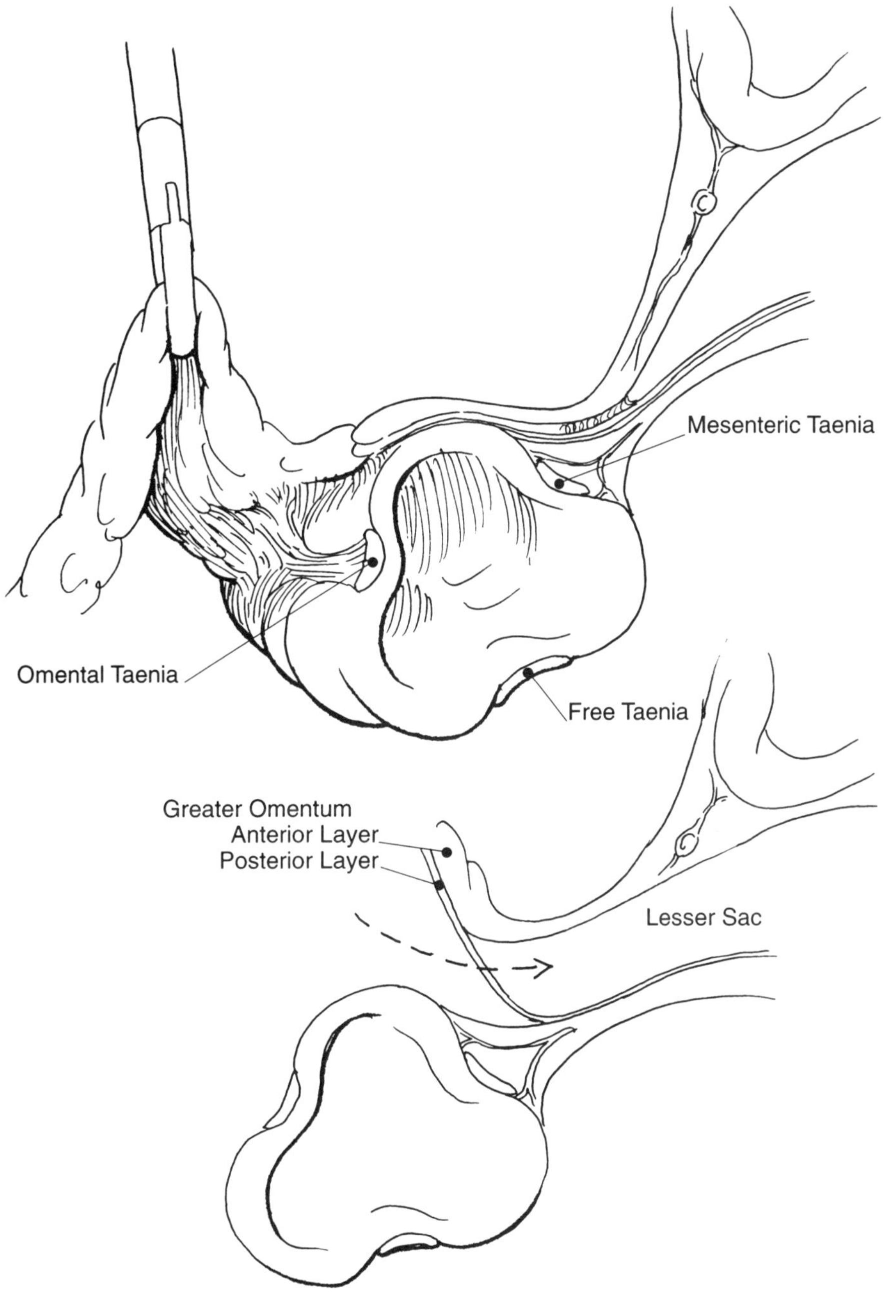

Fig. 6.4

The cecum is commonly (13–32%) mobile (Fig. 6.5A) and often extends into the pelvis (10–20%). Mobility allows sufficient freedom for volvulus in about 10% of individuals. Normal rotation with failure of right-sided fixation results in a common right and transverse mesocolon extending from right lower quadrant to left upper quadrant (Fig. 6.5B). The position of the colon is occasionally affected by incomplete rotation, more rarely by hyper- or reverse rotation (Fig. 6.5C).

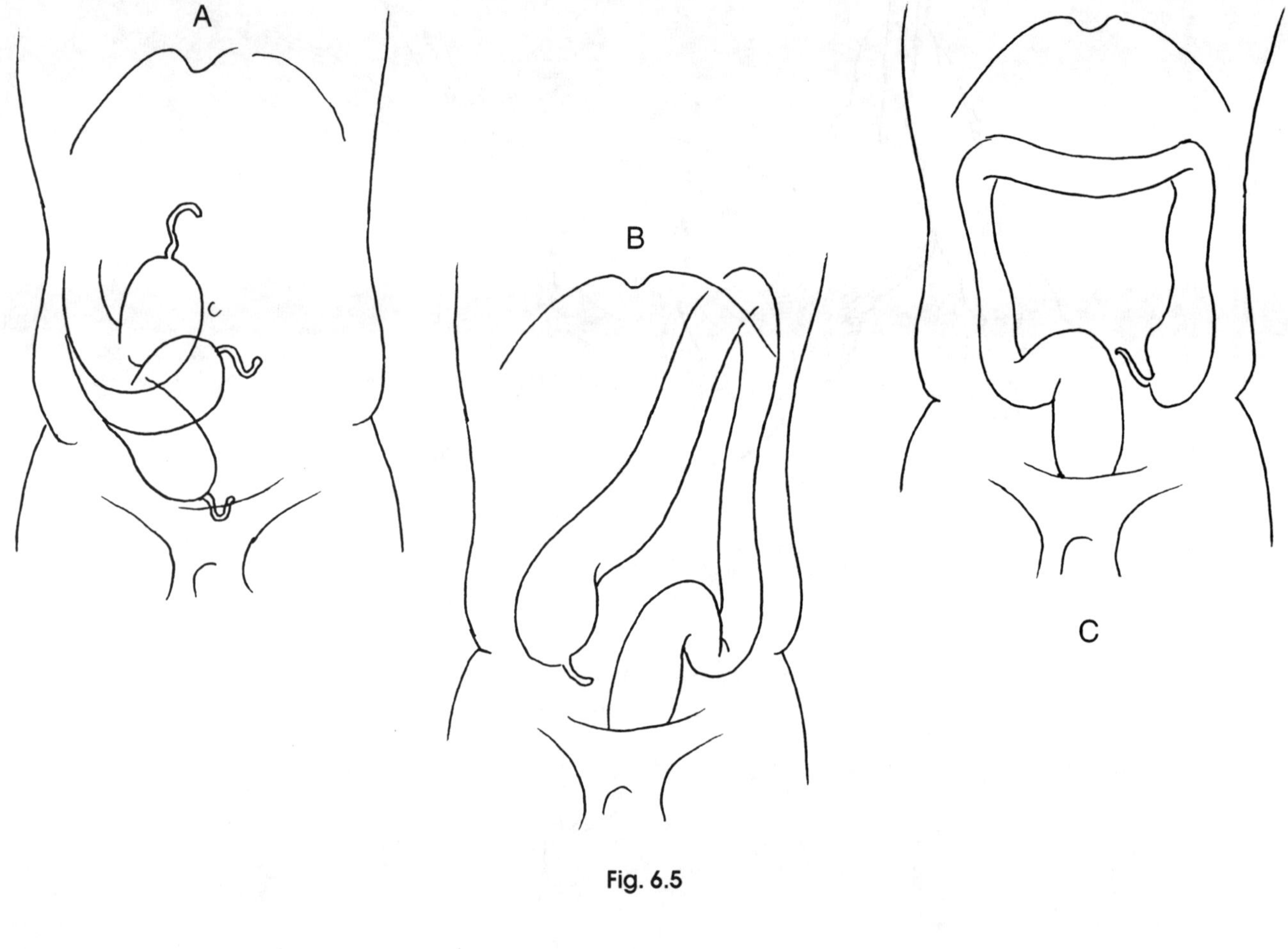

Fig. 6.5

About 5% of the time the cecum is found in a subhepatic location (Fig. 6.6A). With incomplete rotation, bands (Ladd's) between the cecum and the right lateral abdominal wall may compress and partially obstruct the duodenum. In 5% of individuals the cecum is completely fixed and may be covered by a membrane (Jackson's), making mobilization difficult (Fig. 6.6B). Most patients undergoing colon surgery will have such positional variations identified during the preoperative workup.

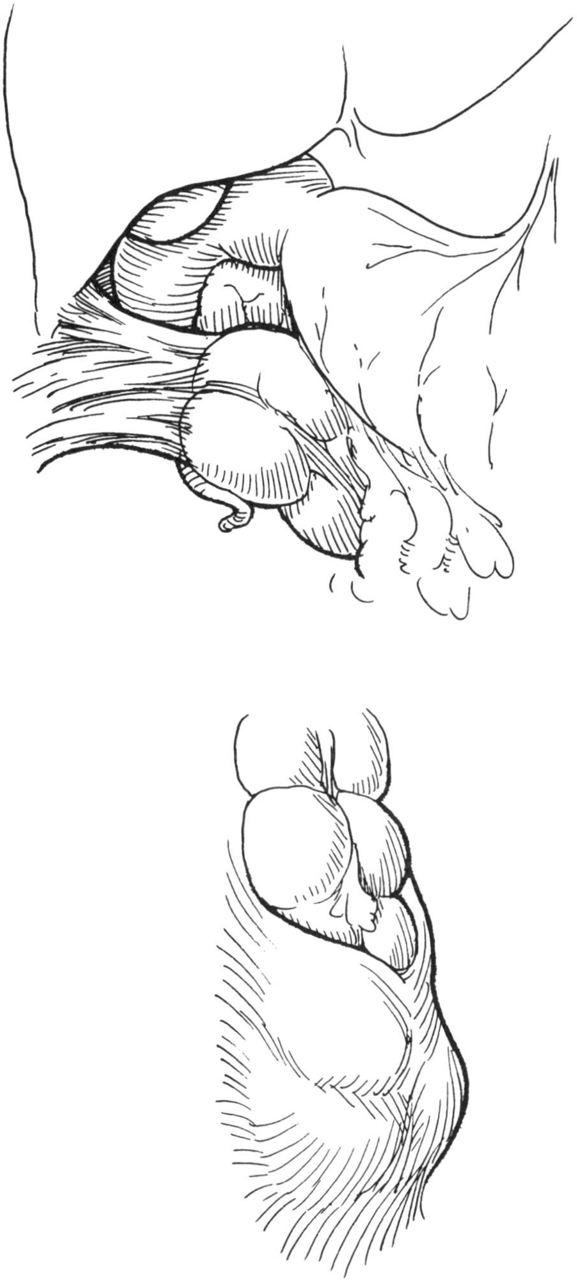

Fig. 6.6

ANATOMY

Colon Mesenteries and Relationships

The structure of the posterior abdominal wall is the key to understanding the relationships of the colon. The endoabdominal fascia covers the muscles of the posterior body wall and is the outer limit of the abdominal cavity (Fig. 6.7). The great vessels and urinary structures lie in their original position between the fascia and posterior parietal peritoneum, enclosed in an intermediate layer of fascia (Gerota's). Note the ureters lying high on the psoas muscles in the lumbar region, close to the vertebral bodies, and crossing the bifurcation of the common iliac vessels.

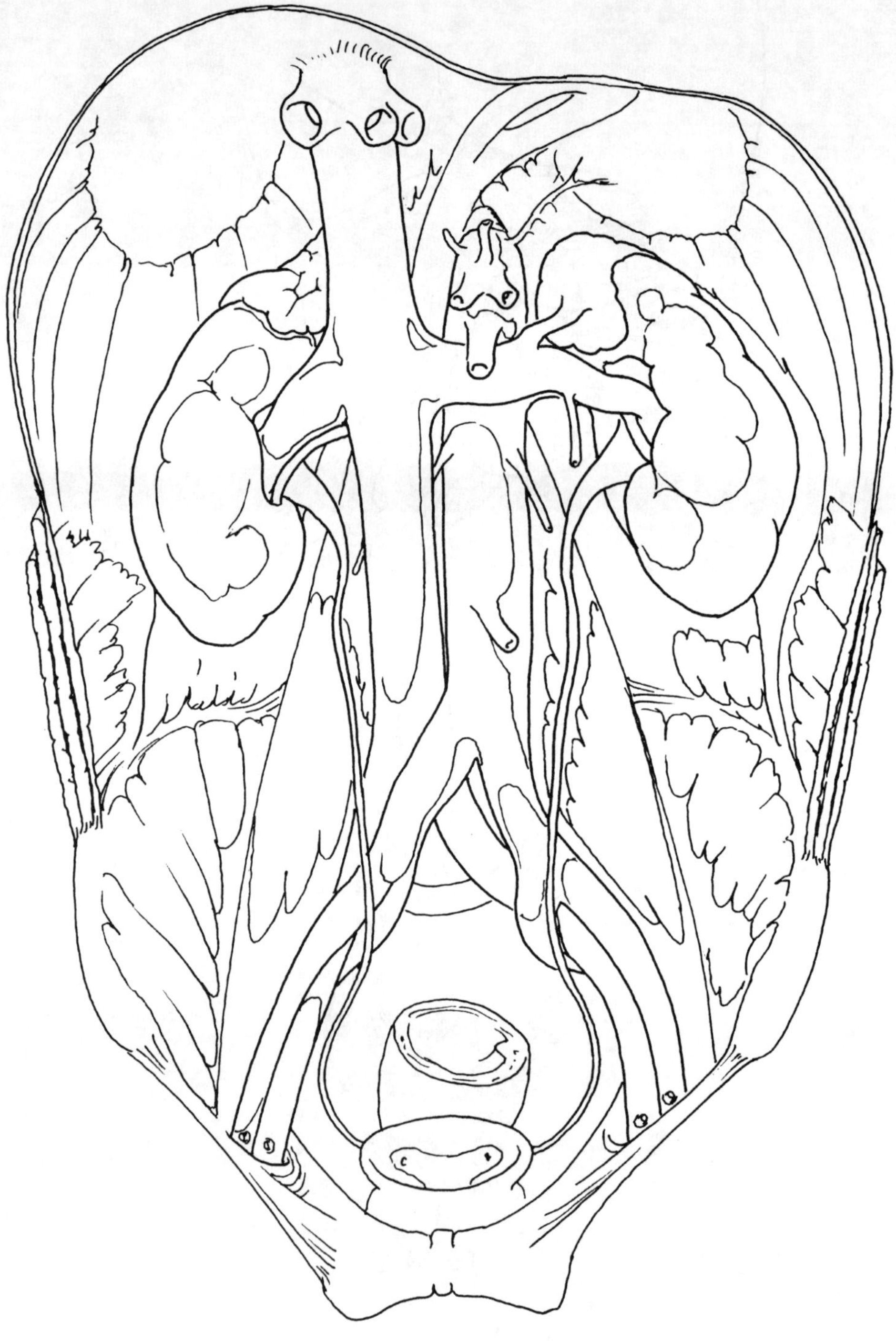

Fig. 6.7

The duodenum and pancreas are secondarily layered on these structures during the formation of the omental bursa and the rotation of the midgut (Fig. 6.8). The fixation of the rotated colon to these underlying structures

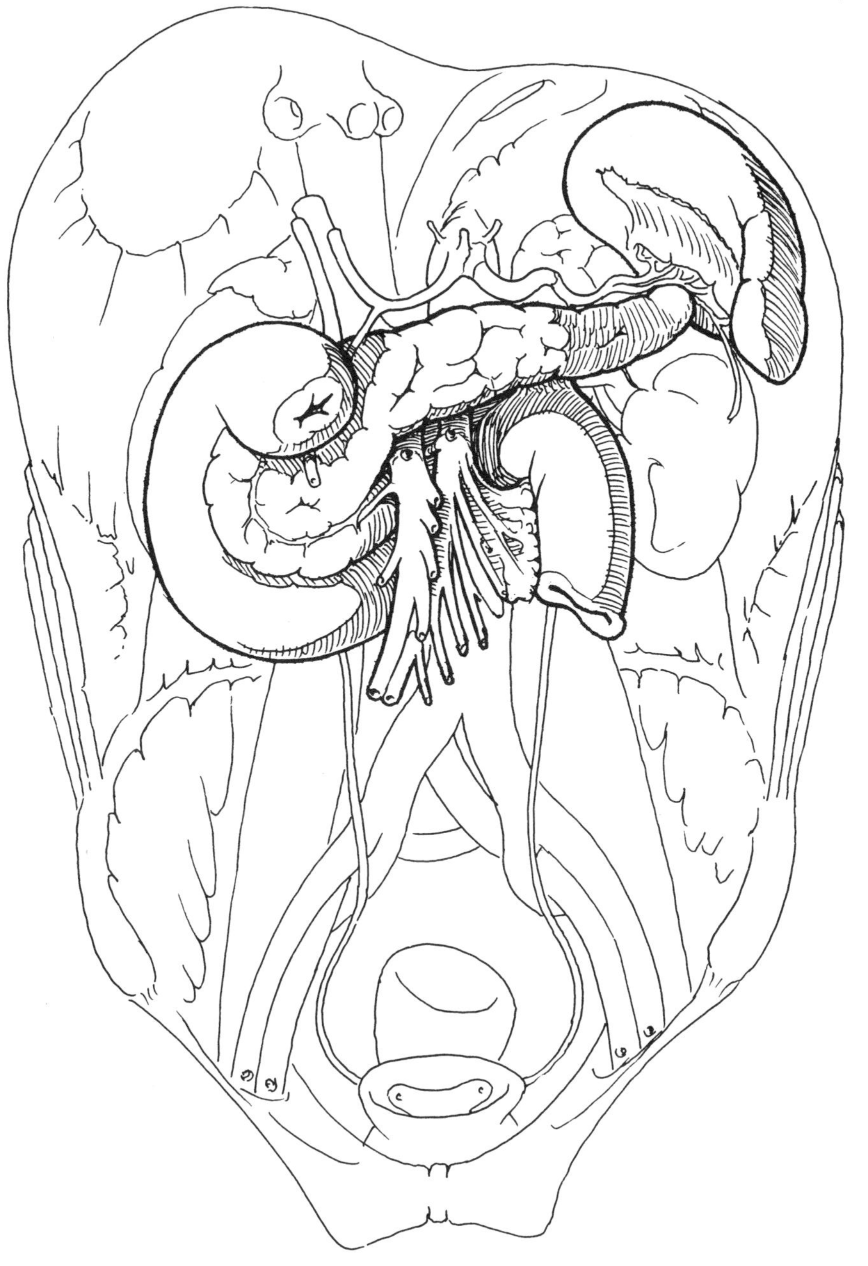

Fig. 6.8

results in two delta-shaped areas of fusion fascia on the right and left and a diagonal attachment of the transverse mesocolon across the second part of the duodenum and across the pancreas (Fig. 6.9). The root of the sigmoid mesocolon crosses the iliac vessels and the left ureter.

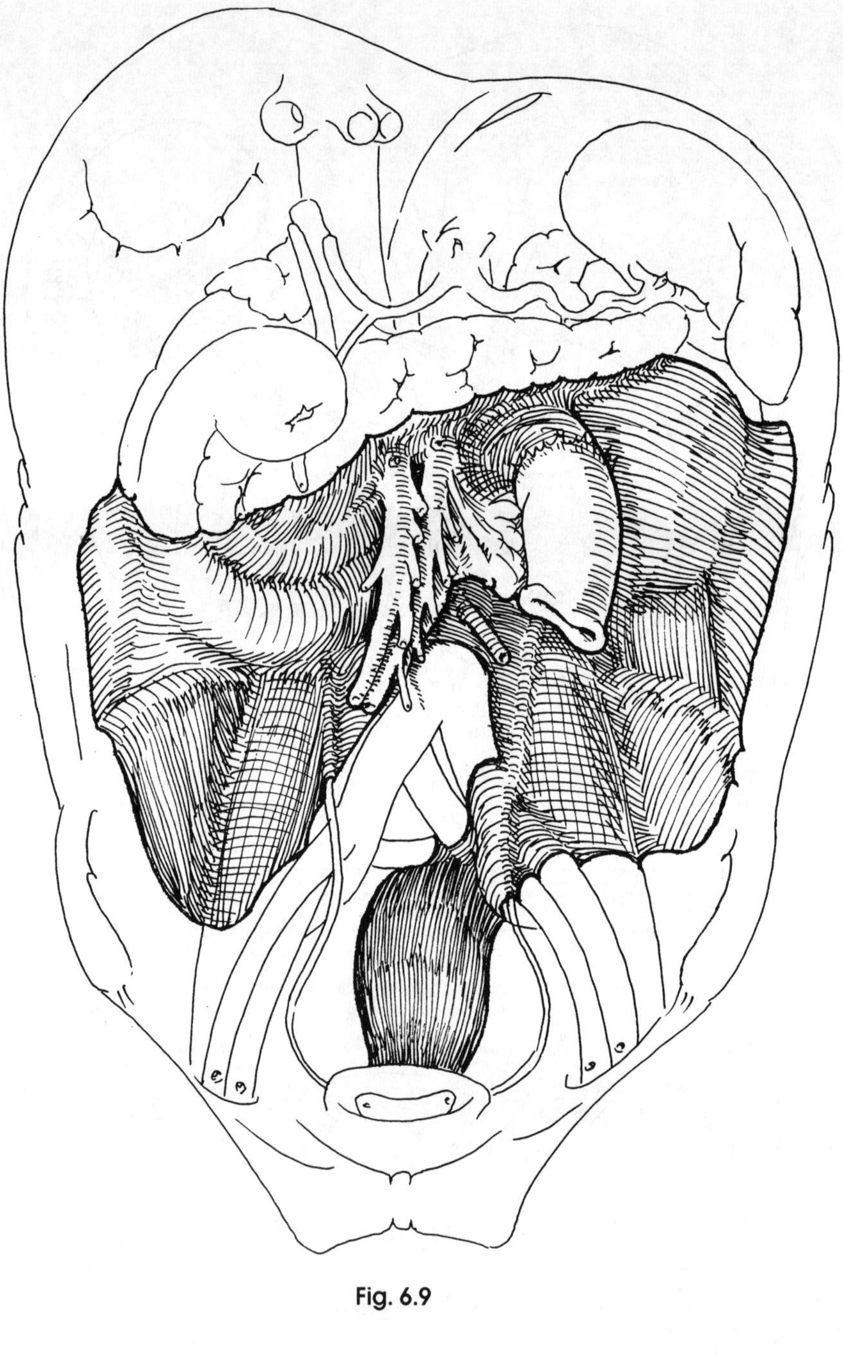

Fig. 6.9

The transverse mesocolon is shortest near the right and left colic flexures and drapes outward centrally, allowing the transverse colon to hang down when an individual is upright (Fig. 6.10). This broad shelf is over-

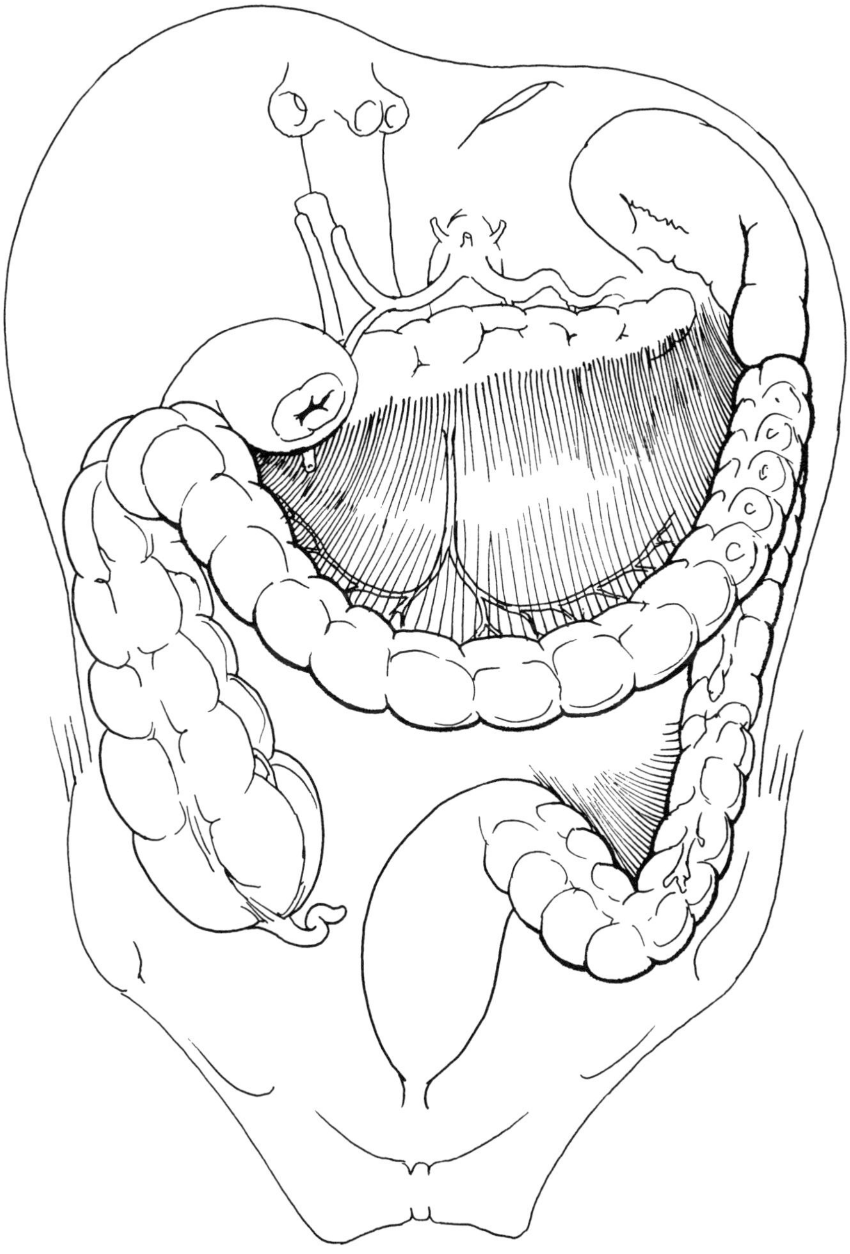

Fig. 6.10

laid by the pendent portion of the distal stomach (Fig. 6.11). The gastrocolic ligament is formed by the anterior layers of the greater omentum containing the gastroepiploic arcade.

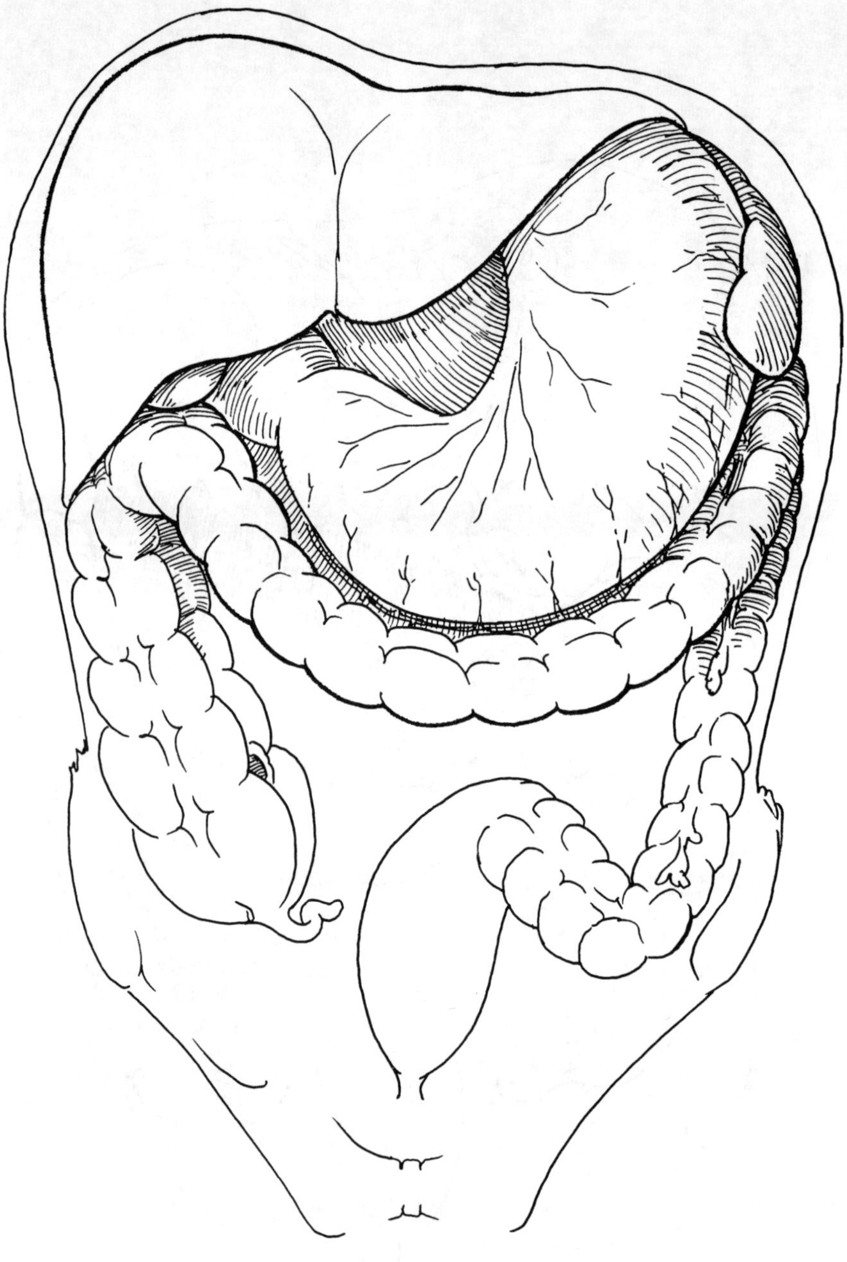

Fig. 6.11

The best appreciation of colon anatomy and relationships is gained from a cross-sectional perspective (Fig. 6.12). The splenic flexure, while variable (Chapter 5), is more cephalad than the hepatic flexure as seen in this reconstruction. Laparoscopic ports placed for left colon mobilization must take into account the extra reach necessary to mobilize this area. The transverse colon is ptotic in this individual and the sigmoid colon is short and direct, but the latter is also often long and redundant. Redundancy of either loop complicates laparoscopic manipulation. The distal transverse colon lies anterior to the proximal descending colon. The cecum lies within the wing of the right iliac bone in direct contact with the iliacus and psoas muscles (sections F and G) explaining the occurrence of psoas abscess from inflammation of the terminal ileum or the appendix which is commonly retrocecal. Note the positions of the ureters on either side in relation to the plane for surgical remobilization of the right and left colon mesenteries.

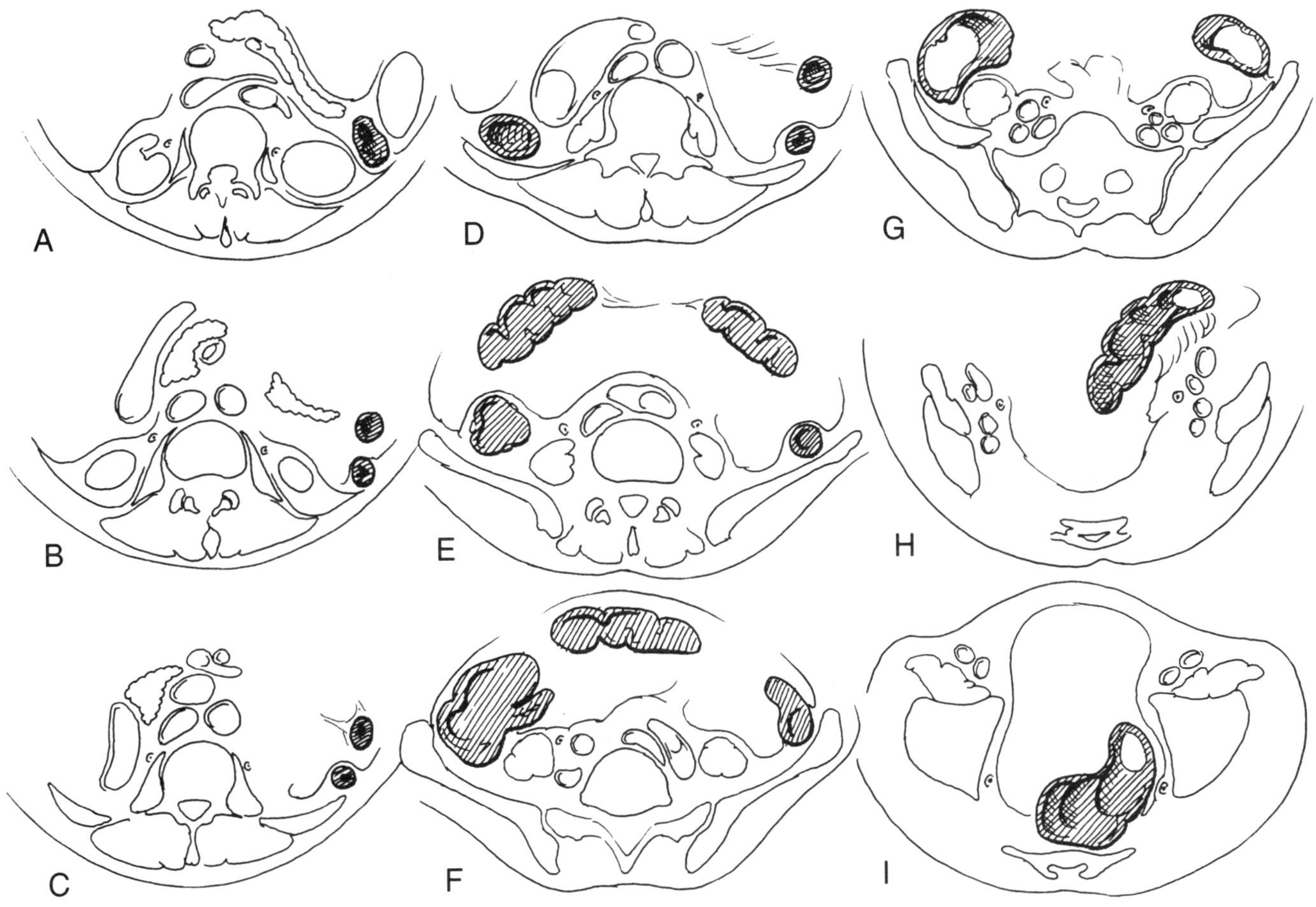

Fig. 6.12

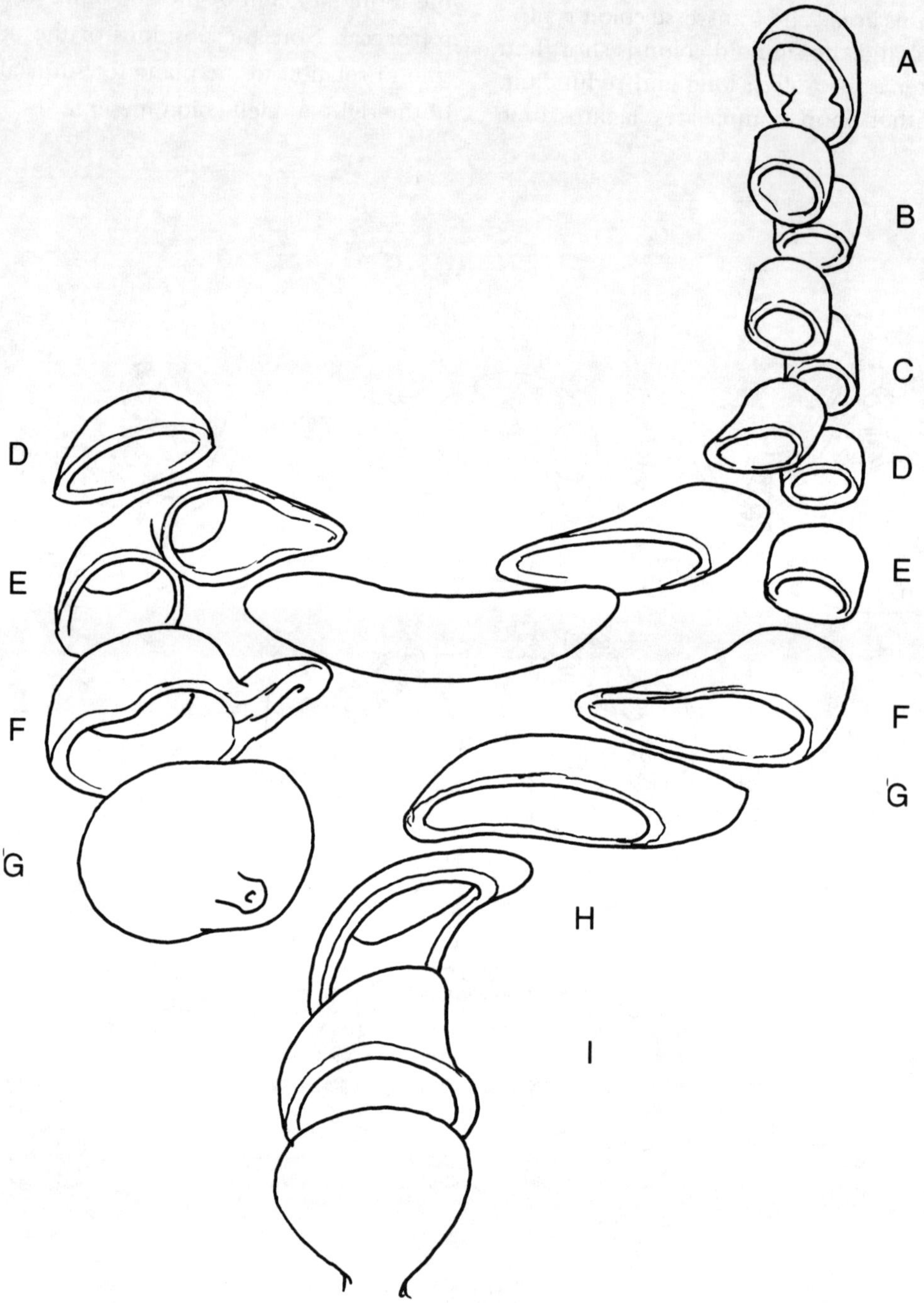

Fig. 6.12 key

Colonic Vessels

The colonic blood supply is derived from the superior and inferior mesenteric arteries, the watershed area at the distal transverse colon defining the division between embryonic midgut and hindgut. The patterns of branching from these two major trunks exhibit moderate variability and are best described by elevating the transverse colon to eliminate the overlap seen in the normal anatomic position (Figs. 6.13A, B).

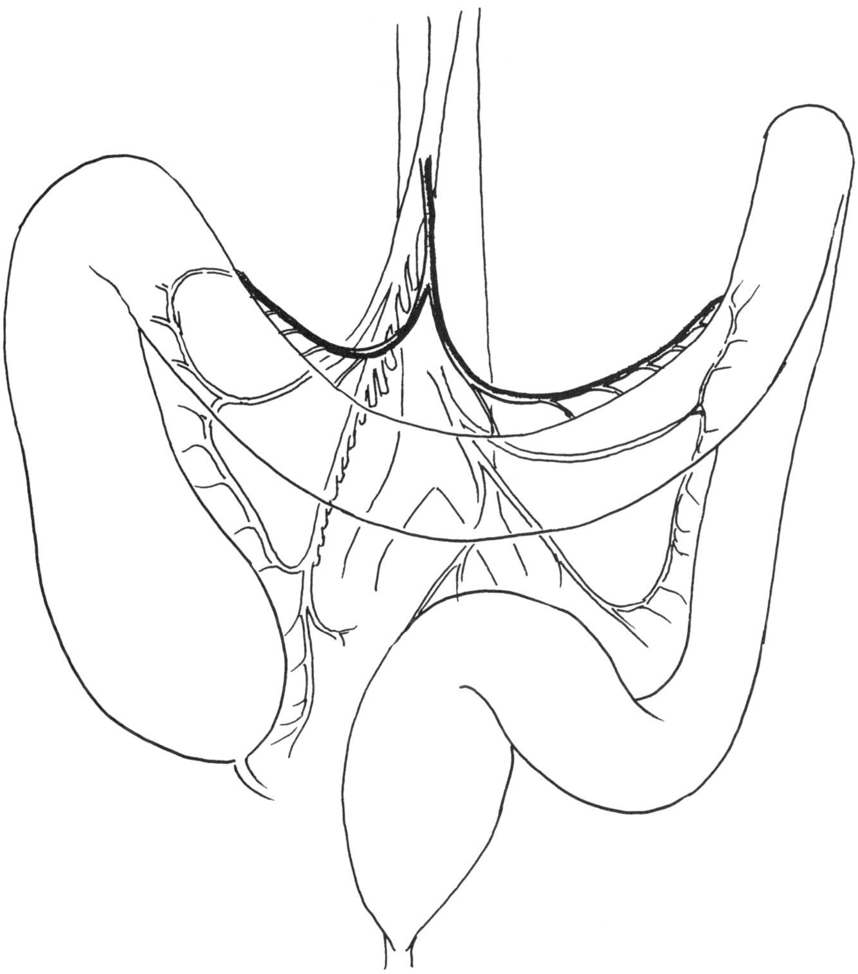

Fig. 6.13A

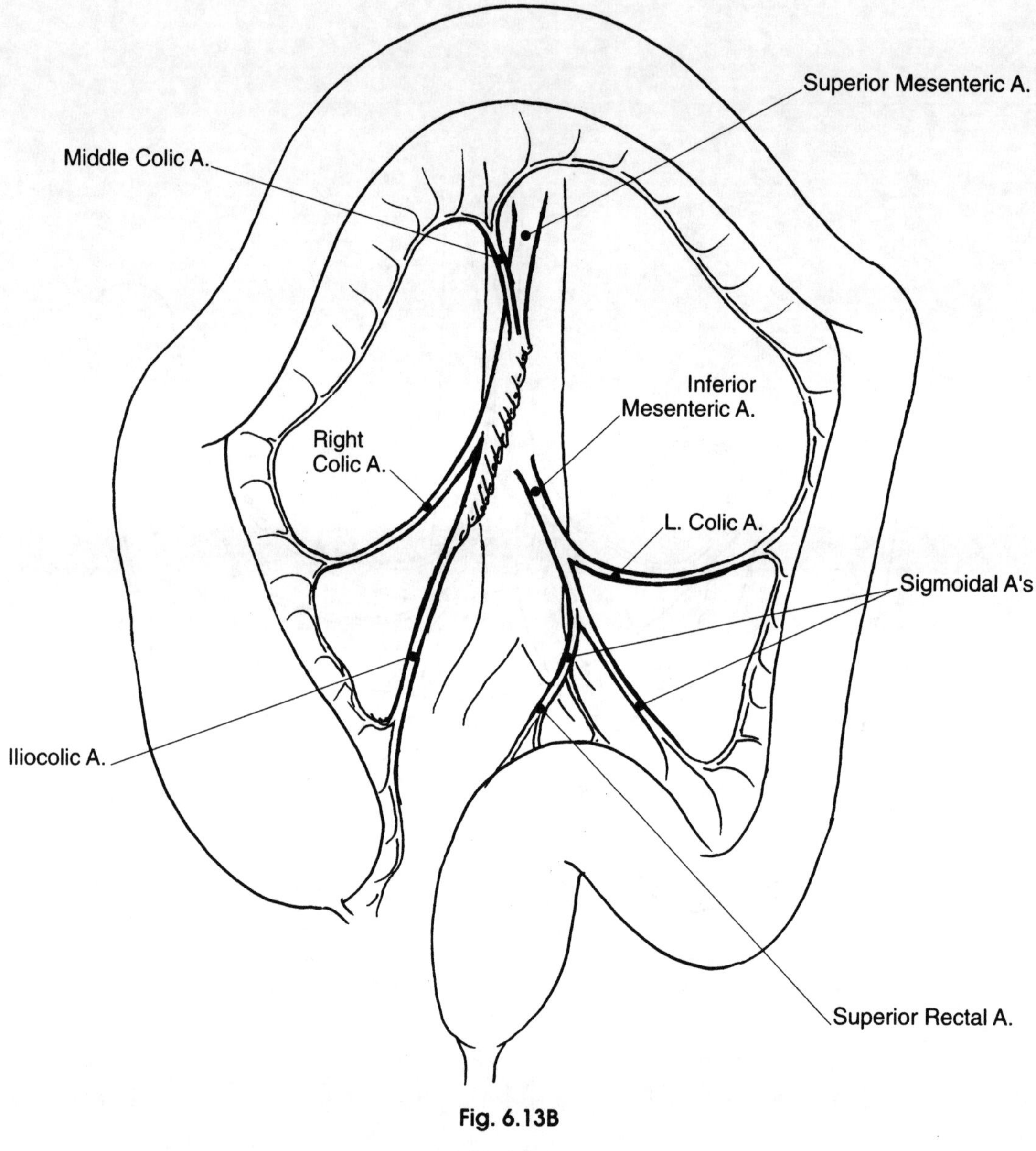
Superior Mesenteric A.
Middle Colic A.
Inferior Mesenteric A.
Right Colic A.
L. Colic A.
Sigmoidal A's
Iliocolic A.
Superior Rectal A.

Fig. 6.13B

Normal communication occurs between colonic vessels around the margin of the mesentery. There are both peripheral and central anastomoses within the mesentery (Fig. 6.14). In the normal state, the small peripheral channel is most evident and is usually referred to as the marginal artery (of Drummond, who described both central and marginal anastomoses in 1913). The central channels become prominent in pathological states where the superior or inferior mesenteric artery is stenosed or occluded. The resulting pressure gradient from one territory to another enlarges existing central connections, often to impressive proportions. Such vessels have been called meandering mesenteric arteries (arc of Riolan, who described such an arcade in the 17th century).

The variations of the superior mesenteric artery at its origin are not directly relevant to a discussion of colon resection except that the surgeon should be aware of the rare common origin of the inferior mesenteric artery with this vessel. Understanding the peripheral branch patterns informs the surgeon about where to expect major vascular pedicles during mobilization and transection of the mesentery.

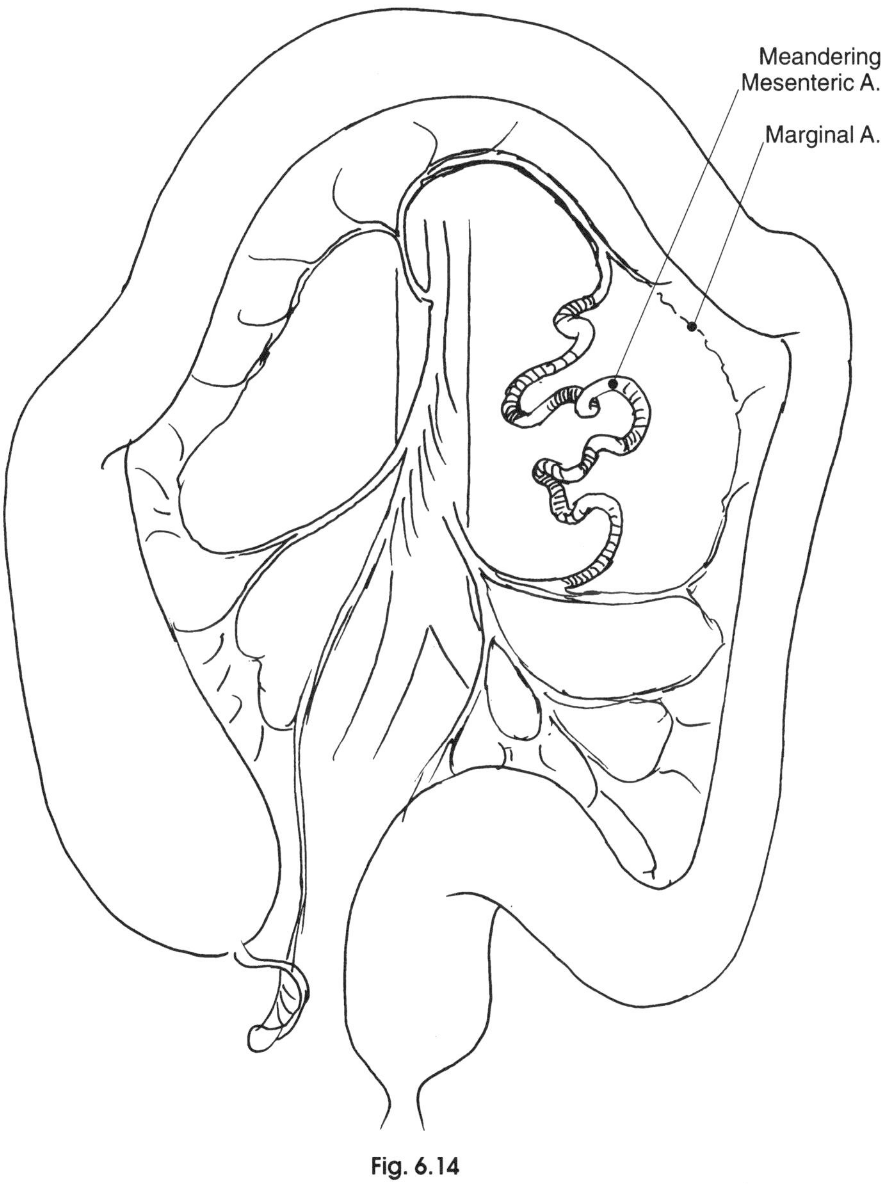

Fig. 6.14

The three usual branches of the superior mesenteric artery, the middle, right and ileocolic arteries (Fig. 6.15) are of equal importance. The middle colic artery arises from the anterior wall of the superior mesenteric artery as it emerges from beneath the neck of the pancreas and passes between the leaves of the transverse mesocolon toward the colon. Approximately two thirds of the time it is an independent vessel and a quarter of the time it has a common origin with the right colic artery. The right colic artery arises independently from the superior mesenteric artery only about a quarter of the time, more commonly arising as a branch of the middle colic or ileocolic artery. It is absent 13% of the time. The ileocolic, like the middle colic, is independent two thirds of the time and shares an origin with the right colic about one third of the time. After giving off cecal and ileal branches, the ileocolic artery terminates in the appendiceal artery which runs deep to the terminal ileum to reach the mesoappendix.

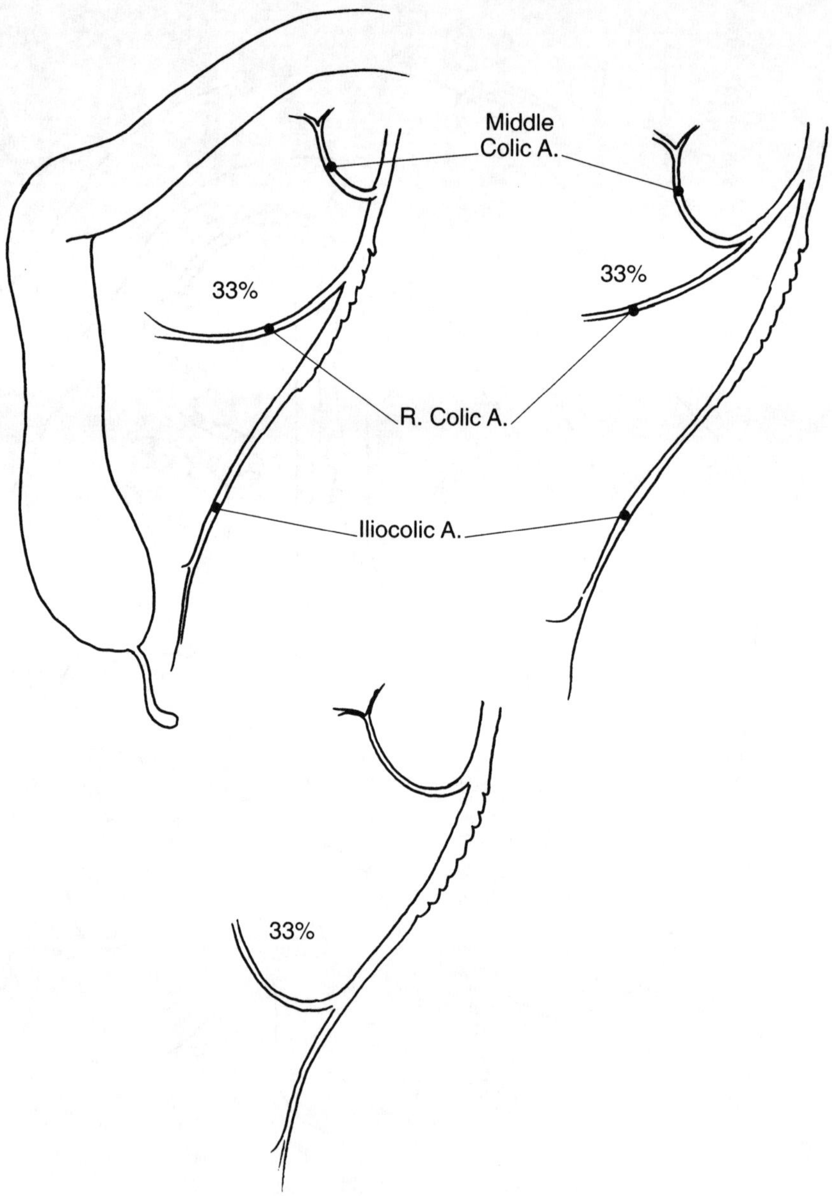

Fig. 6.15

The inferior mesenteric artery gives off a left colic branch, sigmoidal branches, and terminates as the superior rectal artery (Fig. 6.16) The left colic artery may encroach on what is normally superior mesenteric artery territory or may be replaced by a branch of the superior mesenteric artery. The superior rectal artery is the most important source of rectal blood supply. It divides into two branches posterior to the rectum and the branches course downward and anteriorly around the rectum. The branches anastomose with middle rectal branches from the internal iliacs (sometimes only one middle rectal). The inferior rectal branches from the pudendal arteries are of minor significance.

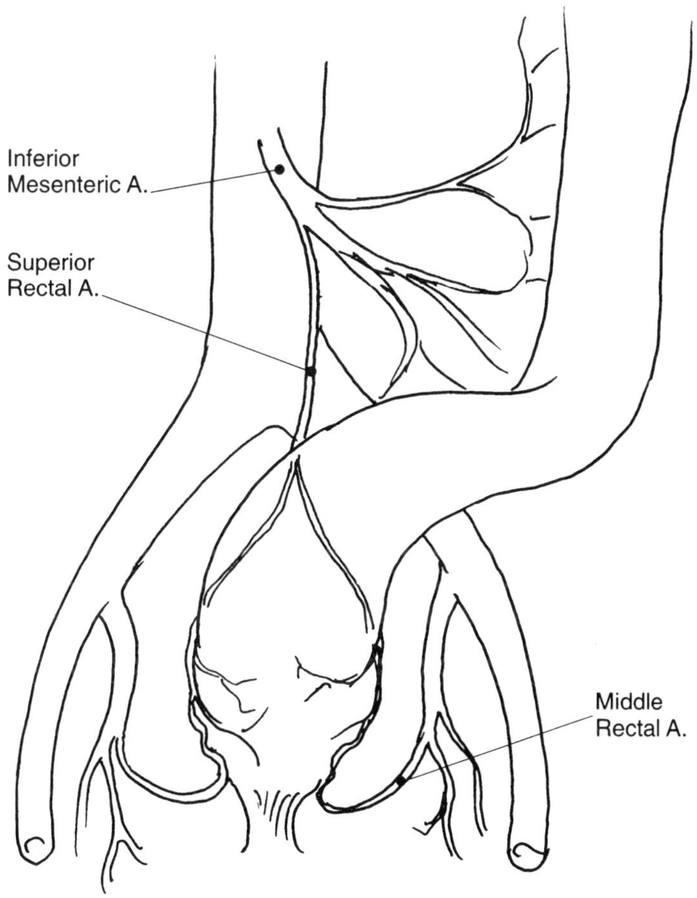

Fig. 6.16

The superior mesenteric vein draining the right and transverse colon follows the superior mesenteric arterial branches (Fig. 6.17). On the left, the inferior mesenteric vein lies in the left mesocolon fusion plane and runs toward the base of the transverse mesocolon independent of the inferior mesenteric artery. It most commonly joins the splenic vein beneath the pancreas. Occasionally it joins the superior mesenteric vein or the junction of superior mesenteric and splenic vein. The lymphatics draining the colon follow the arteries in the reverse direction.

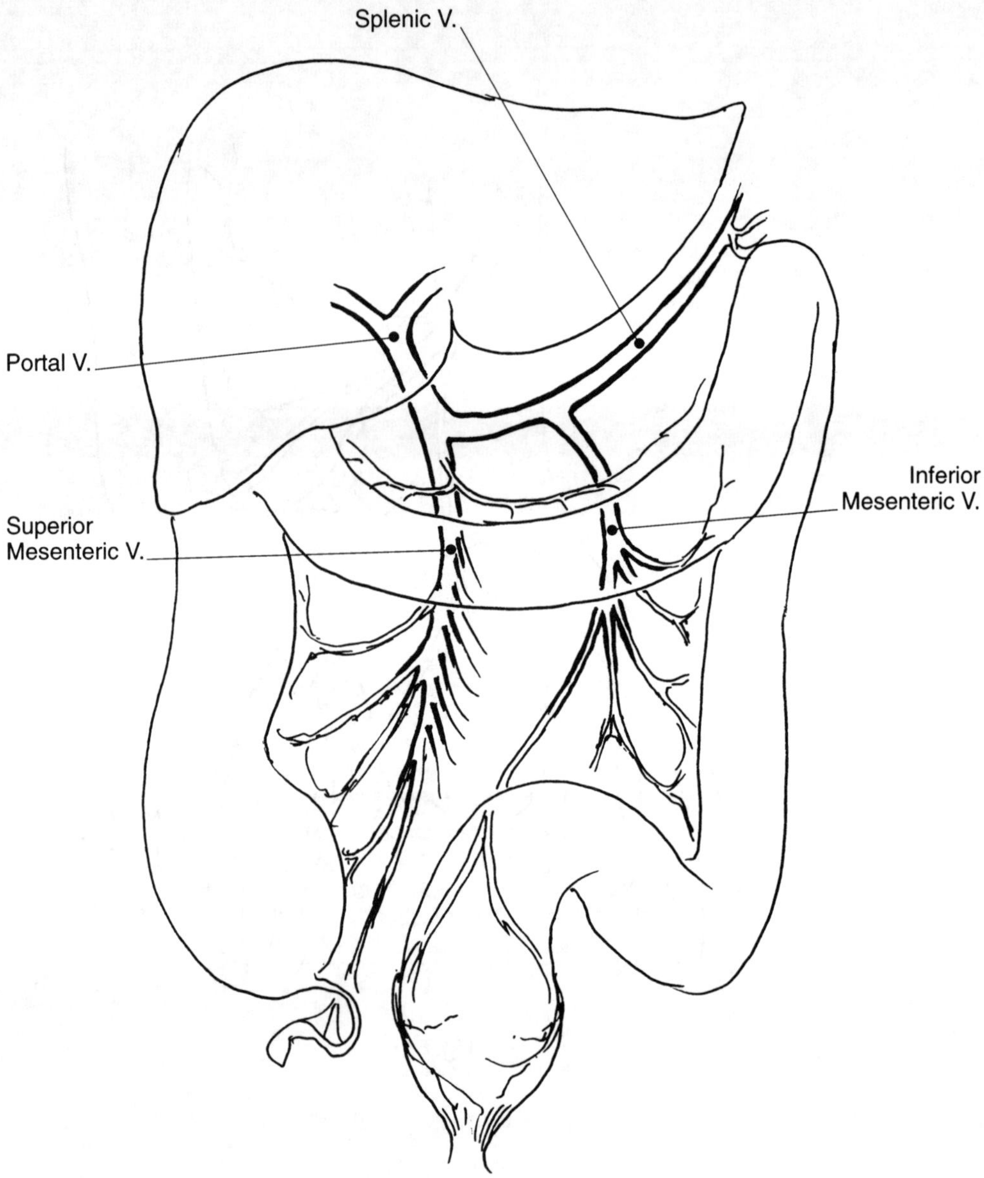

Fig. 6.17

The appendix is supplied by the terminal branch of the ileocolic artery which runs behind the terminal ilium to reach the mesoappendix (Fig. 6.18). The terminal ilium is the only part of the small bowel that has an antemesenteric appendage of fat (crista galli/cock's comb) which identifies it and helps locate the appendix. The base of the appendix is found at the confluence of the three taeniae. More than half of individuals have a retrocecal appendix, either free behind a floppy cecum or retroperitoneal behind a more fixed cecum.

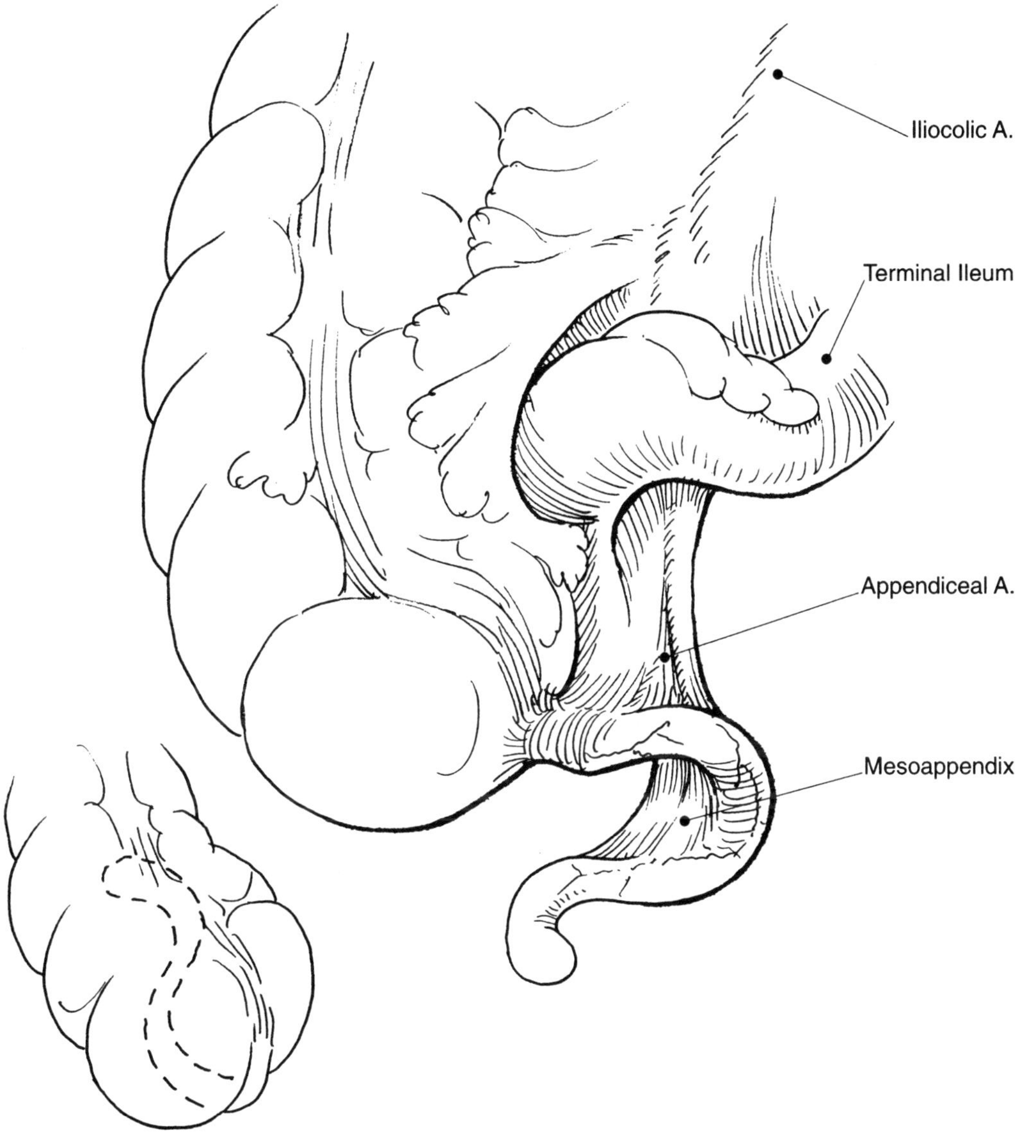

Fig. 6.18

SURGERY

Appendectomy

Laparoscopic appendectomy, first done in association with gynecological procedures, has now been shown in several large series to be equal if not superior to open appendectomy in outcome. Advantages include lower wound morbidity and discomfort, more precise visualization and dissection, the ability to explore the rest of the abdomen and lavage pockets of fluid collection, and possibly fewer adhesions. The latter is especially important in young women who can have a later incidence of infertility of up to 20 to 30%. These are weighed against the simplicity of open appendectomy and the complexity and cost of laparoscopic technology.

Umbilical insufflation and camera (30 or 45° telescope) placement allow initial exploration. The findings dictate the placement of the remaining ports (Fig. 6.19). A large (12mm) port is placed over the appendix for manipulation and extraction. An additional 5mm lower abdominal port (suprapubic, lower midline, or left lower quadrant) is then placed. Placement of a 10mm port in the left lower quadrant at the lateral edge of the rectus allows the camera to be moved to a less constrained position and the surgeon operates through the umbilical and suprapubic ports with the camera in the ideal position between the instruments. The right lower quadrant port is used initially to retract the cecum.

The appendix is mobilized from lateral to medial to avoid damaging the mesentery. The frequent (more than

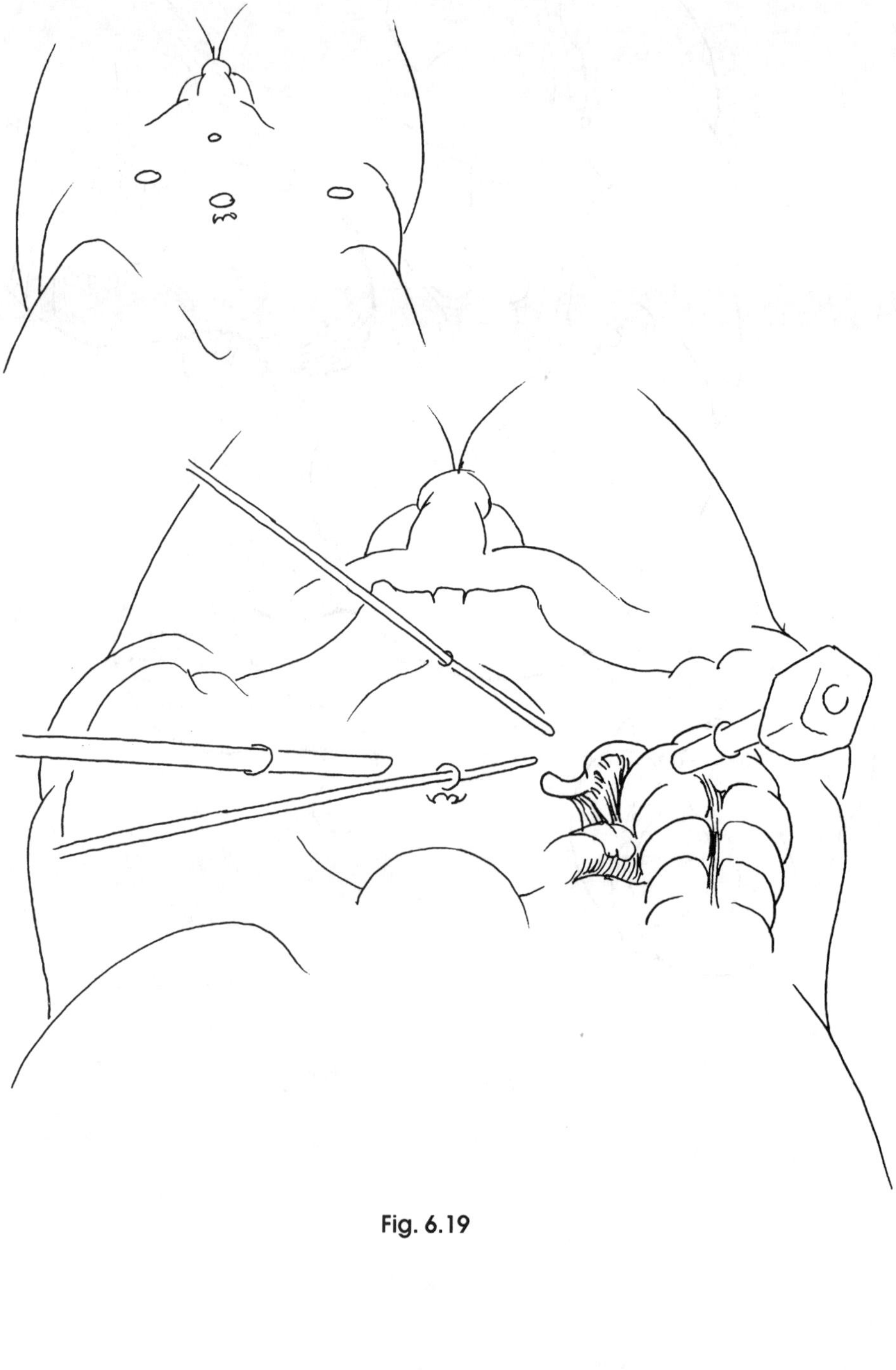

Fig. 6.19

50%) retrocecal appendix may require antegrade dissection. There are several good ways of removing the appendix. The mesentery can be opened at the base of the appendix and the appendix cauterized with the bipolar coagulator (Fig. 6.20) (Semm). A loop ligature is then placed over the folded mesoappendix and secured and a second loop is placed on the appendiceal stump. The appendix is removed through the right lower quadrant port.

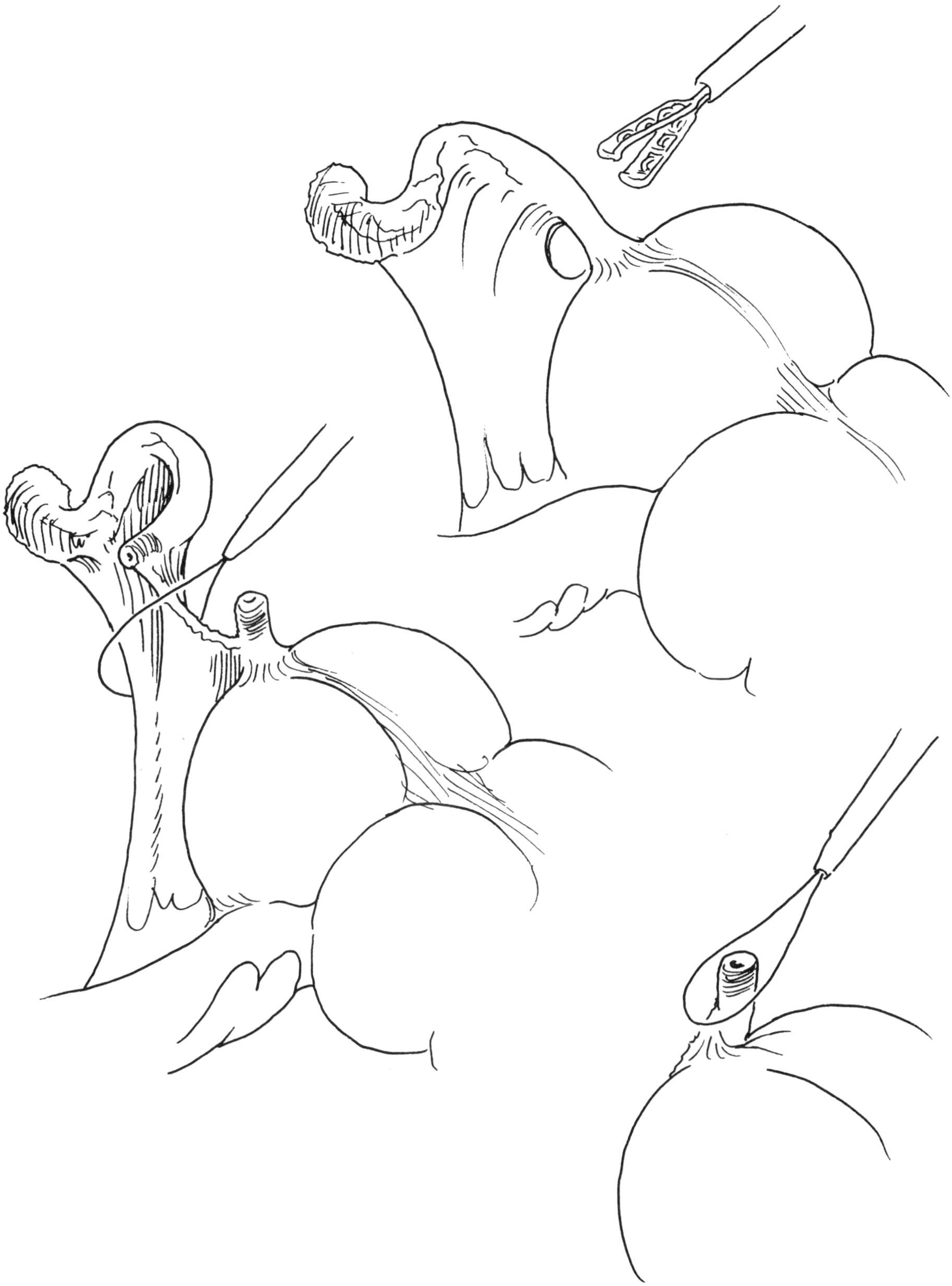

Fig. 6.20

The mesoappendix and the appendix itself can also be secured with a linear stapler (Fig. 6.21). This is the most costly option and makes laparoscopic appendix less competitive with the simplicity of open appendectomy.

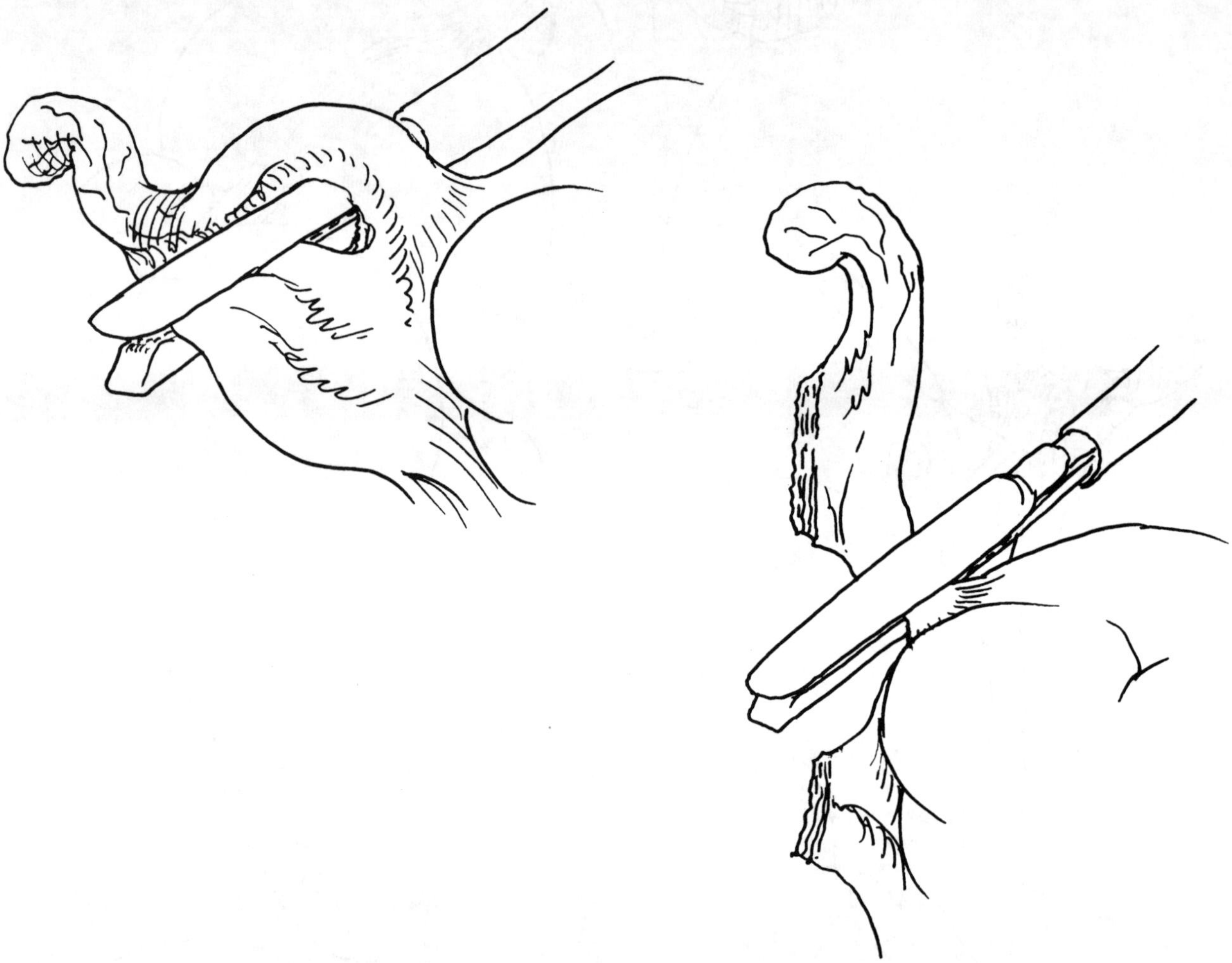

Fig. 6.21

Another option is to cauterize the fine terminal vessels along the mesenteric border (Fig. 6.22). Then no mesenteric ligatures are necessary and the absence of the bulky mesentery makes extraction easier. The appendix is usually withdrawn within the large cannula which serves as a protective sheath against wound contamination. A plastic bag can also be used for the same purpose.

If the mesentery is divided along the appendiceal border, the appendix may also be exteriorized through the 12mm port and the base ligated extracorporeally (Dudai). This eliminates the cost of a stapler and simplifies the procedure. Wound infection has not been a problem. The port is then replaced, and the abdomen is reinflated for final check and lavage.

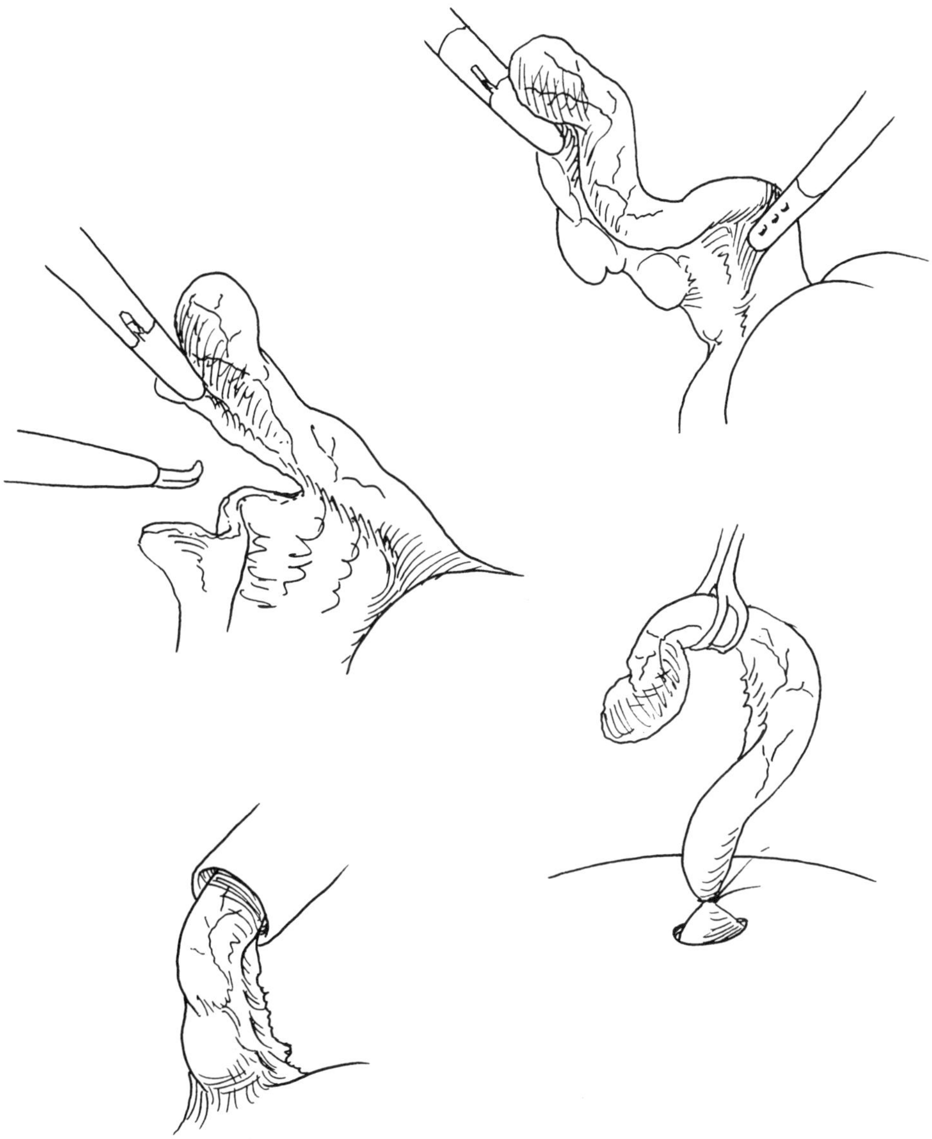

Fig. 6.22

Colon Resection

Assisted laparoscopic colon resection involves laparoscopic dissection and mobilization combined with a minilaparotomy through which the specimen is extracted (or through the perineal wound in abdominal perineal resection). The anastomosis is most often performed on the exteriorized bowel ends. There are advantages and disadvantages compared to open technique. The smaller incision is less painful and the decreased bowel manipulation seems to reduce ileus and allow earlier feeding and discharge.

The adequacy of margins possible with laparoscopic dissection for malignancy is not proven at this time. A length of mesentery containing greater than 13 lymph nodes has been correlated with a 90% accuracy rate in staging for metastatic disease and a 5 cm distal margin seems to be a critical distance below which recurrence rate increases significantly (6.9% vs. 20%). Early reports seem to indicate that these limits can be safely accomplished laparoscopically. There have been reports of peritoneal and port site spread. A theoretical advantage to laparoscopy is the decreased trauma and resulting immunosuppression of open surgery. Currently, it is recommended that laparoscopic colon resection for malignancy be done only as part of prospective, randomized controlled trials.

Benign indications such as diverticular disease, inflammatory bowel disease, polyposis, dysmotility and volvulus are less controversial. Adjunctive endoscopy can help localize lesions not visible from outside the bowel wall since tactile localization is not possible through the laparoscope.

Four ports are used (Fig. 6.23), two or three of which are large (10–12 mm). A central camera position is appropriate for right or left sided resections and the additional ports are placed as needed. The ports are placed in a semicircular pattern opposite the lesion. A second telescope and light source introduced from the side opposite the camera is very useful for transilluminating the mesentery and identifying vessels. Lithotomy position is used for low resections which require transanal EEA application. The table is tilted and rotated as needed to slide viscera out of the area of dissection.

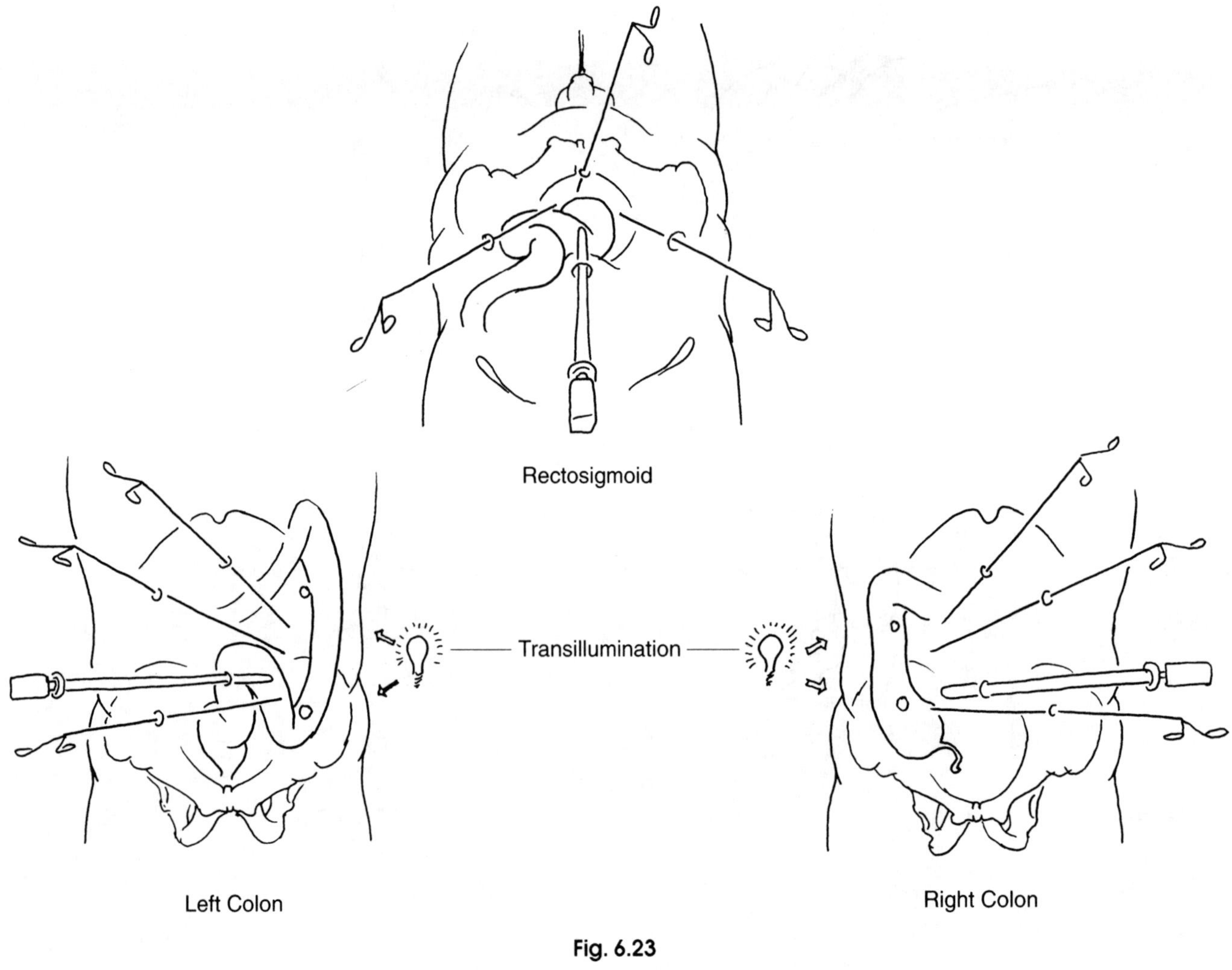

Fig. 6.23

Redundancy of sigmoid and/or transverse colon hamper visualization and dissection as does a fat laden omentum.

Mobilization of right and left colon is started along the peritoneal reflections (Fig. 6.24). As either side is mobilized medially, the retroperitoneal areolar tissue is swept downward off the recreated mesocolon in order to avoid elevating the ureter. Dissection at the hepatic and splenic flexures (Chapters 2, 5) must be done carefully to avoid injuring adjacent structures. If the omentum is to be removed with the specimen, the gastrocolic portion is divided between clips.

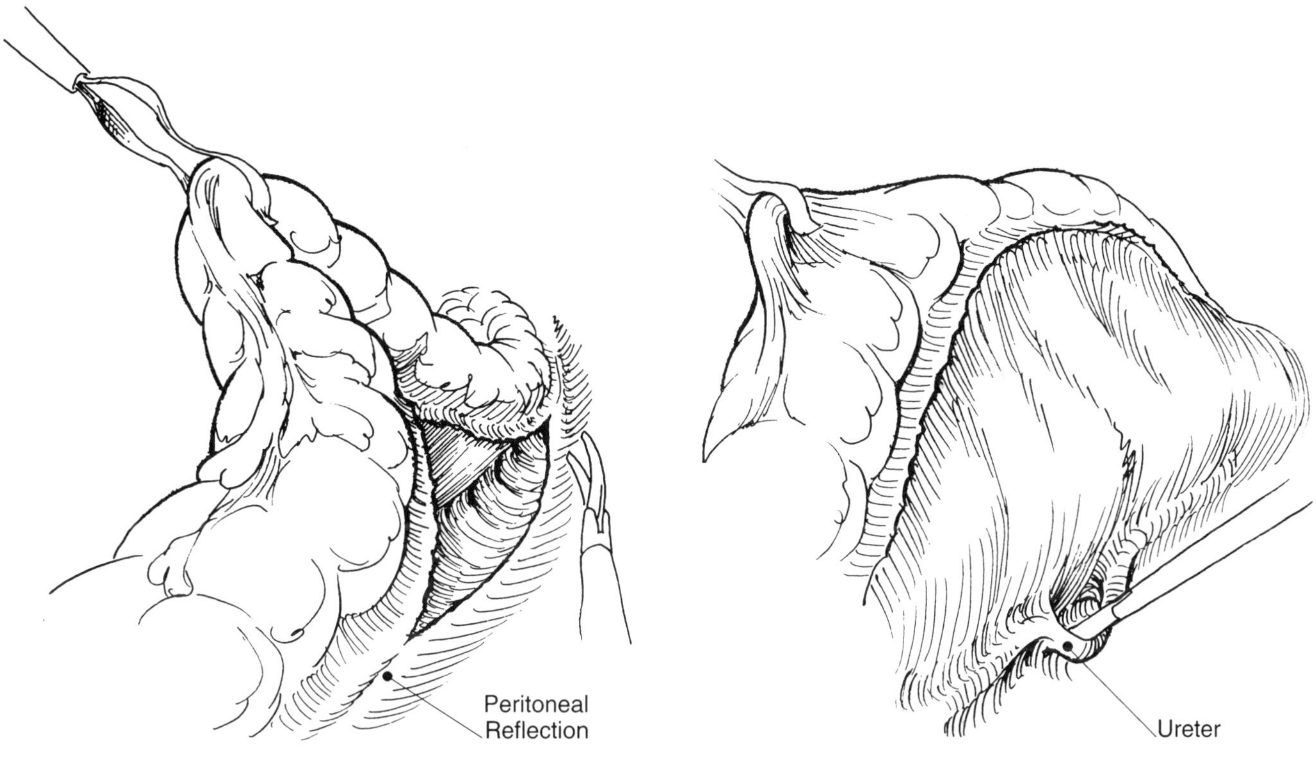

Fig. 6.24

The second light source is used to identify major vessels (Fig. 6.25A). Openings are made on either side of the vascular pedicles. A linear stapler with a vascular load is used to secure the mesentery, supplemented with clips, loops and bipolar cautery where necessary for complete hemostasis (Fig. 6.25B). If there is adequate length of bowel around the lesion, the bowel to be resected is exteriorized through a small incision, usually a

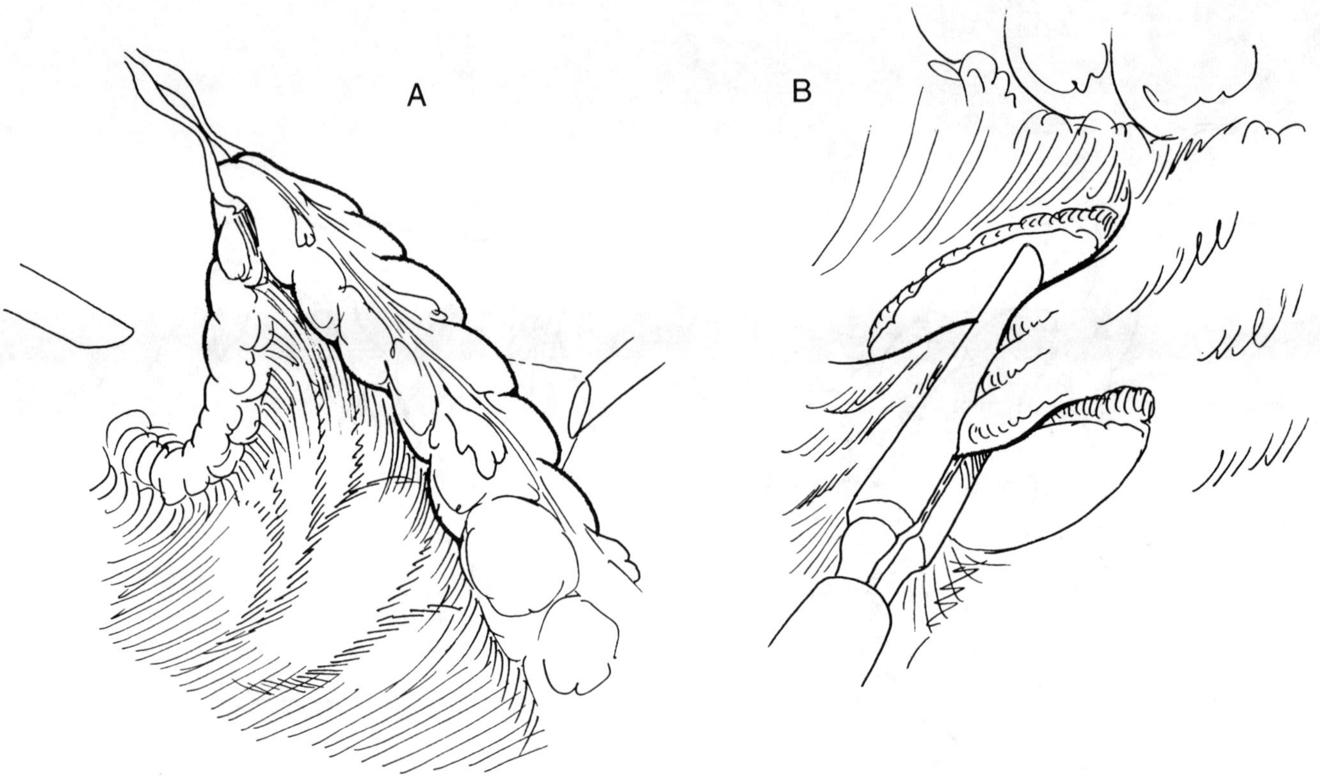

Fig. 6.25

McBurney type, or at the umbilicus. The bowel is divided and anastomosed in a standard manner (Fig. 6.26A). The anastomosis is replaced in the abdomen, the incision is closed, and pneumoperitoneum is reestablished to check for hemostasis.

For a low anastomosis, the proximal end of the colon is exteriorized after resection and the EEA anvil is secured in the end (Fig. 6.26B). The anvil is replaced in the abdomen, the incision is closed, and the abdomen is reinflated. The EEA stapler is passed through the rectum, the stapler ends are mated, and the rectum is joined to the proximal colon under laparoscopic guidance. A longer EEA stapler is available for sigmoid and left colon anastomoses. The anastomosis can be checked by proximal clamping with an atraumatic clamp and insufflating air with the pelvis filled with fluid, or dye can be injected.

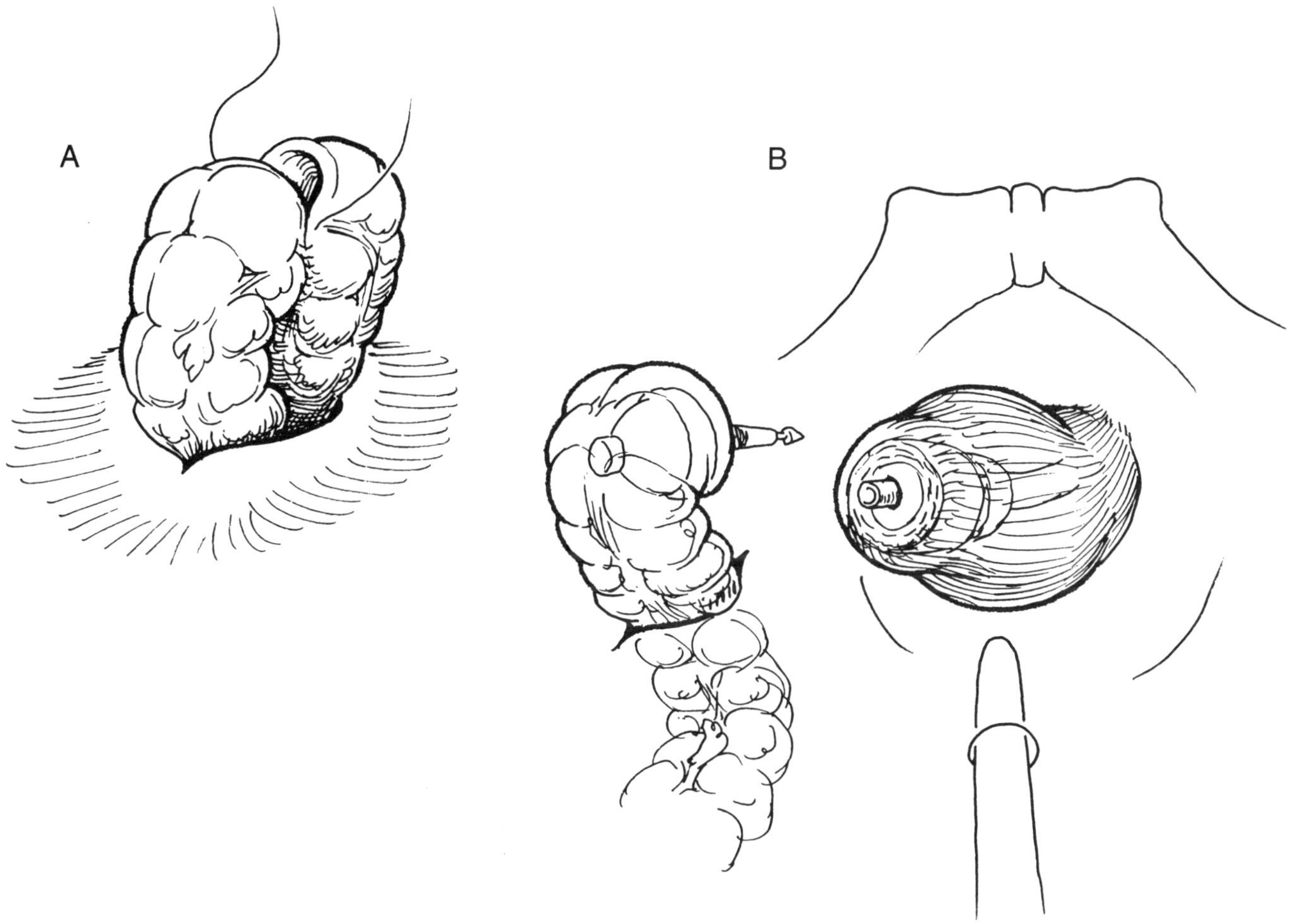

Fig. 6.26

Chapter 6: The Colon

EMBRYOLOGY

Skandalakis JE, Gray SW. Embryology for Surgeons. Williams & Wilkins, Philadelphia. 1994:184-275.

ANATOMY

Bergmann RA, Thompson SA, Afifi AK, et al. Compendium of Human Anatomic Variation. Urban & Schwarzenberg. Baltimore, 1988:79,83,167.

Gray H, Clemente C. Anatomy of the Human Body, Philadelphia: Lea & Febiger, 1985:740,741,1482.

Koritke JG, Sick H. Atlas of Sectional Human Anatomy. Urban & Schwarzenberg. Baltimore, 1988:260-280.

Moskowitz M, Zimmerman H, Felson B. The meandering mesenteric artery of the colon. Am J Radiol 1964; 92:1088-1099.

O'Connor CE, Reed WP. In vivo location of the human vermiform appendix. Clin Anat 1994;7:139-142.

Picken G, et al. The normal vermiform appendix at computed tomography: visualization and anatomical location. Clin Anat 1993;6:9-14.

VanDamme JP. Behavioral anatomy of the abdominal arteries. Surg Clin North Am 199373:699-725.

APPENDECTOMY

Bonanni F, et al. Laparoscopic versus conventional appendectomy. J Am Coll Surg 1995;179: 273-278.

Dudai M, et al. Simple, fast and inexpensive technique of laparoscopic appendectomy (abstract). 4th World Endoscopic Congress, Japan, 1994.

Nowzaradan Y, Westmorland J, Mc Carver CT, et. al. Current techniques in laparoscopic appendectomy. Surg Laparosc Endosc 1993;3:470-476.

MacFayden BV, et al. Laparoscopic management of the acute abdomen, appendix and small and large bowel. Surg Clin North Am 1992;72:1170-1183.

Pier A, Gotz F, Bacher C. Laparoscopic appendectomy in 625 cases: from innovation to routine. Surg Laparosc Endosc 1991;1:8-13.

Richards W, et al. A review of the results of laparoscopic versus open appendectomy. Surg Gynecol Obstet 1993; 177:473-480.

Saye WB, Rives DA, Cochran EB. Laparoscopic appendectomy: three years' experience. Surg Laparosc Endosc 1991;1:109-115.

Valla JS, Limonne B, Valla V, et. al. Laparoscopic appendectomy in children: report of 465 cases. Surg Laparosc Endosc 1991;1:166-172.

COLECTOMY

Darzi A, et al. Laparoscopic abdominoperineal excision of the rectum. Surg Endosc 1995;9:414-417.

Dean PA, et al. Laparoscopic-assisted segmental colectomy: early mayo clinic experience. Mayo Clin Proceed 1994;69:834-840.

Elftmann TD, et al. Laparoscopic-assisted colectomy: surgical techniques. Mayo Clin Proceed 1994;69:825-833.

Fielding GA, Stitz RW. Laparoscopic colorectal surgery. in Paterson-Brown S, Garden J, eds. Principles and Practice of Surgical Laparoscopy, London: W.B. Saunders Co Ltd., 1994:211-224.

Franklin ME Jr, et al. Prospective evaluation of laparoscopic colon resection versus open colon resection for adenocarcinoma. Surg Endosc 1995;9:811-816.

Lointier PH, Lautard M, Massoni C et. al. Laparoscopically assisted subtotal colectomy. J. Laparoendoscopic Surg 1993,3:439-453.

MacFayden Jr. BV, Wolfe BM, McKernan JB. Laparoscopic management of the acute abdomen, appendix and small and large bowel. Surg Clin North Am 1992;72:1169-1183.

Monson JRT, et al. Prospective evaluation of laparoscopic-assisted colectomy in an unselected group of patients. Lancet 1992;340:831-833.

Phillips EH, et al. Laparoscopic colectomy. Ann Surg 1992; 216:703-707.

Quattelbaum Jr. JK, Flanders HD, Usher III CH. Laparoscopically assisted colectomy. Surg Laparosc Endosc 1993;3:81-87.

Ramos JM, et al. Laparoscopy and colon cancer. Arch Surg 1994;129:897-900.

Semm K. Operative Manual for Endoscopic Abdominal Surgery. Chicago, Year Book Medical Publishers Inc. 1987:216.

Senagore AJ, et al. Open colectomy versus laparoscopic colectomy: are there differences? Am Surg 1993;59: 549-554.

Sundin JA, Wasson D, McMillen MM et. al. Laparoscopic assisted sigmoid colectomy for sigmoid volvulus. Surg Laparosc Endosc 1992;2:353-358.

7

The Pelvis

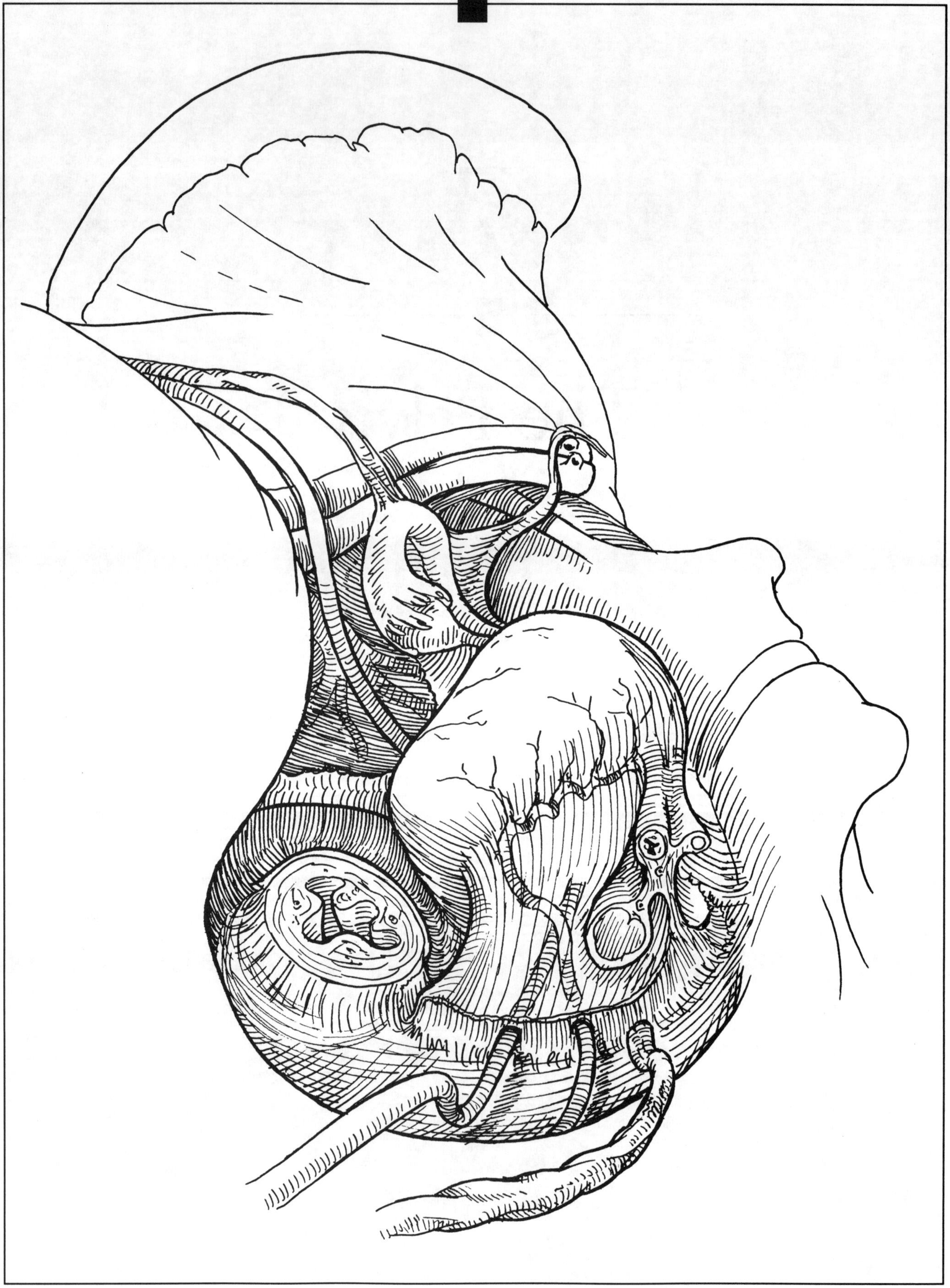

7

The Pelvis

Pelvic anatomy is relevant to the general surgeon, the urologist, and the gynecologist. This chapter focuses on general pelvic and genitourinary embryogenesis and anatomy. Clinical applications in gynecology (hysterectomy) and pelvic lymph node dissection for staging genitourinary malignancy are presented as examples of applied anatomy. This perspective should be cross referenced to the chapters on inguinal anatomy (Chapter 3), the colon (Chapter 6), and the urologic system (Chapter 8).

EMBRYOLOGY

During the embryonic period (the first 8 weeks of gestation), growth, differentiation and remodelling establish a pelvis that is close to the adult configuration. The majority of this development takes place while the embryo is between 4 and 30 mm in crown-rump length (Fig. 7.1). The genital and urinary structures arise from common elements and are so intimately related they must be viewed together. The differentiation and posi-

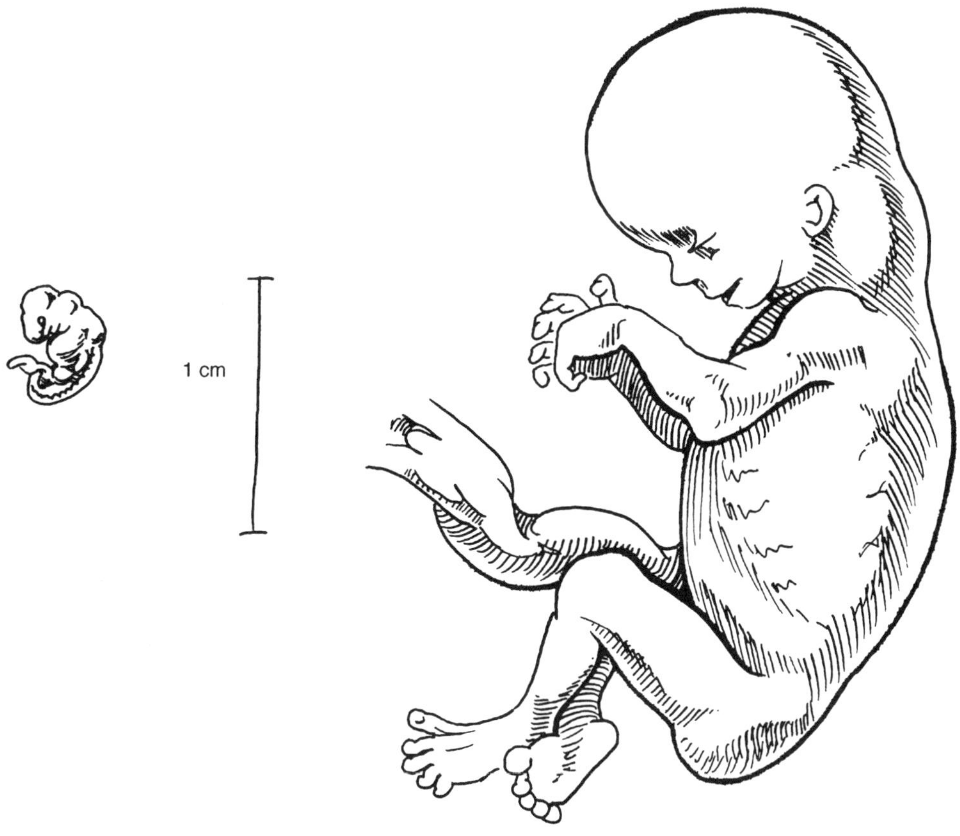

Fig. 7.1

tioning of the gonads continues through the fetal period.

In the fourth week of gestation, the umbilical arteries, which arise from the fused caudal portion of the aorta (Fig. 7.2), anastomose with adjacent dorsal intersegmental arteries. The anastomoses quickly become dominant, and the original aortic roots of the umbilical arteries regress. The new aortic roots will become the common iliac arteries, their continuations toward the lower extremity becomes the external iliac arteries, and the proximal trunks of the umbilical arteries will become the internal iliac arteries, with branches supplying the lower pelvic structures. The umbilical arteries lie on either side of the bladder on their way to the umbilical cord. Their postnatal remnant, the medial umbilical ligaments, are important surgical landmarks. They are a guide for entry and dissection of the retropubic space for bladder neck suspension, they help to avoid bladder injury in dissecting the groin for laparoscopic hernia repair and they lead to the superior vesicle arteries. The continuation of the aorta beyond the iliac trunks regresses, leaving the middle sacral artery. Lymphatics develop in parallel with the vascular structures.

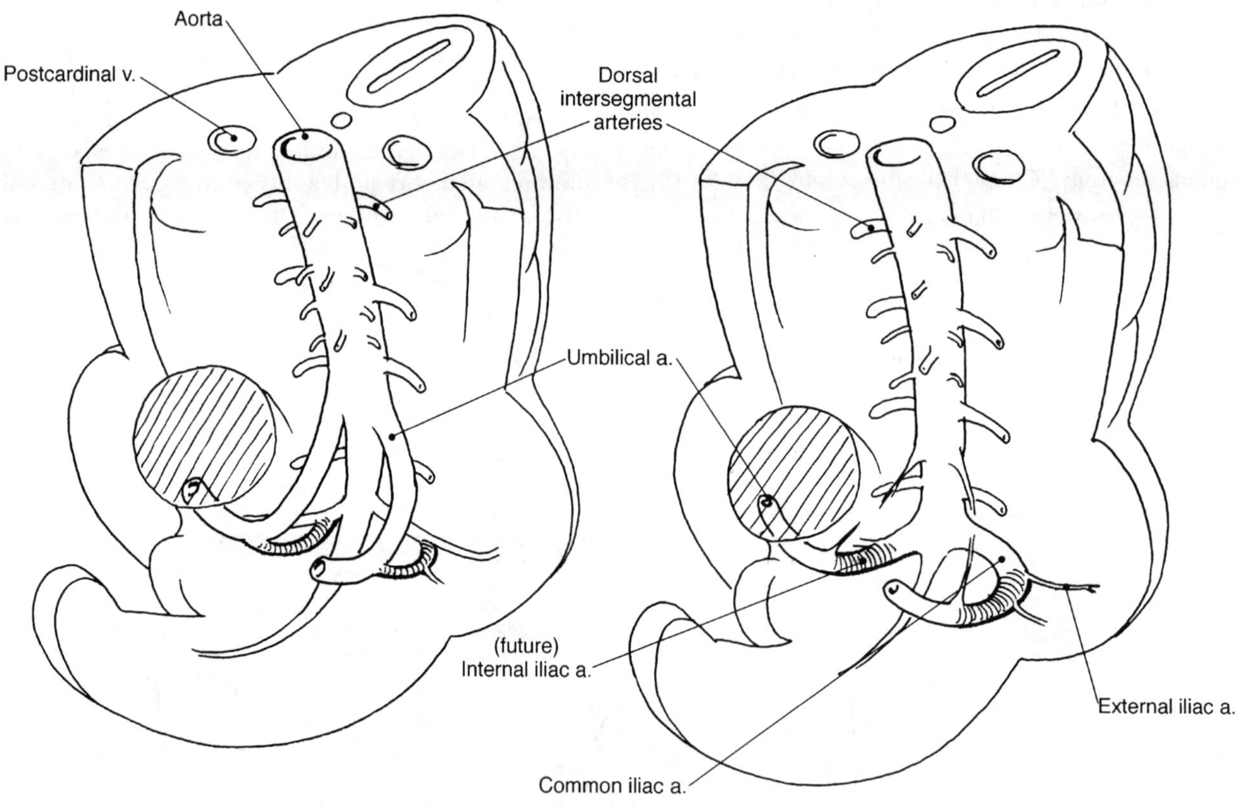

Fig. 7.2

Early in embryonic development the terminal hindgut is incorporated into the infolding tail region and at about 2 weeks develops a ventral diverticulum, the allantois (Fig. 7.3). The junction of allantois and hindgut becomes the cloaca and is closed off by a two layer (endoderm and ectoderm) membrane of anterior body wall. The dorsal hindgut mesentery contains multiple ventral aortic branches until one becomes dominant as the inferior mesenteric artery and supplies the hindgut. Umbilical (future internal iliac) branches supply the rectum. The tailgut caudal to the cloaca regresses in the fifth week. The cloaca is then progressively divided by a mesodermal septum, forming the rectum posteriorly and the urogenital sinus anteriorly. The anal musculature coalesces around the terminal gut tube, forming the external sphincters.

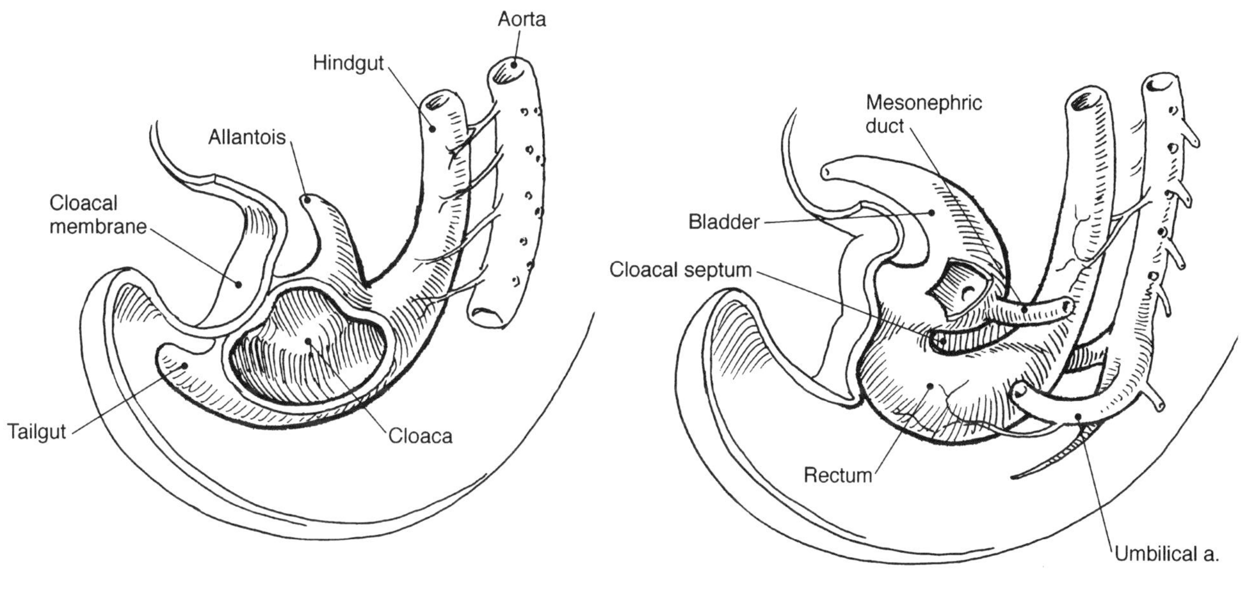

Fig. 7.3

During the third week of gestation, bilateral urogenital ridges fed by lateral segmental arteries develop from intermediate mesoderm in the lower cervical and upper thoracic dorsal body wall and grow in a caudal direction (Fig. 7.4). While nephrogenic elements develop and regress from cranial to caudal within these ridges, bilateral tubular structures (mesonephric/Wolffian ducts) form in parallel and reach the cloaca at the end of week

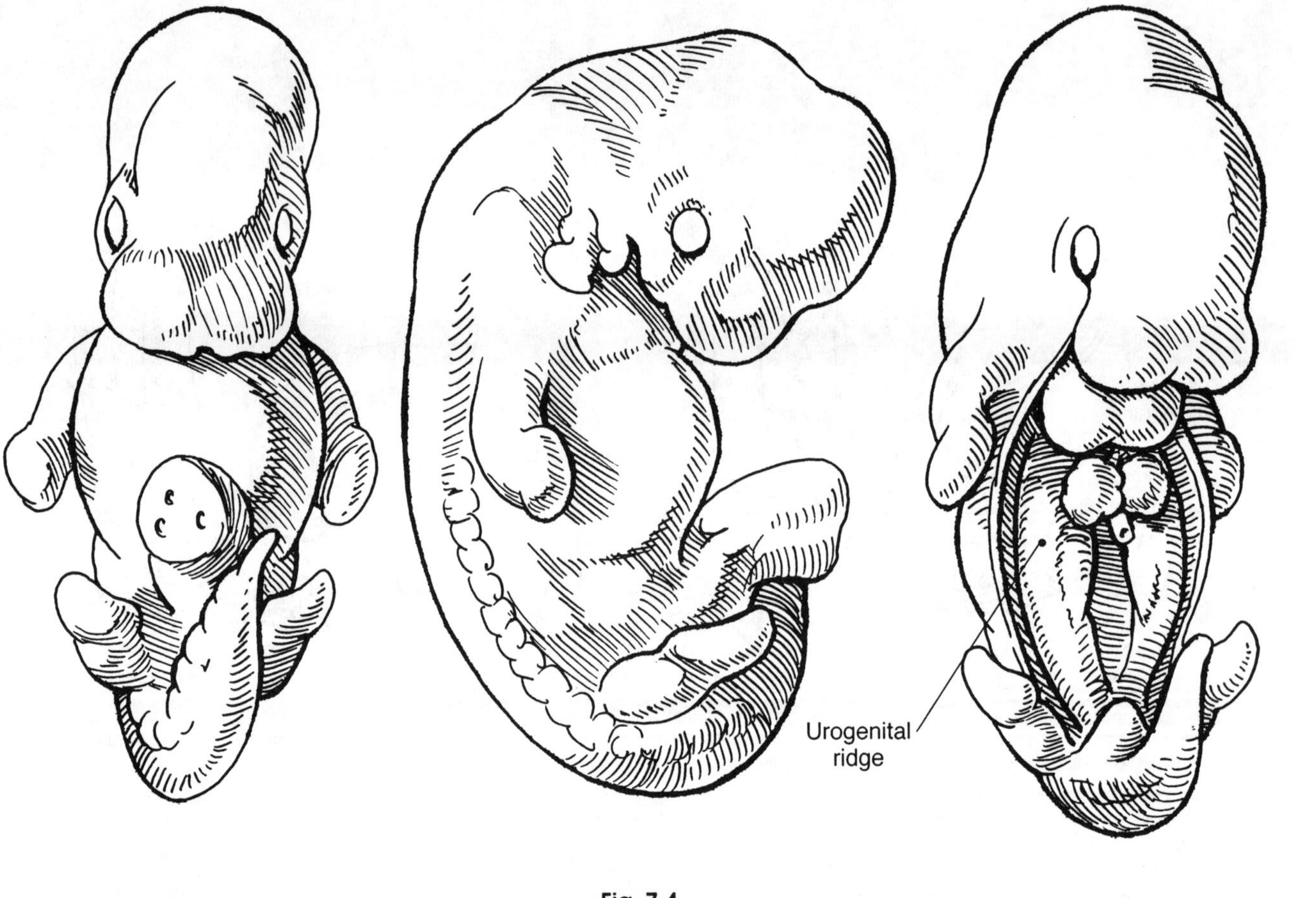

Fig. 7.4

five (Fig. 7.5). The most caudal portion of the nephrogenic cord evolves last and becomes the metanephros, the definitive kidney. At about the time the mesonephric duct reaches the cloaca, a dorsal bud near its terminal end, the future ureter, grows into the developing metanephros. In the ensuing 6 weeks, the mesonephric kidneys regress and the metanephric kidneys ascend in the retroperitoneum relative to body

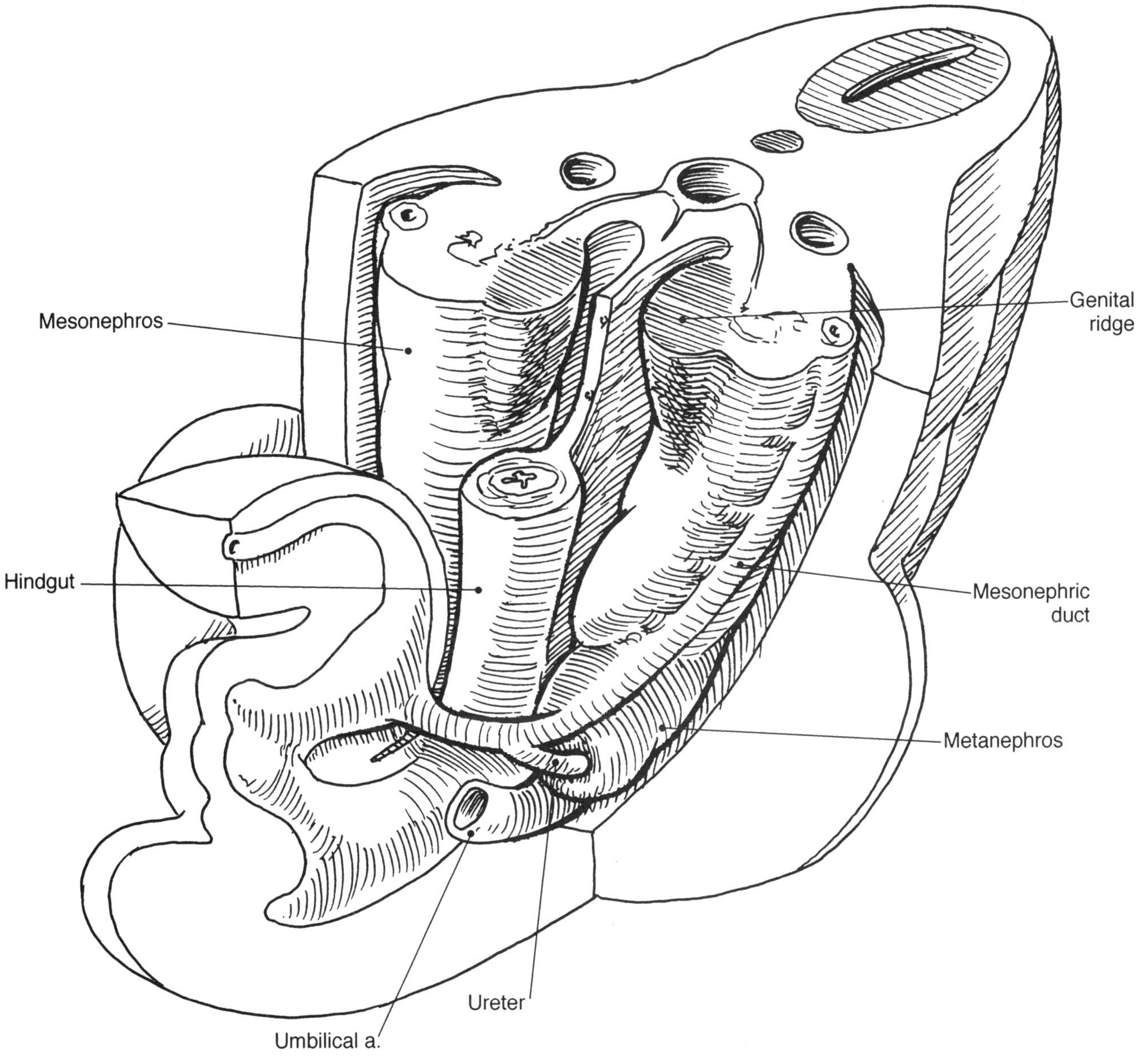

Fig. 7.5

growth (Fig. 7.6), approaching the developing adrenal glands (Chapter 8). The ureters elongate and the orientation of the renal hila changes from anterior to anteromedial. The kidneys acquire successively higher lateral segmental aortic branches as they ascend. Incomplete arterial regression leaves supplemental renal arteries in some individuals.

During this same period, gonadal ridges are developing on the ventromedial portions of the urogenital ridges and the adrenal glands are forming at the cranial ends. About the sixth week, another set of ducts, the paramesonephric (Müellerian) ducts, develop posterior to the mesonephric ducts. The paramesonephric ducts play a key role in the development of the female repro-

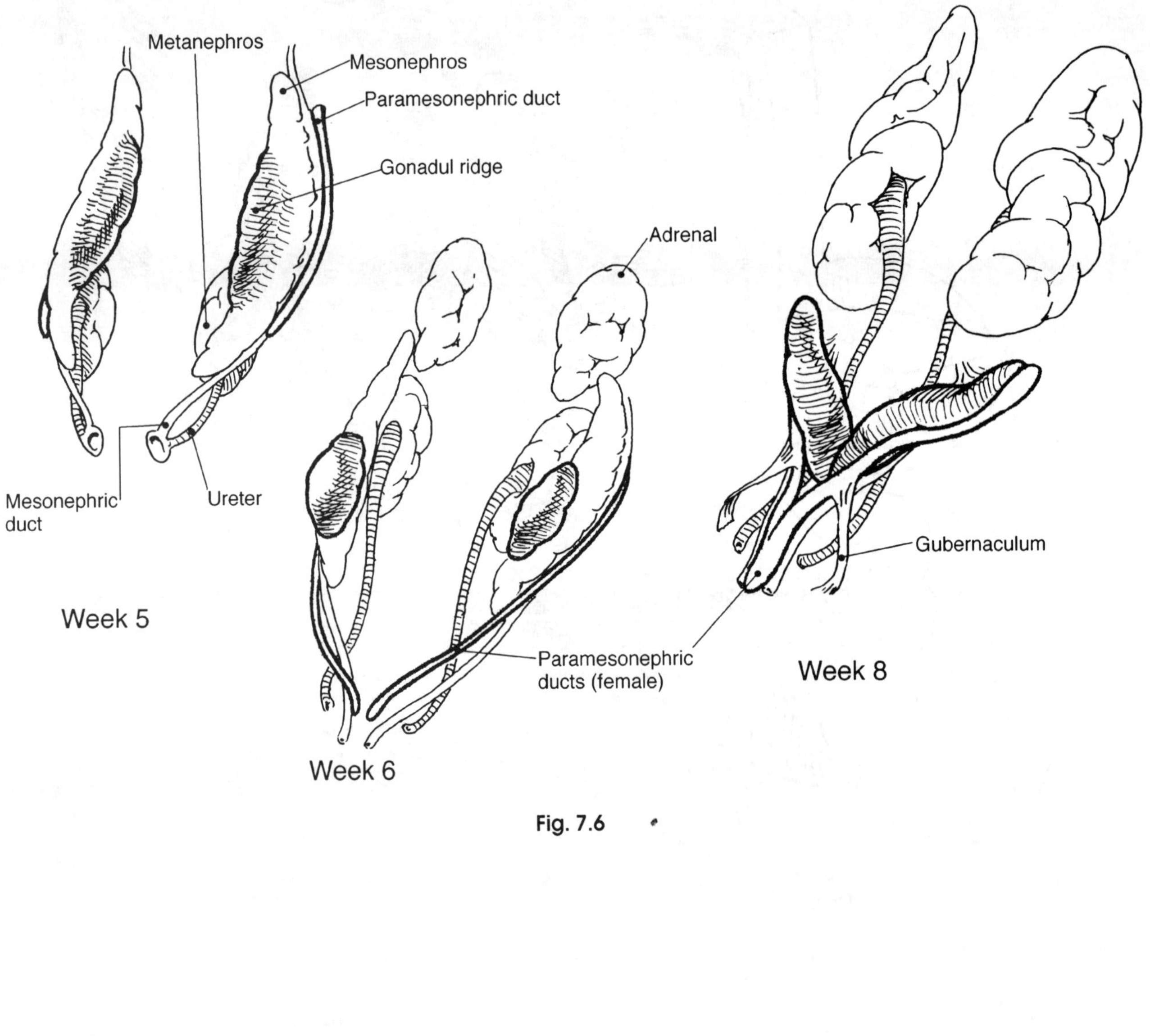

Fig. 7.6

ductive organs while the mesonephric ducts contribute to the male sexual apparatus.

Sexual differentiation of the gonads begins about the seventh week of gestation and continues through the third month (Fig. 7.7). The regressing mesonephroi leave filmy bands that connect the gonads to the diaphragm above and to the inguinal region below. During week eight, an additional thickening, the gubernaculum, forms in the edge of the inguinal fold. In both sexes, the lower ends of the paramesonephric ducts fuse and join the Müellerian tubercle on the dorsal wall of the cloaca. The fates of the two sets of ducts diverge after week eight.

In the male, rete cords of the testis join with about a dozen mesonephric tubules which drain into the mesonephric duct, forming the efferent ductules and epididymis. The continuations of the mesonephric ducts form the vas deferens, seminal vesicles and ejaculatory ducts. The paramesonephric ducts in the male regress by three months. The gubernaculum attaching the lower poles of the testes to the scrotal swellings (Chapter 3) grows little relative to the elongation of the body, resulting in the positioning of the testes at the deep inguinal ring by week 28 of gestation. Descent of the testes through the inguinal canal posterior to the processus vaginalis occurs in the seventh month. The testicular vessels from the abdominal aorta are carried into the inguinal canal as the internal spermatic vessels. Passage of the testes to the superficial ring takes only a few days, but descent into the scrotum takes four more weeks.

In the female, the paramesonephric ducts continue to develop, forming the Fallopian tubes, uterus and upper portion of the vagina. The mesonephric ducts regress by the end of the third month. During the 12th week, the ovaries "descend" below the pelvic brim and the mid portions of the gubernacula attach to the junction of the uterus and fallopian tubes, forming the ovarian ligament above and the round ligament of the uterus below. The round ligament of the uterus runs through the inguinal canal and is attached to the labial swelling. The blood supply to the ovaries from the abdominal aorta runs in the peritoneal folds at the cephalad poles of the ovaries, forming the infundibulopelvic ligaments.

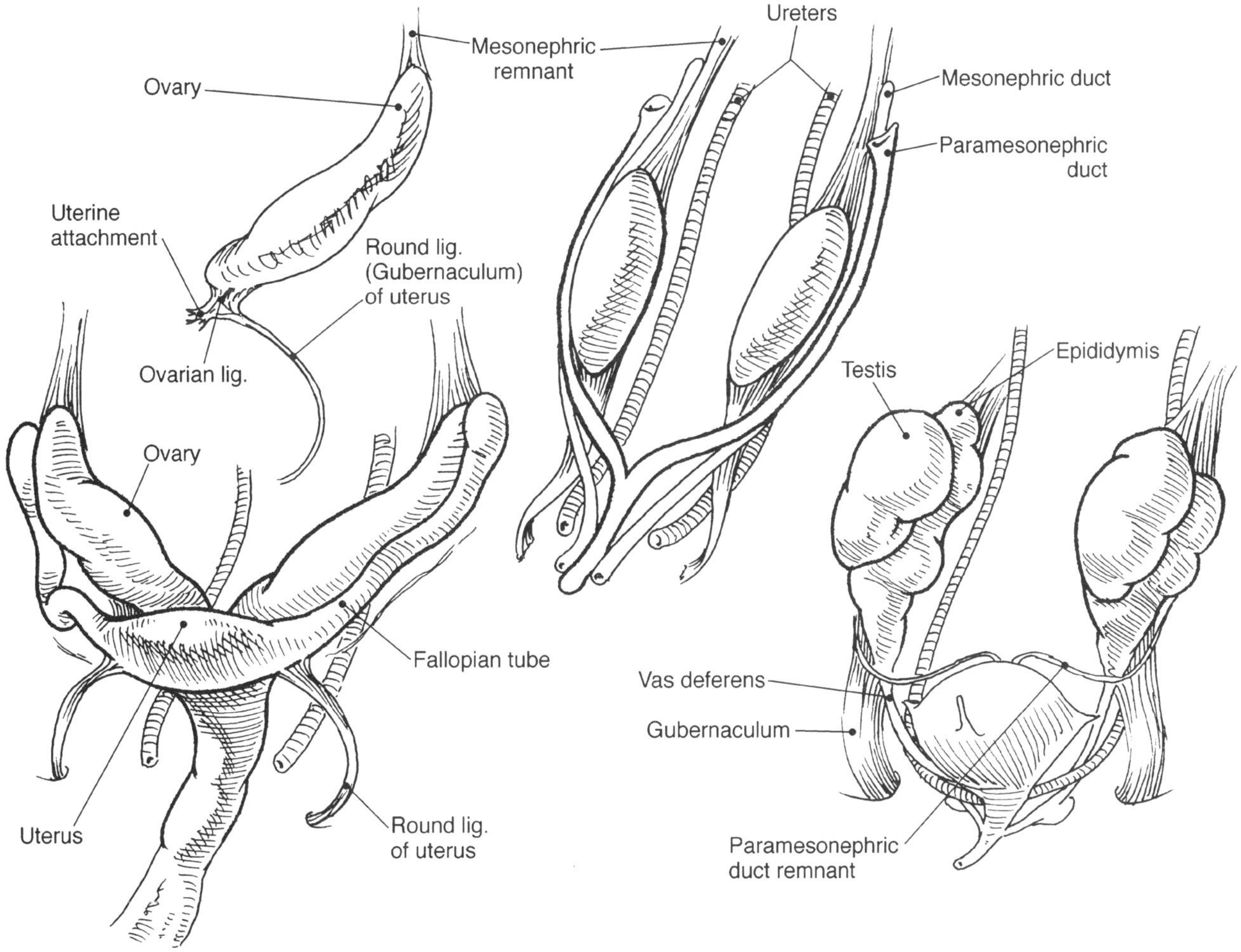

Fig. 7.7

ANATOMY

Musculoskeletal Framework

The bony pelvis formed by the innominate bones (ilium, ischium, and pubis) and sacrum forms two superimposed bowls, the broad, shallow lesser pelvis above the ileopectineal line and the deep, narrow, posteriorly angulated true pelvis below (Fig. 7.8). The pelvic ring is bound together by cartilage and ligaments at the sacroiliac junctions and at the pubic symphysis. The lower sacral and coccygeal segments are joined to the ischium by two strong bands, the sacrospinous and sacrotuberous ligaments. The sacrospinous ligament bounds the greater sciatic foramen above and the lesser sciatic foramen below. The large bony obturator foramina are closed by dense membranes with a small cephalad opening (obturator canal) for passage of the obturator nerve and vessels to the adductor compartment of the thigh.

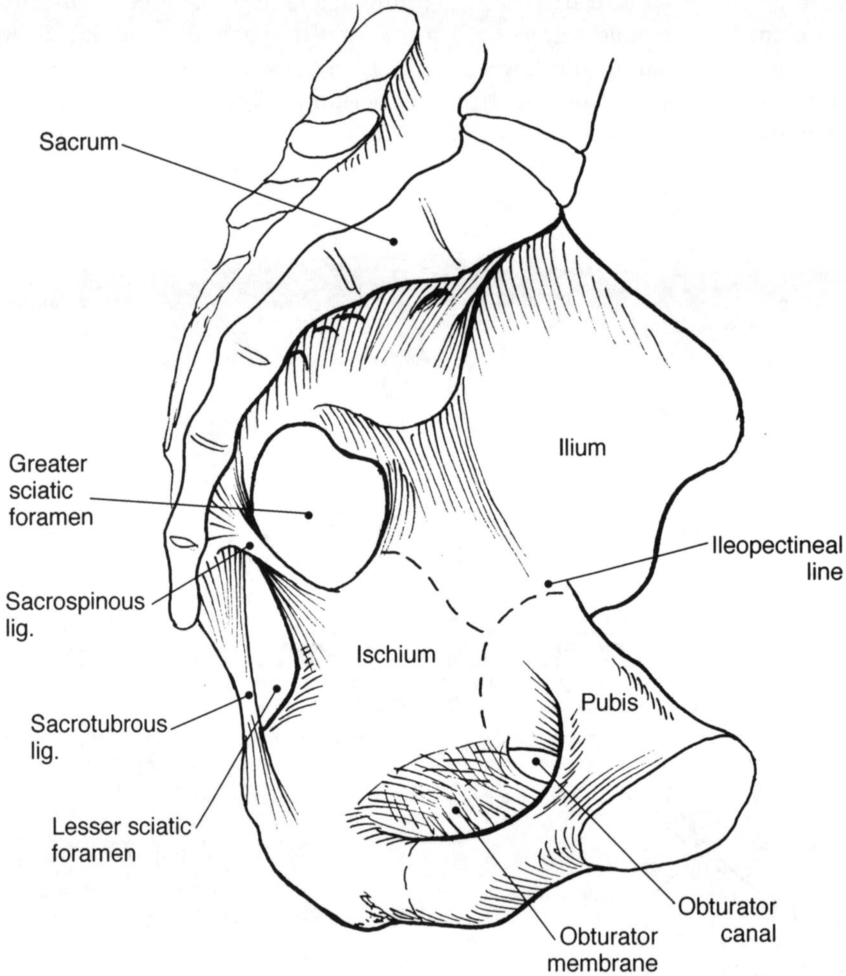

Fig. 7.8

Three muscles close the lateral walls of the true pelvis (Fig. 7.9): the obturator internus, piriformis, and coccygeus. The obturator internus has a broad origin below the rim of the true pelvis and over the obturator foramen and exits the pelvis through the lesser sciatic foramen to reach the greater trochanter of the femur. The piriformis originates along the inner rim of the mid sacrum and exits the pelvis through the greater sciatic foramen on its way to the greater trochanter. The coccygeus lies anterior to the sacrospinous ligament between the inner rim of the lower sacrum and the spine of the ischium. The inner surfaces of these muscles are covered by the continuation of the investing layer of abdominal fascia which in this region is called the endopelvic fascia.

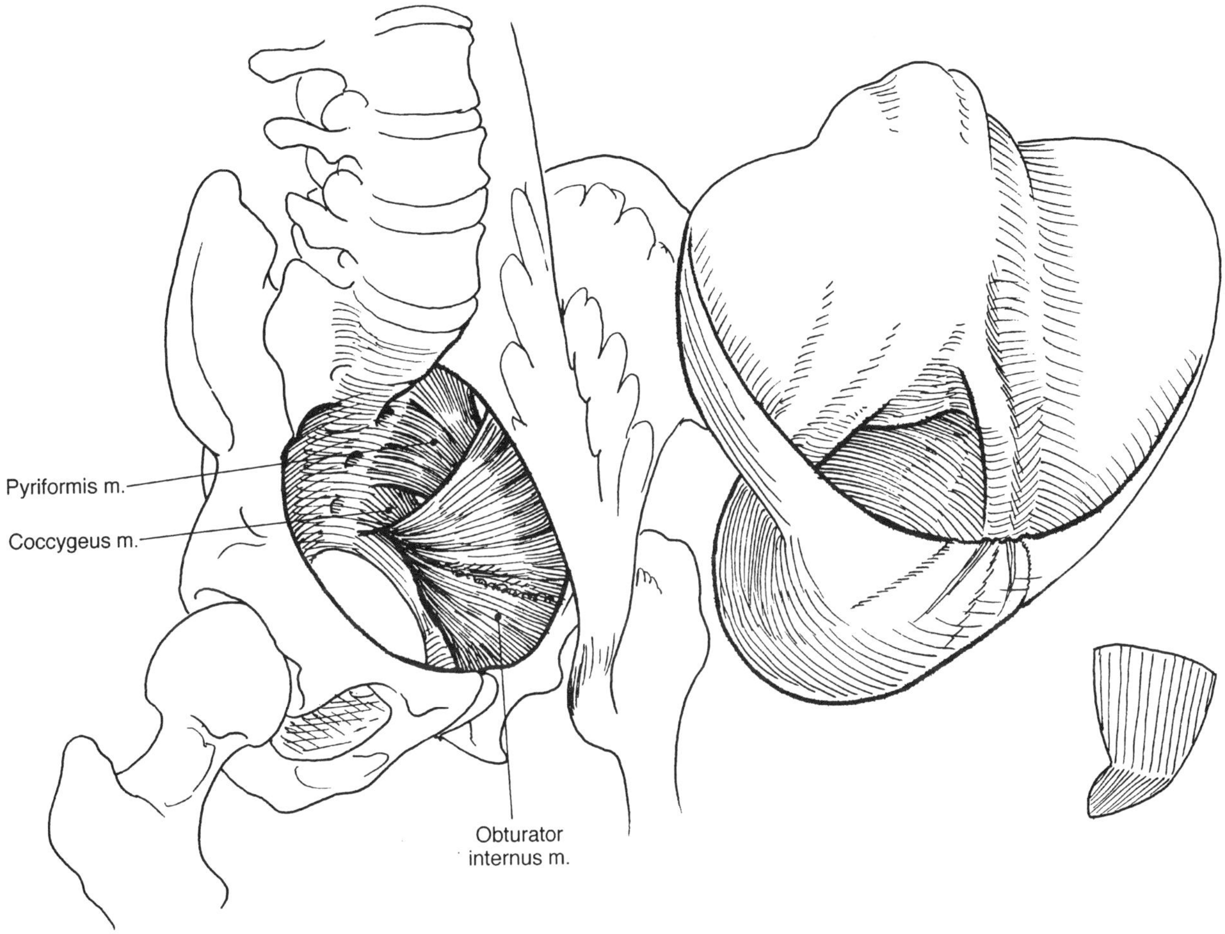

Fig. 7.9

From the laparoscopic viewpoint, the true pelvis appears as a rearward projecting bowl at the caudal end of the abdominal cavity. The slope of the pubic bones and the hollow of the sacrum angulates the axis of the pelvis 45 degrees posterior to the long axis of the body. The pelvic outlet is capped by the muscular pelvic and perineal diaphragms. The bowl of the lesser pelvis is covered by the fused iliopsoas muscles, which exit between the iliopubic rami and the lateral portions of the inguinal ligaments (Fig. 7.10). The round profile of the psoas muscles forms a yoke-like collar around the rim of the true pelvis. A triangular sheet of muscle, the urogenital diaphragm, fills the angle between the inferior pubic rami. The major component of this triangle, the flat deep transverse perineus muscle, acts as a sphincter around the membranous urethra and surrounds the introitus of the vagina. Fusiform superficial transverse perinei and ischio- and bulbocavernosus muscles border the superficial surface of this perineal diaphragm.

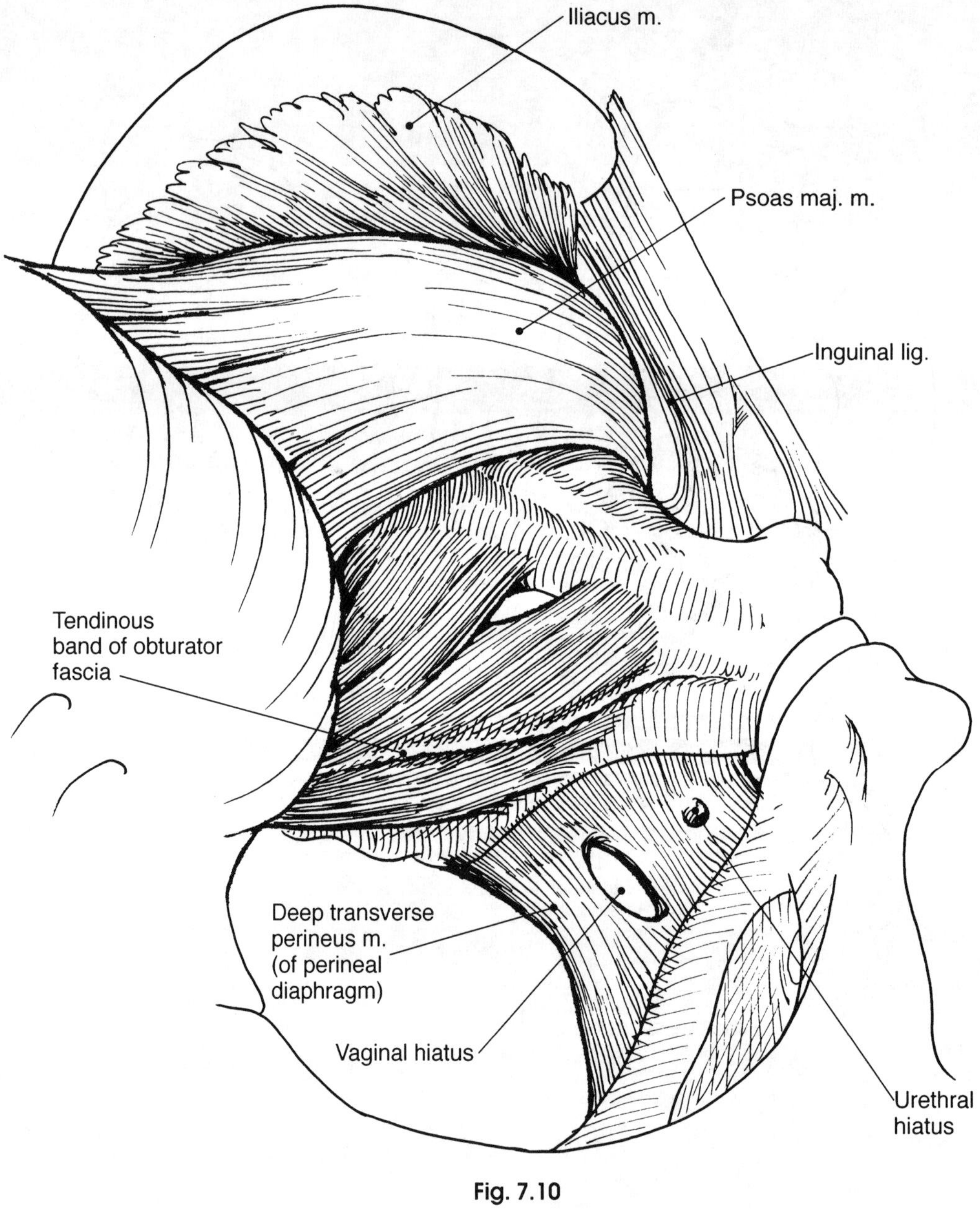

Fig. 7.10

Above the perineal diaphragm, the inferior pelvic aperture is covered by a concave muscular diaphragm, the levator ani (Fig. 7.11). The posterior portion of the levator ani is formed by two broad muscular sheets, the iliococcygei, which run from the thickened central band of obturator fascia (tendinous arc) to the inner surface of the coccyx. Anterior to the coccyx, the two muscles interdigitate and fuse in the midline (anococcygeal raphe). The anterior portion of the levator is formed by the pubococcygeus muscles. The central portion of the pubococcygeus is penetrated by the rectum and the anterior limbs form a V-shaped hiatus through which the urethra and the vagina in the female pass. Anterior to the rectum, the pubococcygei fuse with each other and with the central tendinous point of the perineum. Lateral to the central point on either side, a cleft, the ischiorectal space, lies between the urogenital diaphragm and the levator ani. The most medial bands of the pubococcygei encircle the lower rectum just above the external anal sphincters, forming the puborectalis sling which creates an anorectal angulation important in fecal continence.

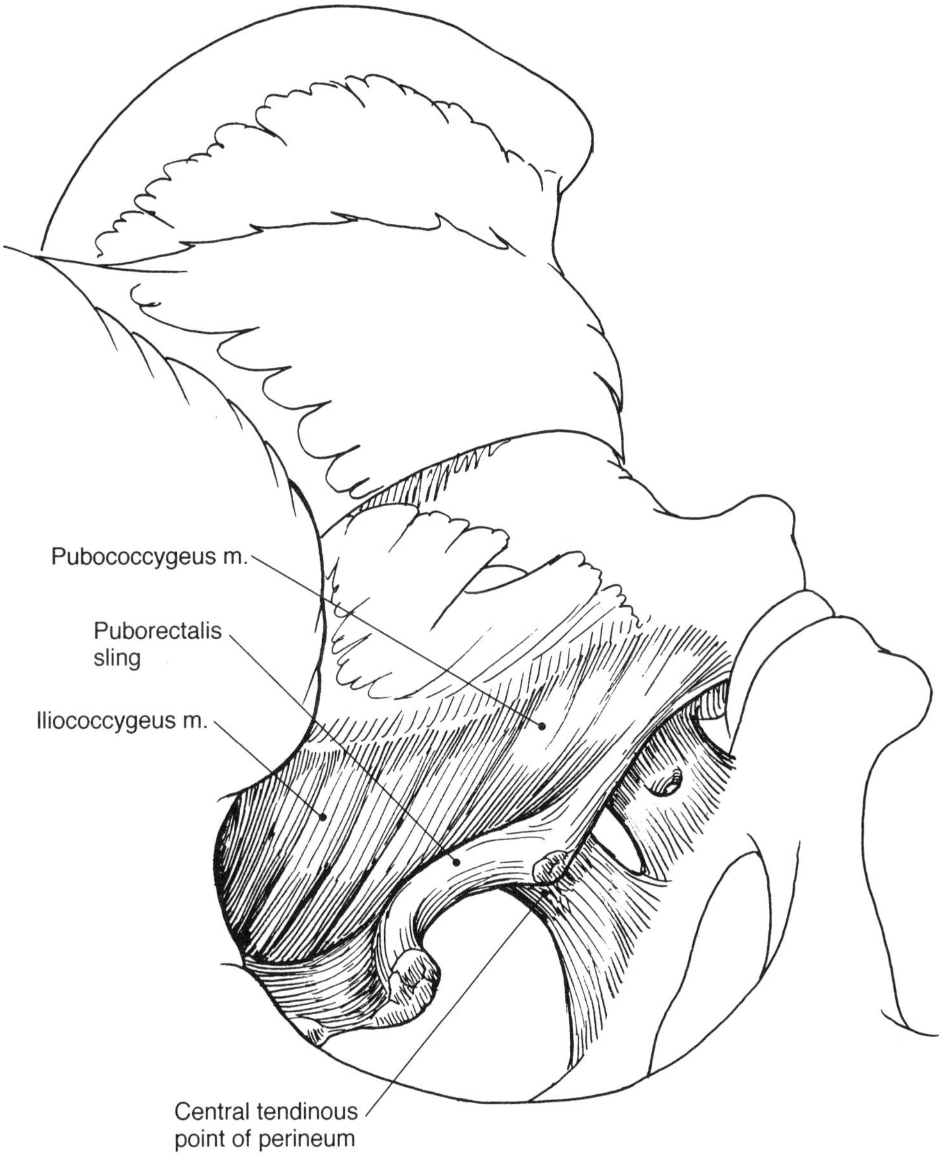

Fig. 7.11

The Pelvic Neurovascular Space

The walls of the true pelvis are lined by a layer of nerves and blood vessels lying between the endopelvic fascia and the pelvic peritoneum. The deep layer of nerves consists of the ventral sacral nerve roots posterolaterally and the sympathetic chains lying medial to the sacral foramina (Fig. 7.12). The two lower lumbar nerves (L4 and L5) and the sacral nerves exchange fibers to form the sacral plexus over the piriformis and coccygeus muscles. Sympathetic gray rami join the sacral nerve roots near the sacral foramina and branches of the lower sacral nerves descend over the levator ani to supply splanchnic innervation to the pelvic viscera. The sacral plexus nerves converge in the hiatus between piriformis and coccygeus muscles to form the sciatic nerve exiting the pelvis through the greater sciatic foramen along with the superior gluteal vessels.

The blood vessels of the pelvis consist of the splayed out internal iliac branches and associated lymphatics. The common and external iliac vessels lie at the inner rim of the psoas muscles like a yoke rimming the inlet of the true pelvis. Within a short distance of the aortic and caval bifurcations, the common iliacs divide into external and internal iliac branches and the internal iliac trunks dive posterolaterally into the bowl of the pelvis.

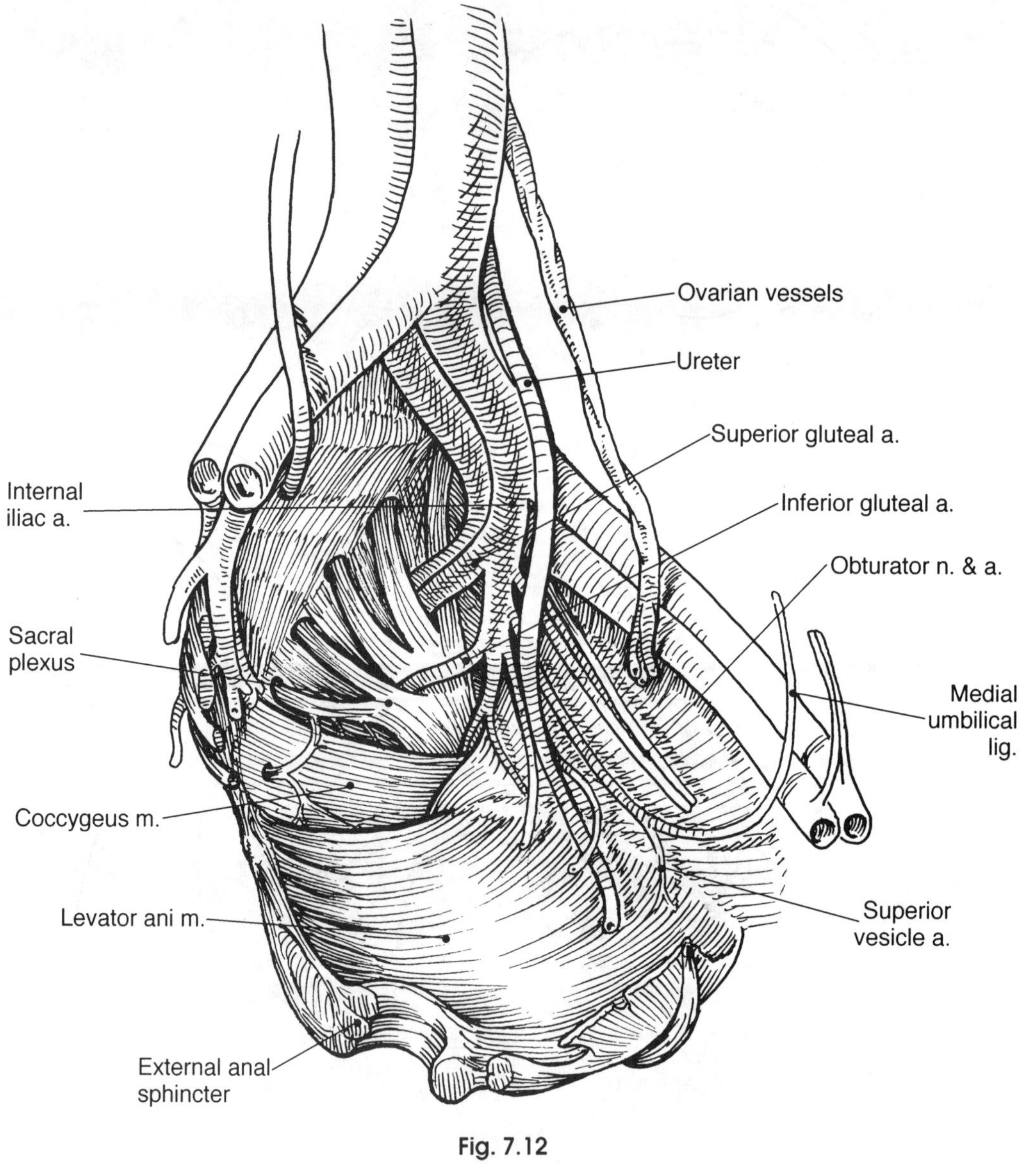

Fig. 7.12

The branches of the internal iliac arteries splay out in fan-like manner and are highly variable (Fig. 7.13). The most common branching pattern (75%) is into a posterior division whose major branch is the superior gluteal artery and an anterior division with a common stem giving rise to the inferior gluteal and internal pudendal arteries and multiple smaller pelvic visceral branches arising separately. The posterior division includes two smaller parietal branches, the iliolumbar and lateral sacral arteries. The small branches of the anterior division include the obturator artery (25% of the time this vessel arises from the inferior epigastric artery) and internal pudendal arteries to muscles of the pelvis and adductor thigh (obturator), and visceral branches to the rectum, uterus, and bladder. The most anterior of the anterior division branches are the obliterated umbilical arteries, which ascend toward the umbilicus on the anterior abdominal wall on either side of the bladder (Chapter 3). The pelvic venous drainage parallels the arterial pattern but the veins are more numerous and interconnect in plexi around the pelvic viscera.

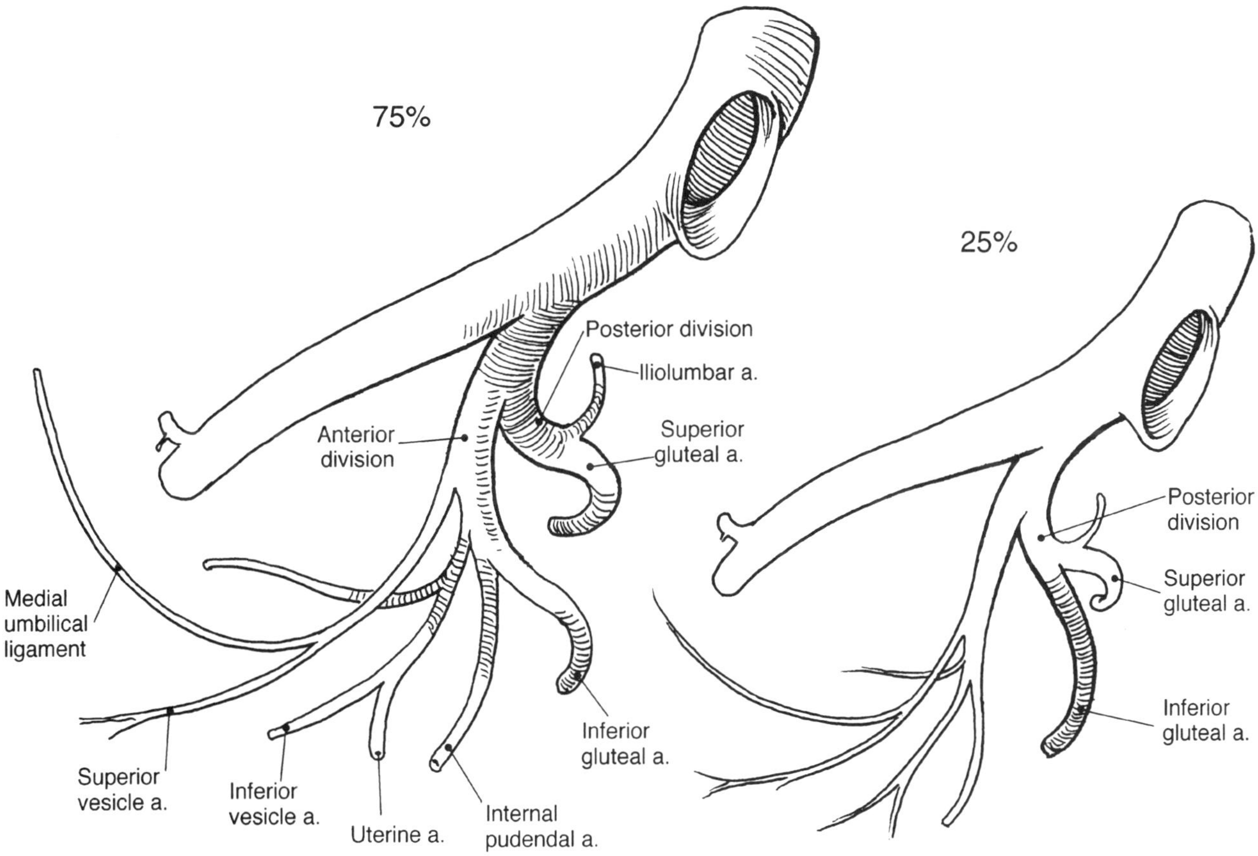

Fig. 7.13

The pelvic lymphatic channels and lymph nodes lie along the course of the blood vessels and drain the viscera supplied by those vessels (Fig. 7.14). Lymphatic drainage patterns are discussed in detail below in relation to pelvic lymph node dissection.

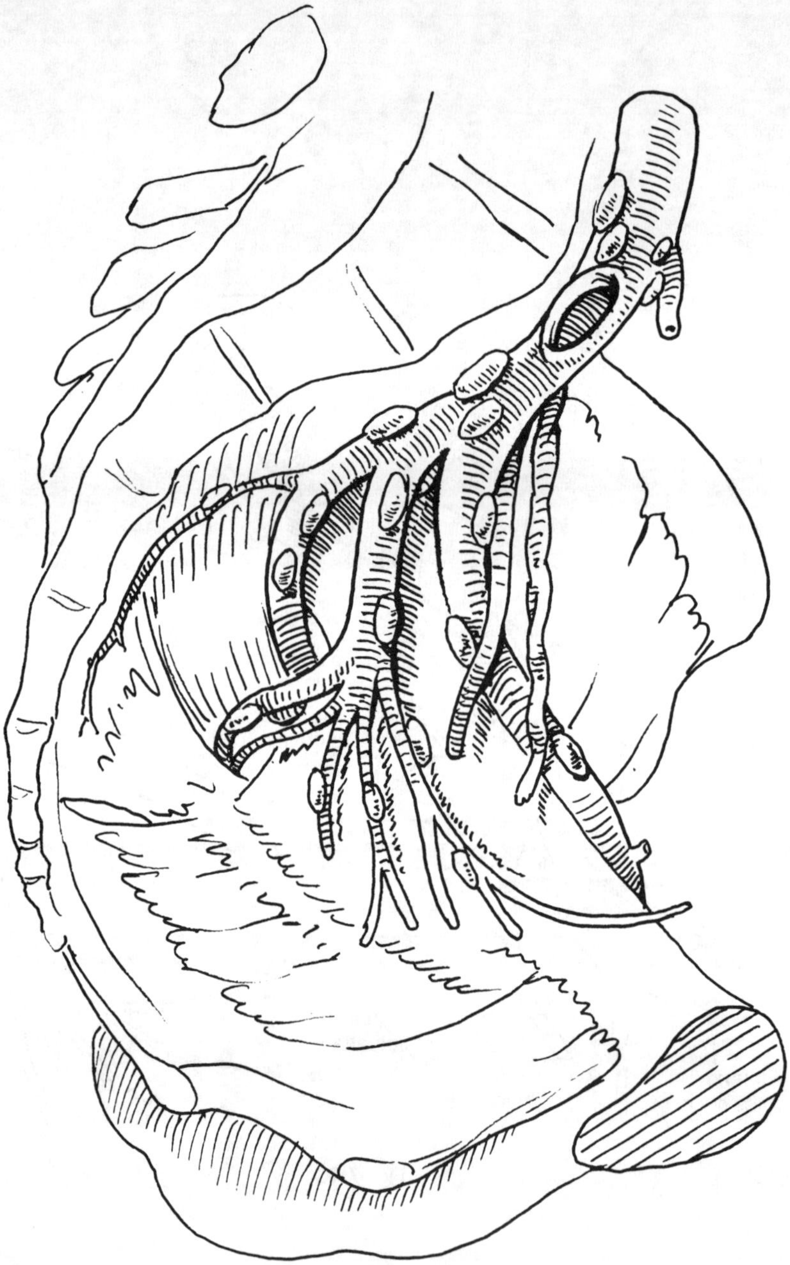

Fig. 7.14

Networks of fine autonomic nerves run on the arteries to the pelvic viscera (Fig. 7.15). Autonomic fibers descending from the aortic plexus form the superior hypogastric plexus on the sacral promontory below the aortic bifurcation. Bilateral inferior hypogastric nerve bundles descend to the pelvic plexi on the pelvic sidewalls in the area of the tendinous arc of the levator. The pelvic plexi receive splanchnic branches from the sacral plexus on each side. Autonomics from the pelvic plexi extend along the blood vessels to the walls of the pelvic viscera forming rectal, uterovaginal, and vesical plexi.

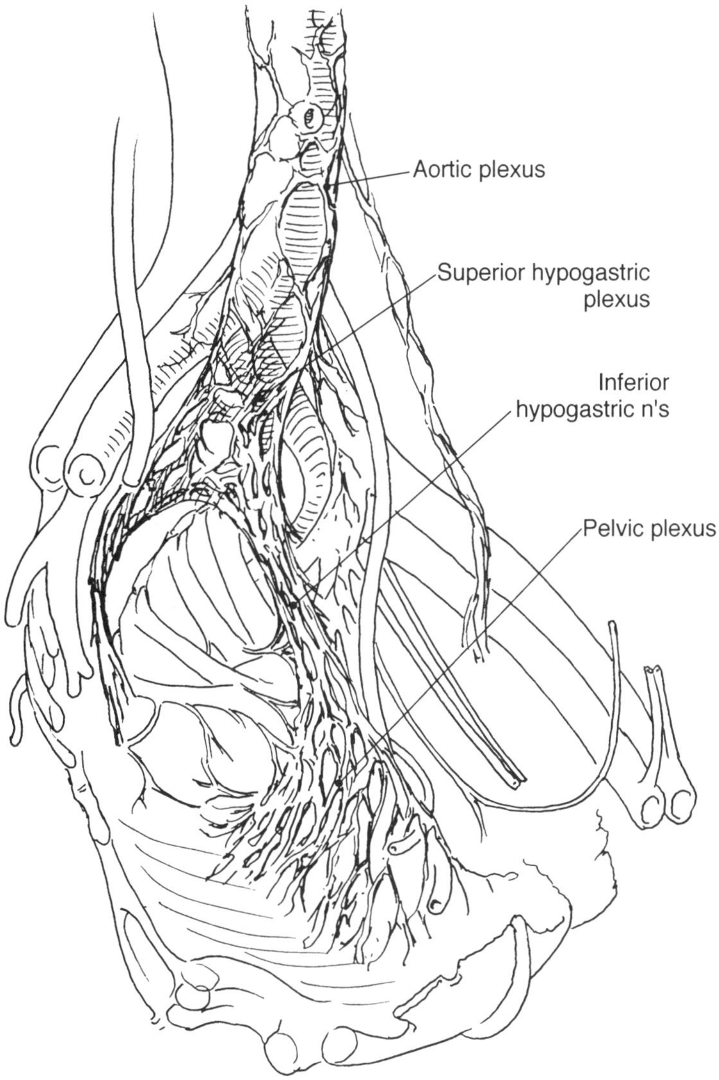

Fig. 7.15

The Pelvic Viscera

The rectum and genitourinary organs are cradled in the pelvic basin above the levator ani (Fig. 7.16). The ureters descend into the pelvis in the retroperitoneum ensheathed in a continuation of the renal fascia (Chapter 8). They cross over the external iliac arteries just beyond the takeoff of the internal iliacs. After crossing the raised collar formed by the external iliac arteries, the ureters follow the contours of the pelvic bowl and diverge laterally before turning anteromedially toward the bladder.

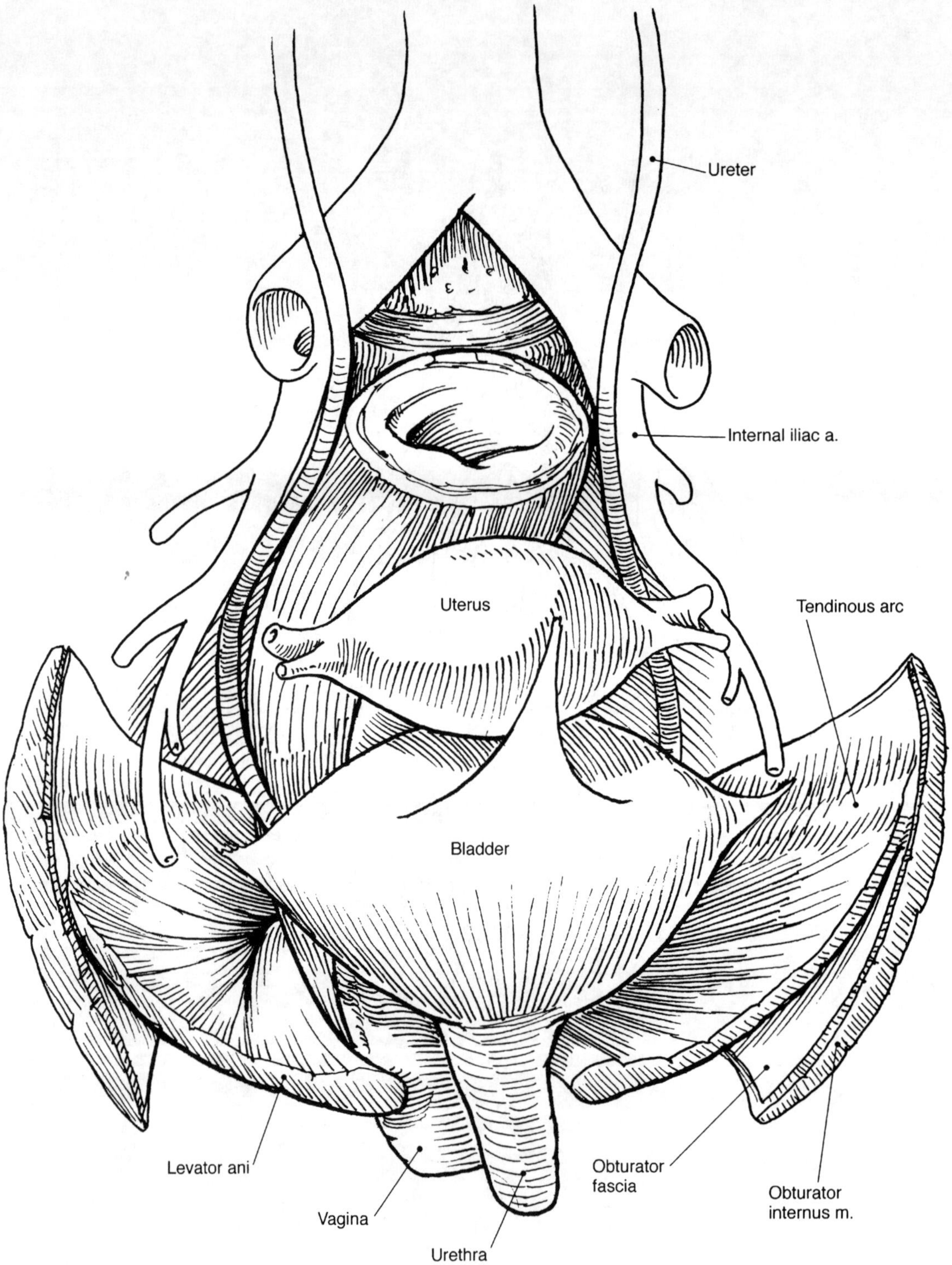

Fig. 7.16

The relationships of the pelvic organs are best seen in sagittal section (Fig. 7.17). The volume of the pelvic basin occupied by the bladder and rectum at any time depends on the distention of these organs. The remaining pelvic volume is filled with loops of bowel and omentum. In the male, the posterior surface of the bladder and prostate directly abut the anterior rectal wall and the most dependent point of the peritoneal cavity is the rectovesicle recess. In women, with the uterus and vagina interposed between bladder and rectum, the rectovaginal recess (pouch of Douglas) is most dependent.

The ureters enter the bladder posterolaterally, tunnel diagonally through the wall and enter the base of the bladder forming a trigone with the urethral orifice. The urethra in the male passes through the prostate and perineal diaphragm before entering the corpus spongiosum of the penis. In the female, the proximal urethra is surrounded by extensions of the bladder musculature above the perineal diaphragm. The bladder is supplied by superior and inferior vesicle arteries. The inferior bladder surface is surrounded by the vesicle venous and nerve plexi.

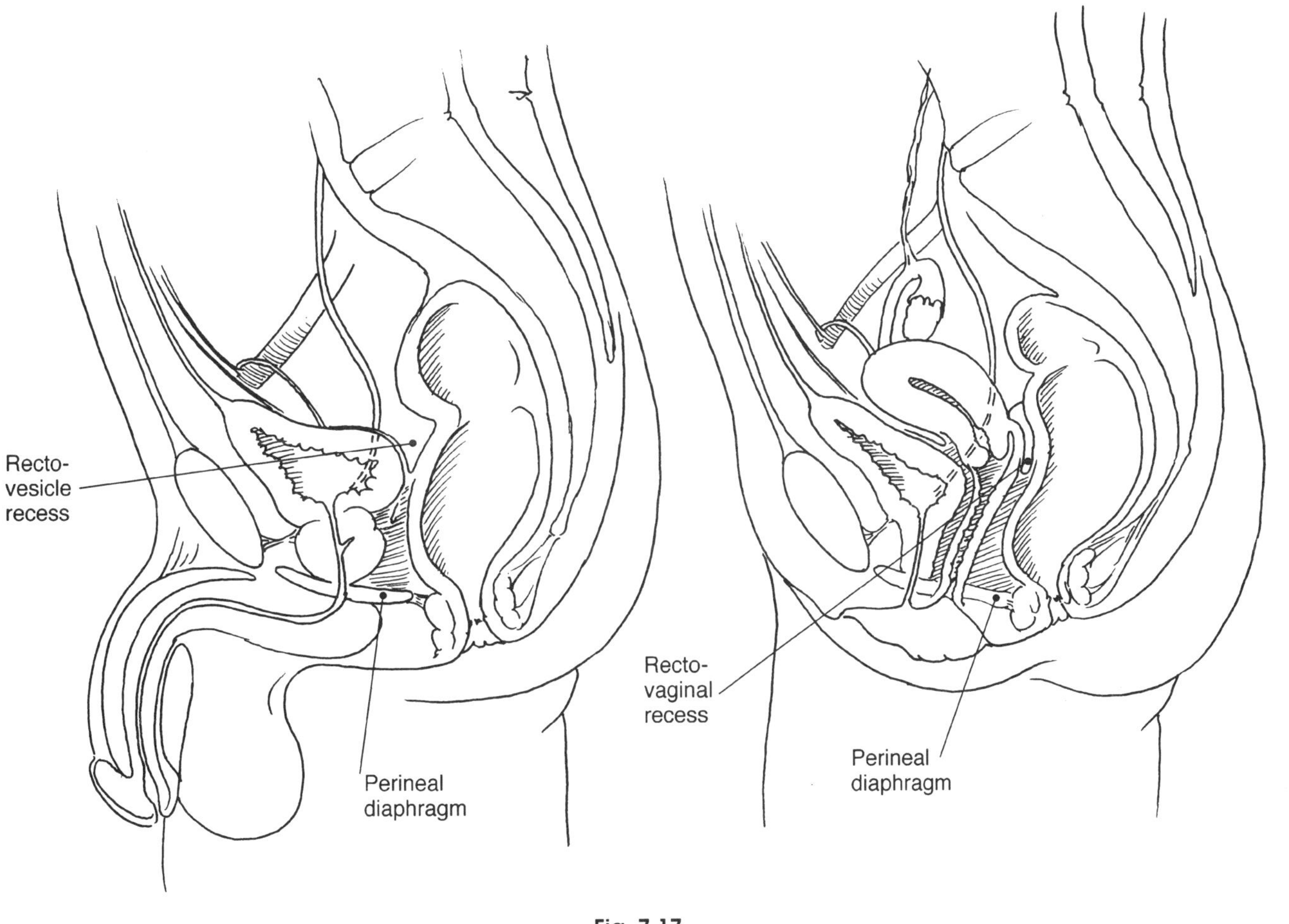

Fig. 7.17

When the bladder is empty, it lies flat against the slope of the inner surface of the anterior abdominal wall and pubis (Fig. 7.18). In this condition, the lateral extent of the bladder wall is difficult to discern and is subject to injury. The obliterated umbilical artery (medial umbilical ligament) on either side is a good guide to these margins. The obliterated urachus (median umbilical ligament) tapers upward toward the umbilicus from the anterior dome of the bladder adjacent to the abdominal wall.

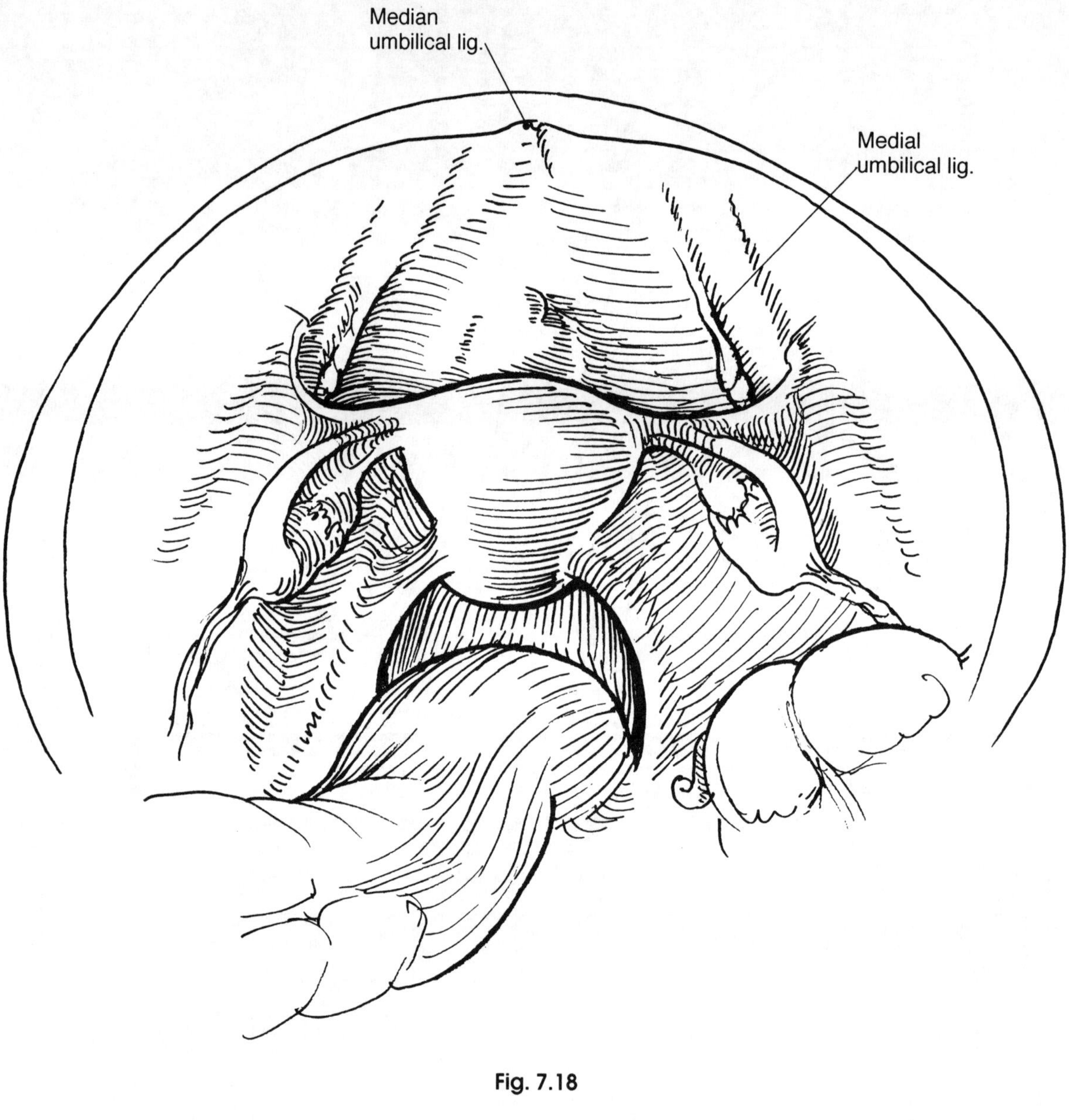

Fig. 7.18

The uterus, in its usual anteverted position lies on the dome of the bladder and is displaced according the distention of the bladder (Fig. 7.19). The peritoneal reflection between uterus and bladder does not extend down to the cervix, whereas the posterior peritoneal reflection extends down beyond the attachment of posterior vaginal wall to the cervix, allowing transvaginal access to the peritoneal cavity through the posterior cul-de-sac.

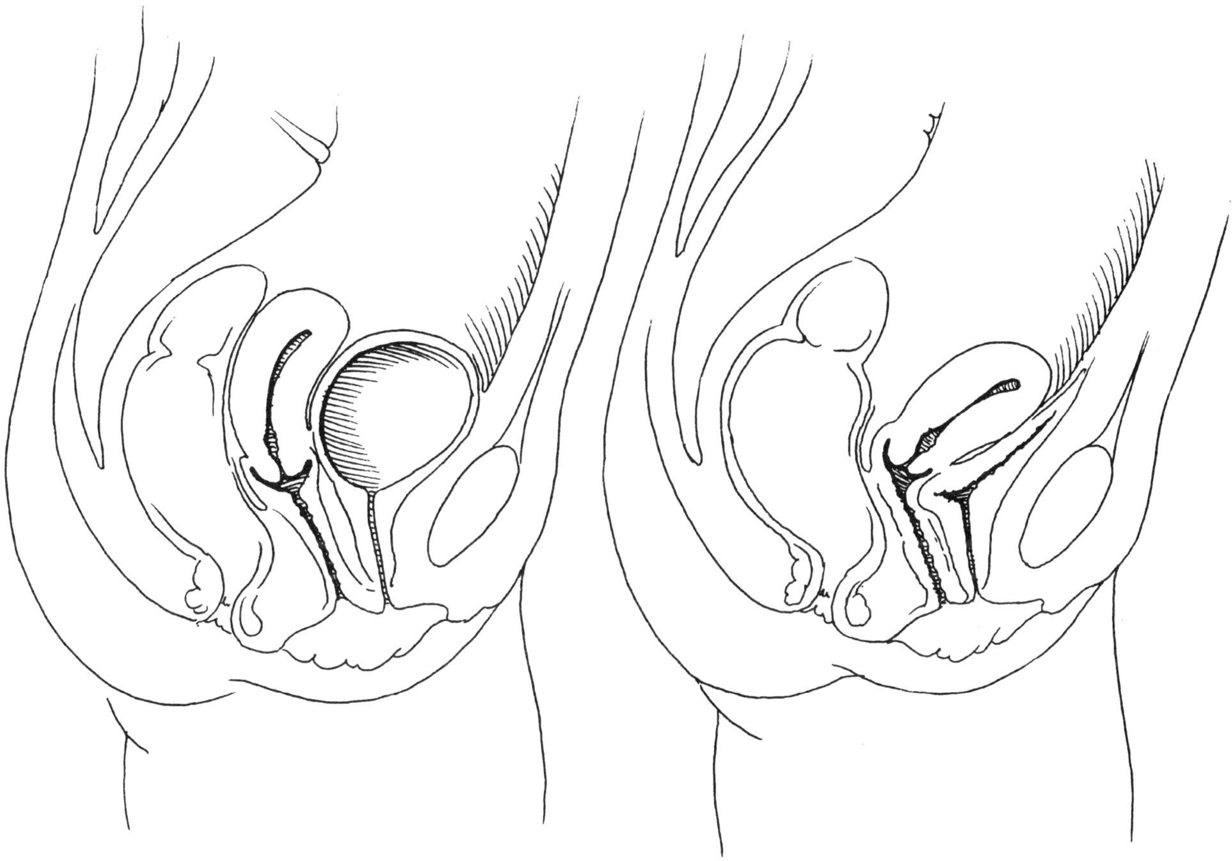

Fig. 7.19

The body of the uterus is a truncated triangle with the base at the fundus and tapers down to a narrowed isthmus between body and cervix (Fig. 7.20). Three structures attach to each corner of the uterus. The round ligament (remnant of the lower segment of gubernaculum) follows a curved course anterolaterally to the deep inguinal ring. The fallopian tube extends laterally and upward to the pelvic wall, then arches over posteriorly just below the external iliac vessels. The ovarian ligament (the remnant of the proximal segment of gubernaculum) attaches to the inferior pole of the ovary. The ovary is suspended from its superior end by the ovarian vessels and the covering fold of peritoneum, the infundibulopelvic ligament. The ovarian vessels run between ovary and Fallopian tube and descend along the lateral borders of the uterus to anastomose with the ascending uterine arteries. The uterine arteries reach the uterus near the cervix by passing medially in the plane above the pelvic diaphragm. They pass over the ureters as the ureters descend diagonally close to the cervix. The uterine venous and nervous plexi extend from the pelvic floor up along the uterus.

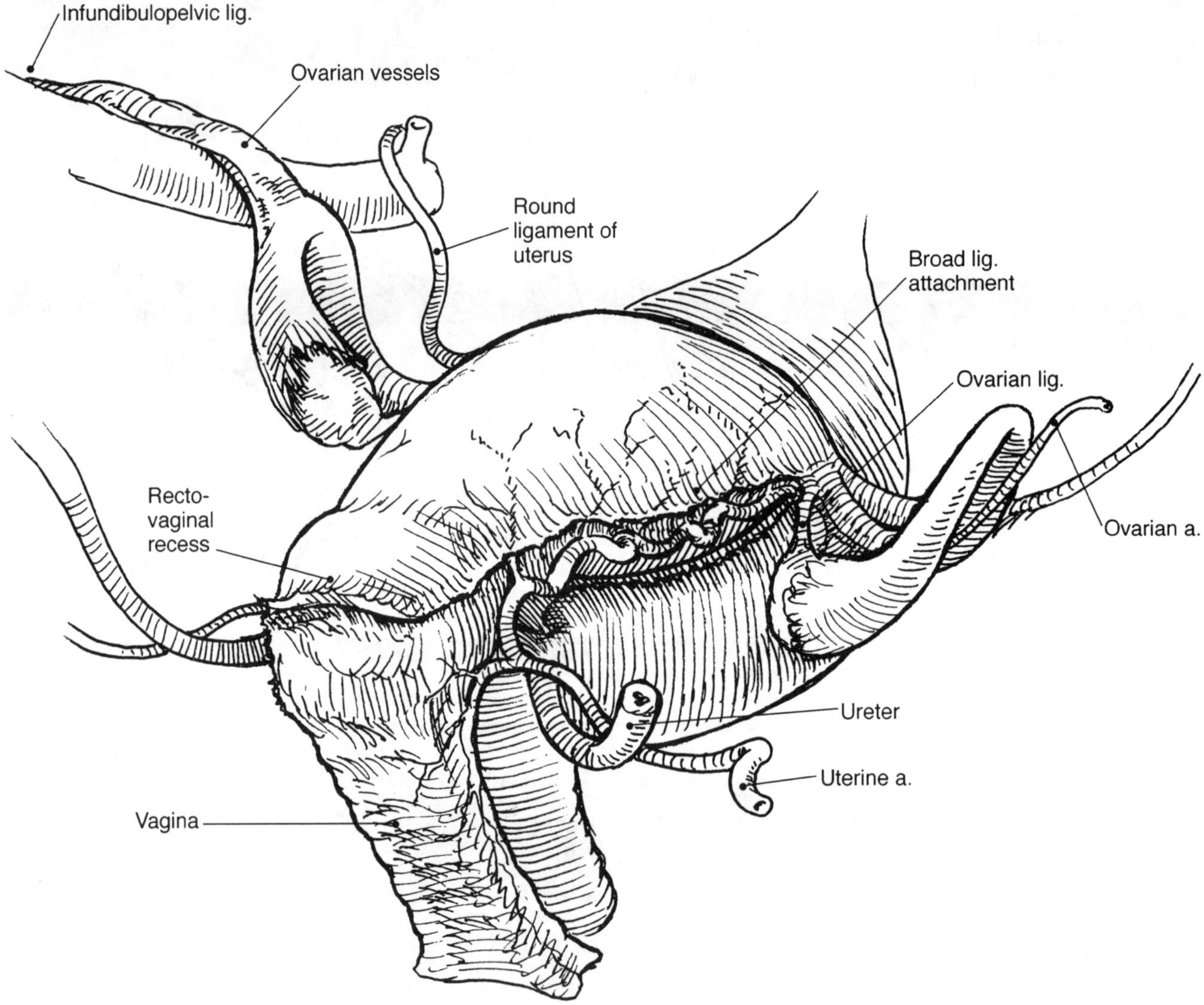

Fig. 7.20

The posterior wall of the rectum covers the majority of the sacral hollow and a portion of the anterior rectal wall is covered by visceral peritoneum above the recto-vaginal or rectovesical recess (Fig. 7.21). Thus the line of the rectal peritoneal reflection is almost vertical, leaving a portion of anterior rectum above the reflection.

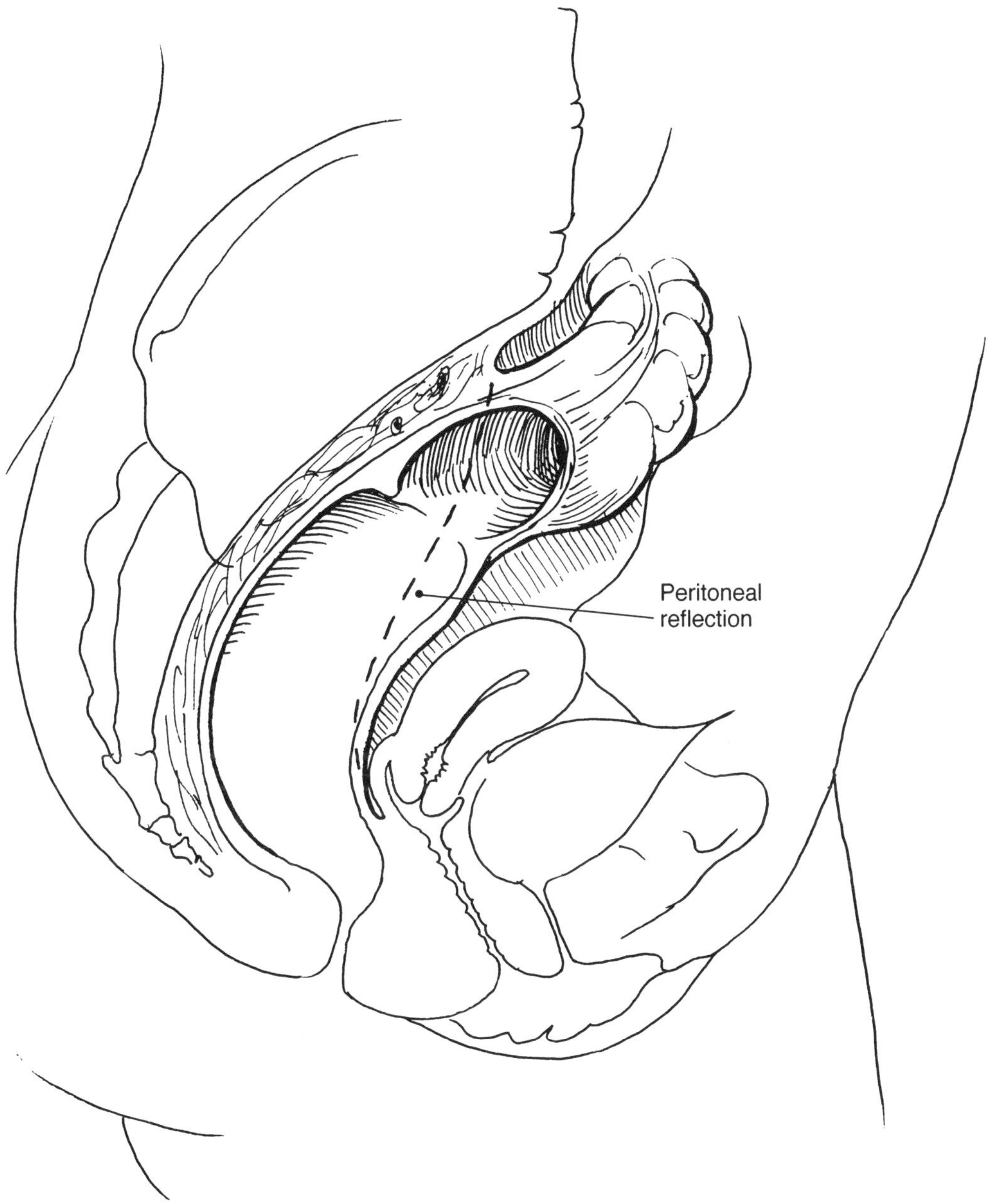

Fig. 7.21

The Pelvic Connective Tissue

The structures between the pelvic diaphragm and the pelvic peritoneum are encased in connective tissue (Fig. 7.22). While this layer is continuous, some areas are thickened to form sheets and bands of connective tissue that connect to and help support the pelvic organs. The major pelvic "ligaments" are the broad ligaments, the

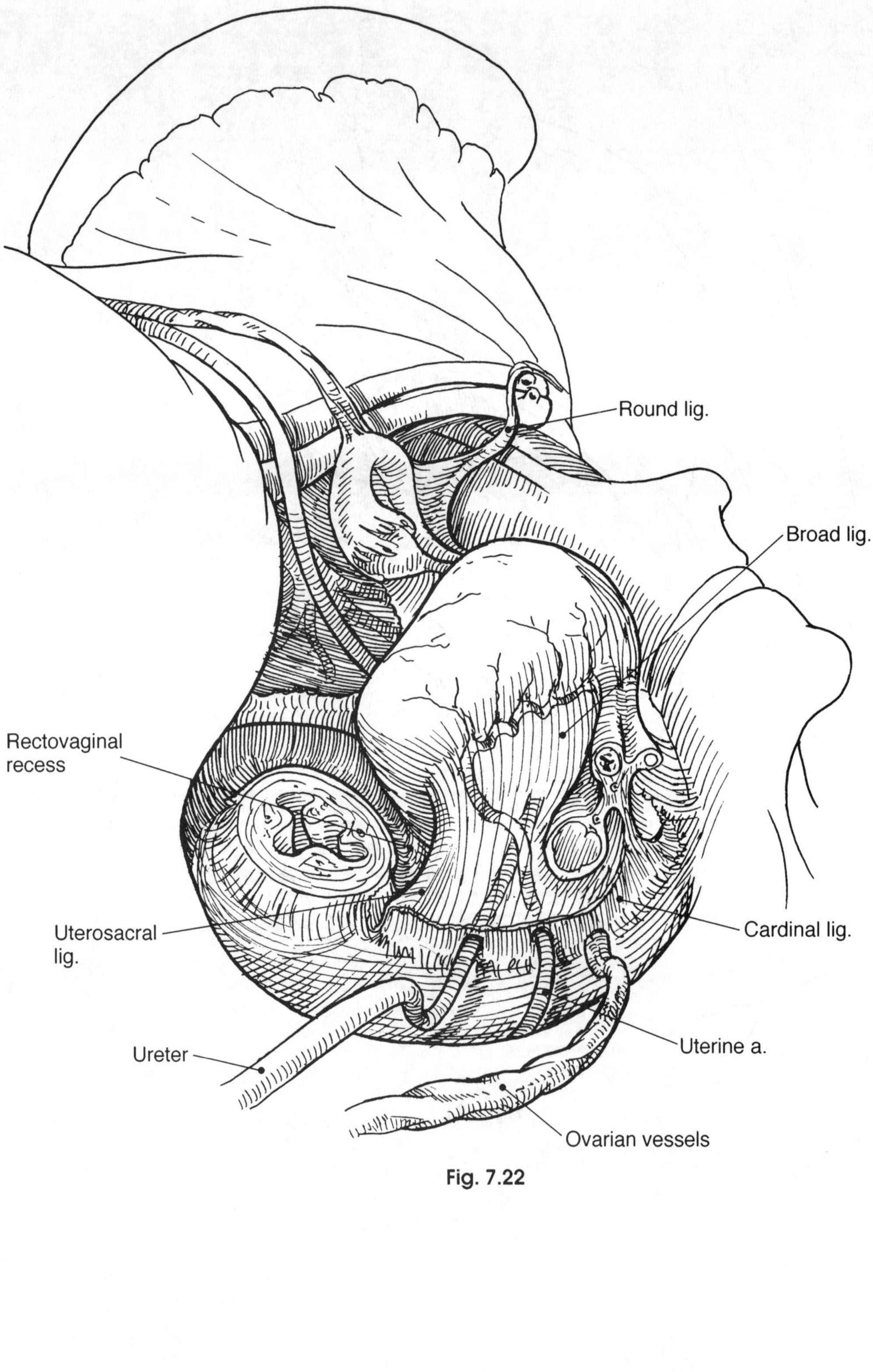

Fig. 7.22

cardinal ligaments, and the uterosacral ligaments (Fig. 7.23). The broad ligaments extend from the lateral borders of the uterus to the pelvic side walls and enclose the Fallopian tubes in their free cephalad margins. The round ligaments diverge anteriorly near the upper portion of this layer, creating tent-like folds. A shelf-like mesentery extending from the posterior surface of the broad ligaments support the ovaries. At the base of the broad ligaments, the pelvic connective tissue fans out anteriorly and laterally above the plane of the pelvic diaphragm as the cardinal ligaments, attaching the cervix broadly to the pelvic floor. The continuation of this sheet posteriorly forms two sharp folds which extend to the sacrum, the uterosacral ligaments. These straddle the rectum and deepen and define the rectovaginal recess. This same connective tissue layer extends into and reinforces the infundibulopelvic ligament. The ureters run through the connective tissue adjacent to the uterosacral ligaments and pass through the cardinal ligaments at the base of the broad ligaments to reach the bladder. This is a critical anatomic relationship crucial to the correct performance of a number of advanced gynecologic procedures including uterosacral nerve ablation, fulguration of endometriosis, laparoscopic hysterectomy, and sacral colpopexy.

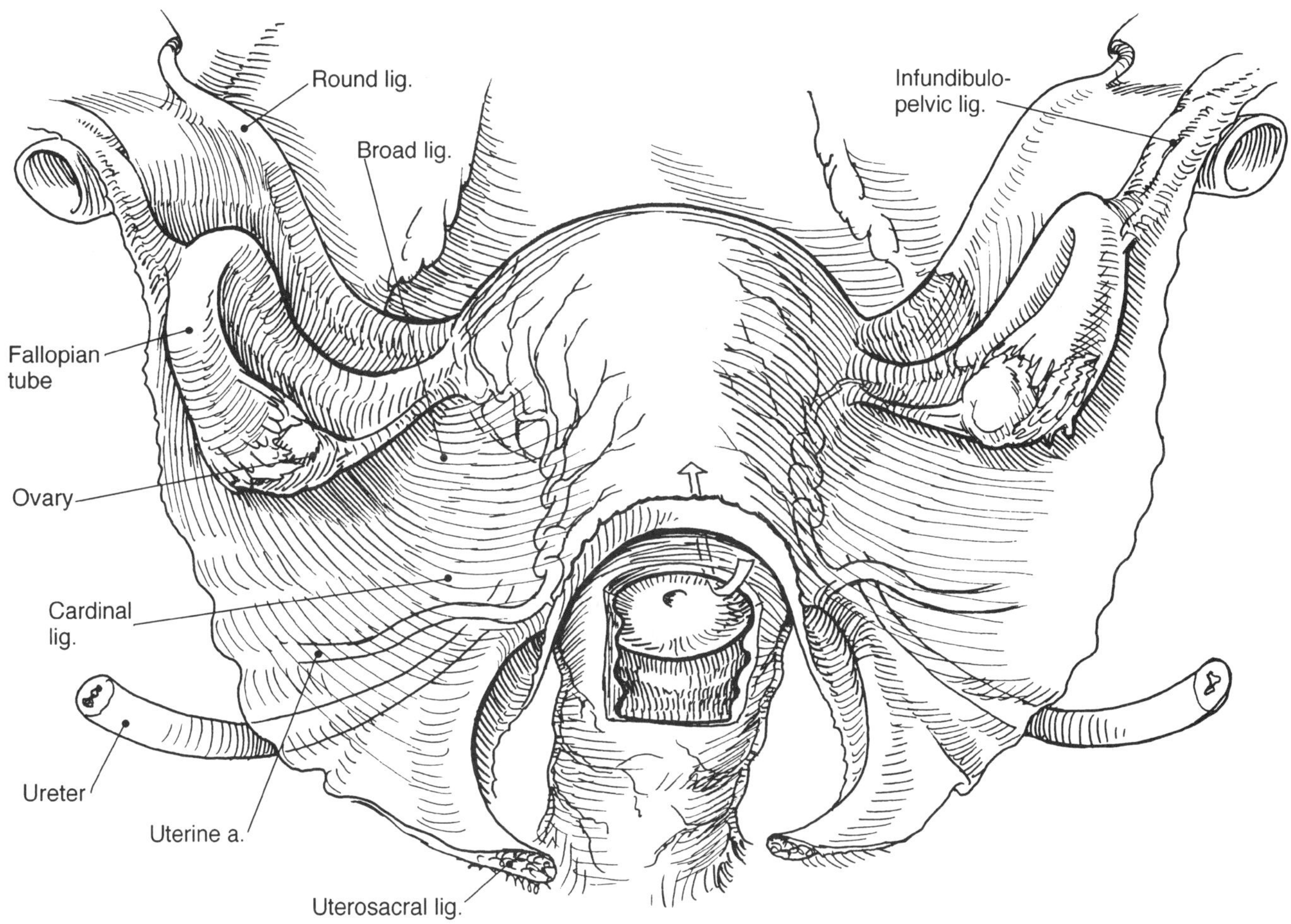

Fig. 7.23

The Laparoscopic View of the Pelvis

Visualization of the pelvic floor and pelvic organs during laparoscopy is obtained by decompressing the bladder with a Foley catheter and evacuating omentum and bowel loops from the pelvic basin by putting the patient in Trendelenburg position (Fig. 7.24). Preoperative bowel preparation with an electrolyte solution is recommended for extensive procedures such as pelvic and periaortic lymphadenectomy. The rectosigmoid junction covers the posterior part of the visible pelvis and extends up and to the left over the sacral promontory.

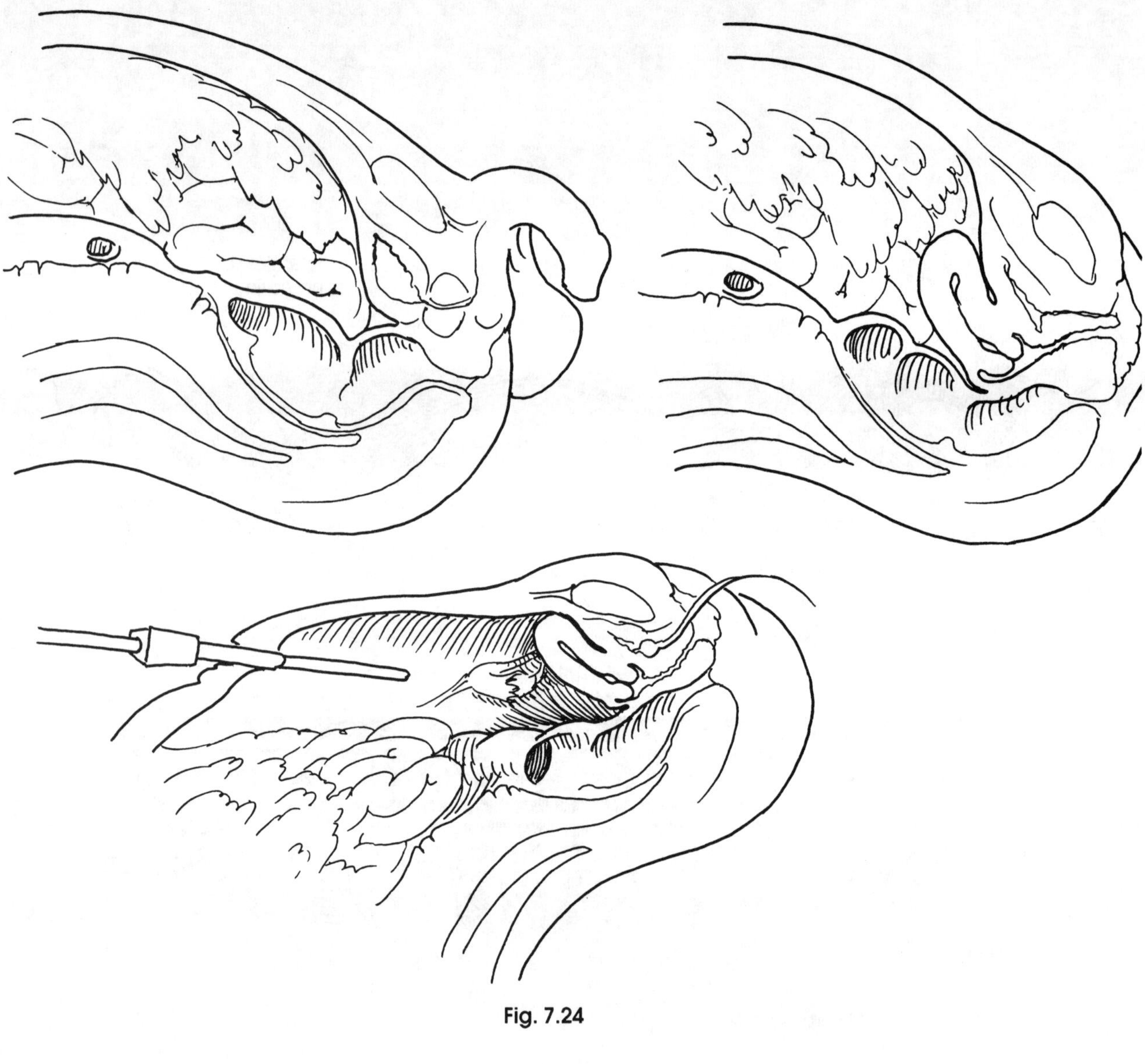

Fig. 7.24

The Foley balloon identifies the base of the bladder anteriorly, the remainder of the flattened bladder being indistinguishable from the lower anterior abdominal wall (Fig. 7.25). The medial umbilical ligaments (obliterated umbilical arteries) cross the deeper pectineal (Cooper's) ligaments in the inguinal region on either side. The margin of the true pelvis is marked by the ridge of the external iliac vessels.

In the male, the vas deferens can be seen beneath the pelvic peritoneum rising up from the base of the bladder, over the distal iliac vessels and turning the corner around the inferior epigastric vessels into the deep inguinal ring (Chapter 3). Posterolaterally on the right, the ureter can sometimes be seen crossing the junction of common and external iliac artery. On the left the ureter lies beneath the root of the sigmoid mesentery. The deepest point of the male pelvis is the rectovesicle recess.

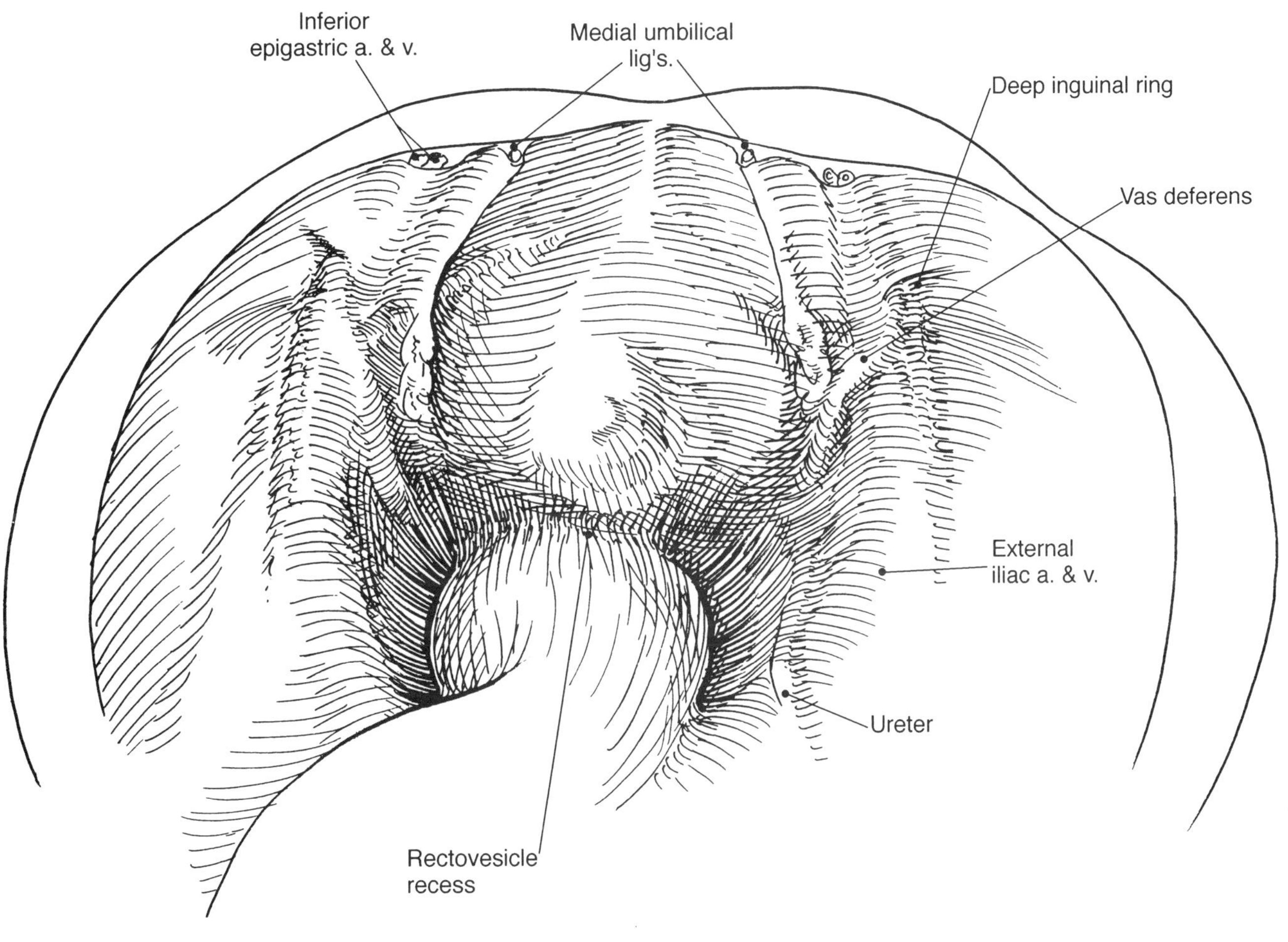

Fig. 7.25

In the female (Fig. 7.26), the uterus and adnexa are interposed between the rectum and bladder. The broad ligaments divide the pelvic space into anterior and posterior parts. The ovaries and distal Fallopian tubes are suspended on the lateral pelvic walls by the infundibulopelvic ligaments containing the ovarian vessels and autonomic nerves. The rectovaginal cul-de-sac (pouch of Douglas), the deepest point of the female pelvis, is bounded bilaterally by the sharp ridges of the uterosacral ligaments.

SURGERY

Overview

For many years laparoscopy has been a standard gynecological diagnostic and treatment tool for a variety of pelvic conditions. The advent of videolaparoscopy and the pioneering work of Semm and others has extended the application of laparoscopic techniques to more major procedures both in gynecology and other abdominal surgery.

Laparoscopic hysterectomy in the true sense requires the completion of the entire procedure through the laparoscope. This requires greater physician operating expertise, operating time and possibly patient risk. These limiting factors generally lead most gynecologic surgeons to perform laparoscopic assisted hysterectomy, doing the majority of dissection laparoscopically and completing the procedure vaginally. Laparoscopic assisted hysterectomy has been offered to a variety of patients with both benign and malignant disease. Selection of patients for laparoscopic assisted hysterectomy should exclude those who can be done by vaginal hysterectomy alone.

Two examples of pelvic laparoscopic surgery, laparoscopic hysterectomy and pelvic lymph node dissection demonstrate applied pelvic laparoscopic anatomy.

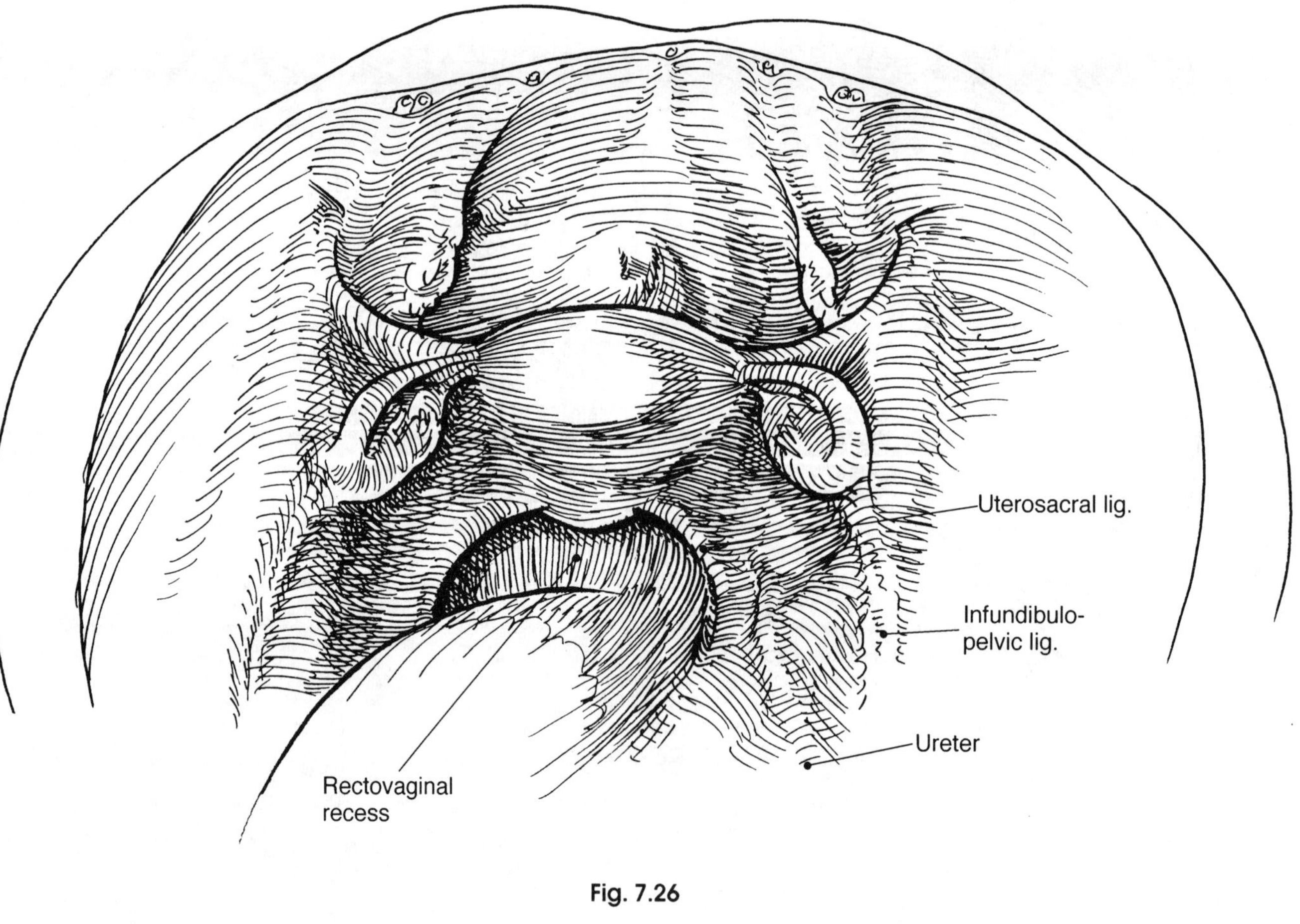

Fig. 7.26

Laparoscopic Hysterectomy

The patient is placed in a modified lithotomy position with the arms tucked at the sides and with a Foley catheter in place. The anatomic landmarks noted are the aortic bifurcation and the anterior superior iliac spines. After direct Hasson or Veress needle insufflation, a large camera port is placed at the umbilicus. Two lateral ports and one suprapubic port are placed under direct vision (Fig. 7.27). A manipulator is placed into the

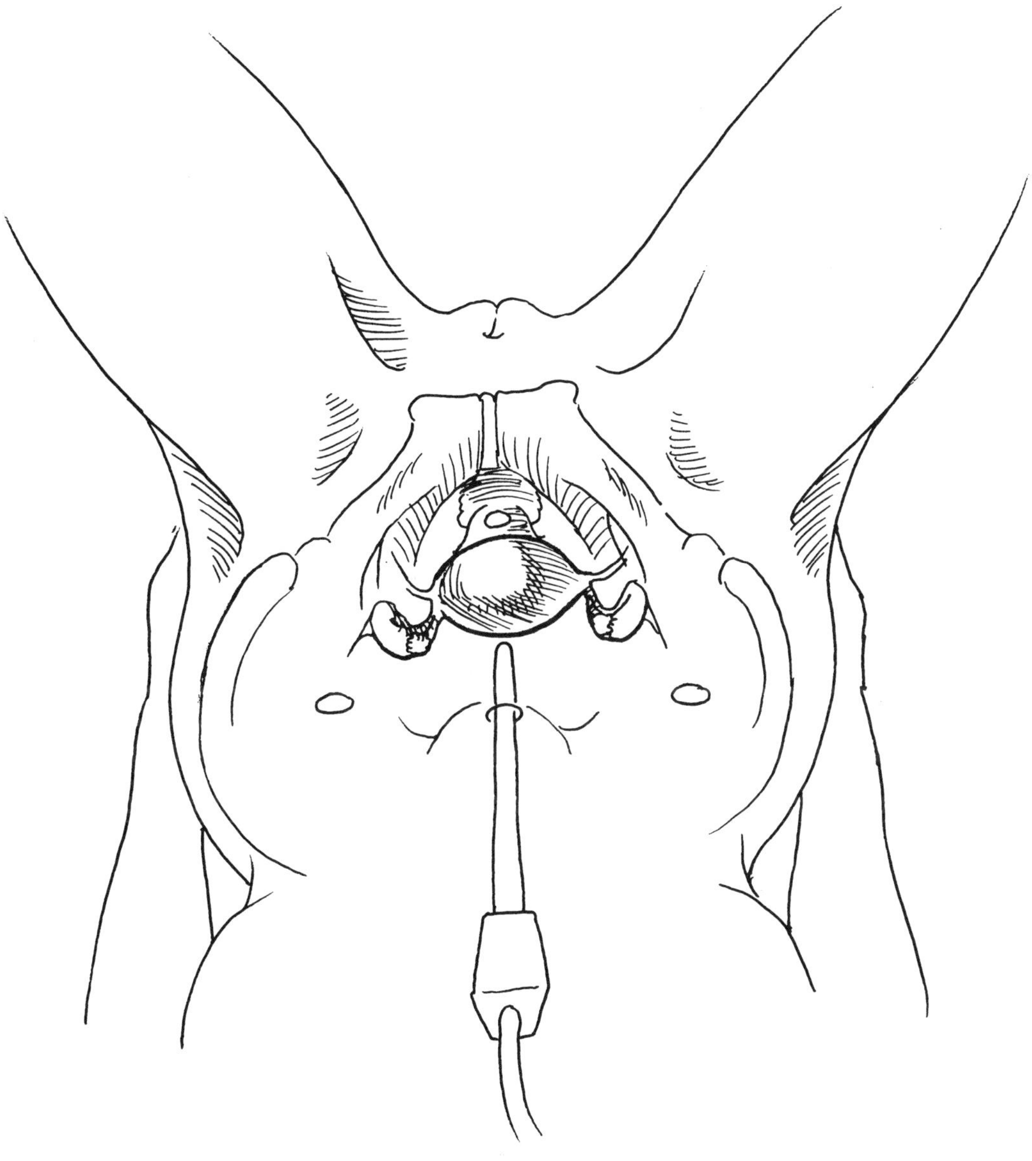

Fig. 7.27

uterus transvaginally to facilitate pelvic visualization and dissection. After general abdominal examination, the patient is placed in Trendelenburg position to slide bowel and omentum out of the true pelvis and the pelvic organs are inspected (Fig. 7.28). The courses of the ureters from the iliac vessels toward the bladder are identified. Ureteral catheters may be placed to help prevent injury in patients at high risk (extensive adhesions, endometriosis or bulky gynecological pathology).

The round ligaments of the uterus are dessicated with

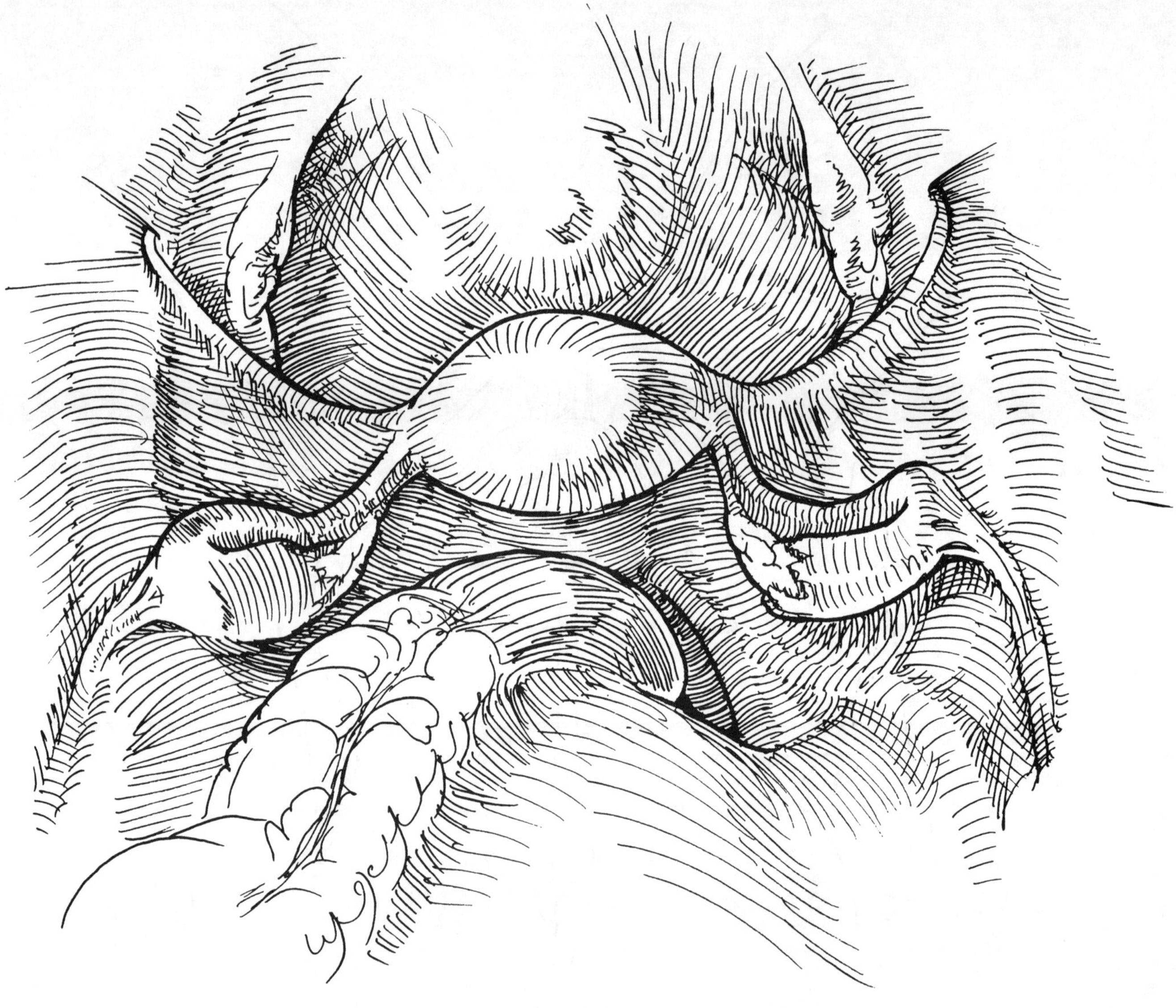

Fig. 7.28

the bipolar coagulator and transected far enough from the uterus to leave an adequate length to grasp as a handle (Fig. 7.29). Starting at the point of transection, the anterior leaf of the broad ligament is opened down to the vesicouterine reflection. Visual confirmation of the location and courses of the ureters is required at this point in the dissection. This may require opening the peritoneum on the posterior surface of the broad ligament above the ureters.

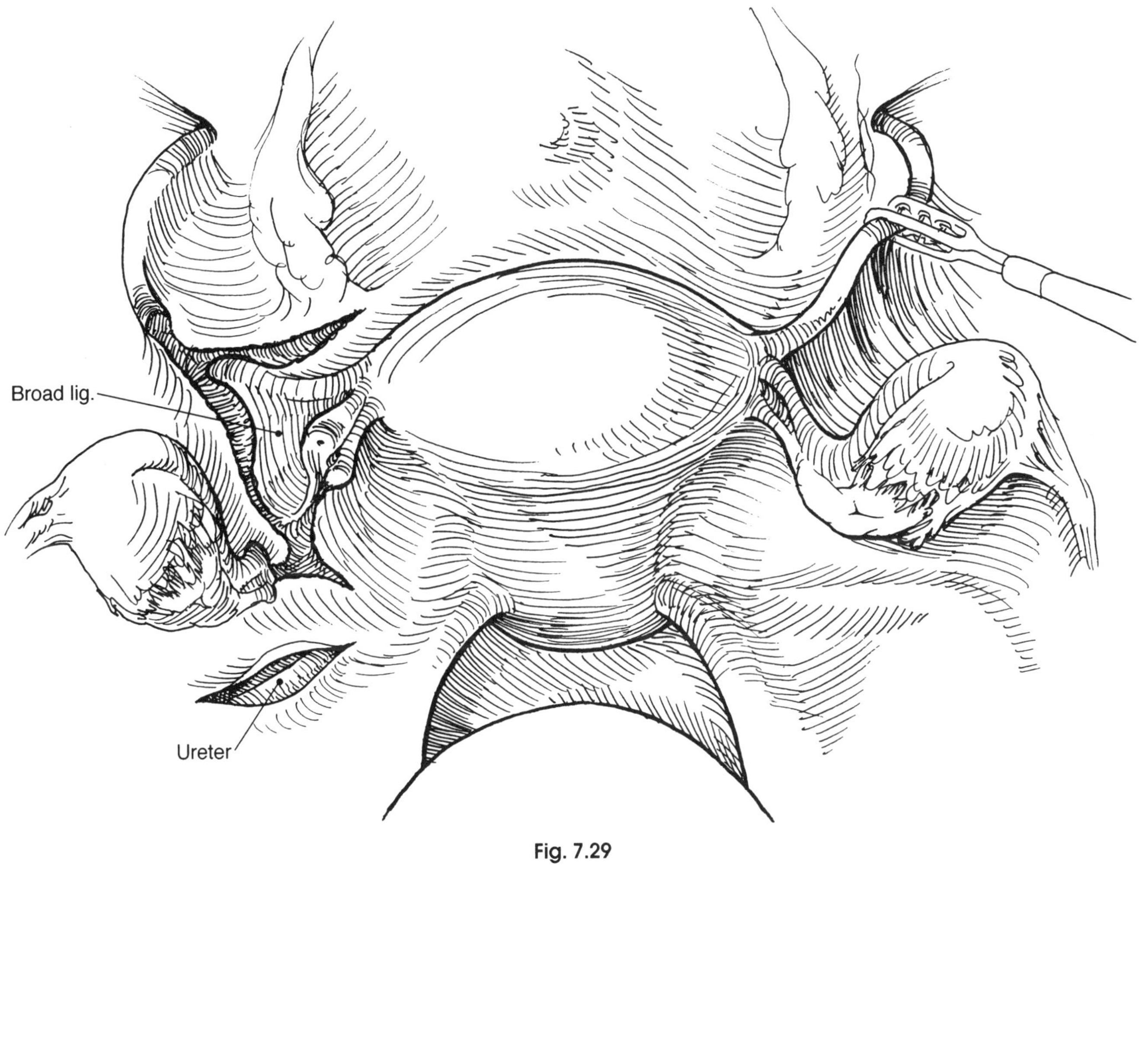

Fig. 7.29

If the adnexa are to be left, the fallopian tubes and utero-ovarian ligaments are divided next. If the adnexa are to be taken, the infundibulopelvic ligaments are dessicated with bipolar current and divided (Fig. 7.30). A linear stapler can be used as an alternative. The adnexa are mobilized by dividing their attachments toward the broad ligaments.

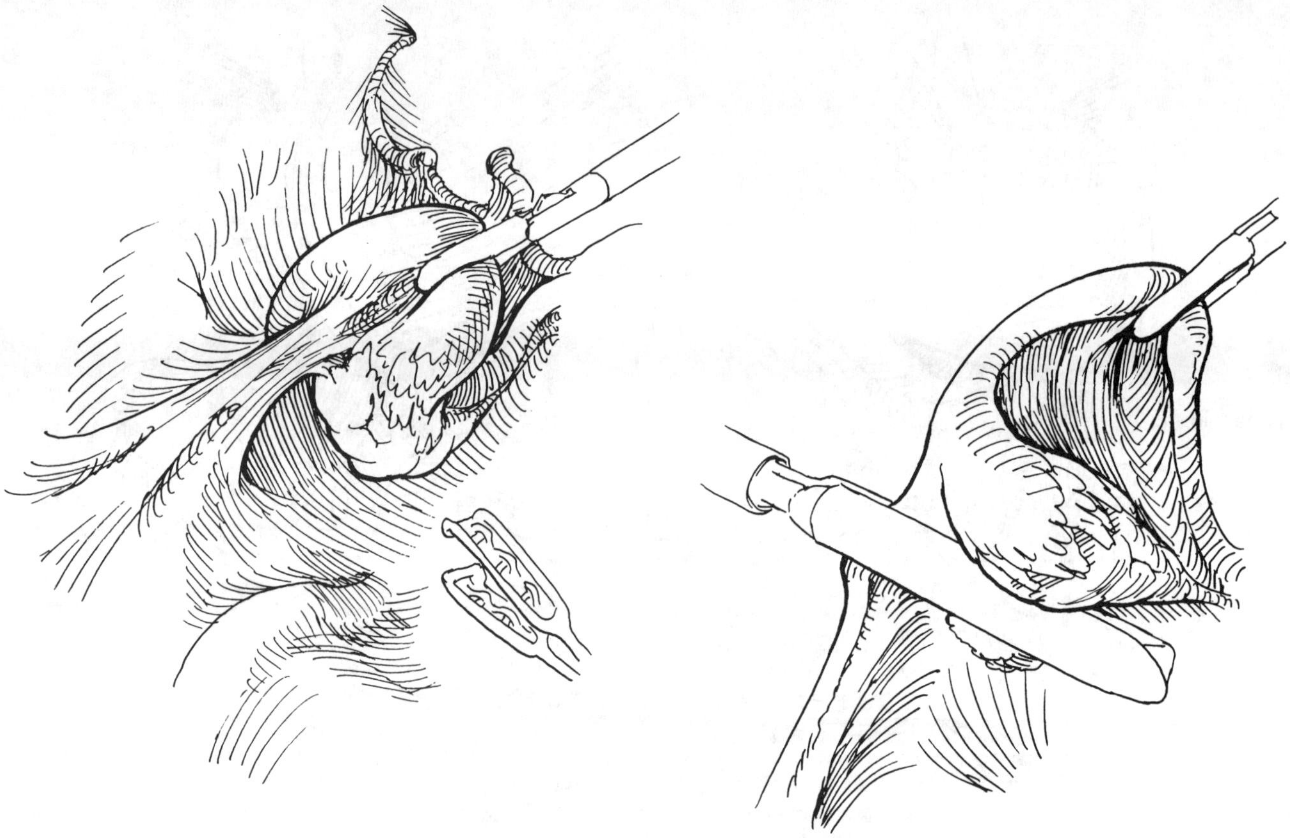

Fig. 7.30

The anterior incisions are connected across the vesicouterine recess (Fig. 7.31). A combination of hydrodissection, blunt, and sharp dissection are used to separate the bladder from the cervix until the upper portion of the anterior vaginal wall is exposed.

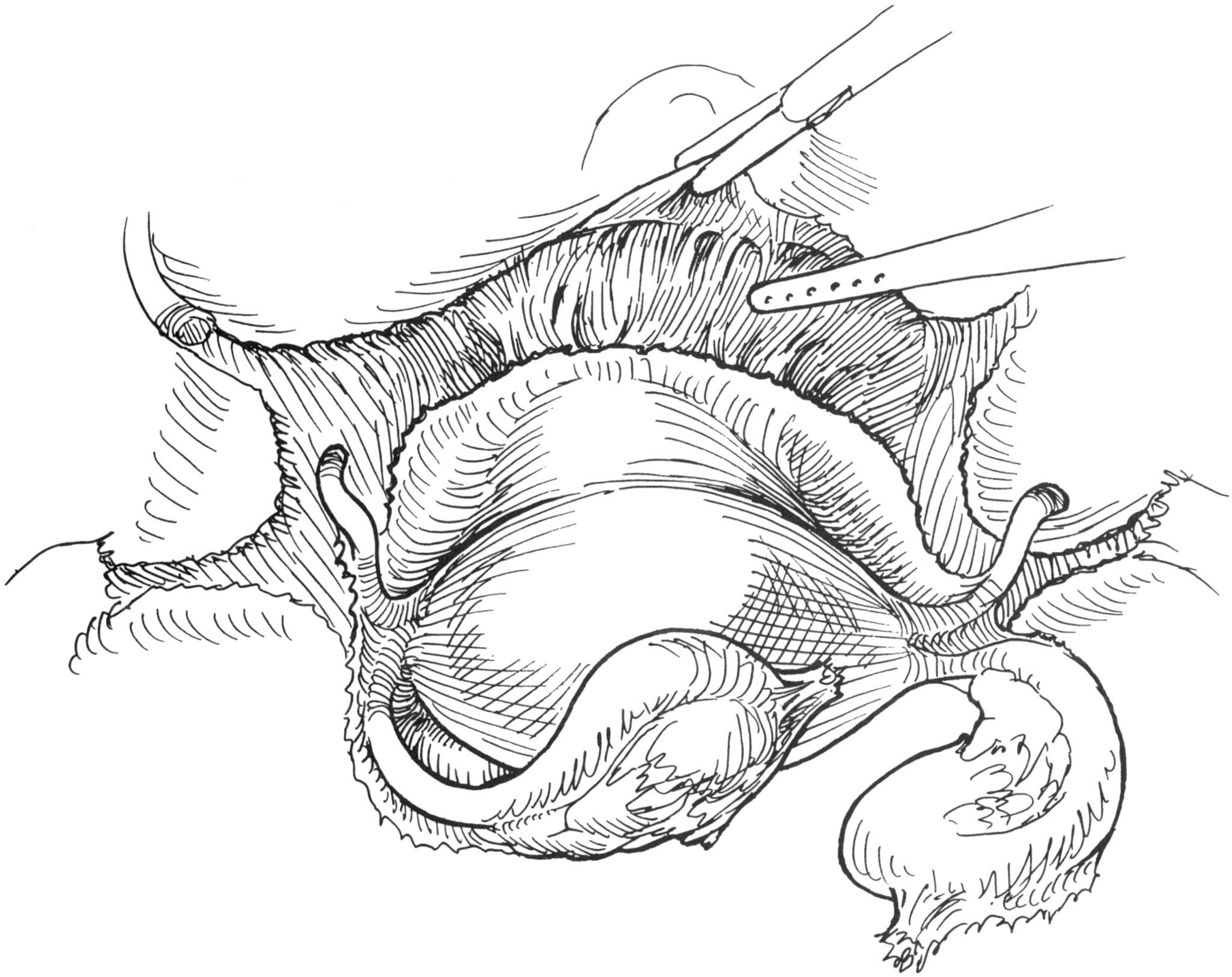

Fig. 7.31

The uterine vessels are next identified on either side a few centimeters lateral to the cervix and carefully dissected free (Fig. 7.32). The course and location of the ureters beneath the vessels are clearly identified during this dissection. When free, the vessels are dessicated and divided. Alternately, the uterine arteries are skeletonized lateral to the cervix where the anterior division may be dissected, or the entire vessel may be ligated subsequently from below.

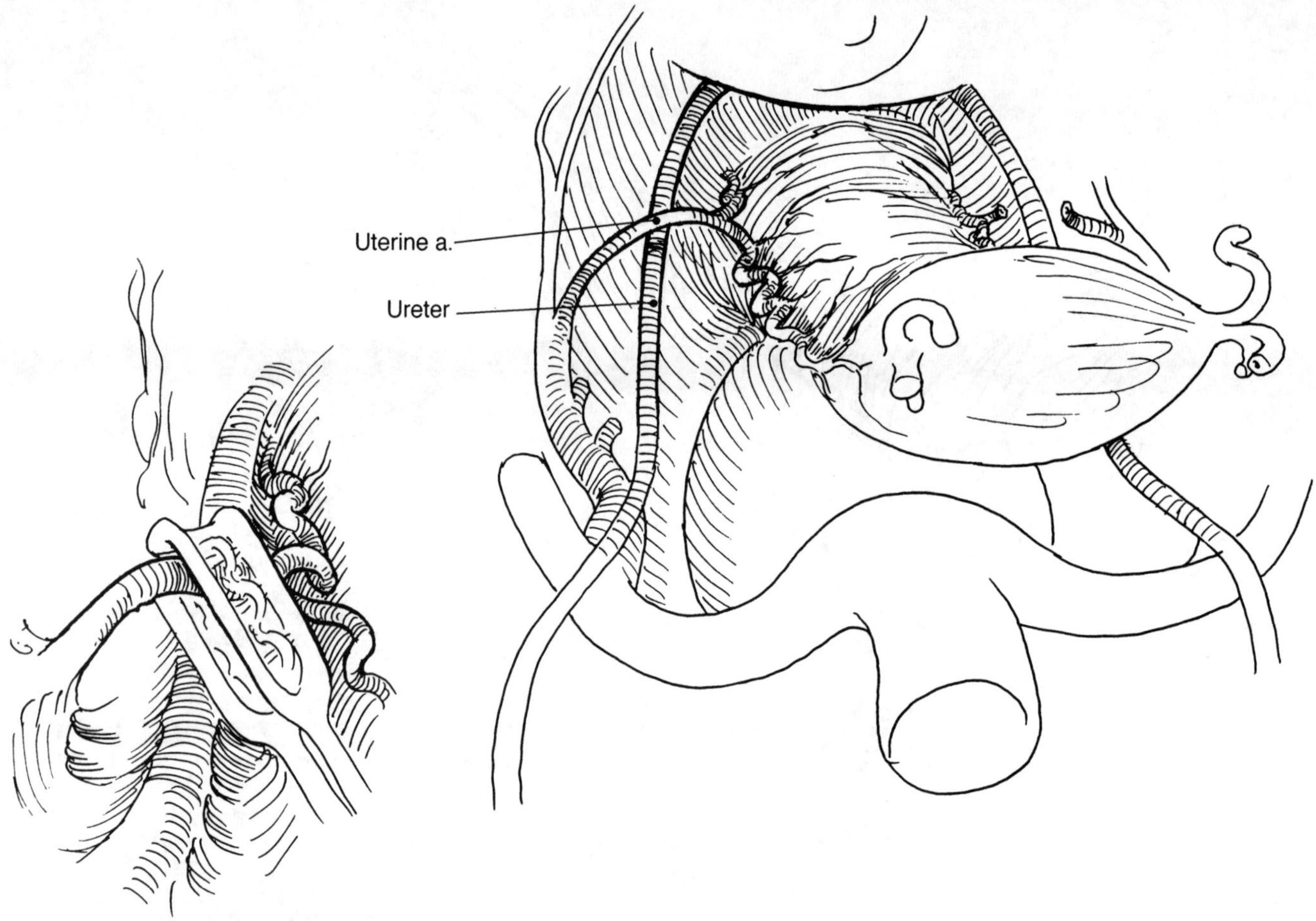

Fig. 7.32

The posterior peritoneal incision is completed across the rectovaginal recess (pouch of Douglas) (Fig. 7.33). With the uterus retracted to the opposite side, the cardinal and uterosacral ligaments attaching the uterus to the pelvic floor may be carefully divided with a linear stapler. The location of the ureter must be clear prior to this step. The posterior vaginal wall is exposed in the cul-de-sac.

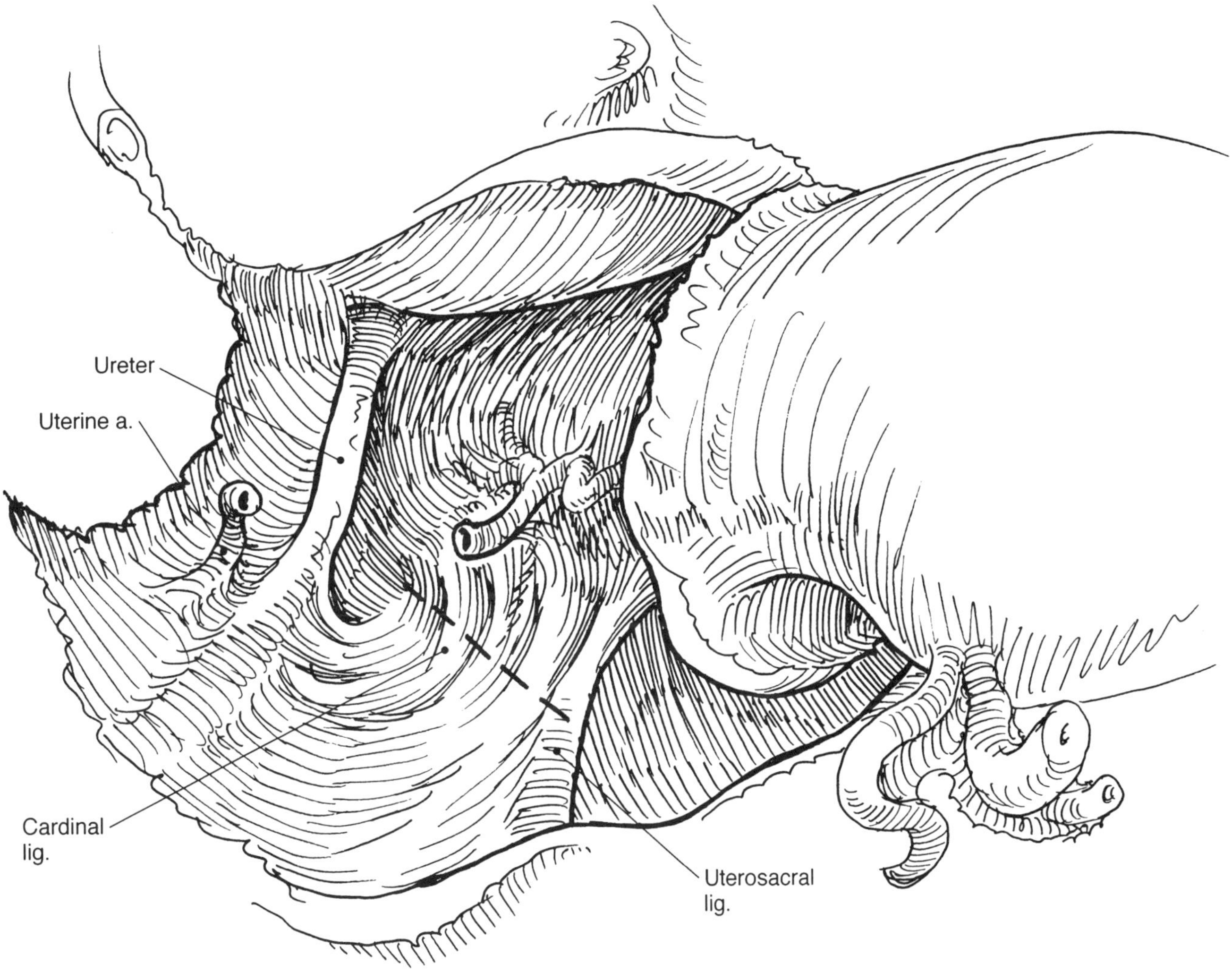

Fig. 7.33

With a vaginal sponge forceps tenting the vaginal wall, the vagina is opened transversely anteriorly and posteriorly using unipolar cautery (Fig. 7.34). The vaginal transection is completed around the lateral walls. The specimen is removed intact through the vagina if small enough or is morcellated if necessary. Alternatively, if there is adequate mobility, the anterior and posterior colpotomies may be performed vaginally. After this, the uterosacral and cardinal ligament complex may be safely clamped, divided, and ligated.

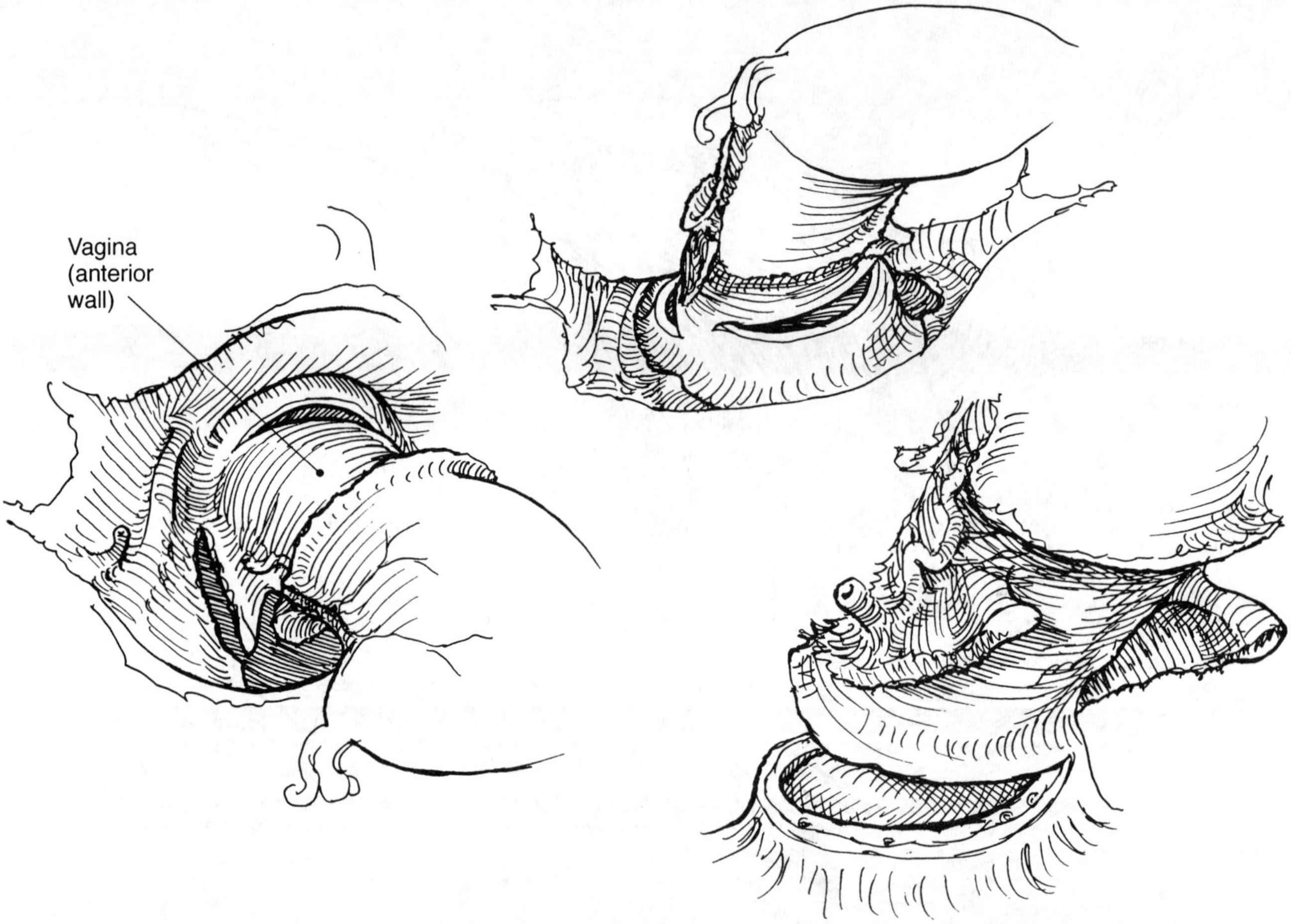

Fig. 7.34

After careful bipolar control of vaginal cuff bleeders, the corners of the cuff are sutured to the cardinal-uterosacral ligament complexes either from above or below and the remainder of the cuff is sutured closed ensuring that the anterior and posterior vaginal mucosa are incorporated (Fig. 7.35).

PELVIC LYMPH NODE DISSECTION

Introduction

Pelvic lymph node dissection is the most accurate means of detecting nodal metastasies from carcinoma of the genitourinary pelvic organs. Lymphangiography, ultrasound, CT, and MRI scans have high false negative and false positive rates. The importance of identifying nodal metastases from the pelvic urological organs, particularly the prostate, and from the gynecological structures in the female, lies in the need for accurate staging. Prognosis and more importantly therapeutic planning are dependent on this knowledge. Pelvic lymph node dissection for staging prostate carcinoma has become the most common urological laparoscopic procedure and pelvic and para-aortic lymph node dissection may be performed in the staging of gynecologic malignancies.

Specific relationships relevant to pelvic lymph node dissection are reviewed below, followed by a description of comprehensive nodal excision. The current emphasis on staging versus therapeutic lymph node dissection has led most practitioners to perform a modified dissection, which is less extensive than that shown. One exception is pelvic and para-aortic lymphadenectomy performed in conjunction with radical hysterectomy for cervical cancer.

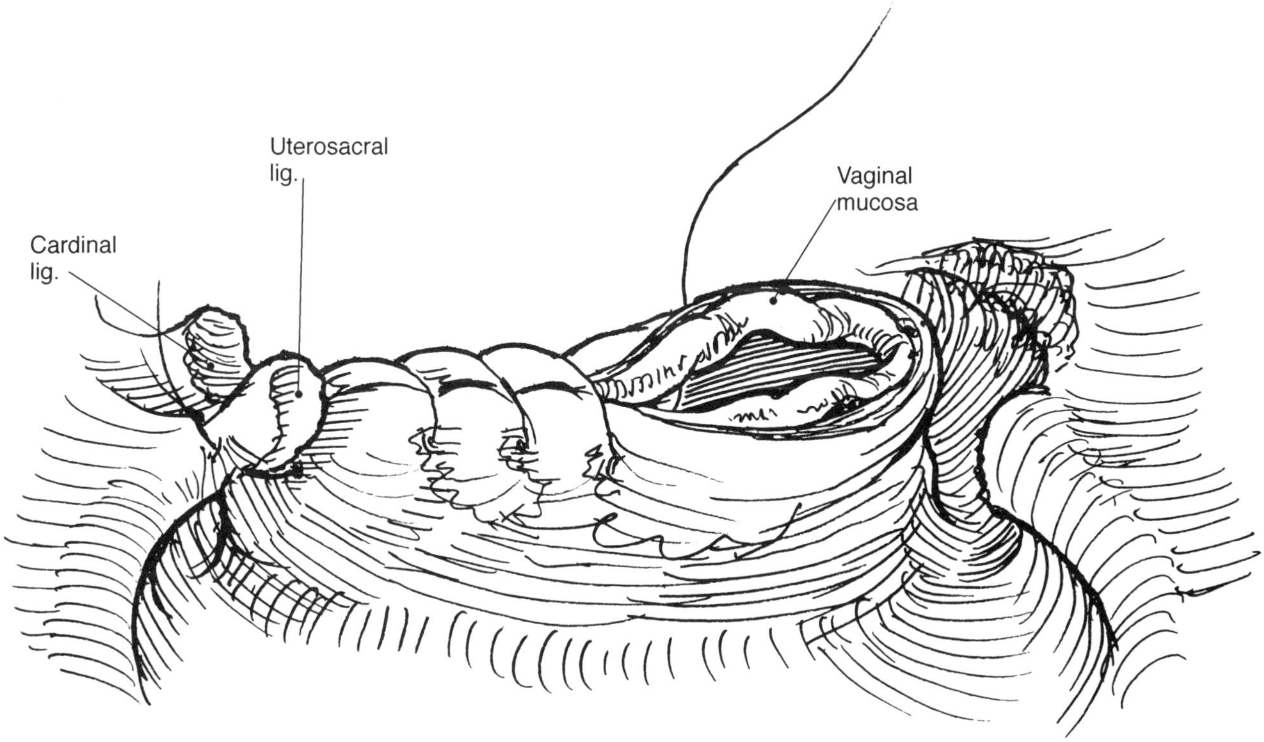

Fig. 7.35

Anatomic Landmarks

Lymphatic sacs that are secondarily colonized by lymphocytes arise from mesenchyme early in embryonic development. The lymphatics develop in close association with the blood vessels and the relationship persists into adult life. Lymphatic drainage from the pelvic organs goes predominantly to the external, internal, and common iliac chains, with minor pathways along the pelvic floor to the presacral nodes (Fig. 7.36). The lymphatic channels around the external and common iliac vessels interconnect, but three dominant pathways have been demonstrated by lymphangiogram. The drainage of an organ or a region of an organ follows the vascular supply.

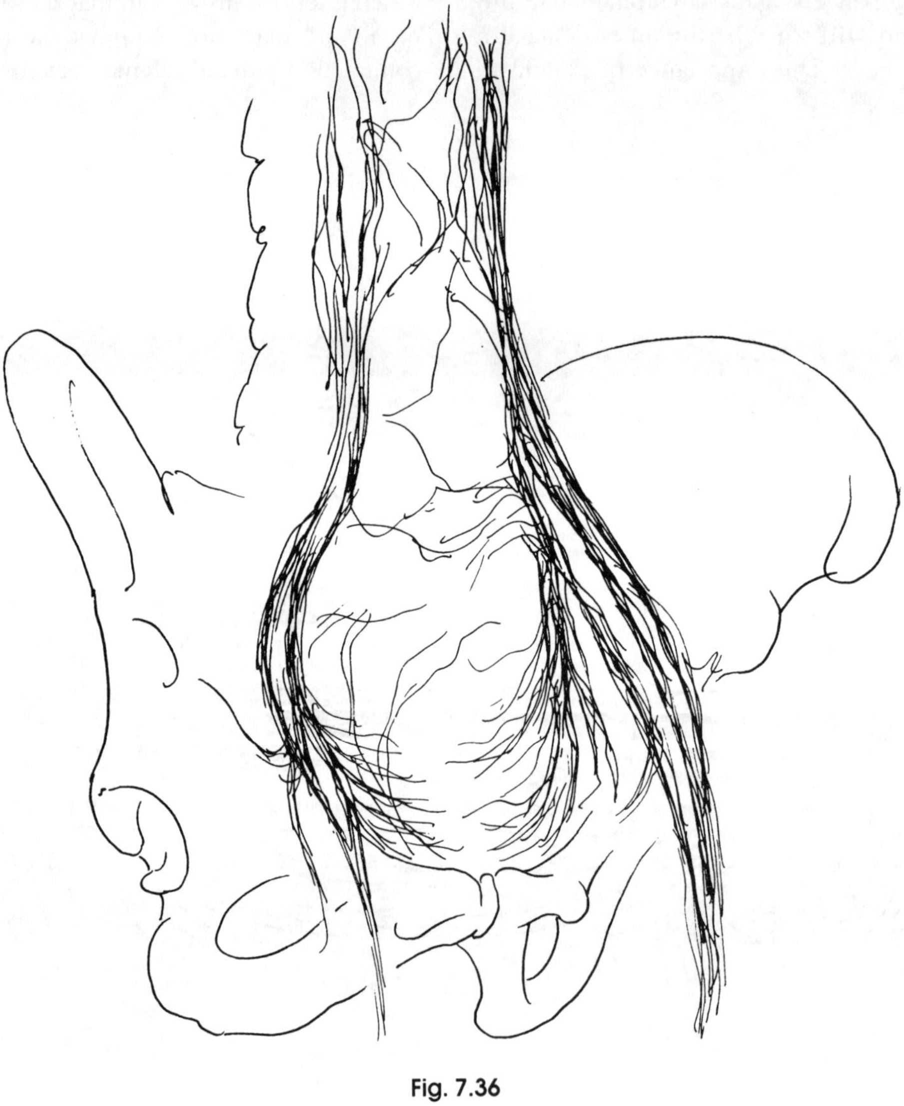

Fig. 7.36

The nodes that are most significant and accessible lie between the inguinal floor below and the common iliac vessels above and between the medial umbilical ligament medially and the genitofemoral nerve laterally (Fig. 7.37)

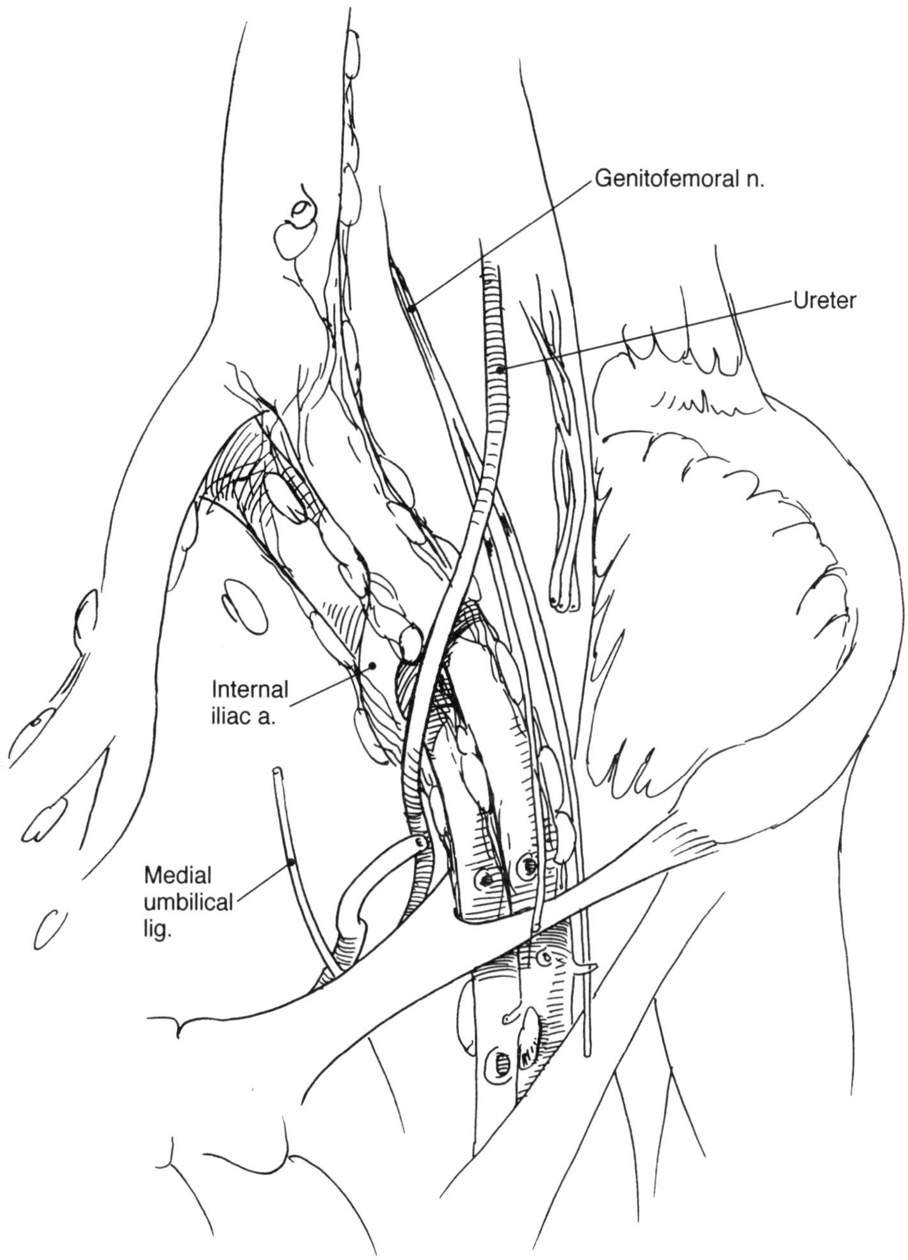

Fig. 7.37

Below the deep inguinal ring lies the transition between external iliac and femoral vessels (Fig. 7.38). Here, the vessels pass through the femoral ring, bounded by the lacunar ligament medially, the iliopubic tract and inguinal ligament above, the superior pubic ramus below and the iliopsoas muscle laterally. The vessels are surrounded by a continuation of the endoabdominal/transversalis fascia (the femoral sheath).

Lymphatics accompany the vessels through the sheath, and on the medial side of the vein one sometimes finds the highest of the deep inguinal lymph nodes (Cloquet's node) at the level of the femoral ring. Technically this node is not part of the pelvic lymphatics and requires meddlesome dissection through the transversalis fascia to remove. On the pelvic side of the transversalis fascia there are two or three retrocrural lymph nodes that mark the beginning of the external iliac chains. These nodes lie on the tributaries of the external iliac vessels at the abdominal wall.

There are normally two preperitoneal tributaries of the iliac vessels at the abdominal wall, the inferior epigastrics and the deep circumflex iliacs. The inferior epigastric vessels arise from the anterior surface of the iliacs and run up toward the umbilicus passing the medial side of the deep inguinal ring. Near their origin, the epigastrics give rise to external spermatic vessels which penetrate the transversalis fascia to accompany the spermatic cord (Chapter 3). They lie between the lateral cremasteric fibers and the cord along with the genital branch of the genitofemoral nerve. The epigastrics also

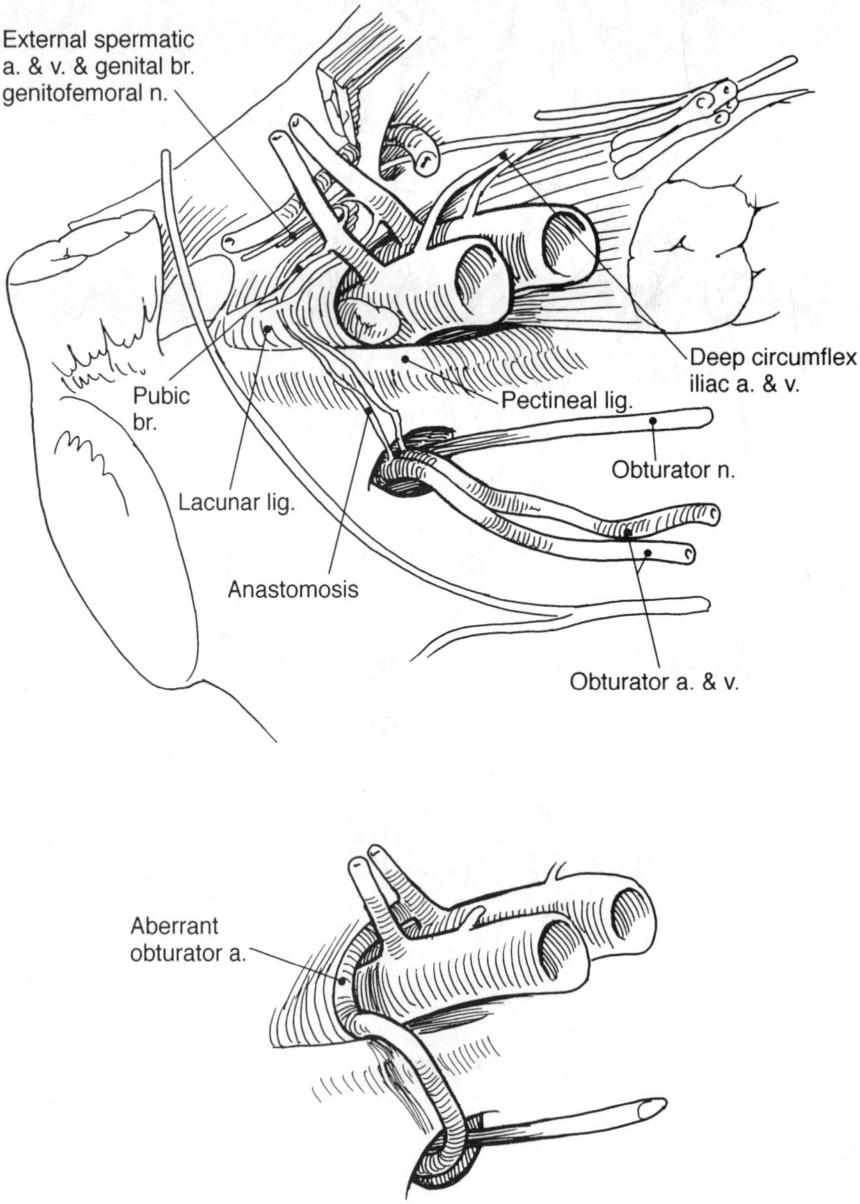

Fig. 7.38

give rise to small pubic branches that run medially. These anastomose with ascending branches of the obturator vessels. In as many as 20% of individuals, this connection takes the form of a dominant aberrant obturator artery, replacing the more common origin from the internal iliac artery. The deep circumflex iliac vessels arise on the lateral sides of the external iliacs and run along the iliopubic tract toward the anterior superior spine of the ilium. They are crossed by both branches of the genitofemoral nerve as the nerves penetrate the transversalis fascia to reach the inguinal canal and the proximal thigh respectively.

The bulky iliopsoas muscle fills the lateral portion of the space between the superior pubic ramus and the inguinal ligament (Fig. 7.39). On its surface, the internal spermatic vessels descend toward the deep inguinal ring in the male and are usually visible beneath the peritoneum on the surface of the external iliac artery near the ring. The medial margin of the muscle supports the external iliac vessels over the rim of the true pelvis and the collar of muscle and vessels overhangs the obturator fossa below.

The internal obturator muscle originates from the obturator membrane and the bony margins of the obturator foramen. The upper part of the muscle and membrane is fenestrated for passage of the obturator nerve and vessels to the adductor compartment of the leg. This foramen lies at the inferior margin of the superior pubic ramus below the external iliac vessels. The deep location of the obturator neurovascular bundle in the hollow of the pelvic sidewall makes access to the obturator lymphatics difficult.

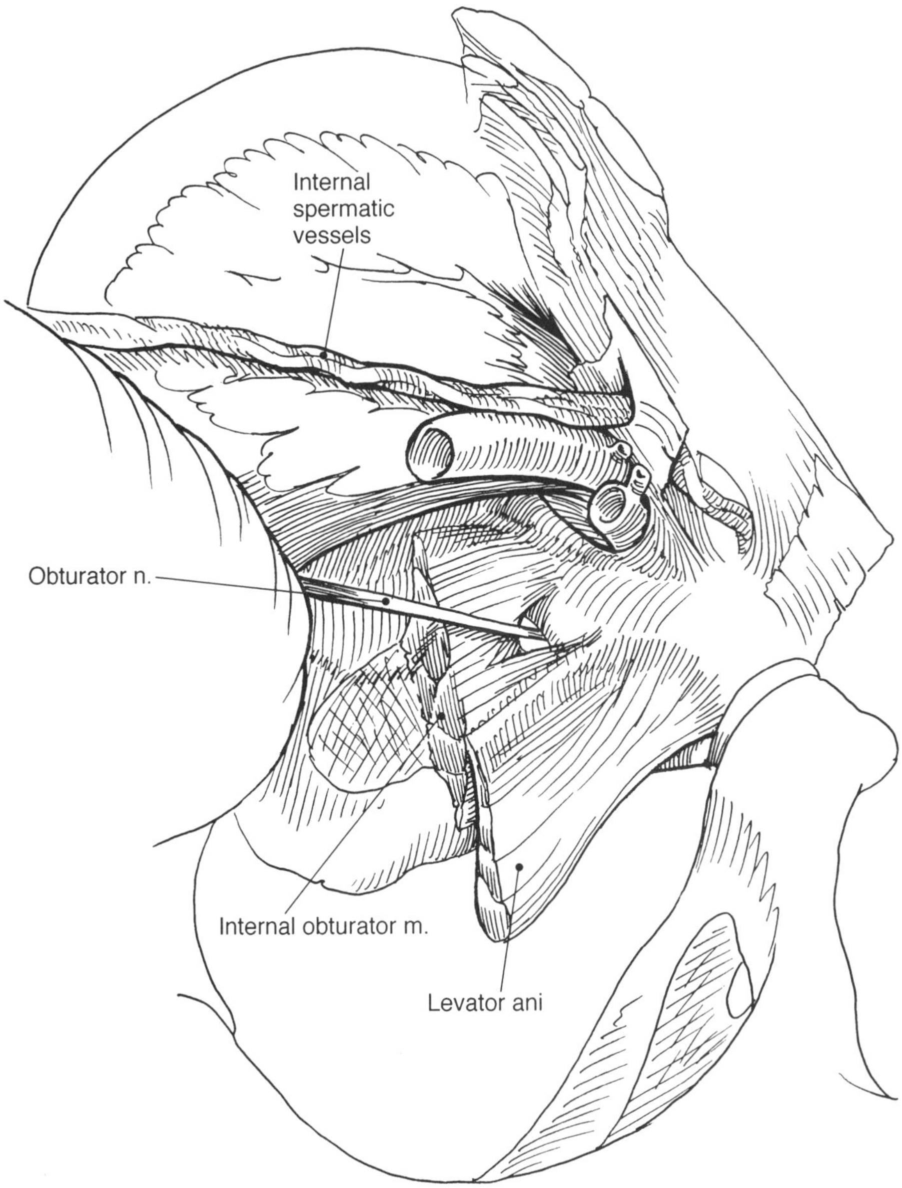

Fig. 7.39

On the sidewall of the true pelvis beneath the overhang of the psoas muscle and external iliac vessels, the hollow of the obturator fossa descends steeply. The levator muscles of the pelvic diaphragm take origin along a horizontal condensation of obturator fascia. The sheets of obturator and levator muscle form the lateral boundary of the paravesical and parauterine space. The obturator nerve originates from the lumbar plexus, descends behind the psoas muscle and emerges beneath the medial border of the psoas at the pelvic brim deep to the common iliac vessels. It passes lateral to the internal iliac vessels and runs along the pelvic sidewall to the obturator canal.

The internal iliac vessels descend into the true pelvis on either side of the sacral promontory (Fig. 7.40). The branching of the internal iliacs is variable, particularly the anterior division. The major division into a posterior division with one major vessel, the superior gluteal, occurs in 75% of individuals. The other 25% have the inferior gluteal also arising from the posterior division rather than the anterior. The other branches, the superior and inferior vesicle, the obturator, the middle rectal and the uterine usually come from the anterior division.

The lymphatic channels and nodes of the pelvis are conveniently grouped according to the vessels they

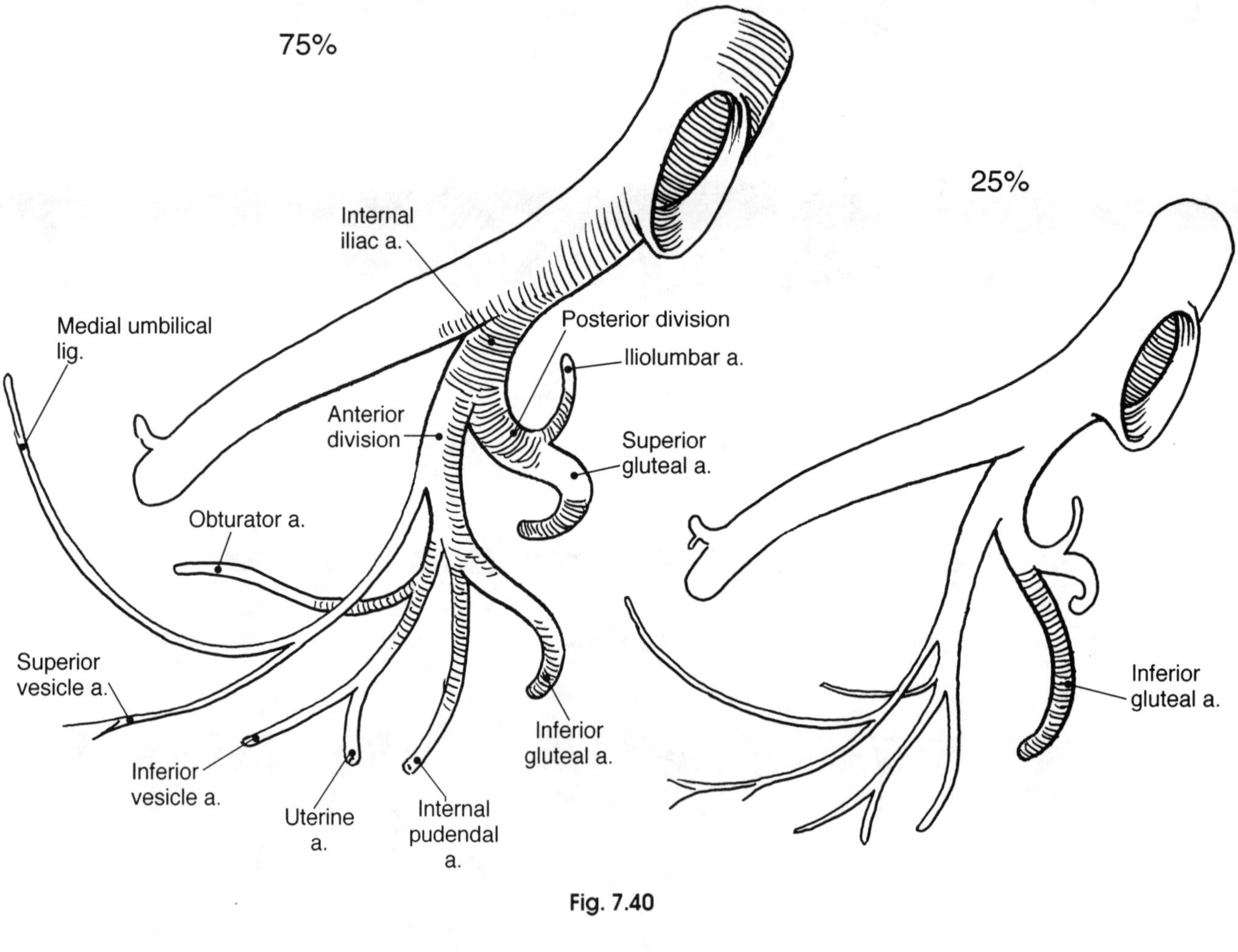

Fig. 7.40

accompany (Fig. 7.41). The external iliac chain has three components. The external group lies lateral to the external iliac artery in the groove between the artery and the psoas muscle. The middle group lies on the anterior surface of the artery and the internal group lies against the pelvic wall beneath the external iliac vein. The internal group is contiguous with the obturator nodes of the internal iliac group below. The obturator nodes lie along the course of the obturator neurovascular bundle against the pelvic sidewall. The ureter descends into the pelvis medial to the obturator chain. The other nodes of the internal iliac group are interspersed among the branches of that vessel and include the lateral sacral nodes near the second and third sacral foramina. The external and internal iliac groups drain into the common iliac chains. The internal group of common iliac nodes communicates with nodes on the sacral promontory below the aortic and caval bifurcations. The common iliac nodes drain into the para-aortic nodes above.

The medial limit of pelvic lymph node dissection is marked by the obliterated umbilical artery, which is represented by the cord-like medial umbilical ligament. In the fetus, the umbilical arteries lay on either side of the bladder and the adult structure is a warning sign of the lateral limit of the bladder. The medial umbilical ligament is usually the continuation of the superior vesical branch of the internal iliac artery. The vas deferens in the male and the round ligament of the uterus in the female cross over the medial umbilical ligament and the external iliac vessels to enter the deep inguinal ring.

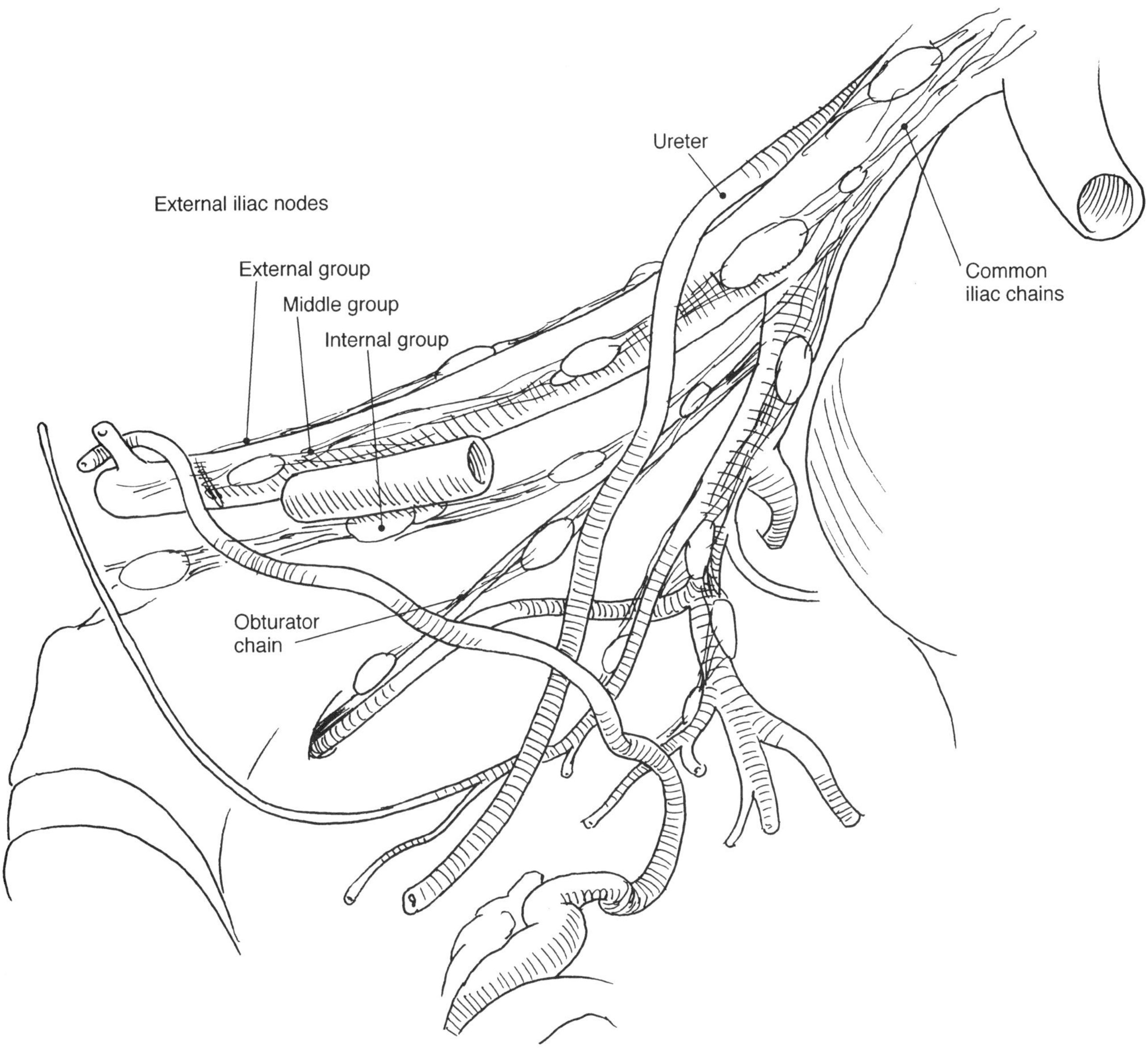

Fig. 7.41

The landmarks around the pelvic brim seen from the laparoscopic perspective are the external iliac vessels, the deep inguinal ring, the inferior epigastric vessels, the vas deferens or round ligament, and the medial umbilical ligament (Fig. 7.42). In thin individuals who do not have a large amount of retroperitoneal fat, the right ureter might be seen crossing the iliac vessels. Similarly, the suggestion of internal spermatic vessels in the male and the ovarian vessels in the female might be seen beneath the peritoneum. The cecum on the right and the sigmoid colon on the left might require some mobilization for exposure.

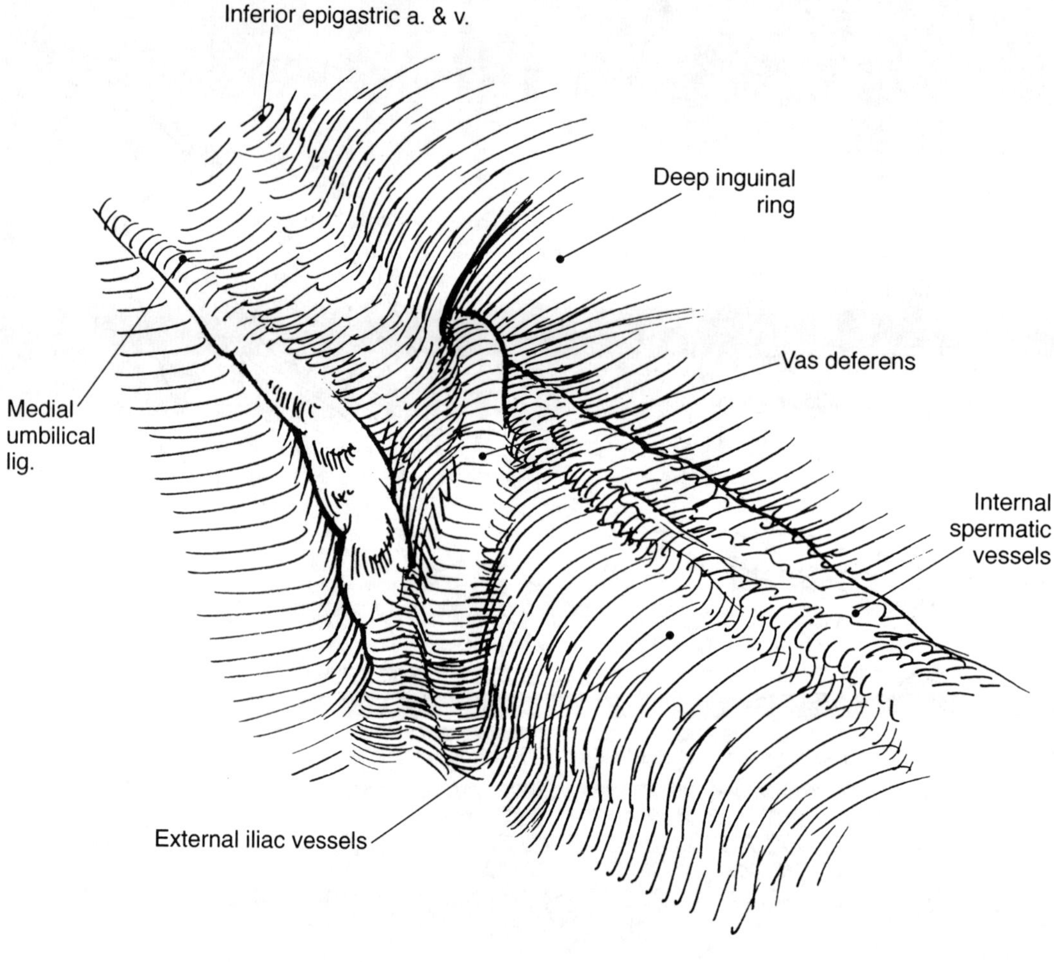

Fig. 7.42

Pelvic Lymph Node Dissection

After insufflation, the camera port is placed at the umbilicus, a second large port is placed at the suprapubic position, and two small ports are placed at the margins of the rectus muscles between umbilicus and anterior superior iliac spines on each side (Fig. 7.43). With the patient in 30° Trendelenburg and 30° rotation to the side opposite the dissection, the cecum or sigmoid is mobilized as necessary. Dissection is begun by retracting the

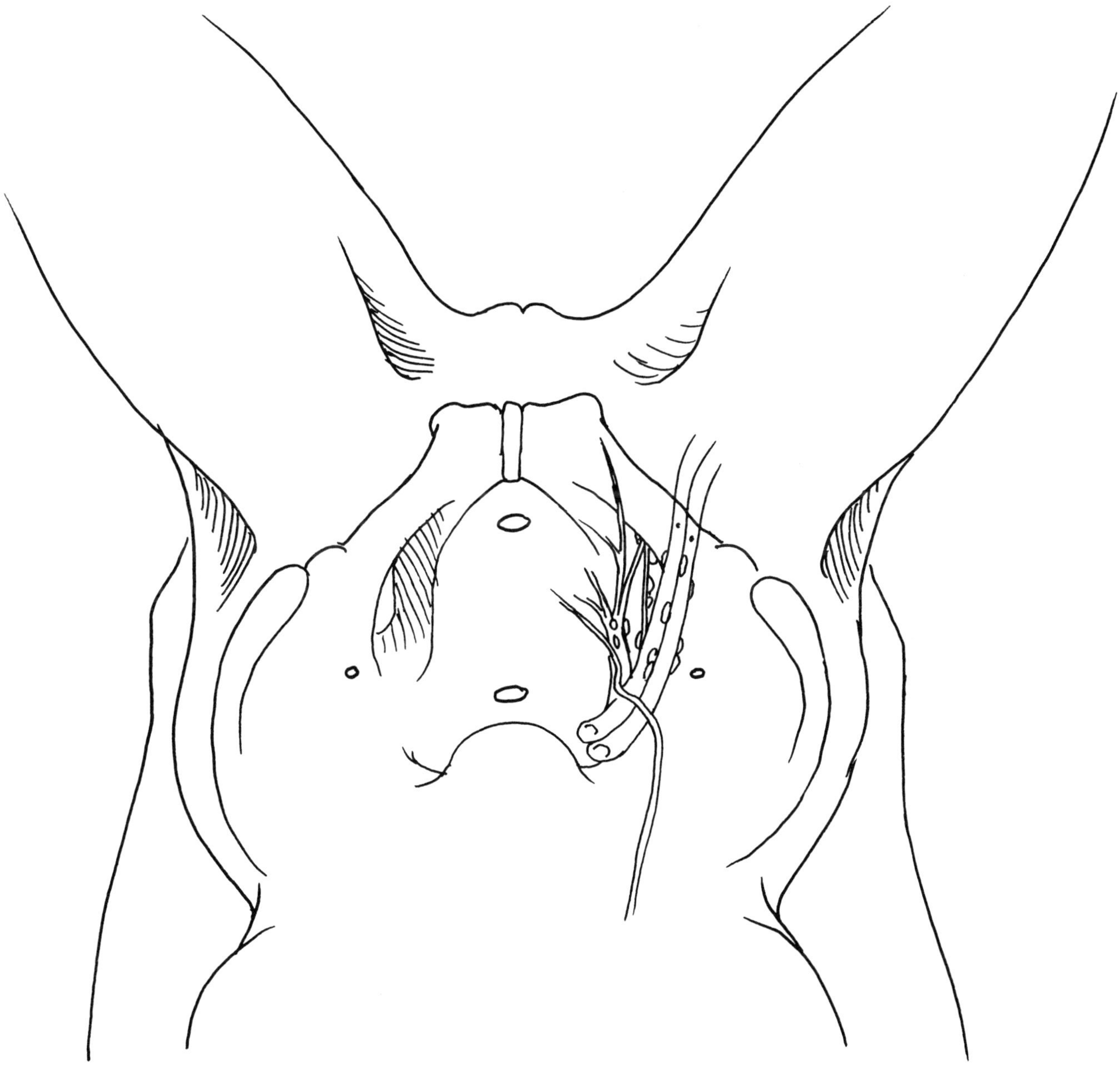

Fig. 7.43

medial umbilical ligament medially and incising peritoneum just lateral to it (Fig. 7.44). The incision is continued proximally along the external iliac artery up to the level of the ureter. Care should be taken to avoid damage to the deep circumflex iliac vessels or an aberrant obturator artery.

The vas is divided in the male for better exposure if clinically appropriate. The lateral flap of peritoneum is mobilized by sweeping retroperitoneal fat off it, leaving the internal spermatic vessels with the flap in the male. Ovarian vessels in the female (infundibulopelvic ligament) crossing the proximal external iliacs are divided if

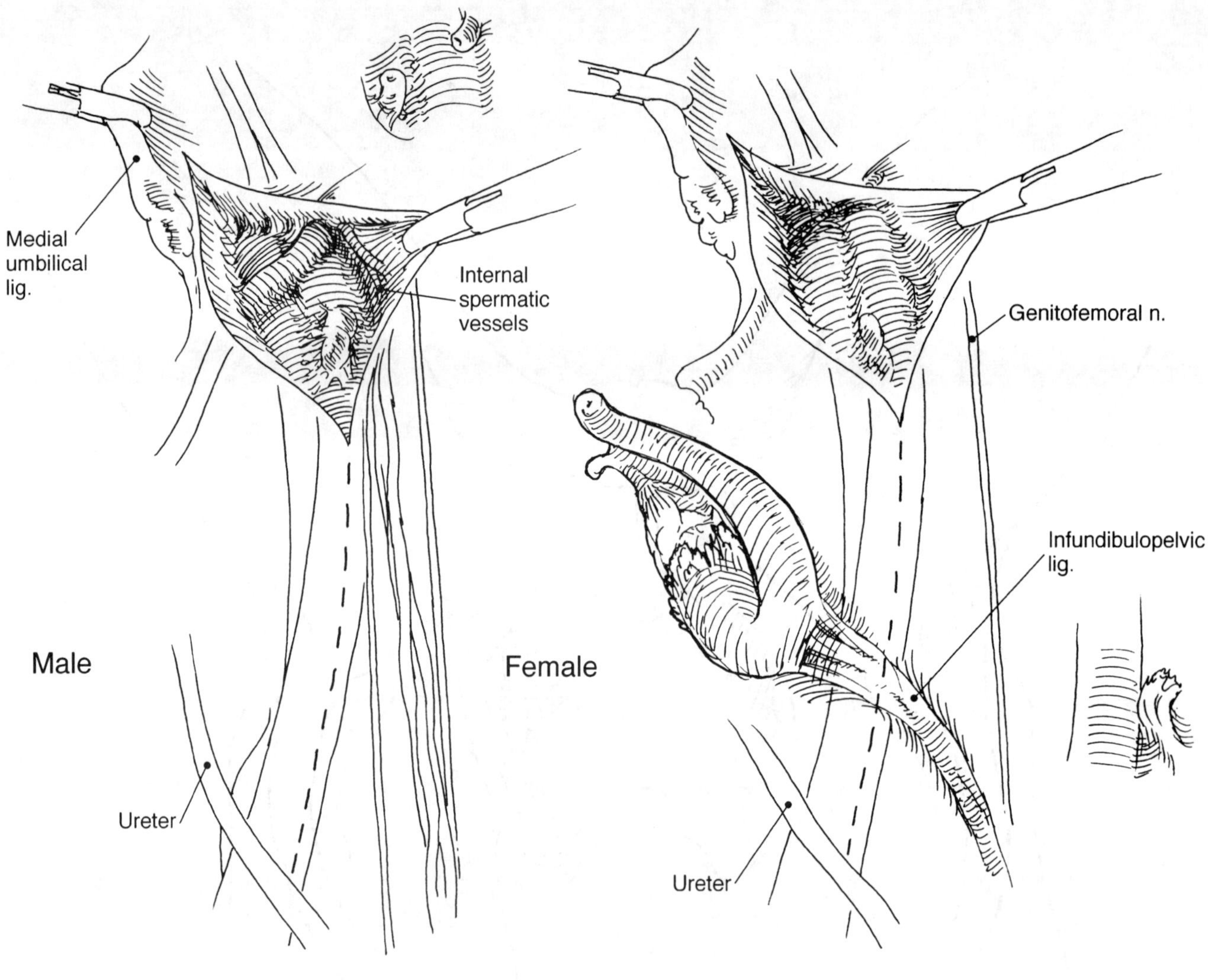

Fig. 7.44

the ovaries are to be removed. If the ovaries are to be left, the tubes and ovaries are mobilized laterally (having been disconnected at the uterine end in the course of hysterectomy) for exposure. The ureter is identified at the proximal end of the dissection (Fig. 7.45). The genitofemoral nerve in identified on the psoas lateral to the external iliac artery and is carefully avoided.

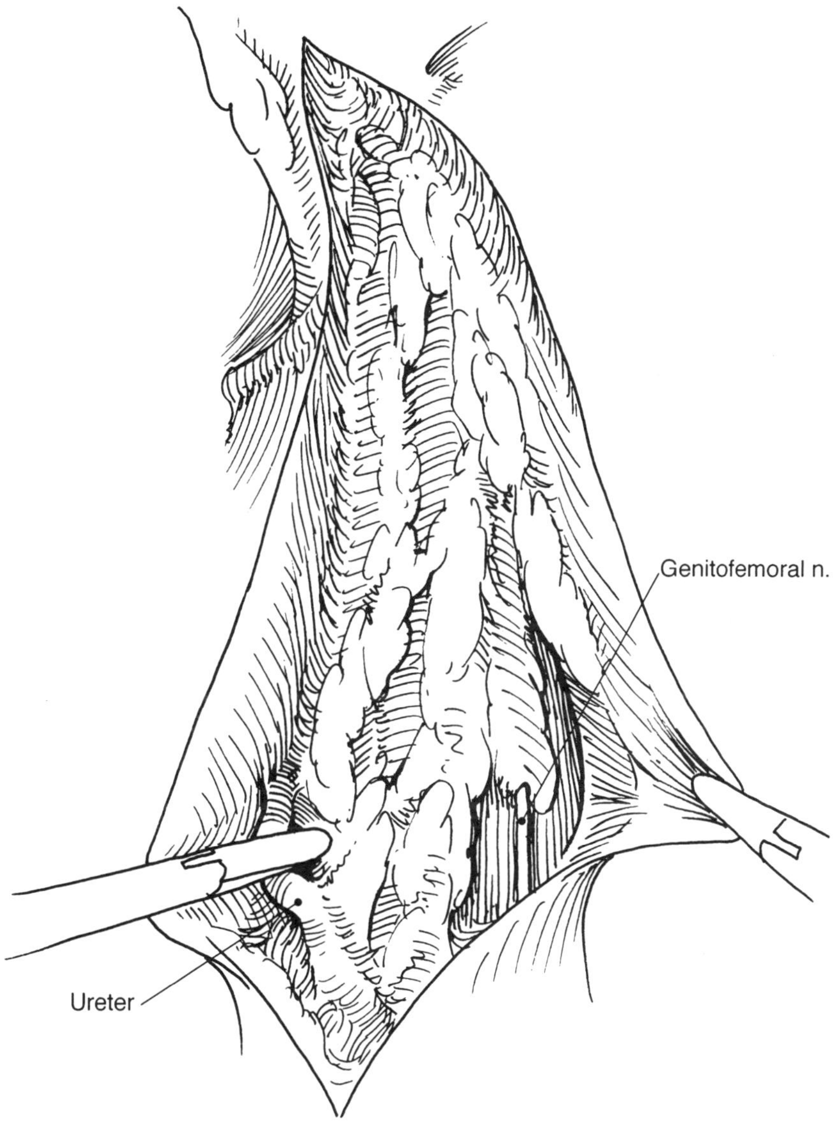

Fig. 7.45

The fibrofatty tissue around the external iliac vessels is sharply and bluntly dissected free, taking care to cauterize major lymphatic channels before cutting (Fig. 7.46). The external iliac vein is identified medial to the artery as a collapsed structure due to the increased intra-abdominal pressure resulting from the pneumoperitoneum.

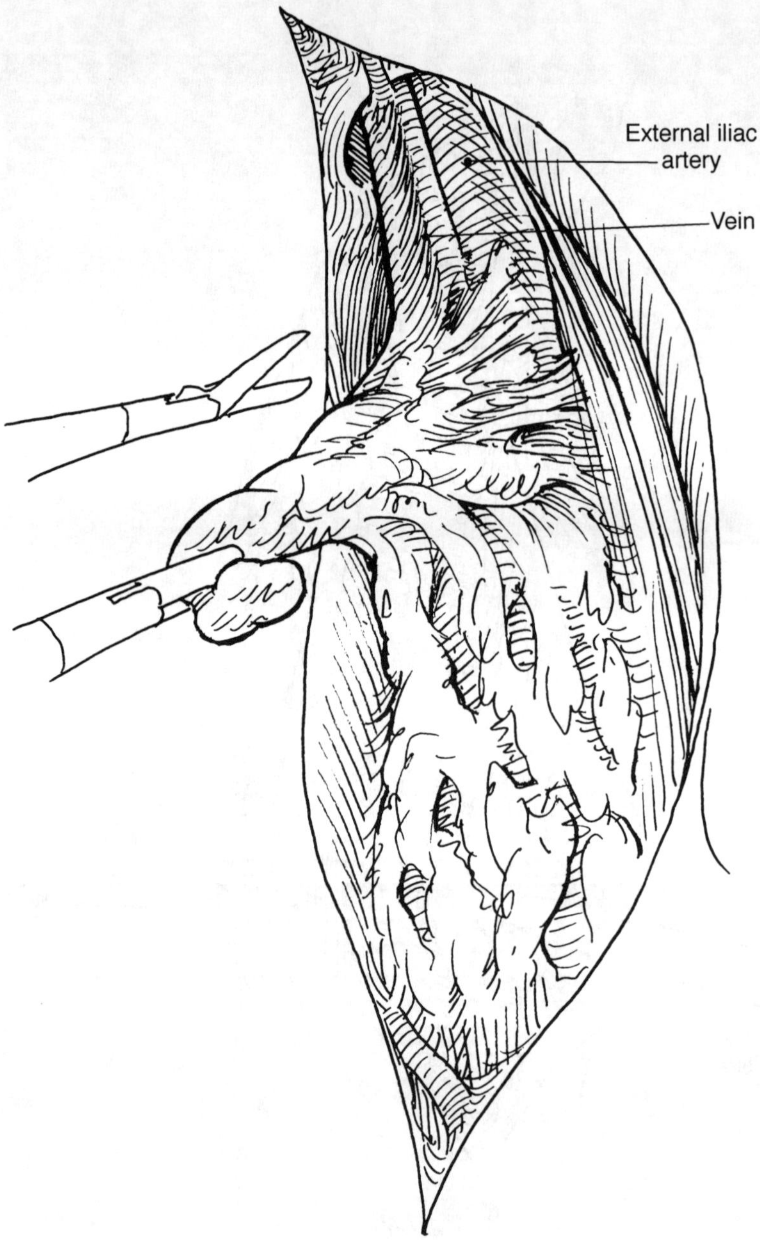

Fig. 7.46

The dissection is carried up to the ureter and the fatty node-bearing tissue is retracted medially (Fig. 7.47). Throughout the dissection, hemostasis may be achieved by monopolar cautery of small vessels and lymph channels. Laparoscopic clips and bipolar cautery should also be available. A 4 x 8 inch sponge may be introduced through a 10 mm port and kept in the pelvis to absorb blood and fluid which may absorb light and decrease visualization. A small branch of the external iliac artery to the psoas muscle is sometimes encountered.

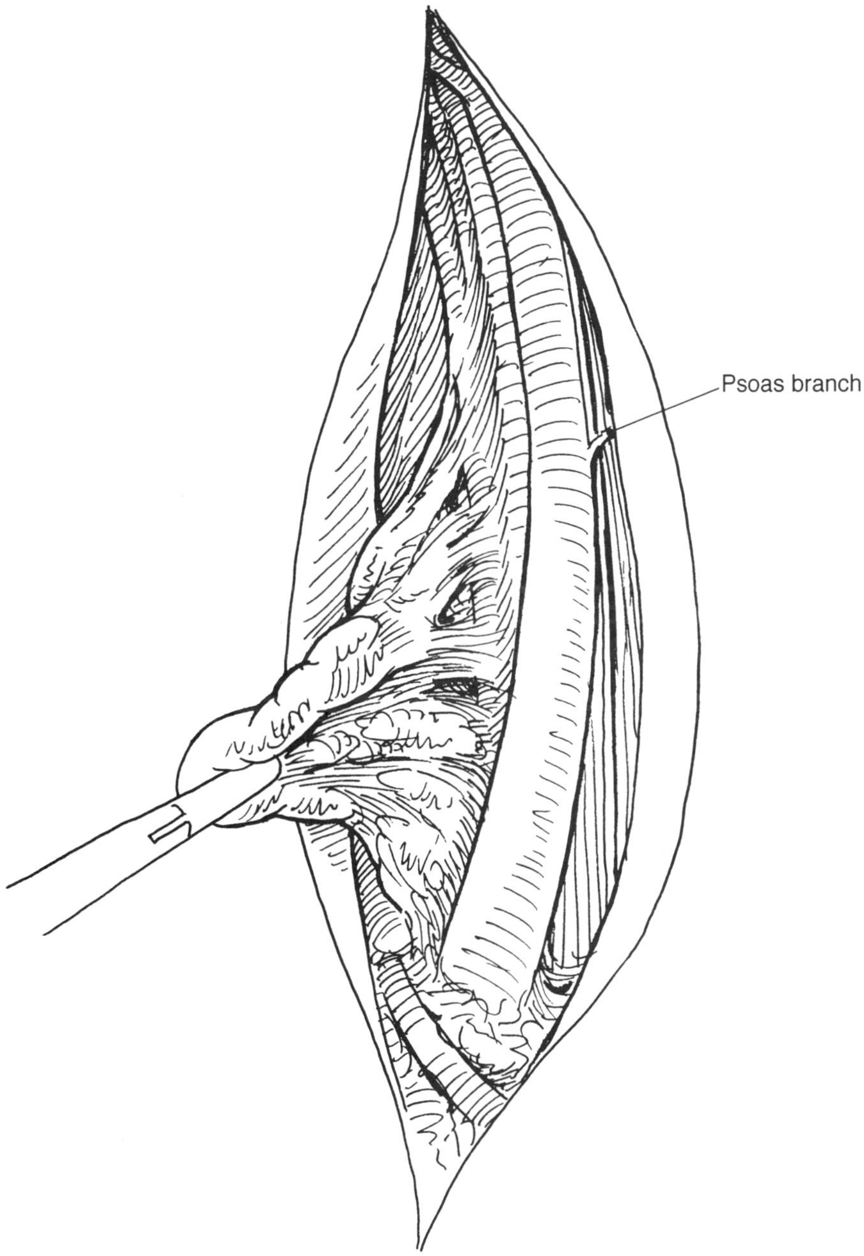

Fig. 7.47

The internal chain of nodes is freed from the medial side of the external iliac vein completing the external iliac dissection and exposing the top of the obturator group of nodes (Fig. 7.48A). Retraction of the external iliac vessels laterally exposes the internal obturator muscle. The operator may elect of remove the nodal groups separately to decrease the bulk of tissue manipulated during further dissection, for ease of removal and for diagnostic localization. The dissection of the obturator group is begun at the pubis taking care not to damage the obturator nerve, which provides motor innervation to the adductor muscles of the thigh.

Additional exposure for a more thorough dissection of the obturator group can be achieved by retracting the external iliac vessels to the medial side (Fig. 7.48B). The nodal tissue is bluntly and sharply dissected free back toward the internal iliac vessels.

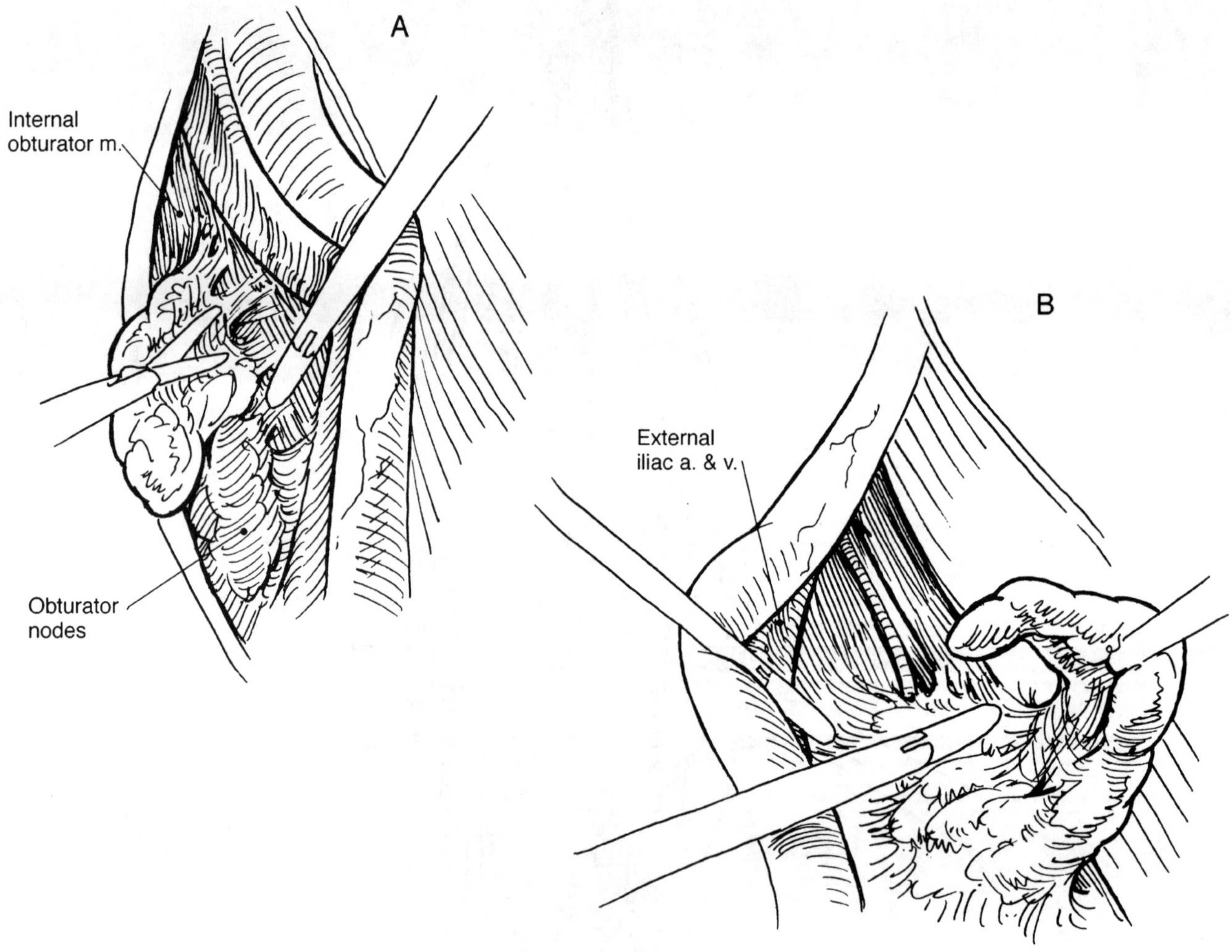

Fig. 7.48

The internal iliac vessels are identified (Fig. 7.49). The sparse internal iliac nodes may be dissected and internal iliac branches divided as necessary if a thorough clean out is indicated. The distal ureter is retracted medially for protection.

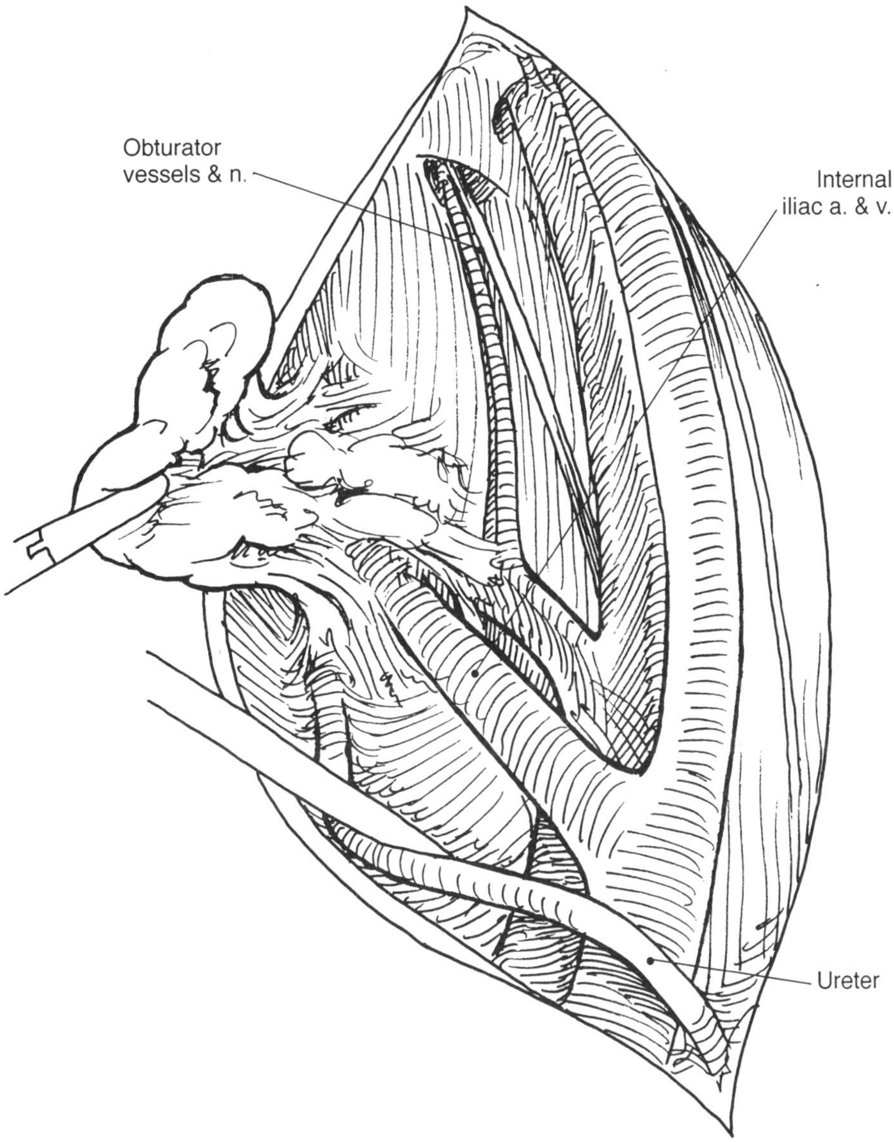

Fig. 7.49

The remaining free nodal tissue is removed with large scoop grasping forceps through the suprapubic port (Fig. 7.50). The peritoneum may be left open to avoid lymphocele formation.

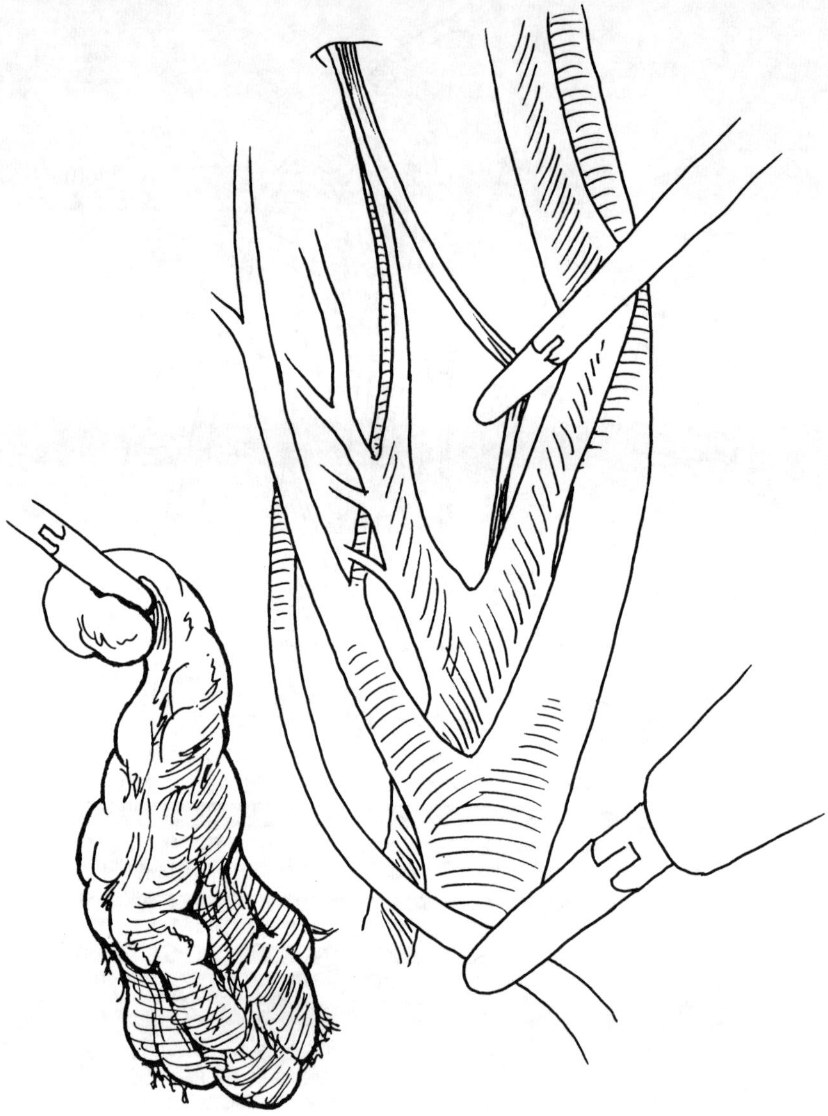

Fig. 7.50

Chapter 7: The Pelvis

EMBRYOLOGY

England MA. Color Atlas of Life Before Birth, Normal Fetal Development. Chicago: Year Book Medical Publishers, 1983:15-24,144,163-166.

O'Rahilly R, Muller F. Human Embryology and Teratology. New York: Wiley-Liss, 1992:207-224.

Skandalakis JE, Gray SW. Embryology for Surgeons. Baltimore: Williams & Wilkins, 1984:594-595,603,737-772,816-847.

ANATOMY

Bergman RA, et al. Compendium of Human Anatomic Variation. Baltimore: Urban & Schwarzenberg, 1988: 173,174,527,528.

Buchsbaum HJ, Schmidt JD. Gynecologic and Obstetric Urology, 3rd ed. Philadelphia 1993:3-60.

Curtis A, et al. The anatomy of the subperitoneal tissues and ligamentous structures in relation to surgery of the female pelvic viscera. SG 1940;643-656.

Fritsch H, Hotzinger H. Tomographical anatomy of the pelvis, visceral pelvic connective tissue and its compartments. Clin Anat 1995;8:17-24.

Ger R. Surgical anatomy of the pelvis. Surg Clin North Am 1988;68:201-1216.

Gray's Anatomy, 13th American Ed., Clemente, C, ed. Philadelphia: Lea & Febiger, 1984:498,748,839,896,906. 1521-1524,1566-1578.

Hinman Jr. F. Atlas of Urosurgical Anatomy. Phila.: WB Saunders Co., 1993:30-32.

Kadir S. Diagnostic Angiography, Philadelphia: WB Saunders, 1986:79-117,259-293.

LAPAROSCOPIC HYSTERECTOMY

Byron J, et al. A randomized comparison of Verres needle and direct trochar insertion for laparoscopy. Surg Gynecol Obstet 1993;177:2595-262.

Grimes DA. Frontiers of operative laparoscopy: a review and critique of the evidence. Am J Obstet Gynecol 1992; 4:1062-1071.

Mettler L, Semm K, et al. Comparative evaluation of classical intrafascial-supracervical hysterectomy (CISH) with transuterine mucosal resection as performed by pelviscopy and laparotomy - our first 200 cases. Surg Endosc 1995;9:418-423.

Nezhat C, et al. Laparoscopic hysterectomy and bilateral salpingo-oophorectomy using the multifire GIA stapler. J Gynecol Surg 1989;6:287-288.

Nezhat F, et al. Complications and results of 361 hysterectomies performed at laparoscopy. J Am Coll Surg 1995; 180:307-316.

Reich H, et al. Laparoscopic hysterectomy. J Gynecol Surg 1989;5:213-215.

Scott-Conner C, Dawson DL. Operative Anatomy. Philadelphia: JB Lippincott Co., 1993:489-495.

Tadir Y, Fisch B. Operative laparoscopy: a challenge for general gynecology? Am J Obstet Gynecol 1993;169:7-12.

Wheeless Jr. CR. Atlas of Pelvic Surgery. Philadelphia: Lea & Febiger, 1988:258-281,290-293,241-255.

LAPAROSCOPIC PELVIC LYMPH NODE DISSECTION

Childers JM, et al. The role of laparoscopic lymphadenectomy in the management of cervical carcinoma. Gynecol Oncol 1992;47:38-43.

Childers JM, et al. Laparoscopic para-aortic lymphadenectomy in gynecologic malignancies. Obstet Gynecol 1993; 82:741-747.

Nelson JH, et al. Anatomy of the female pelvic and aortic lymphatic systems demonstrated by lymphangiography. Am J Obstet Gynecol 1964;88:460-469.

Nelson JH. Atlas of Radical Pelvic Surgery. New York: Appleton-Century-Crofts, 1977:143-155,168,169.

Reich H. Pelvic sidewall dissection. Clin Obstet Gynecol 1991;34:412-422.

Thomas R. Laparoscopic pelvic lymphadenectomy. In: Das S, Crawford E eds. Urologic Laparoscopy. Philadelphia: WB Saunders Co., 1994:165-170.

Vancaille TG, Sheussler WW. Laparoscopic pelvic lymphadenectomy. In: Zucker KA ed. Surgical Laparoscopy. St. Louis: Quality Medical Publishing, Inc., 1993:241-261.

Wheeless Jr. CR. Atlas of Pelvic Surgery. Philadelphia, Lea & Febiger, 1988:421-428.

Winfield HN. Laparoscopic pelvic lymph node dissection: application to genitourinary malignancies. In: Gomella LG, et al eds. Laparoscopic Urologic Surgery. New York: Raven Press, 1994:111-129.

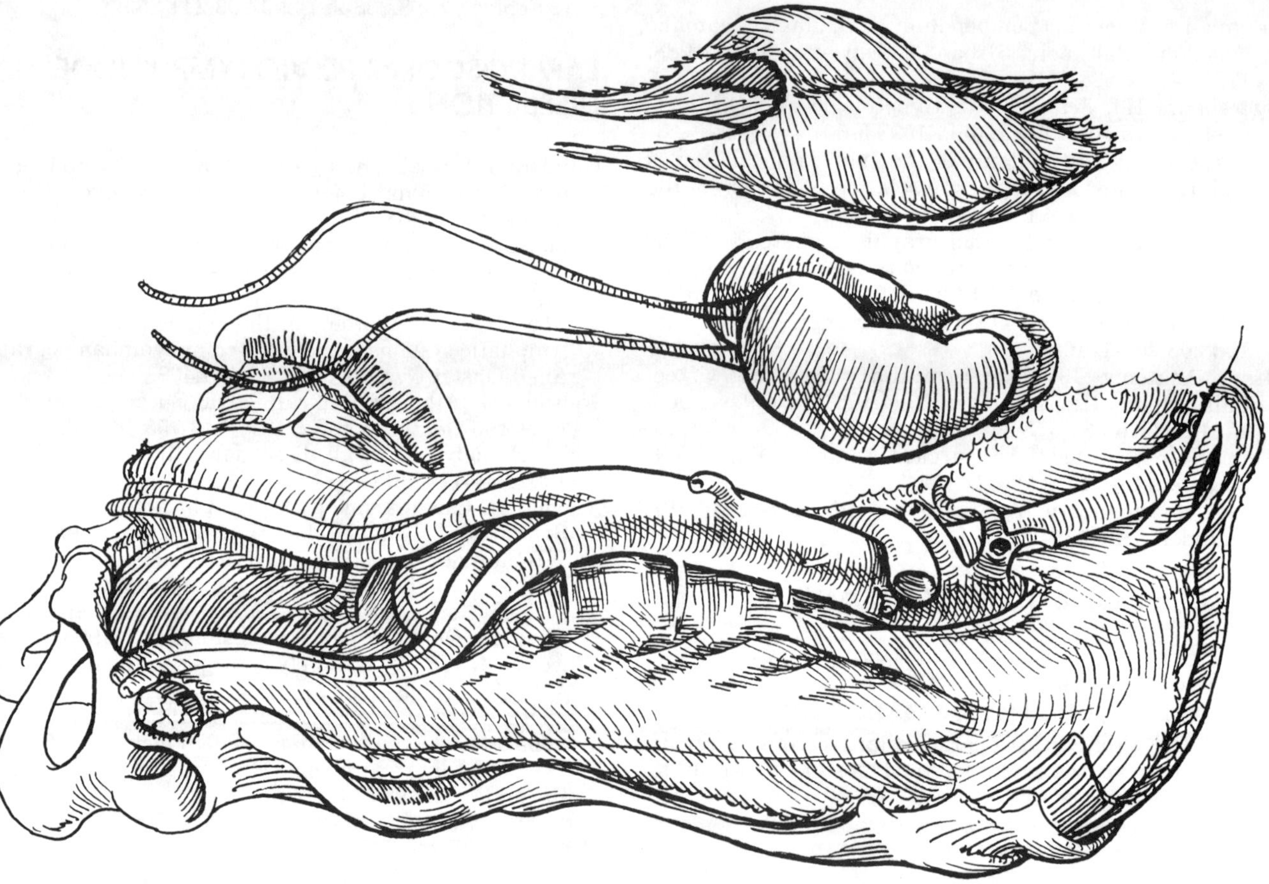

8

The Urologic System

EMBRYOLOGY

At three and a half weeks of gestation, bilateral nephrogenic ridges develop from intermediate mesoderm along the dorsal body wall of the embryo starting from the seventh somite and progressing caudally (Fig. 8.1). Between weeks four and eight, the definitive kidneys (metanephros) and ureters develop at the caudal end of the ridge, the adrenal glands develop at the cephalad ends, and the gonads develop along the anteromedial margins (Chapter 7 for detailed gonadal embryology). The kidneys and gonads shift positions relative to the coelomic cavity during this period, the kidneys approaching the adrenals in a cephalad direction and the gonads descending toward the pelvis.

The nephrogenic ridges generate segmental tubules successively in a cranial to caudal direction, forming the mesonephros. On each side, these tubules connect to a longitudinal channel (Wolffian/mesonephric duct), which develops in parallel with the mesonephros beneath the epithelium of the ridge. At the end of the fifth week, the mesonephric ducts reach the cloaca and

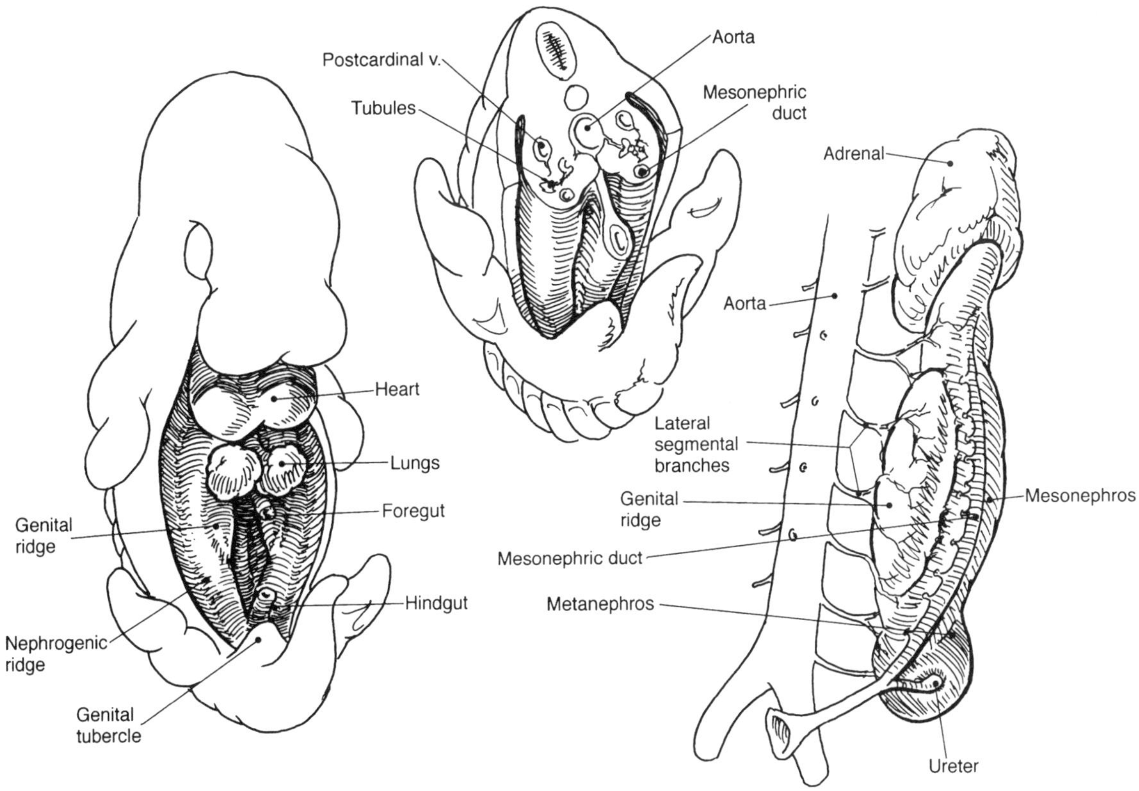

Fig. 8.1

at the same time send dorsal buds to the caudal end of the nephrogenic ridges, the metanephric blastema destined to become the definitive kidneys. The metanephric tissue surrounds the growing ureteral buds and separates from the urogenital ridges and from the mesonephros above. The connections between the metanephroi and the mesonephric ducts become the ureters.

Between the fourth and seventh weeks, the cloaca is divided by an infolding of body wall (the urorectal septum) into the urogenital sinus anteriorly and the rectum posteriorly. After its union with the urogenital sinus, the portion of the mesonephric duct distal to the ureter, the common excretory duct, is incorporated into the wall of the urogenital sinus (Fig. 8.2). As the common channel is absorbed, the ureteral orifice is initially lateral to the mesonephric duct orifice. Growth of mesonephric duct mesoderm in the wall of the urogenital sinus displaces the ureteral orifices cranially and laterally, forming the superficial trigone of the bladder.

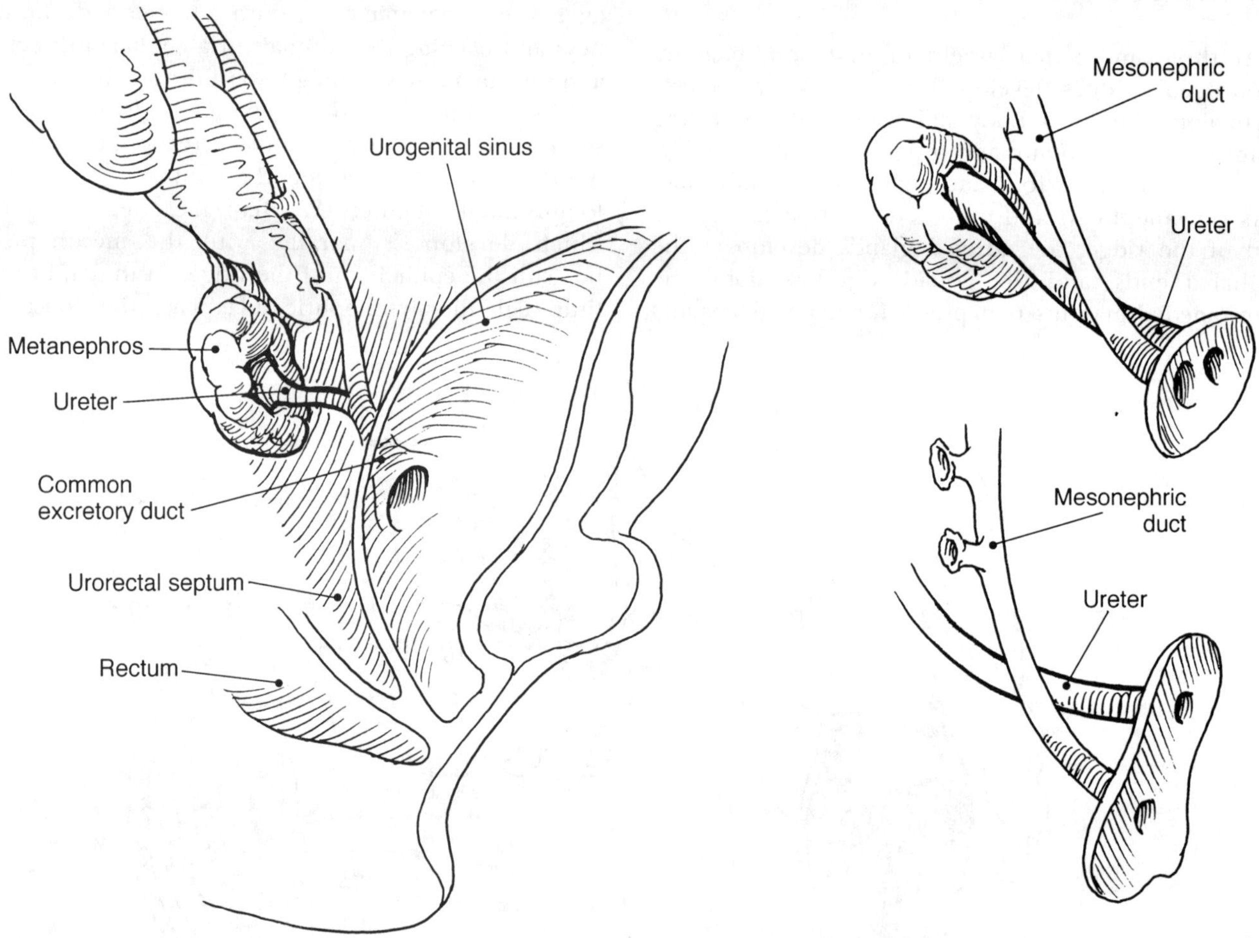

Fig. 8.2

In less than 1% of individuals, the ureteric bud splits before reaching the metanephric blastema, resulting in duplication of the ureter (Fig. 8.3). Early splitting results in a long duplication while a late split may manifest only as a split renal pelvis, the most common form of duplication . When the bifurcation involves the ureter, most such divisions are found in the mid portion of the ureter and are unilateral. Rarely, the split ureteric buds may meet separated metanephric blastema and form duplicate kidneys. Detailed explications of the rare urinary tract anomalies are found in the references cited at the end of the chapter.

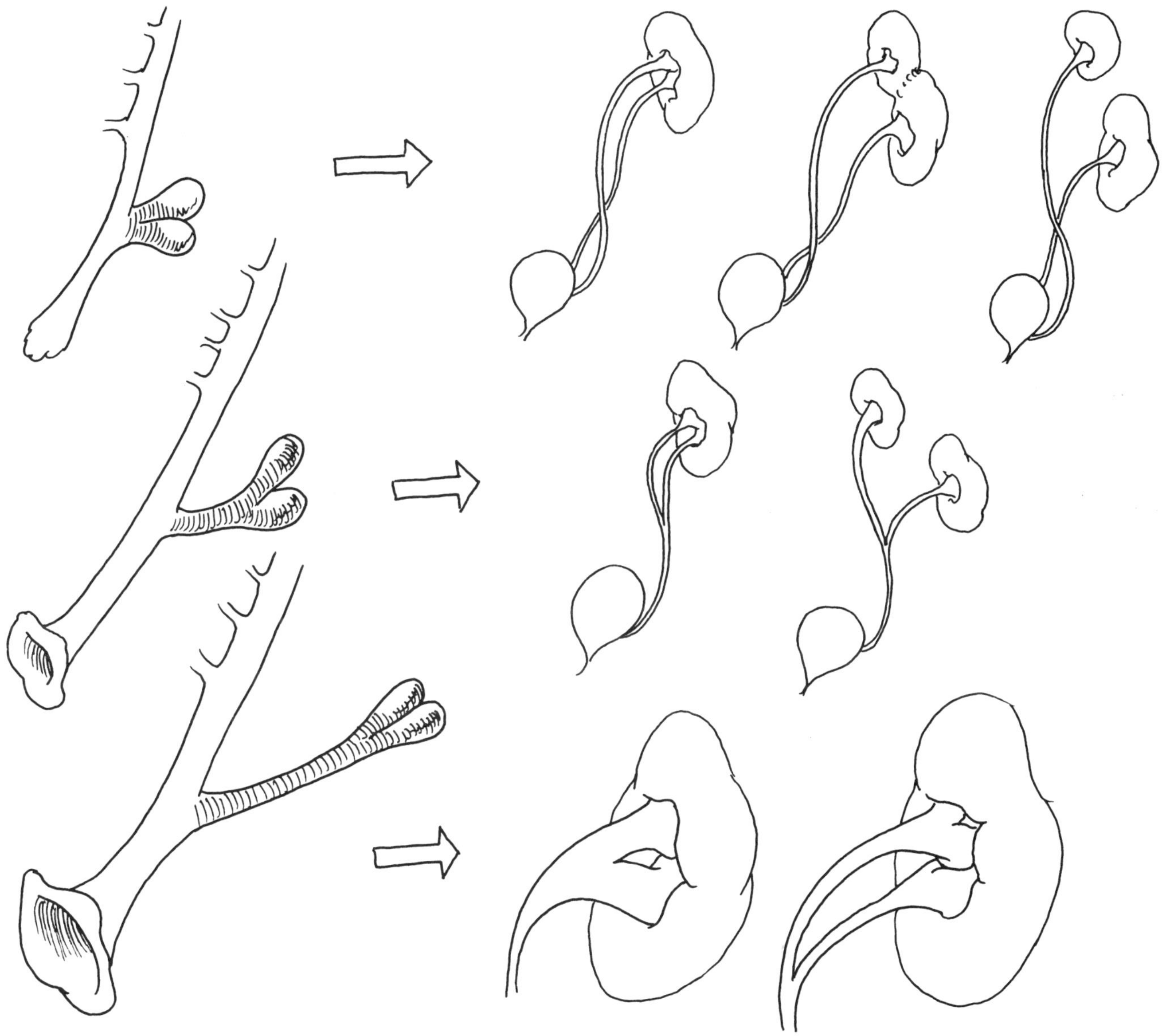

Fig. 8.3

The renal hila rotate from an anterior to an anteromedial position and the kidneys make contact with the lower poles of the adrenal glands by the eighth week (Fig. 8.4). Arrested ascent results in an ectopic kidney that may lie anywhere along the path from pelvis to upper abdomen and derives its blood supply from the vessels at that level, for example the iliacs, inferior mesenteric artery or lower aorta. Failure of an umbilical artery to acquire a normal secondary connection to a dorsal segmental aortic branch (Chapter 7) results in ascent of the kidney behind the future iliac artery, producing the rare retroiliac ureter. Early fusion of the metanephric blastema results in the rare horseshoe kidney, which remains in a pelvic position. and derives its blood supply from pelvic vessels.

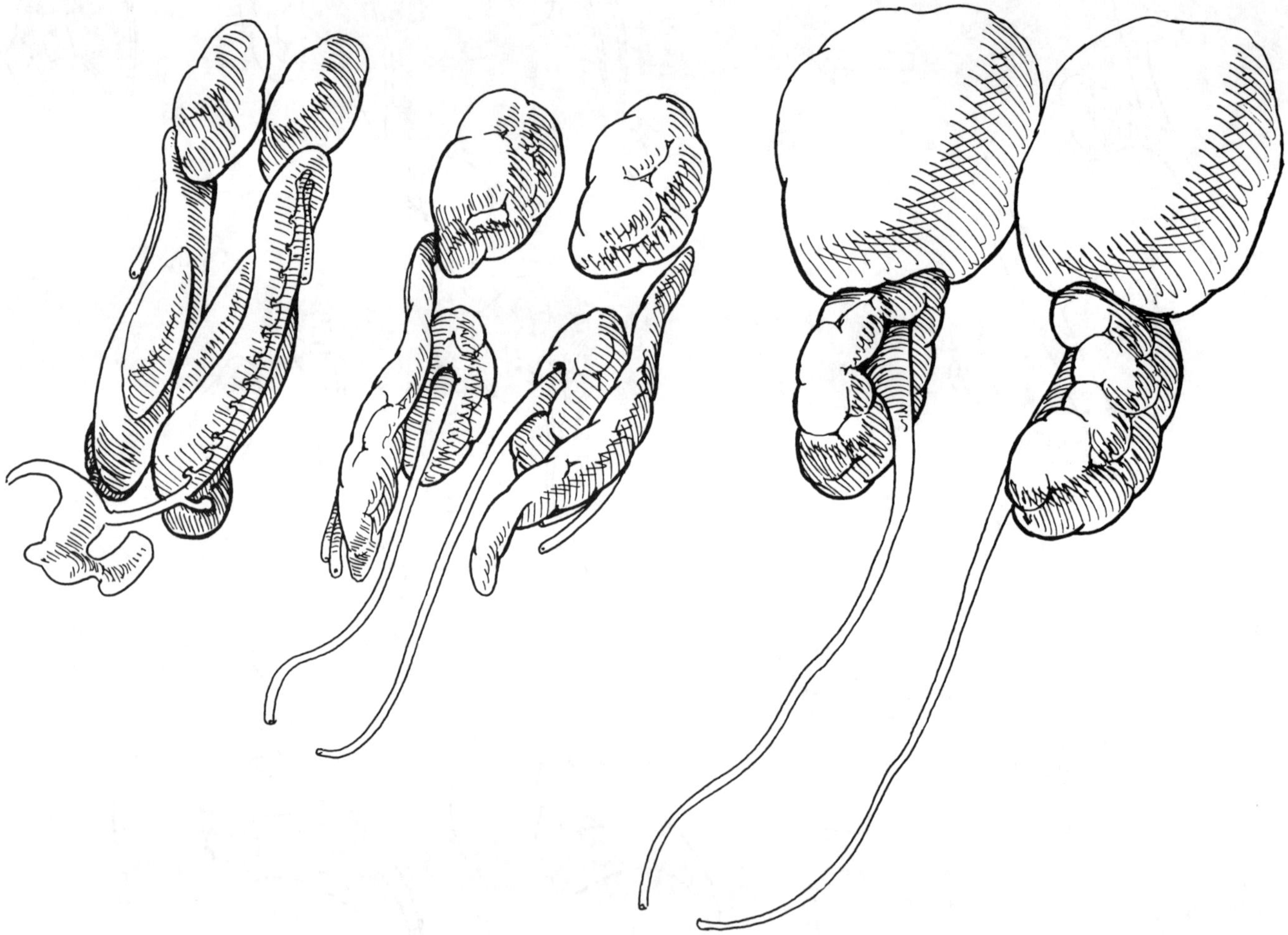

Fig. 8.4

The structures of the urogenital ridges are initially supplied by multiple lateral segmental aortic branches (Fig. 8.5). As the mesonephroi regress and the metanephric kidneys ascend relative to the abdominal cavity, approaching the developing adrenal glands, they acquire their definitive blood supply. Persistence of segmental vessels, particularly the lower ones that regress later, leaves accessory renal vessels in about a third of individuals. An adrenal or gonadal branch may arise from such a vessel.

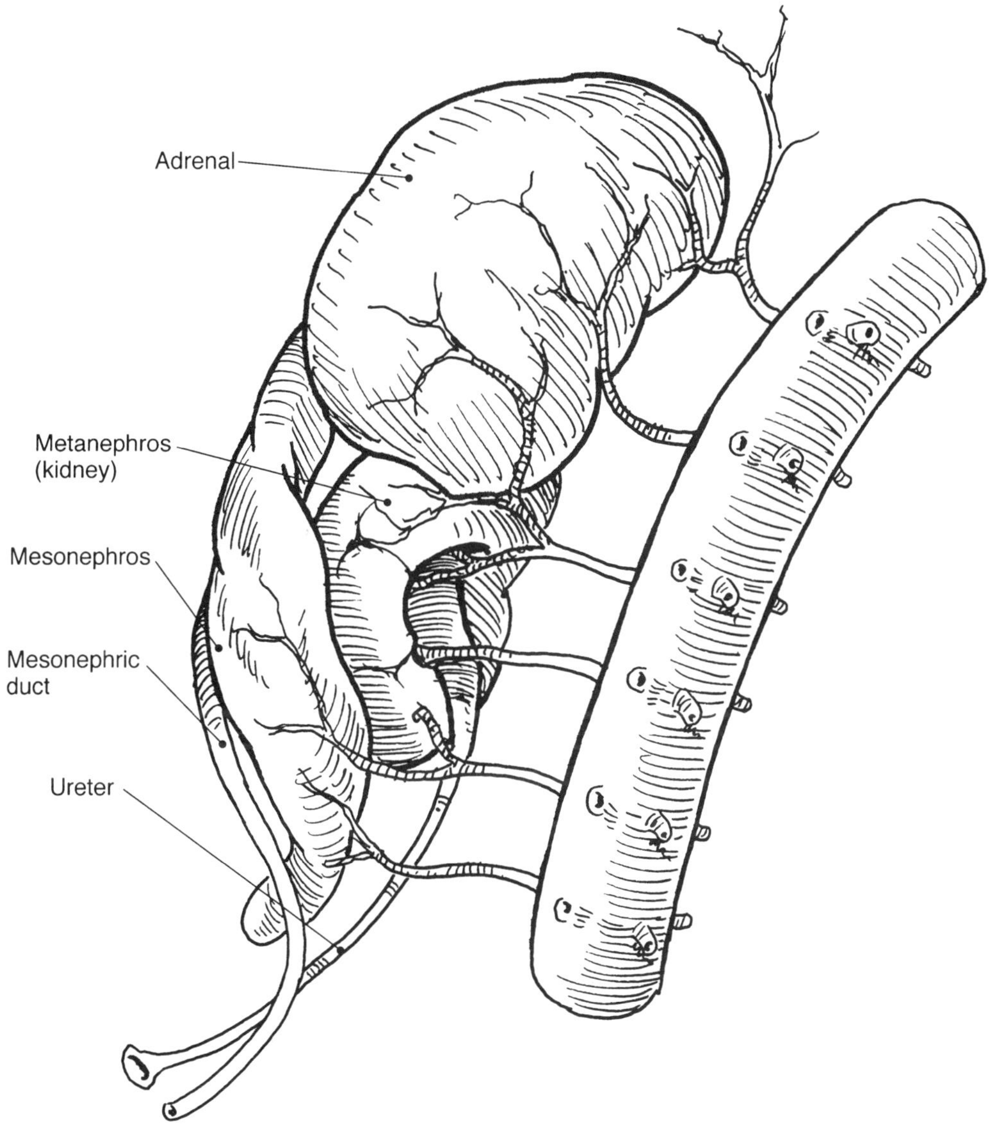

Fig. 8.5

The definitive abdominal venous drainage develops during this period from complex interconnection and selective regression of three paired venous channels, the primitive postcardinal veins, supplemented by the subcardinal and supracardinal veins in that order (Fig. 8.6). The subcardinal veins connect with the postcardinal and supracardinal veins and at 6 weeks, intersubcardinal anastomoses form in the area of the future renal veins. The body of the left renal vein is derived from one of these intersubcardinal anastomoses. The supracardinal veins also anastomose with each other behind the aorta creating a collar. The suprarenal cava is formed from the

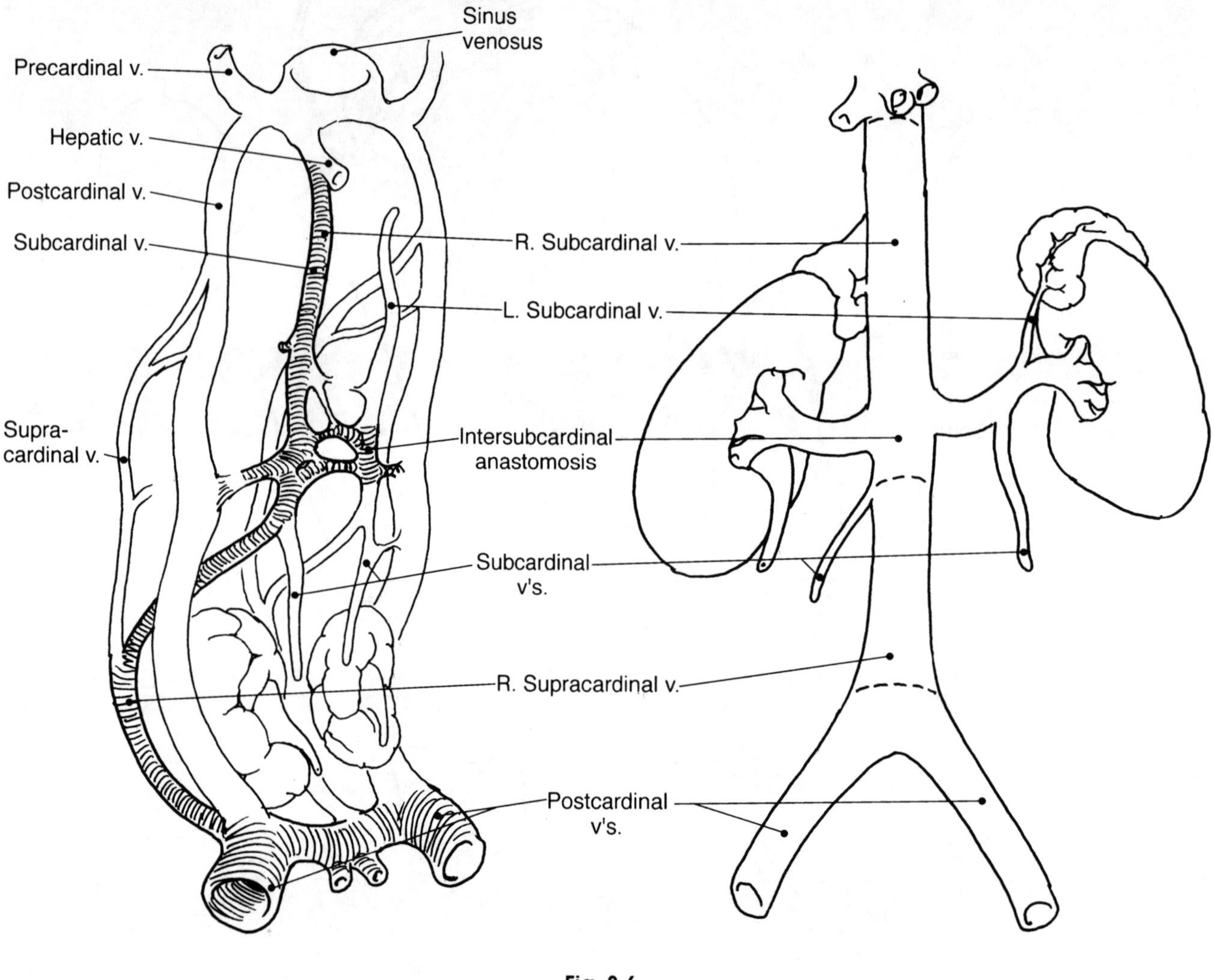

Fig. 8.6

right subcardinal vein. The remnants of the left subcardinal vein are the left adrenal vein above and the left gonadal vein below the left renal vein. The caudal remnant of the right subcardinal is the right gonadal vein. Formation and connection of supracardinal veins followed by selective regression results in the mature inferior vena cava. The infrarenal portion is formed mainly by the right supracardinal vein connecting to postcardinal derivatives at the iliac bifurcation. Persistence of the primitive renal collar results in a circumaortic collar of left renal veins if both anterior and posterior components remain, or a posterior vein alone if only the posterior components remain (Fig. 8.7). Rarely the more ventral right postcardinal vein persists instead of the right

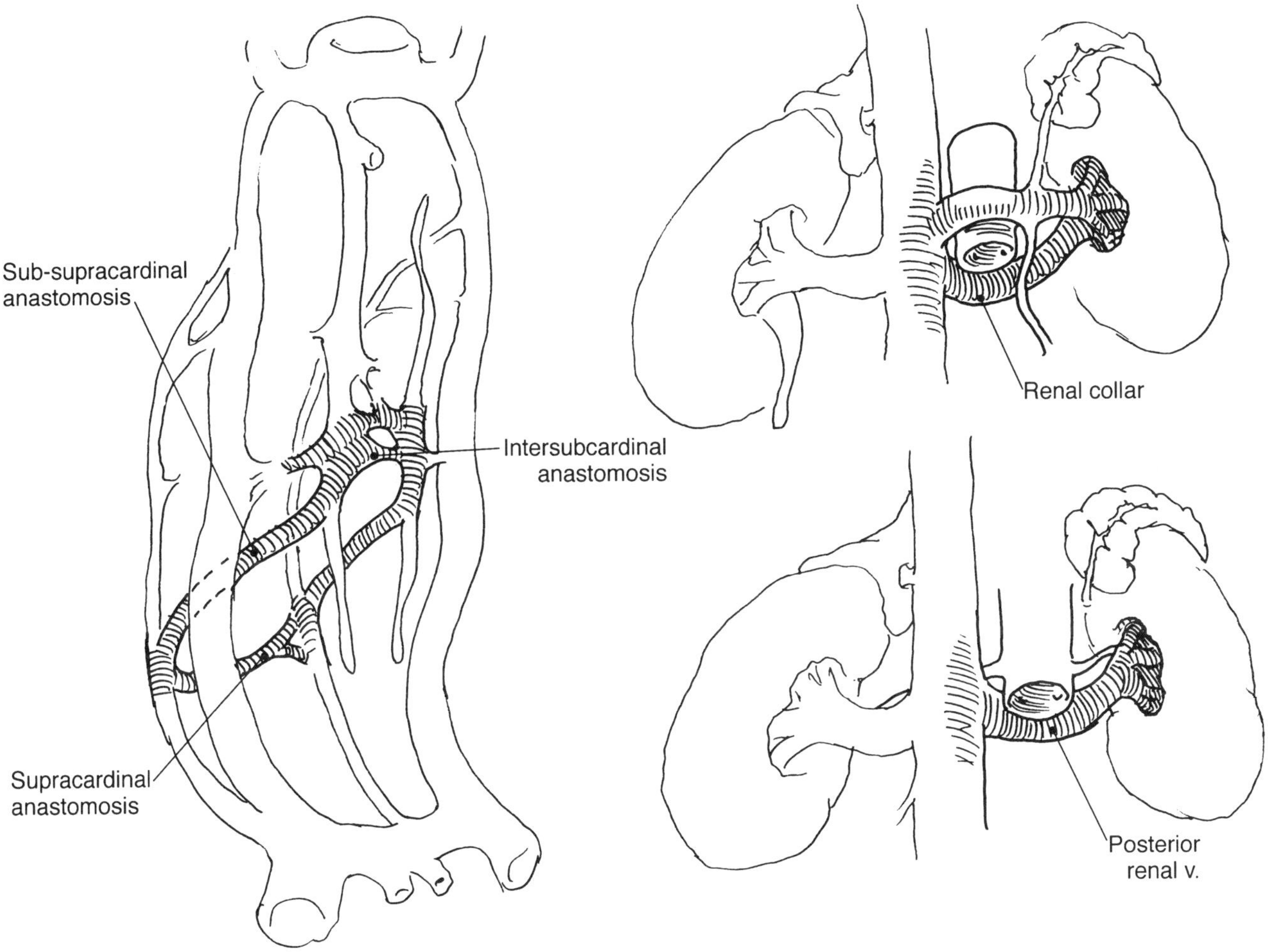

Fig. 8.7

supracardinal, causing the right ureter to lie in a retrocaval position (Fig. 8.8). Persistence of both infrarenal supracardinal veins results in duplication of that portion of the inferior vena cava (Fig. 8.9). If only the left becomes dominant, that portion of the vena cava lies to the left of the aorta.

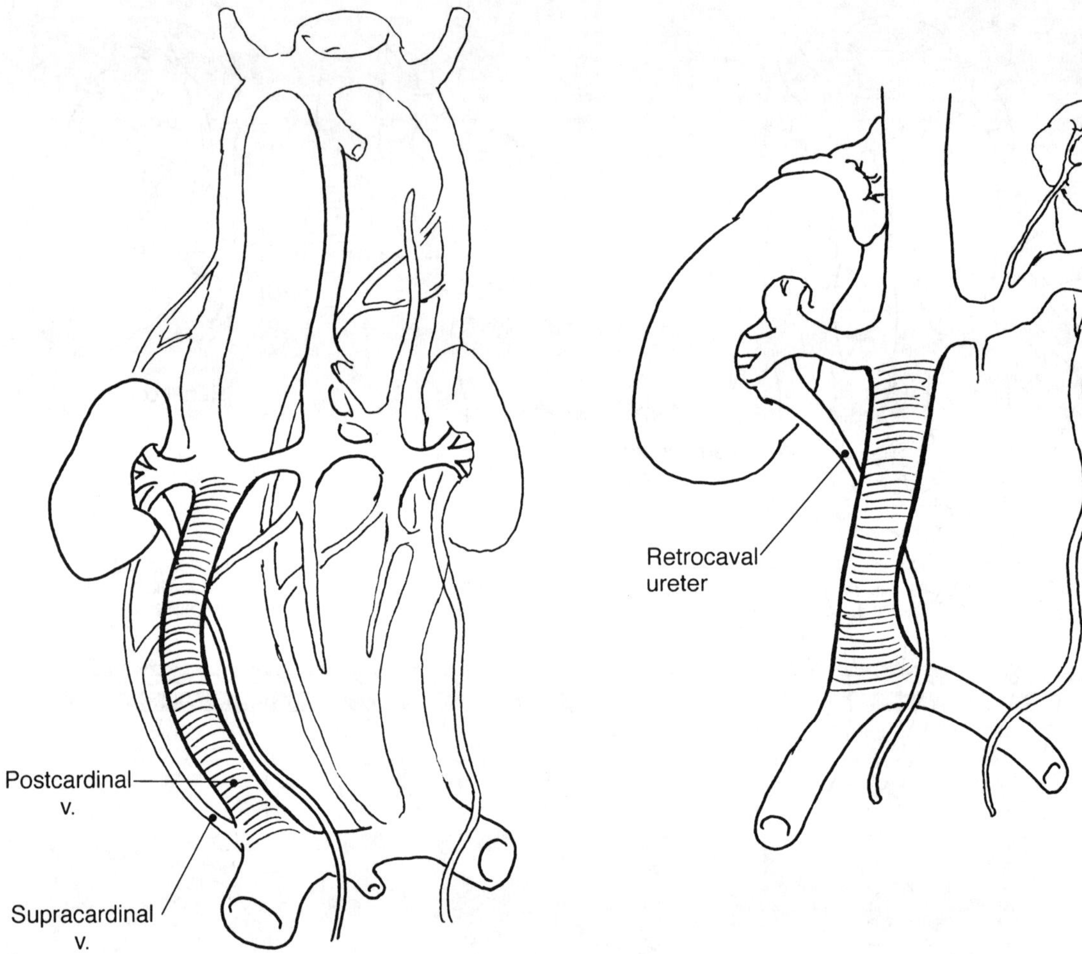

Fig. 8.8

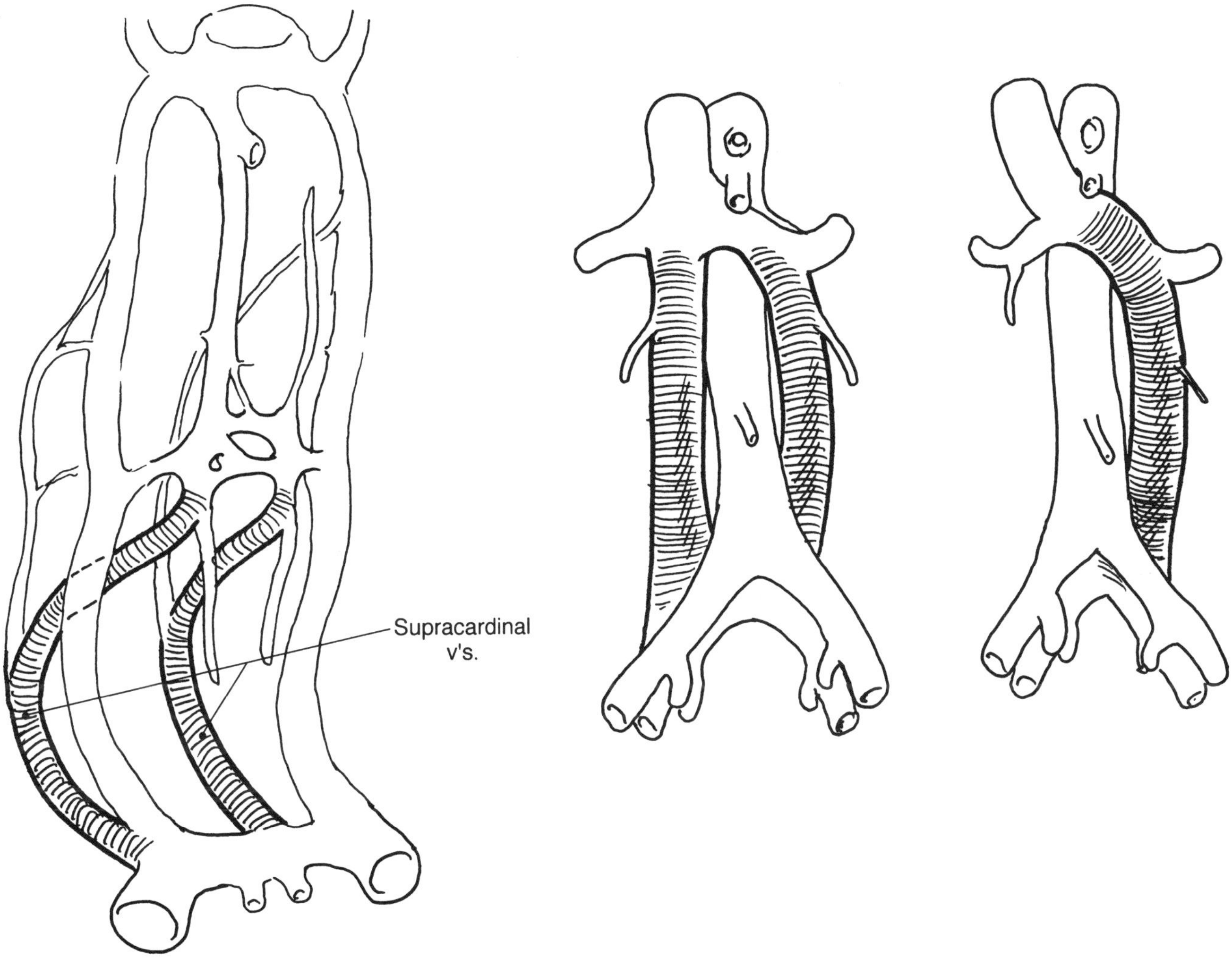

Fig. 8.9

The adrenal glands initially appear in the fifth to sixth weeks of development from the ingrowth of coelomic epithelium (parietal peritoneum) into the underlying mesoderm adjacent to the bowel mesentery at the cranial ends of the mesonephric ridges (Fig. 8.10A). Ectopic adrenal tissue may be found intra-abdominally, retroperitoneally, beneath the renal capsule and associated with the sexual organs. The epithelial cortical primordia of the adrenal glands are invaded starting in the seventh week by neural crest (chromaffin) cells, which are distributed along the aorta. Those cells that invade the adrenal primordia will become the medulla of the glands. Persistence of para-aortic and para-iliac chromaffin cells (as far down as the bladder), particularly the larger aggregates around the inferior mesenteric artery and at the bifurcation of the inferior vena cava (organ of Zuckerkandl), may give rise to extra-adrenal pheochromocytoma (Fig. 8.10B). At the time the metanephric kid-

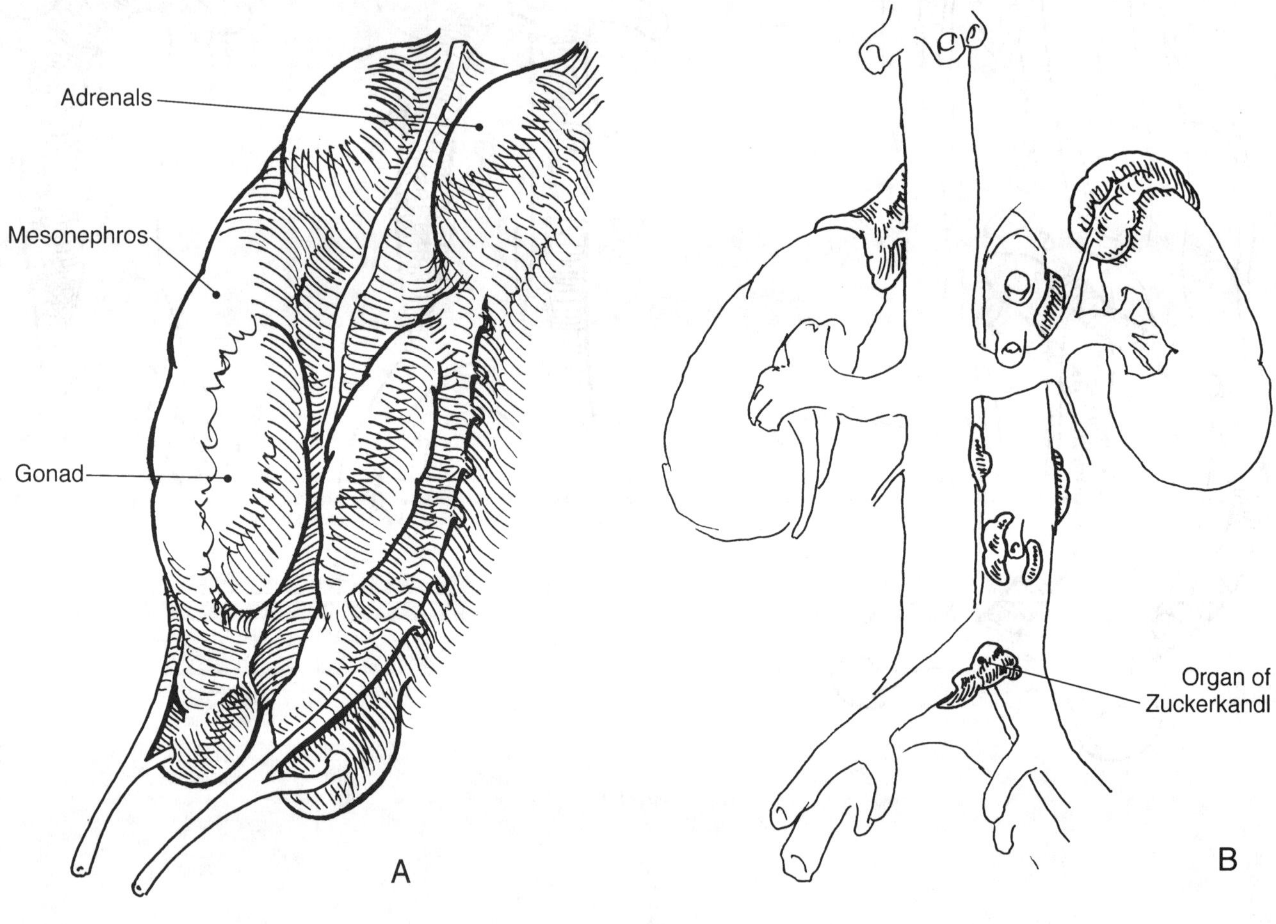

Fig. 8.10

neys reach the adrenals in the upper abdomen, the adrenal glands separate from their peritoneal attachments and are larger than the kidneys due to the bulk of primitive cortical elements (Fig. 8.11). They reach their maximal size about the fourth month of gestation. The primitive cortical tissue regresses in the later fetal period and after birth, leaving the thin permanent cortex.

In addition to direct aortic branches (derivatives of the highest mesonephric segmental branches), the adrenal arterial supply is shared with vessels of the septum transversarum (inferior phrenic arteries), and the kidneys (renal artery). The arterial branches are multiple and fine. Venous drainage does not follow the arterial supply but usually converges into a single channel on each side, draining on the right into the back wall of the inferior vena cava and into the renal vein on the left (due to the regression of the left sided system of veins in the formation of the inferior vena cava).

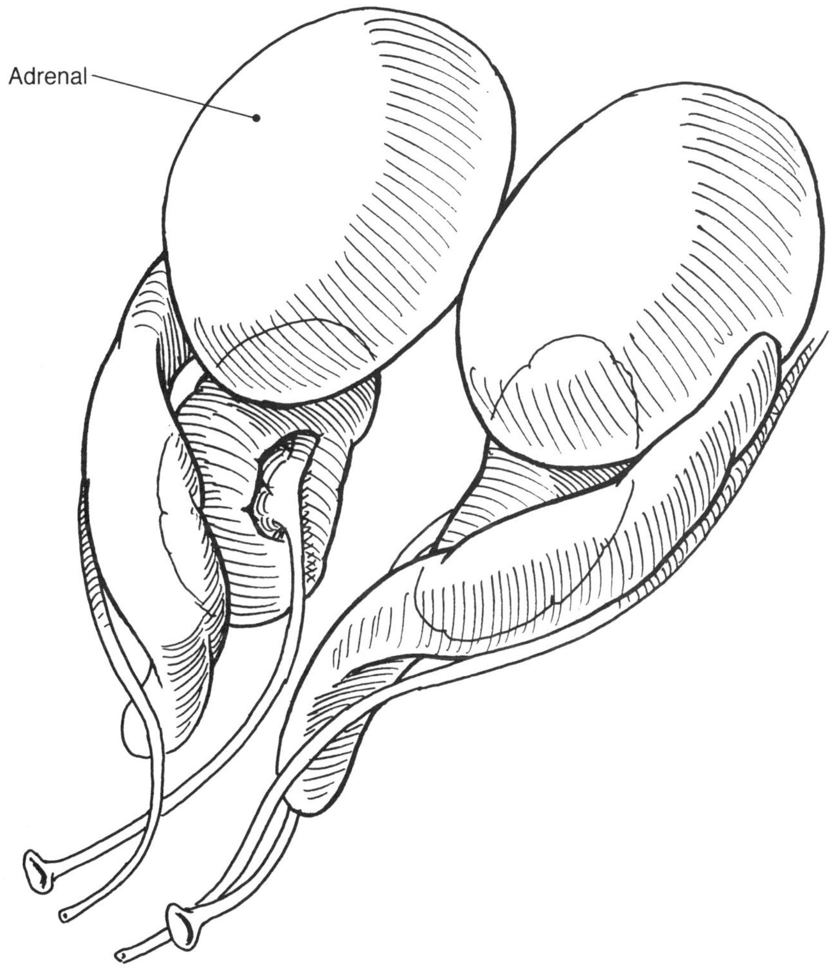

Fig. 8.11

ANATOMY

Fascial Planes

The abdominal cavity is the space bounded by the endoabdominal fascia lining the inner surfaces of the abdominal and pelvic muscles, the diaphragm above and the pelvic floor below (Fig. 8.12). This fascia is named regionally according to the underlying muscles or area, e.g., transversalis, iliopsoas, and endopelvic fascias.

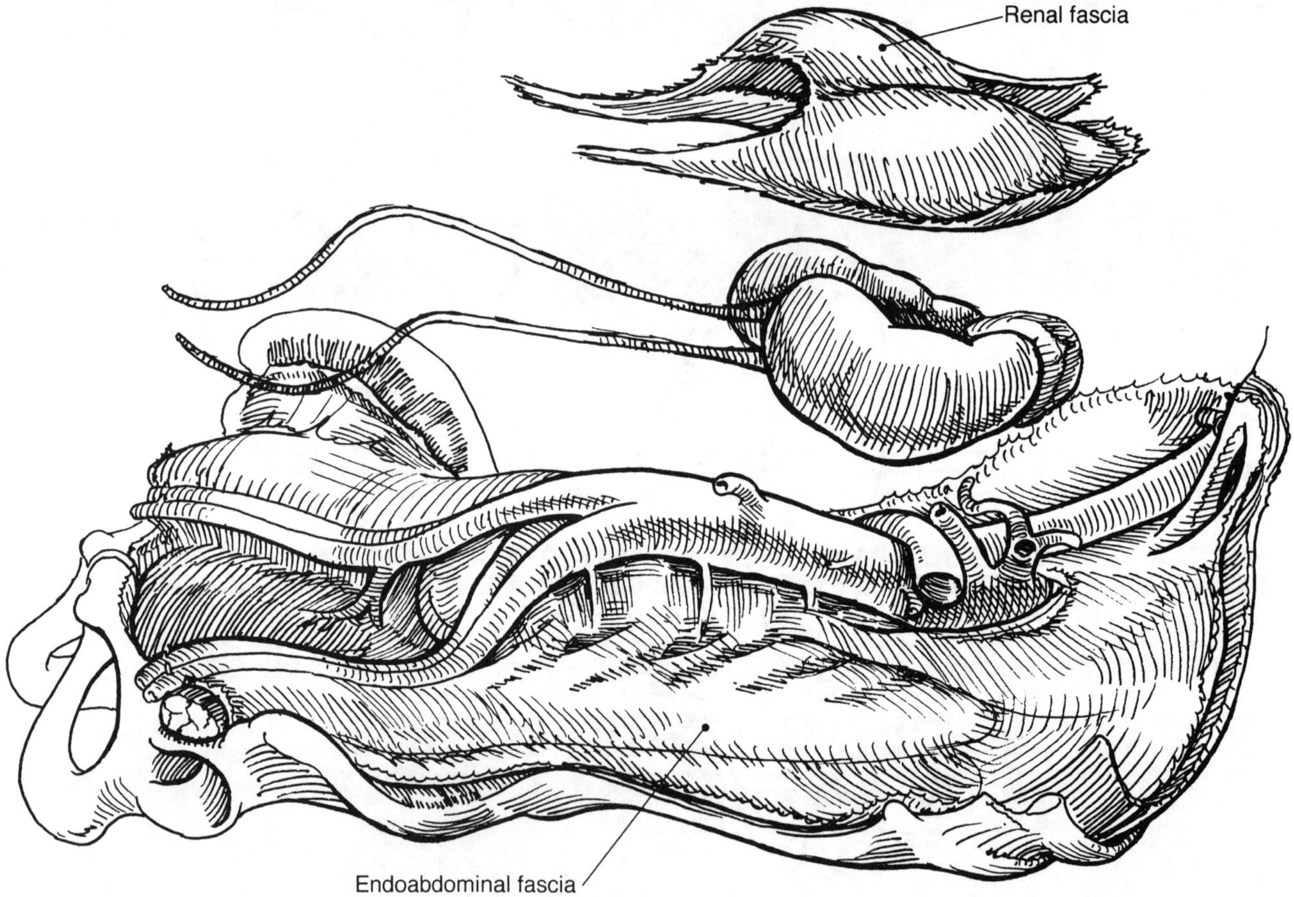

Fig. 8.12

The kidneys, ureters, and adrenal glands develop behind the dorsal parietal peritoneum of the embryo and are found between these layers in the adult. These structures are enclosed in an additional envelope of renal fascia (Gerota's) (Fig. 8.13), which contains a cushioning layer of fat and fine fibrous septae (perirenal space). The fat is most abundant around the margins of the kidneys, extends into the renal hila and encases the adrenal glands. Tapering extensions enclose the adrenal glands above and the ureters below.

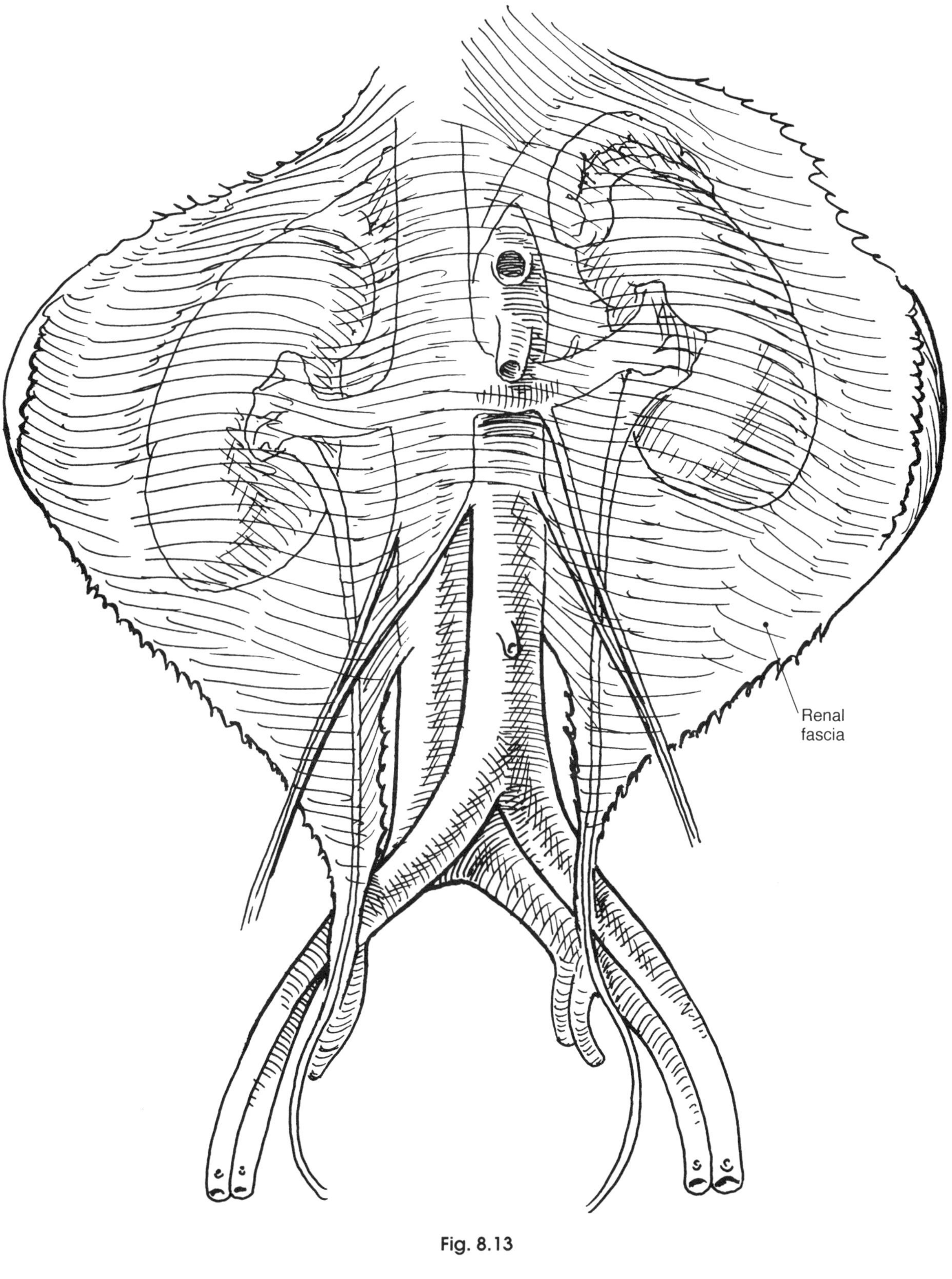

Fig. 8.13

The anterior and posterior laminae of the renal fascia join laterally as the lateroconal fascia and extend medially across the midline anterior and posterior to the great vessels at the level of the renal vessels (Fig. 8.14). Fusion of the medial extensions with the transversalis fascia posteriorly and with the vascular adventitia leaves no effective communication between the perirenal spaces on either side.

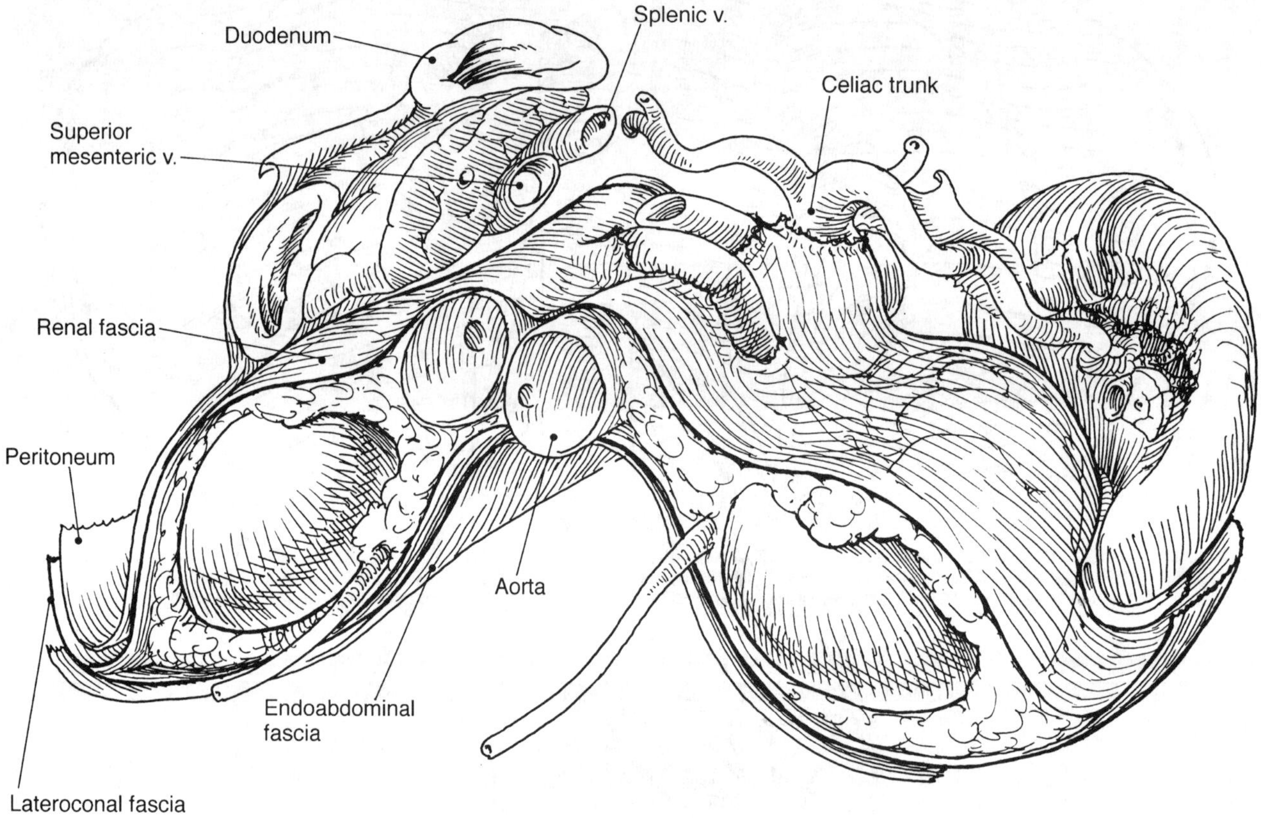

Fig. 8.14

Only the upper pole of the right kidney and the lower part of the right adrenal are covered simply by the renal fascia and parietal peritoneum due to the fusion layers created by formation of the omental bursa and the rotation of the colon (Fig. 8.15). Thus the anterior pararenal space (between renal fascia and posterior peritoneum) on the right includes the head of the pancreas, the second and third portions of the duodenum, the hepatic flexure, and the root of the right side of the transverse mesocolon. On the left are the tail of the pancreas, the fourth portion of the duodenum, the splenic flexure and the root of the left side of the transverse mesocolon.

Access to the kidneys and adrenals is begun by reopening the fusion fascia planes of the right or left colon at the lateral peritoneal reflections (white line of Toldt). Once the pararenal space is entered, the renal fascia must be opened to enter the perirenal space.

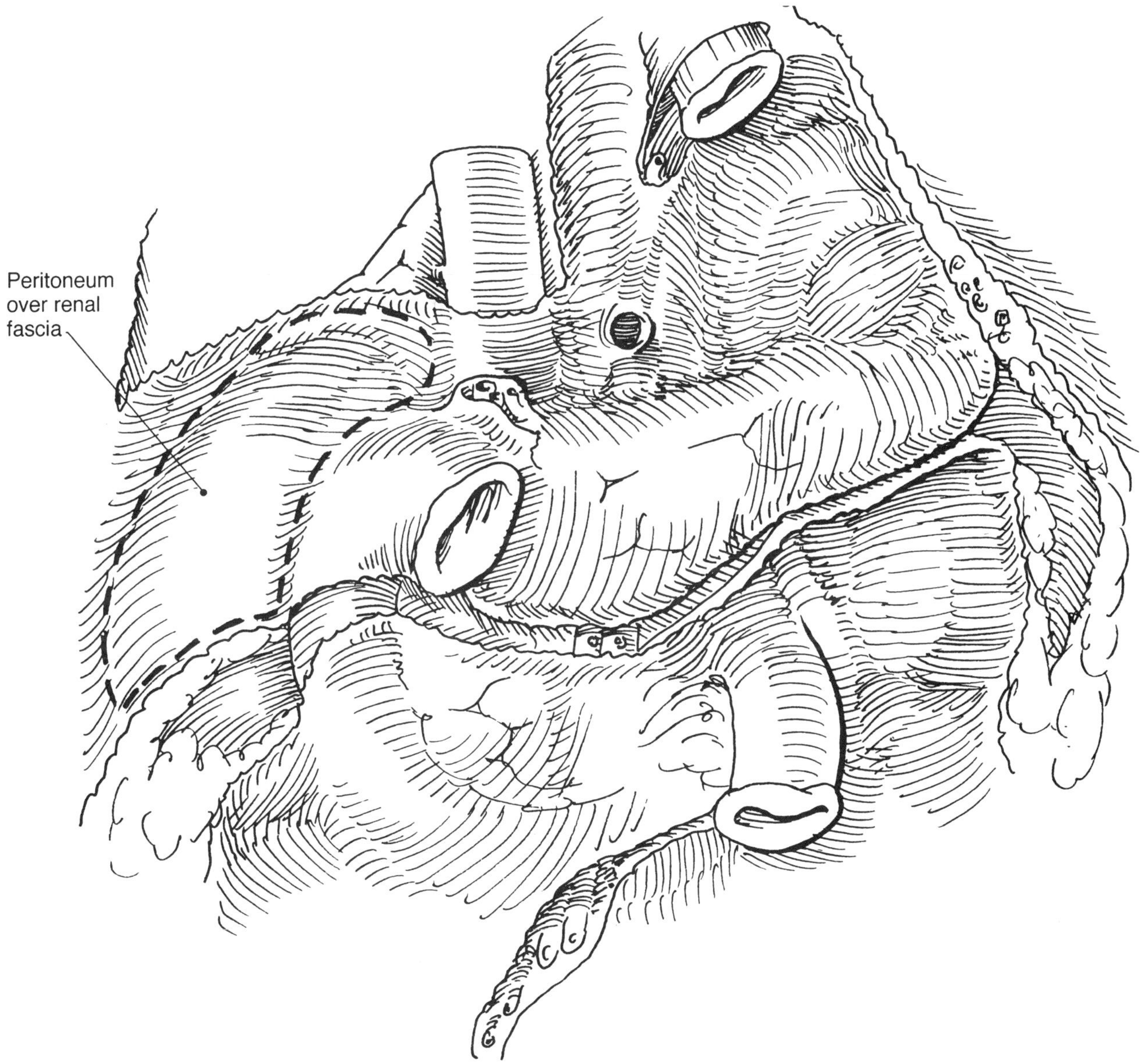

Fig. 8.15

The Kidneys

The kidneys rest in the paravertebral gutters at a level between the upper border of the 12th thoracic vertebral body above and the third lumbar vertebra below (Fig. 8.16). The right kidney is displaced slightly more caudally than the left by the bulk of the liver. The upper poles of the kidneys are adjacent to the crura of the diaphragm on their medial side and lie over the origins of the diaphragm from the lumbocostal arches. Below the lumbocostal arches, the lower portions of the kidneys lie on the psoas muscles medially and the quadratus lumborum muscles laterally.

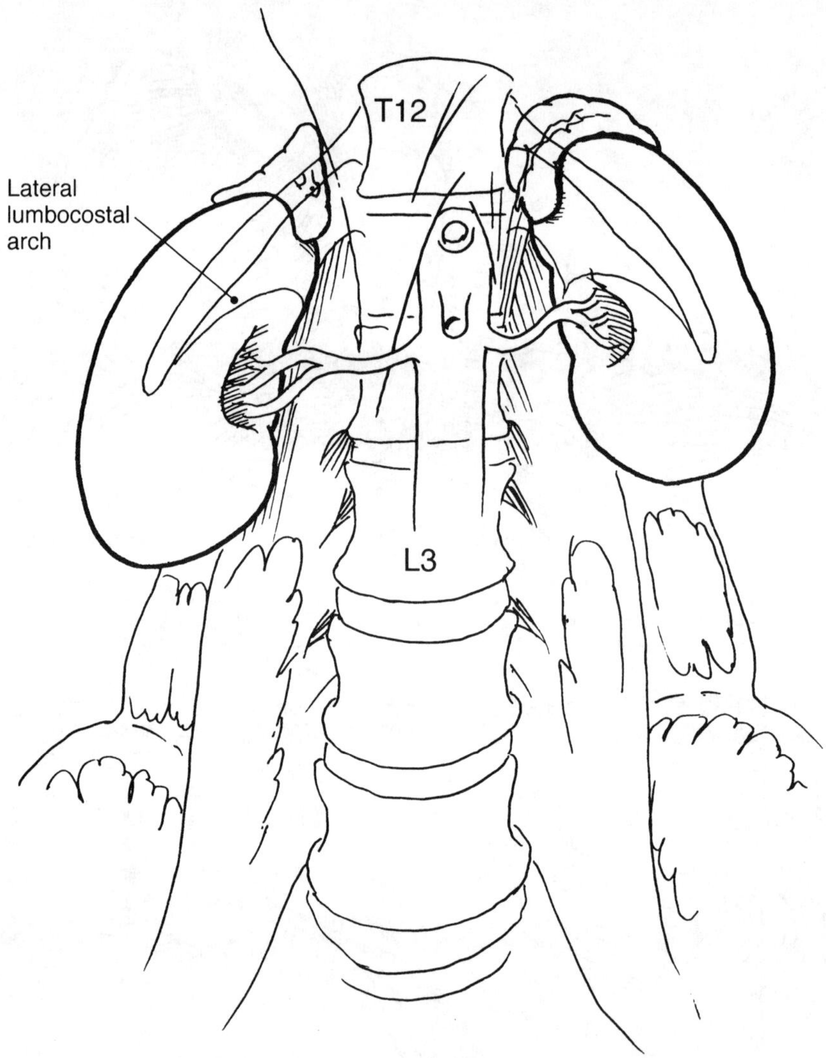

Fig. 8.16

The posterior pleural reflections lie in the diaphragmatic sulcus behind the upper poles of the kidneys (Fig. 8.17). There is some movement of the kidneys possible within the renal fascial envelope independent of the adrenal glands, which are fixed. Excessive descent in the upright position is called ptosis and must be distinguished from an ectopic location due to arrested ascent in the embryo.

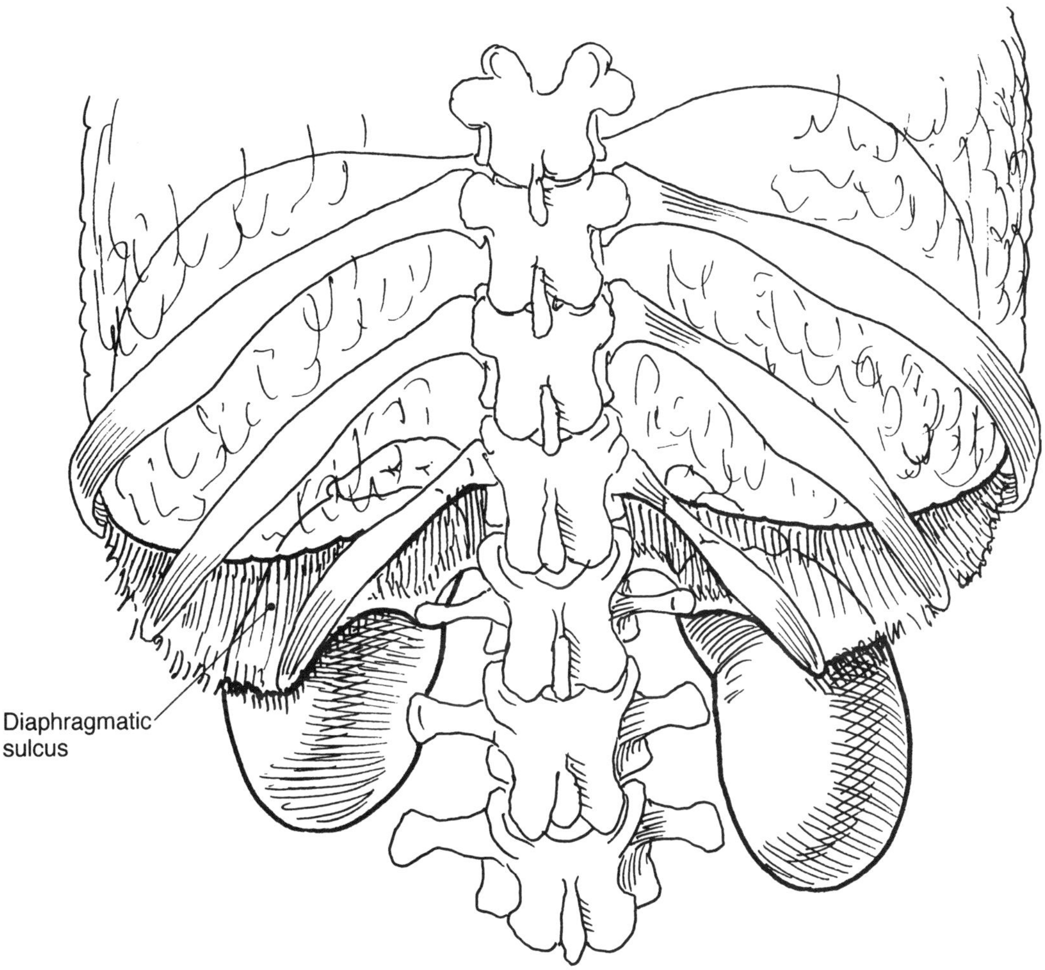

Fig. 8.17

In the frontal plane, the lower poles of the kidneys are slightly more lateral than the upper poles due to the shape of the psoas muscles medially (Fig. 8.18A). In the sagittal plane, the lower poles are slightly more anterior (10°) due to the curve of the lower posterior ribs and the psoas muscles posteromedially (Fig. 8.18B). In cross section, the axis between the hilum and the lateral margin of the kidney is about 30° above the horizontal, due to the slope of the paravertebral gutter (Fig. 8.19).

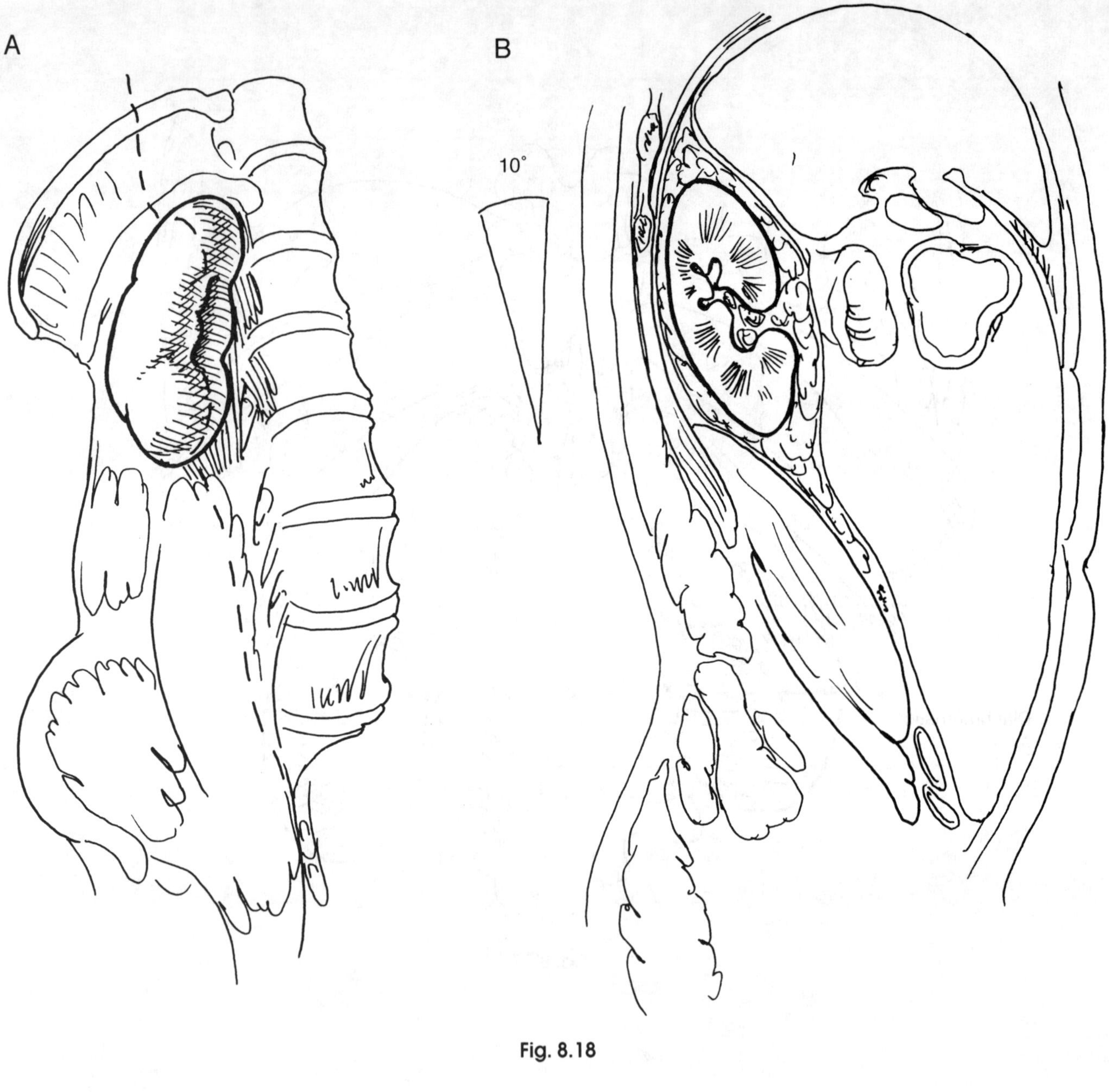

Fig. 8.18

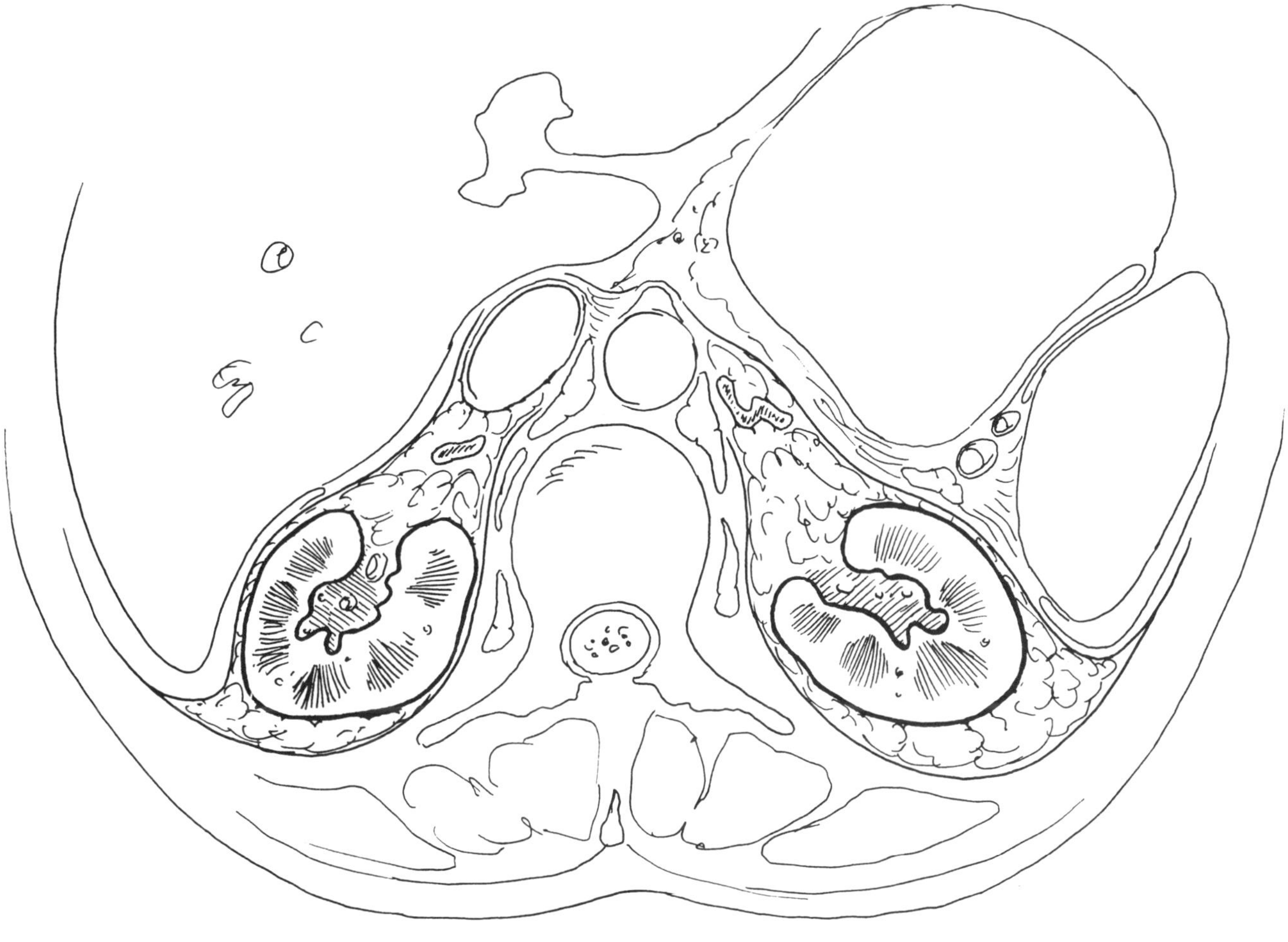

Fig. 8.19

Anteriorly, the kidneys are secondarily covered during embryologic life by the duodenum, pancreas, and spleen in the formation of the omental bursa, and by the colon in the course of its rotation (Fig. 8.20). Viewed from a caudal, laparoscopic perspective (Fig. 8.21A), the kidneys lie in the paravertebral gutters with the great vessels elevated on the ridge of the vertebral bodies. The renal vessels are draped on either side of the vertebrae in their course to the kidneys.

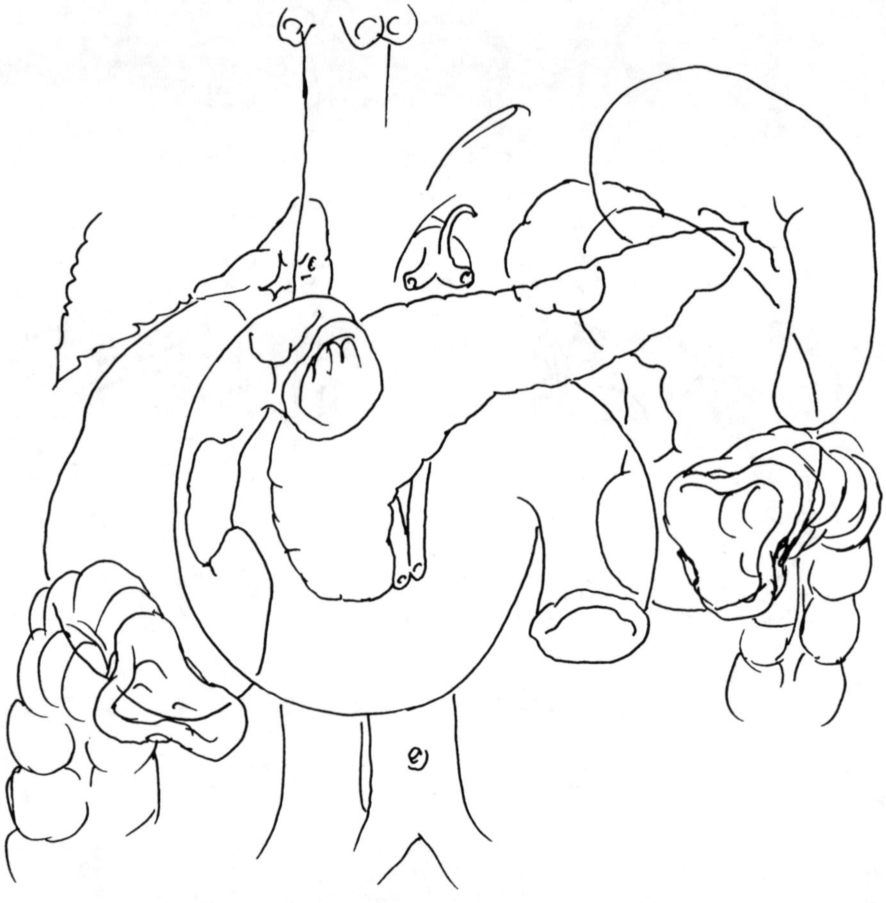

Fig. 8.20

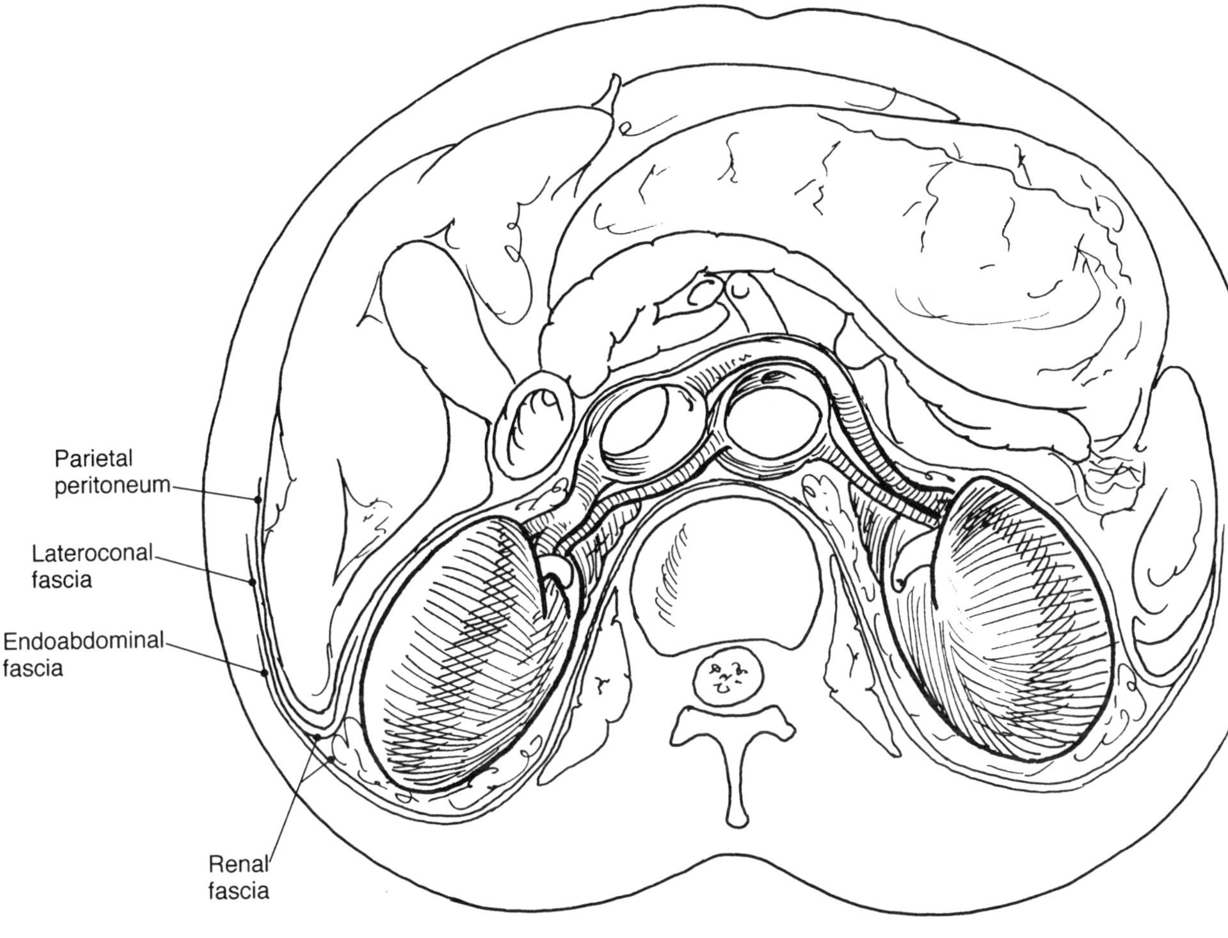
Parietal
peritoneum
Lateroconal
fascia
Endoabdominal
fascia
Renal
fascia

Fig. 8.21A

Viewed from behind (Figs. 8.21B, C), the impressions of the kidneys on the overlying organs is evident. The left kidney is nested behind the spleen, pancreas, stomach and splenic flexure. The right kidney creates an impression behind the liver, duodenum, pancreatic head and hepatic flexure. The upper pole of the right

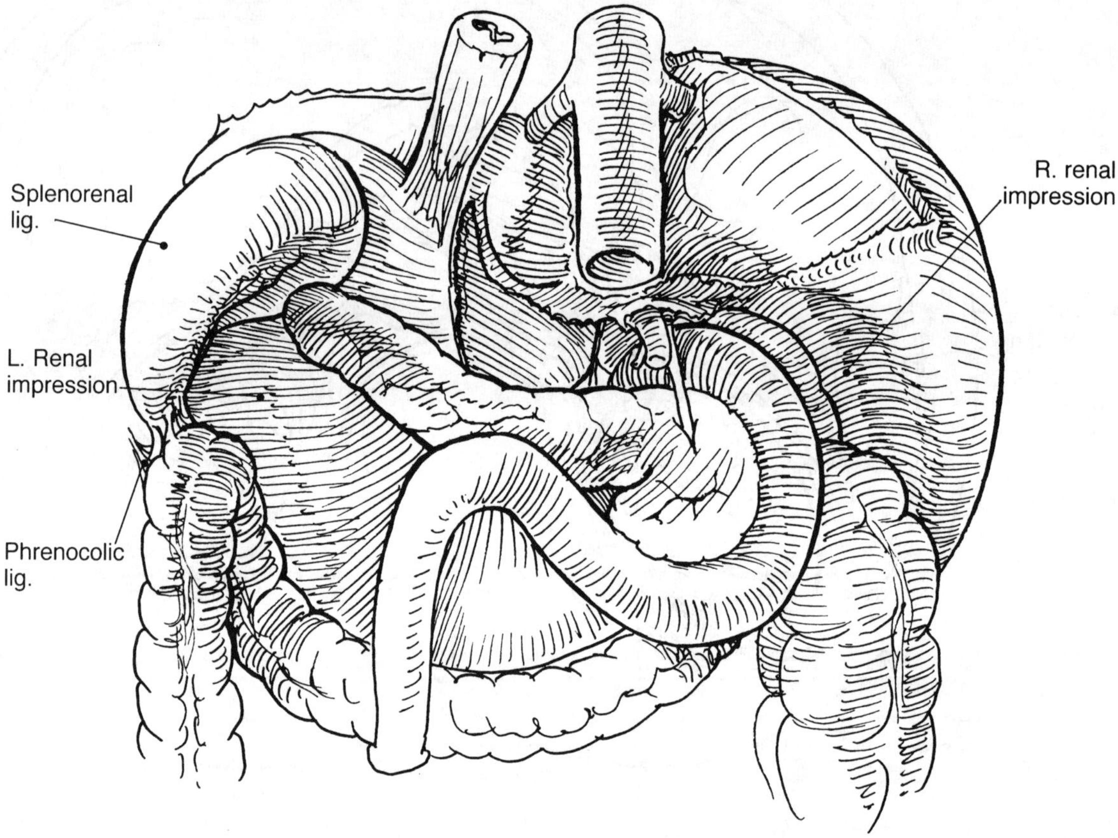

Fig. 8.21B

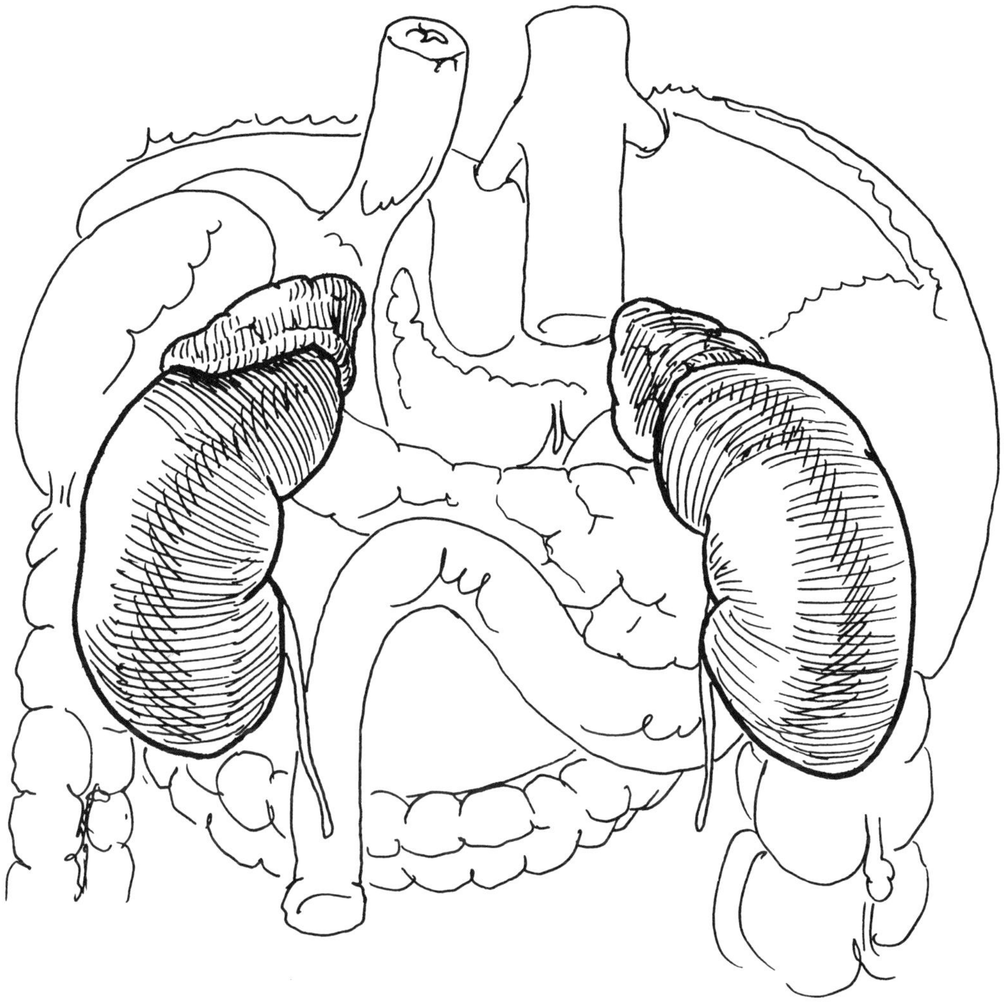

Fig. 8.21C

kidney is partially covered by the inferior margin of the coronary ligament (peritoneal reflection) of the liver (Fig. 8.22) (Chapter 2). This reflection is the deepest point of the hepatorenal recess (Morrison's pouch) between the undersurface of the right lobe of the liver and the anterior surface of the right kidney, where the kidney is most superficial in relation to the general peritoneal cavity.

The organs and peritoneal reflections over the kidneys place the upper pole of the left kidney and the left adrenal beneath the posterior wall of the omental bursa. The lower poles of the kidneys can be felt as bulges beneath the fused mesocolons of the flexures on either side. The spleen covers the cephalad anterolateral portion of the left kidney and the reflection of peritoneum between the two is called the splenorenal ligament (Chapter 5).

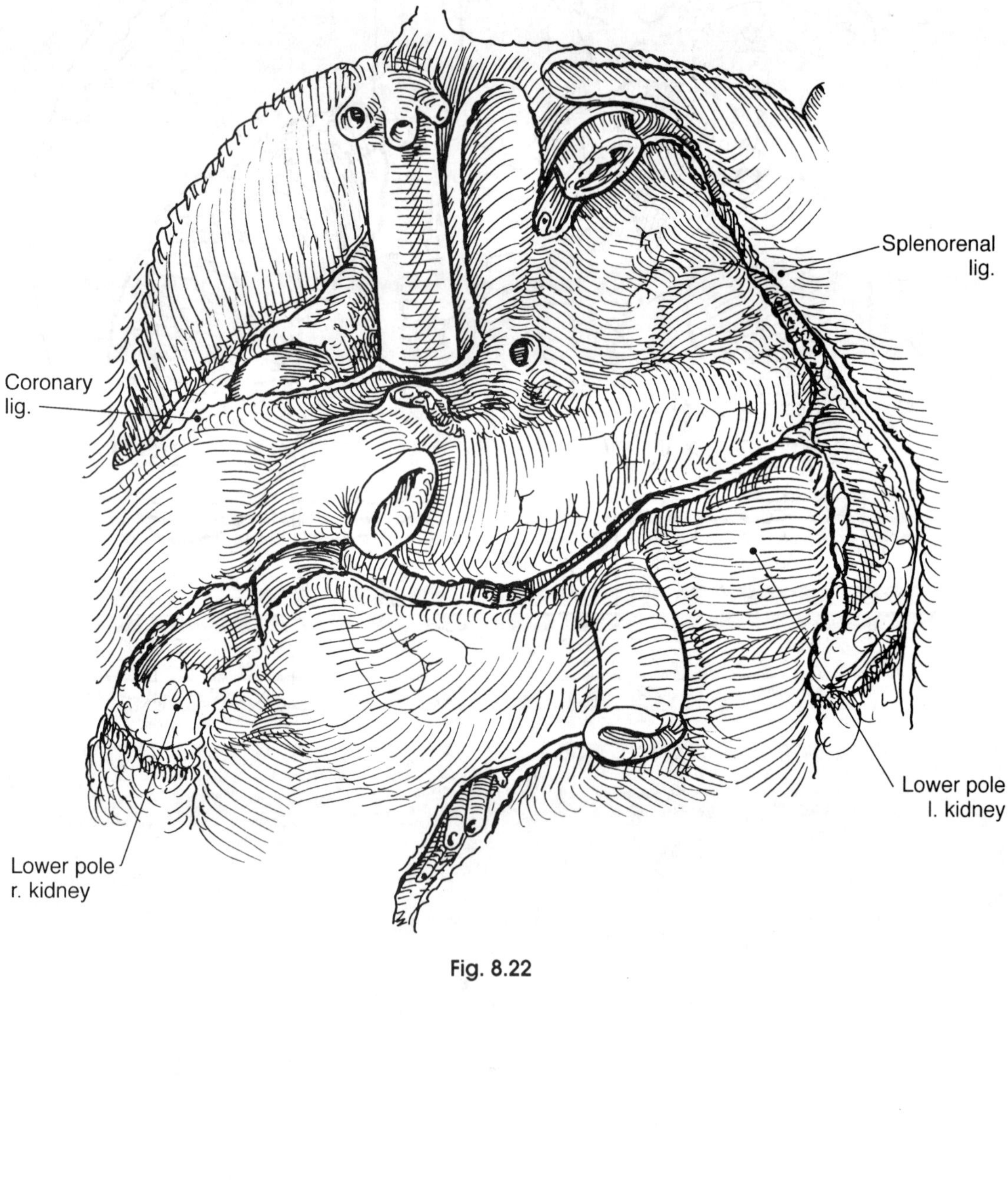

Fig. 8.22

The renal arteries arise from the lateral walls of the aorta slightly below the level of the L1–L2 disk, and the takeoff of the superior mesenteric artery (Fig. 8.23). The right renal artery is usually slightly more caudal and is longer than the left because of the aortic position to the left of the midline. It runs beneath the inferior vena cava where the first branch point is commonly found. Near the hilum of each kidney, the renal arteries divide into four or five branches which lie between the vein branches anteriorly and the renal pelvis posteriorly.

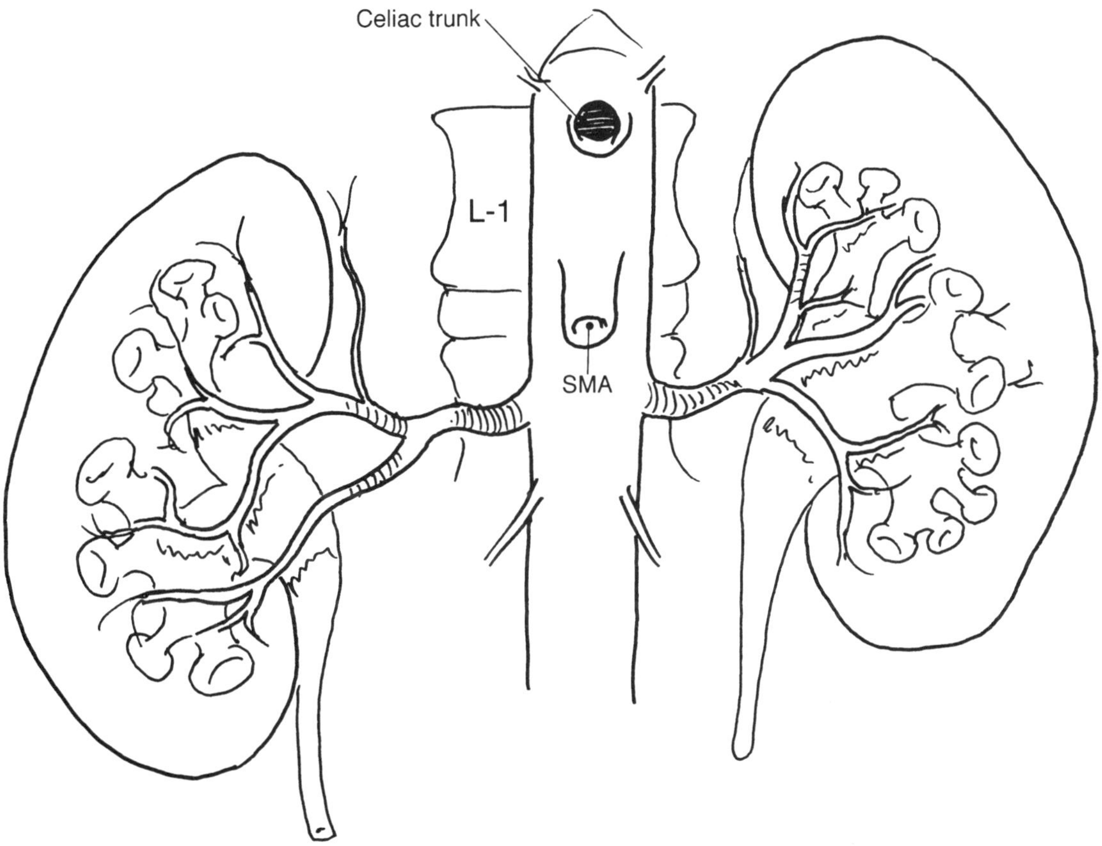

Fig. 8.23

Three quarters of individuals have a single renal artery on each side while accessory vessels are found in one quarter (Fig. 8.24). Accessory vessels may enter the hilum or may directly penetrate one of the renal poles. Accessory lower pole vessels most commonly enter the substance of the kidney directly from the aorta while upper pole branches usually arise from the main renal artery and also supply the adrenal. Accessory arteries can also come from gonadal and superior mesenteric arteries.

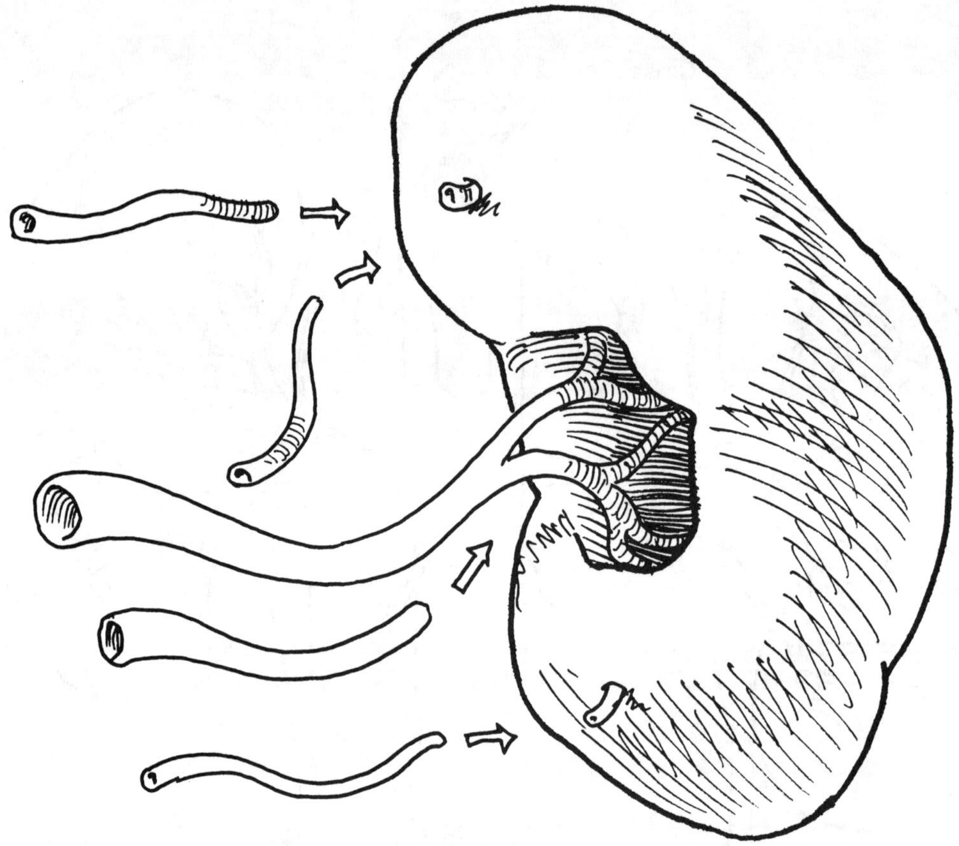

Fig. 8.24

The renal veins lie anterior to the arteries (Fig. 8.25). The longer left renal vein receives the left adrenal and gonadal veins. The left renal artery is most commonly found beneath the upper margin of the renal vein.

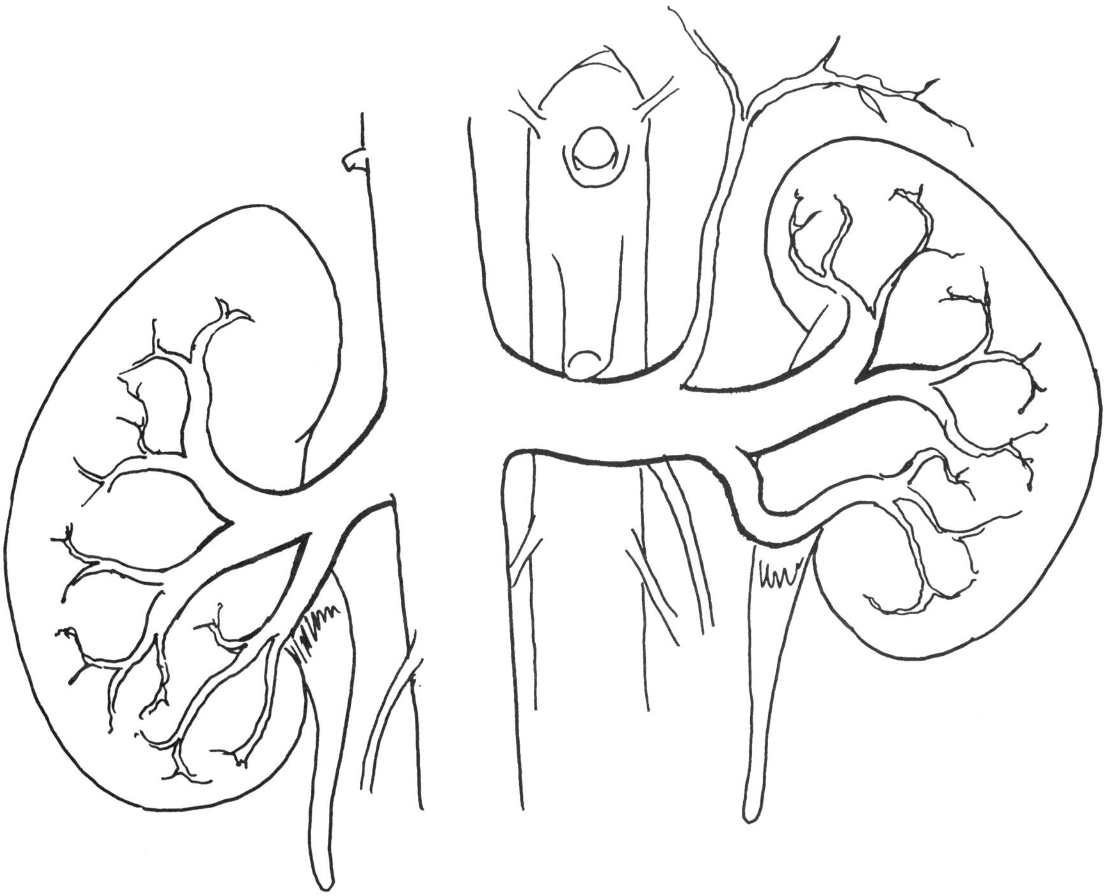

Fig. 8.25

Occasional persistence of posterior supracardinal anastomoses results in a circumaortic renal venous collar or posterior left renal vein (Fig. 8.26). Duplicated or left sided inferior vena cava is a rare finding (Fig. 8.9). Right renal vein duplication may also occur (Fig. 8.27). Both renal veins may anastomose with lumbar veins, posing the threat of bleeding if the renal veins are not isolated near the renal hila.

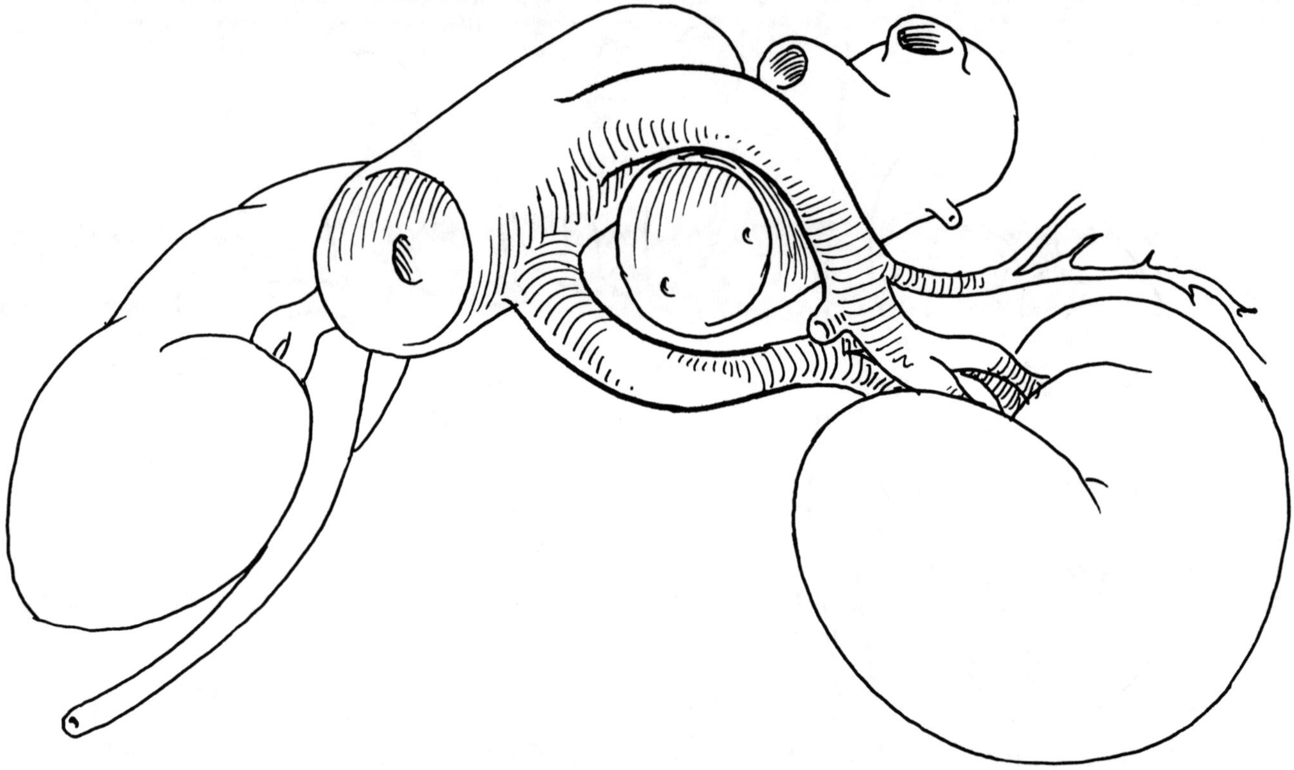

Fig. 8.26

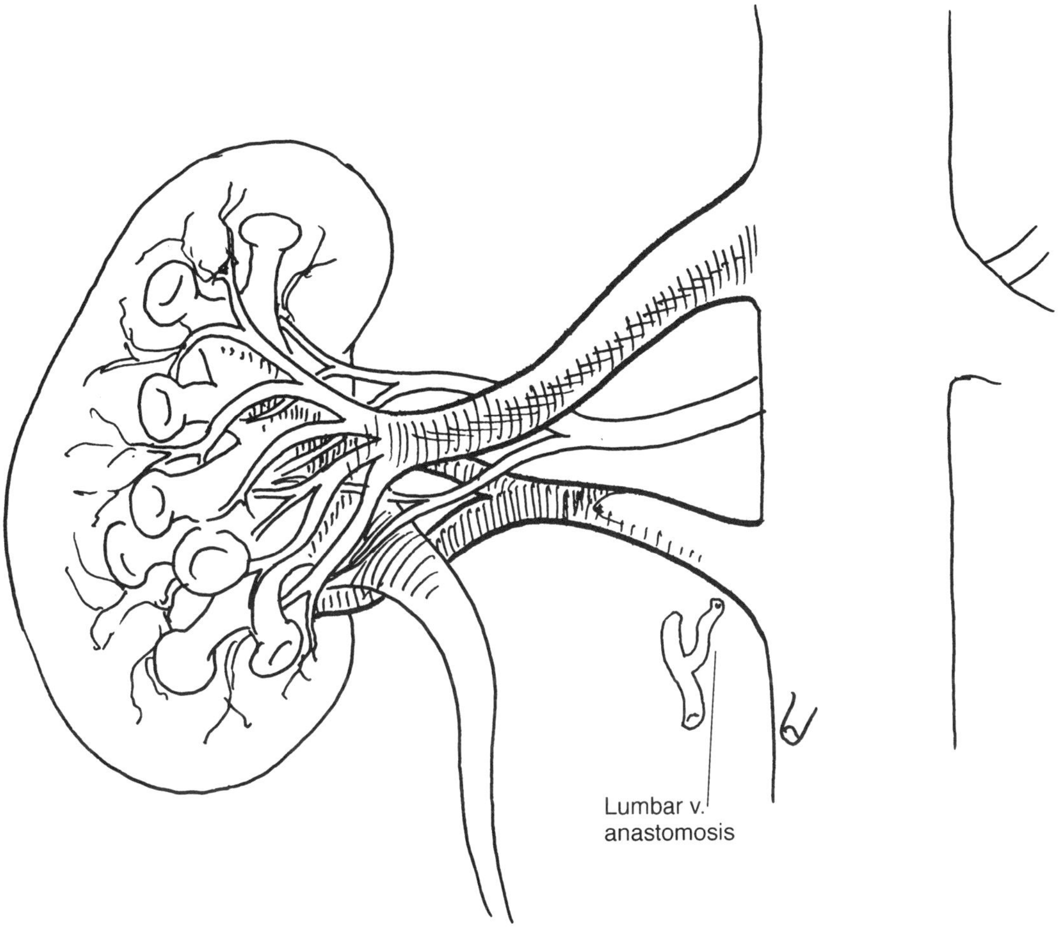

Fig. 8.27

The Ureters

The caudal extension of renal fascia tapers around the beginning of the ureters encased in perirenal fat at the ureteropelvic junction (Fig. 8.13). As the cone of surrounding fat disappears at the lower end of the funnels, the fascia continues as a sheath around the ureters (Fig. 8.28). The sheath is loosely adherent to the back side of the dorsal parietal peritoneum and preferentially stays with that surface when the retroperitoneal plane is dissected. It can be bluntly swept off that layer when the right or left mesocolon is mobilized for colon resection. Near the terminations of the ureters in the bladder, the ureteral sheaths are more prominent and fuse with a sheath (Waldeyer's) derived from the bladder muscle near the deep trigone.

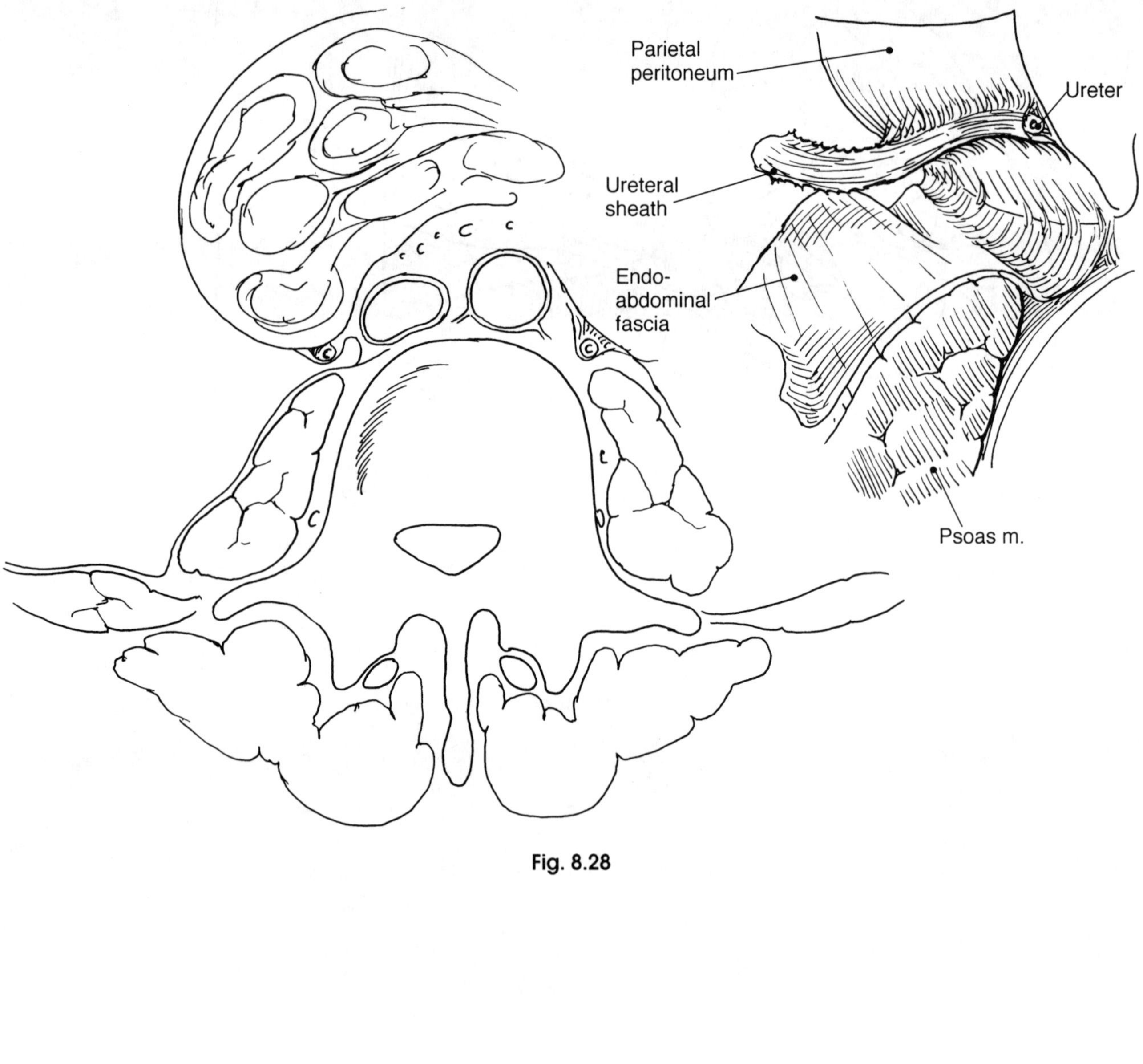

Fig. 8.28

The rich periureteral arterial plexus is supplied by regional vessels and makes the ureters resistant to devascularization when it is mobilized (Fig. 8.29). The proximal ureters receive branches mainly from the renal arteries above with contributions from the aorta and gonadal vessels. The distal ureters are primarily supplied by the vesical arteries with contributions from other internal iliac branches. The less well-vascularized central portions of the ureters receive branches from the aorta and common iliacs with some contributions from the gonadal and uterine arteries. These small arteries run in the subperitoneal plane and send penetrating branches through the ureteric sheath to ramify and interconnect along the course of the ureters. The delicate venous plexus parallels the arterial supply.

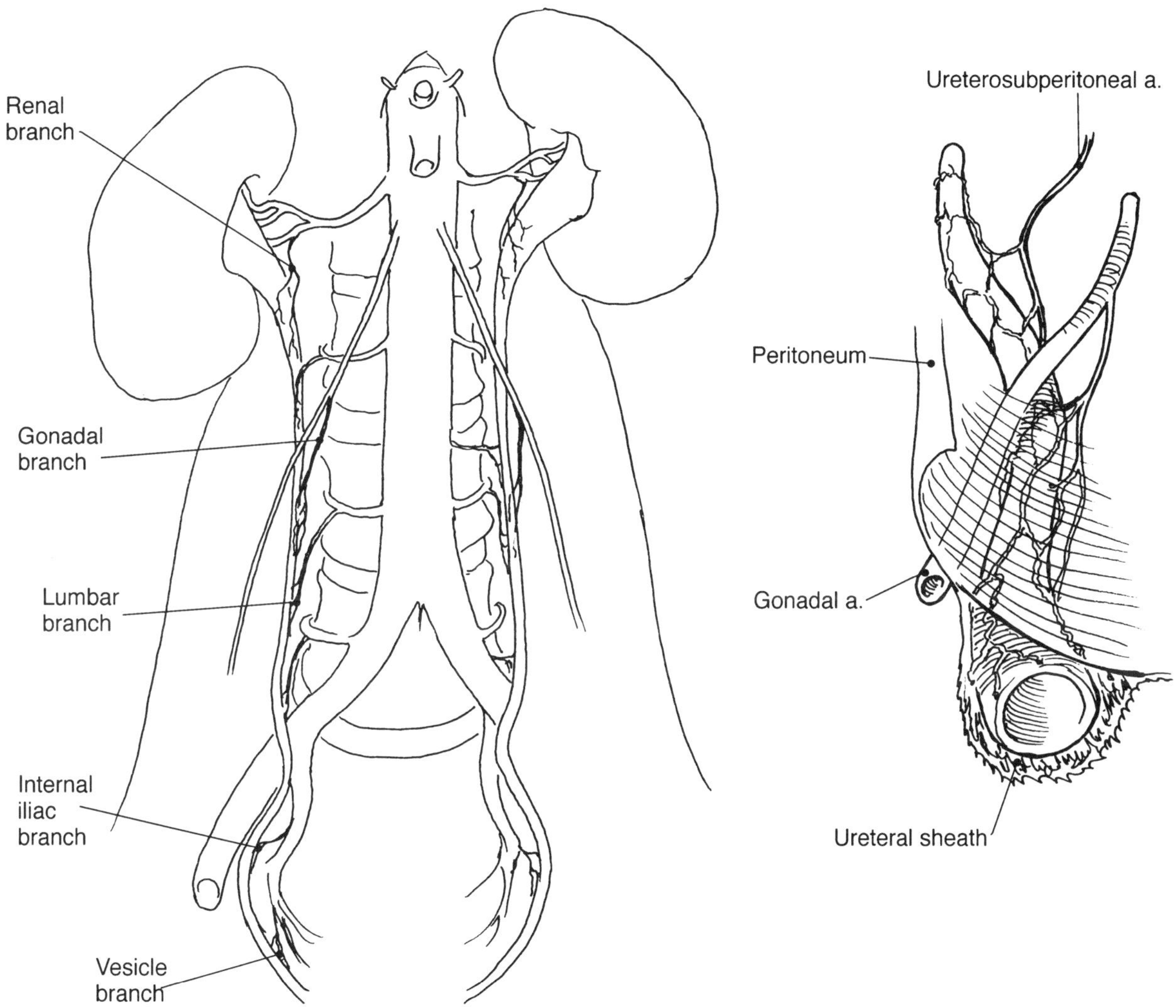

Fig. 8.29

In the lumbar region, the ureters lie on the anterior, paravertebral portions of the psoas muscles a few centimeters lateral to the aorta and vena cava on either side (Fig. 8.30). The colic vessels lie in the plane just anterior to the ureters representing the primitive right and left colonic mesenteries and their fusion fascias. The ureters are crossed anteriorly by the gonadal vessels in the upper part of their course and cross the genitofemoral nerves

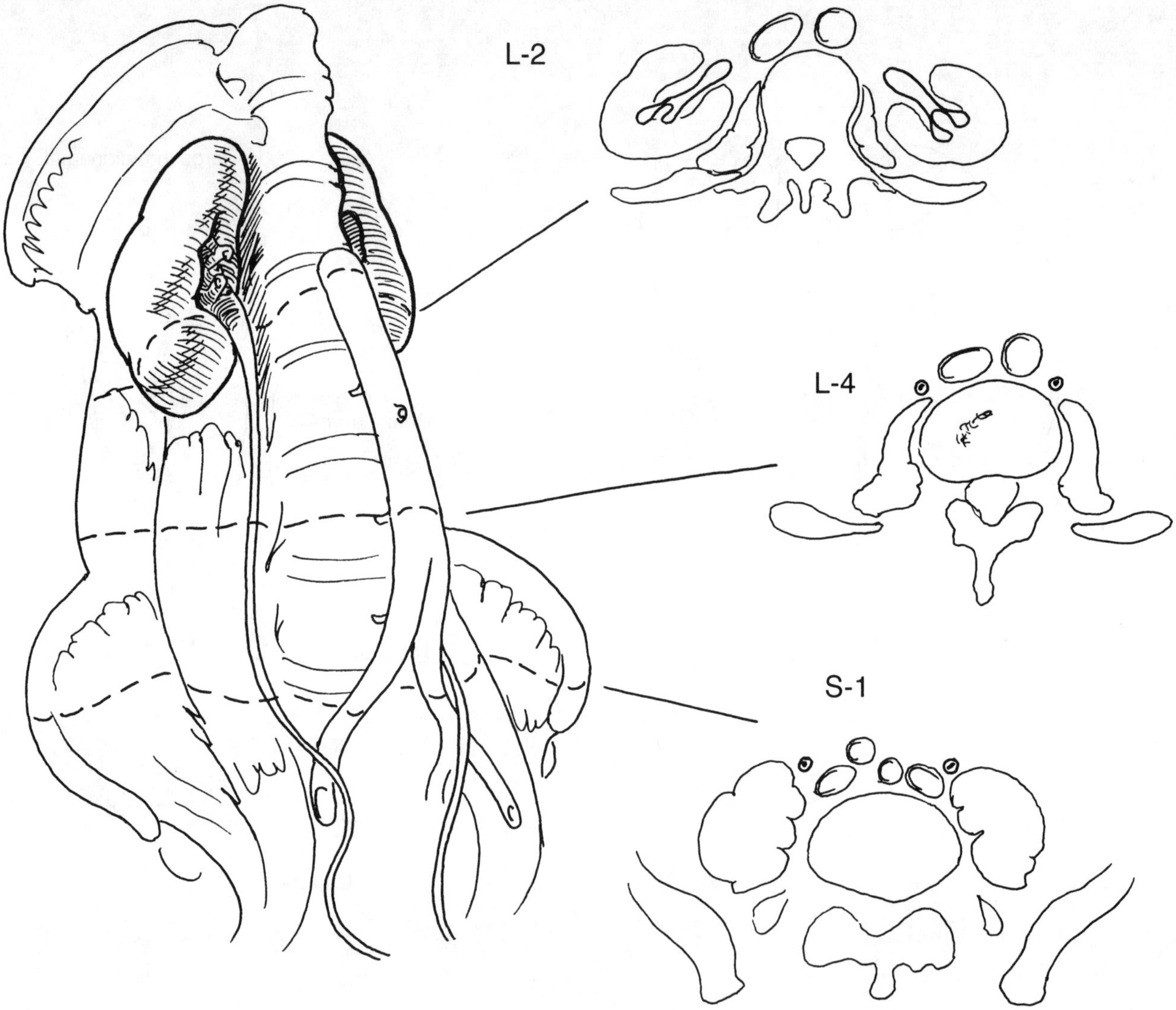

Fig. 8.30

as the latter emerge from the psoas below (Fig. 8.31). The ureters turn slightly medially as they cross the common iliac vessels at the level of the illiac bifurcation. The left ureter lies beneath the root of the sigmoid mesocolon at this level. In the female, the ovarian vessels cross the external iliacs as the infundibulopelvic ligaments just distal to the ureteric crossing. The ureters then turn outward in the subperitoneal plane over the internal iliac vessels to follow the contours of the true pelvis.

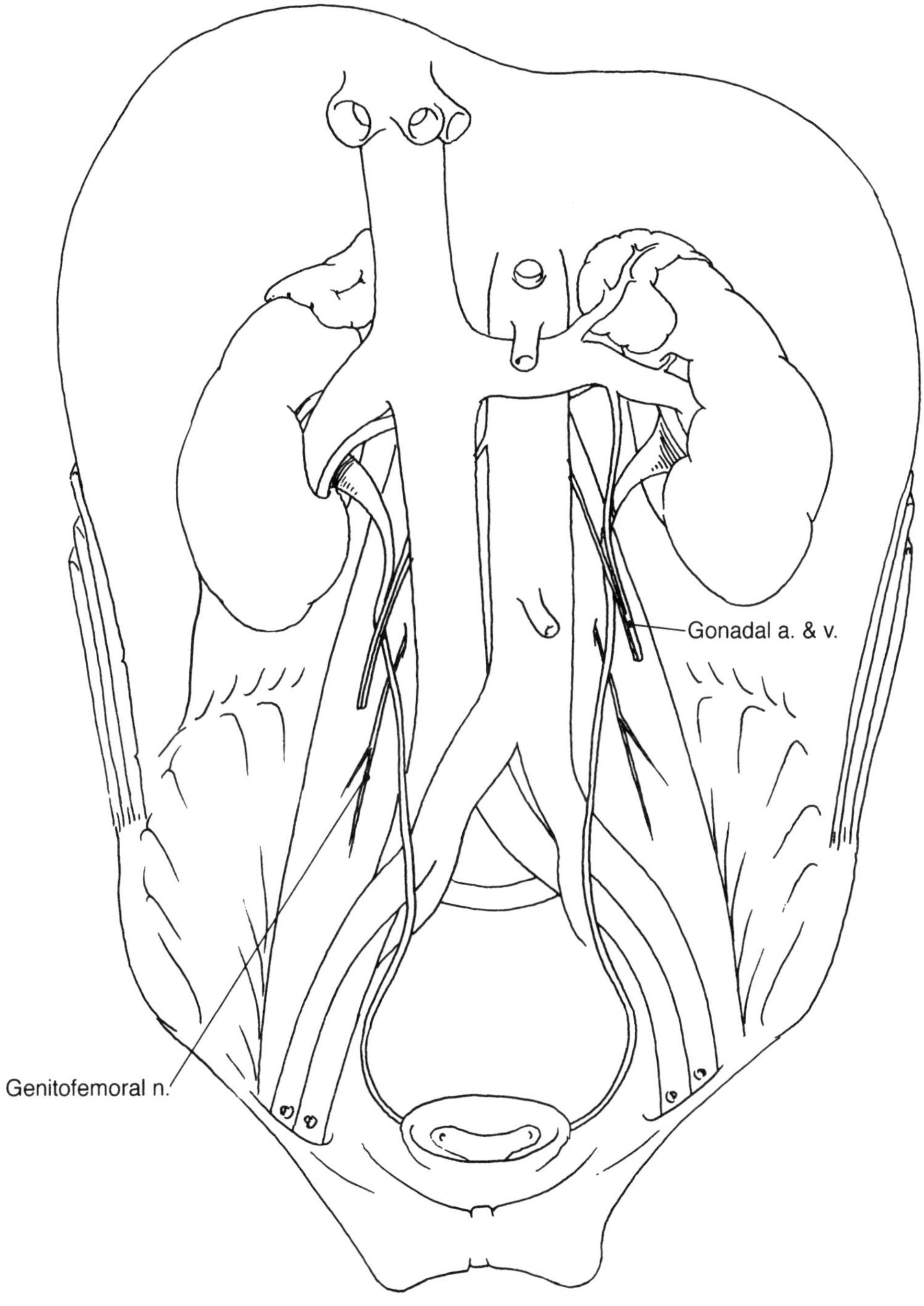

Fig. 8.31

In the male, the ureters pass between the internal iliac vessels and the ascending vas deferens (Fig. 8.32).They then turn anteriorly and pass along the levator ani (pelvic diaphragm), pass through the pelvic/perivesical plexus of veins and penetrate the base of the bladder in front of the upper part of the seminal vesical on each side.

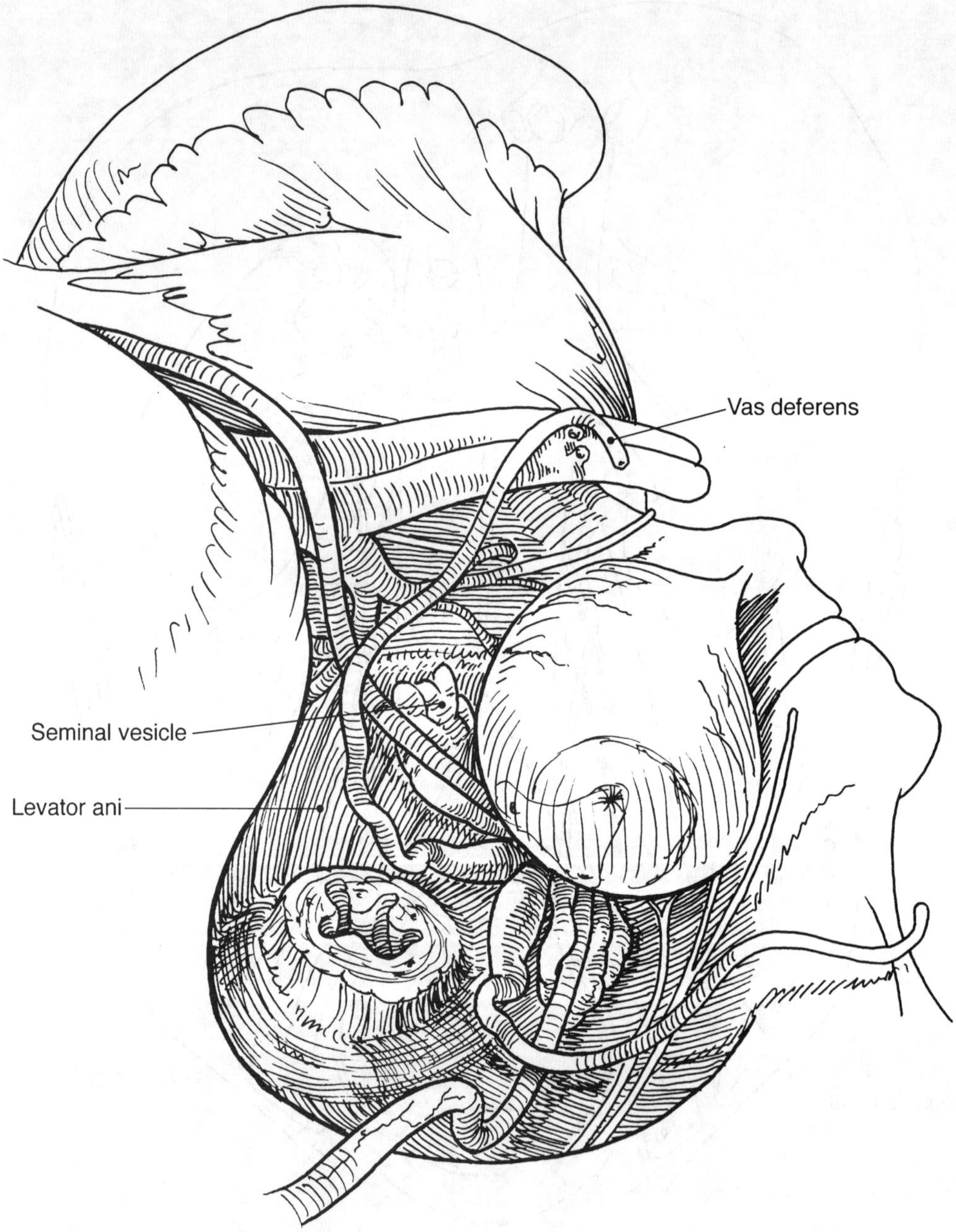

Fig. 8.32

In the female, the ureters cross the iliac bifurcation (Fig. 8.33) and form the posterior borders of the ovarian fossae (Chapter 7). At the pelvic floor, the ureters turn anteriorly on the levator muscles, passing through the uterosacral, cardinal and vesicouterine portions of the pelvic fascia (parametrium) at the base of the broad ligaments. Close to the uterine cervix, the ureters pass under the uterine arteries and through the uterovaginal and vesicovaginal venous plexuses and are vulnerable to injury during gynecologic operations. Limiting dissection to only the medial sides of the pelvic ureters preserves the lateral blood supply and protects the ureters.

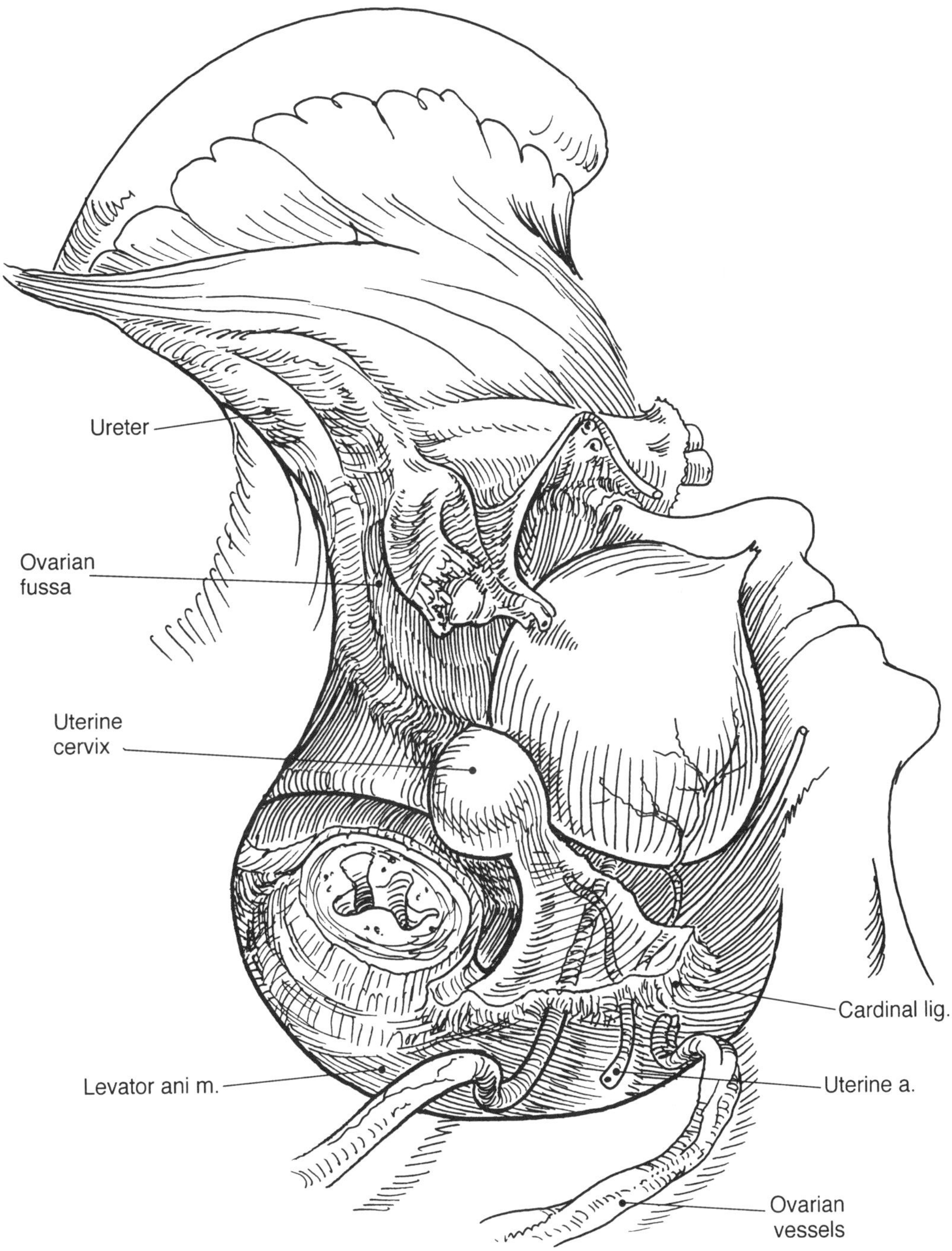

Fig. 8.33

The Adrenals

The adrenals are located at the upper poles of the kidneys encased in perirenal fat within the apex of perirenal fascia on either side (Fig. 8.34). The substance of the adrenal glands is delicate and fragile and easily damaged if handled directly. The adrenals are fixed in position compared with the kidneys, which have some mobility within the renal fascia. The right adrenal gland is shaped like a flattened pyramid with its concave base over the medial portion of the upper pole of the right kidney. Its anteromedial border is a concave trough which fits the back side of the inferior vena cava. The anterolateral surface fits against the underside of the right lobe of the liver (Chapter 2), and the posterior surface faces the diaphragm. The left adrenal gland takes the form of a crescentic leaf with its concave lower margin lying over the curve of the upper pole of the left kidney. It has a broad base medially and tapers laterally. The left adrenal gland lies beneath the posterior peritoneum of the omental bursa partially covered by the spleen laterally and the tail of the pancreas and pancreatic vessels inferiorly. A large tumor of the right gland displaces the upper pole of the right kidney laterally as well as downward, while on the left such a tumor displaces the kidney downward.

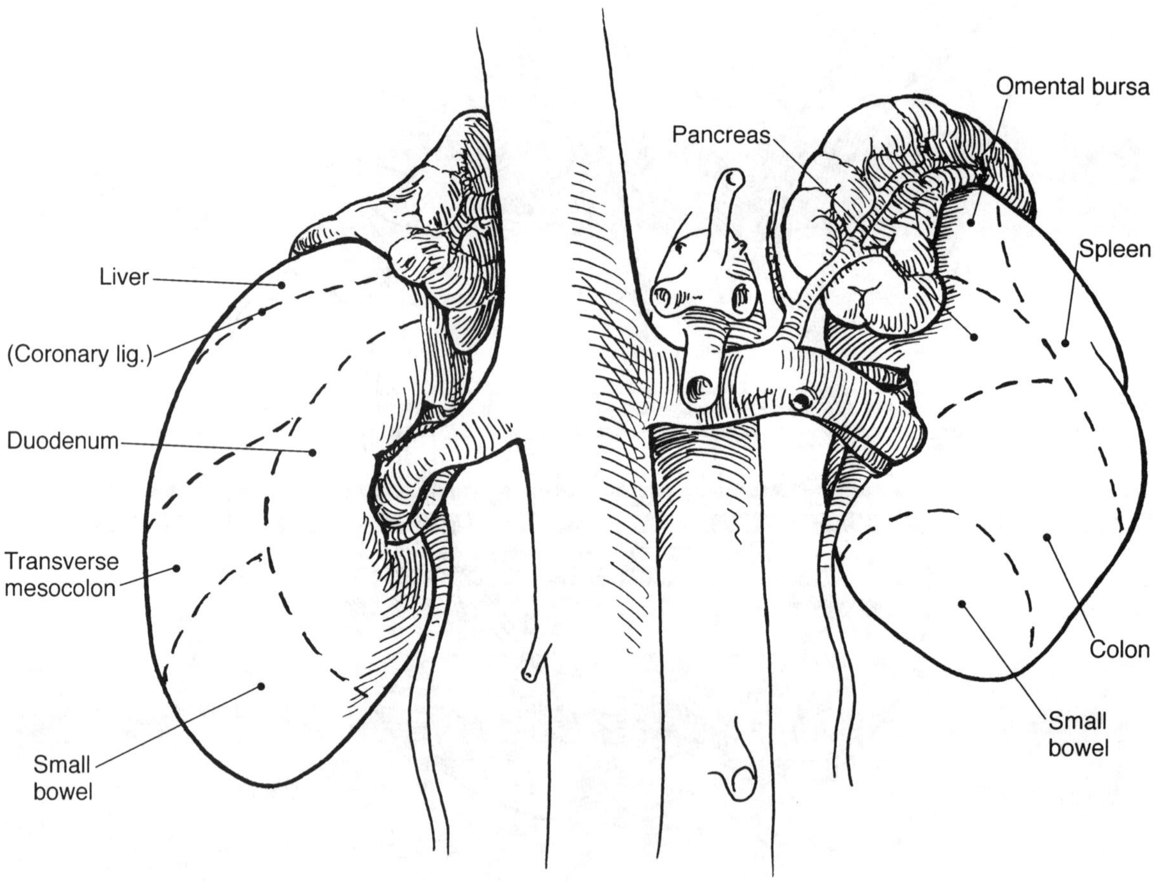

Fig. 8.34

In cross section, the anteromedial positions of the adrenals in the renal fascial envelopes can be seen (Fig. 8.35). The undersurfaces of the adrenals are separated from the kidneys by a layer of perinephric fat. The adrenals lie immediately adjacent to the crura of the diaphragm medially. The posterior gastric wall, separated by the cleft of the omental bursa, lies over the upper anterior surface of the left adrenal.

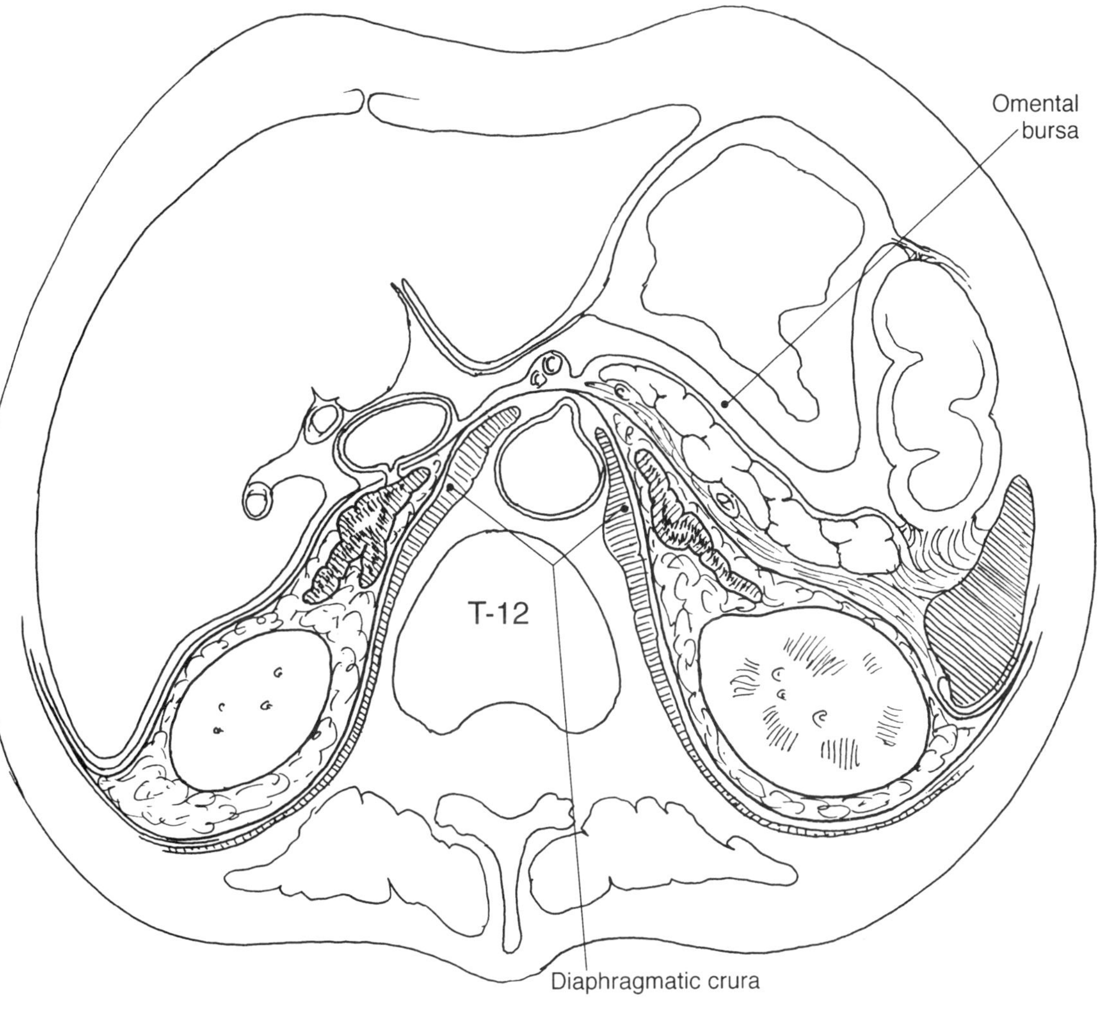

Fig. 8.35

The adrenal glands are supplied by multiple (as many as 60) small peripheral arterial branches arising from the inferior phrenic arteries, the aorta, and the renal arteries (Fig. 8.36). The adrenal gland is covered with a fine pericapsular venous plexus that drains on each side into a single central channel. The venus plexus also communicates via emissary veins with the renal capsular veins. This alternate outflow protects the adrenal from hemorrhage and allows outfolw of catecholamines even if the central vein is ligated. The right adrenal vein is short and empties directly into the posterolateral wall of the inferior vena cava. It may be joined by an accessory hepatic vein. An accessory vein from the lower pole of the gland may join the right renal vein or, rarely, the inferior vena cava. The left adrenal vein, the remnant of the cephalad portion of the left subcardinal vein, forms a linear channel in the long axis of the gland like the central vein of a leaf, and drains into the left renal vein. It often receives drainage from the inferior phrenic vein. The latter also drains across the anterior border of the esophageal hiatus (Chapter 4) toward the inferior vena cava at the caval hiatus. Variations of the left adrenal drainage are rare.

SURGERY

Nephrectomy

Laparoscopic nephrectomy is performed at selected centers for benign disease (e.g., renovascular hypertension, small nonfunctioning kidney, chronic infection) of the kidney at the present time. Although not the most commonly performed urologic laparoscopic procedure, nephrectomy is presented here as a good example of the applied regional anatomy. Its use in malignancy is very controversial due to issues of adequacy of margins, limitations of staging and fear about seeding of tumor cells.

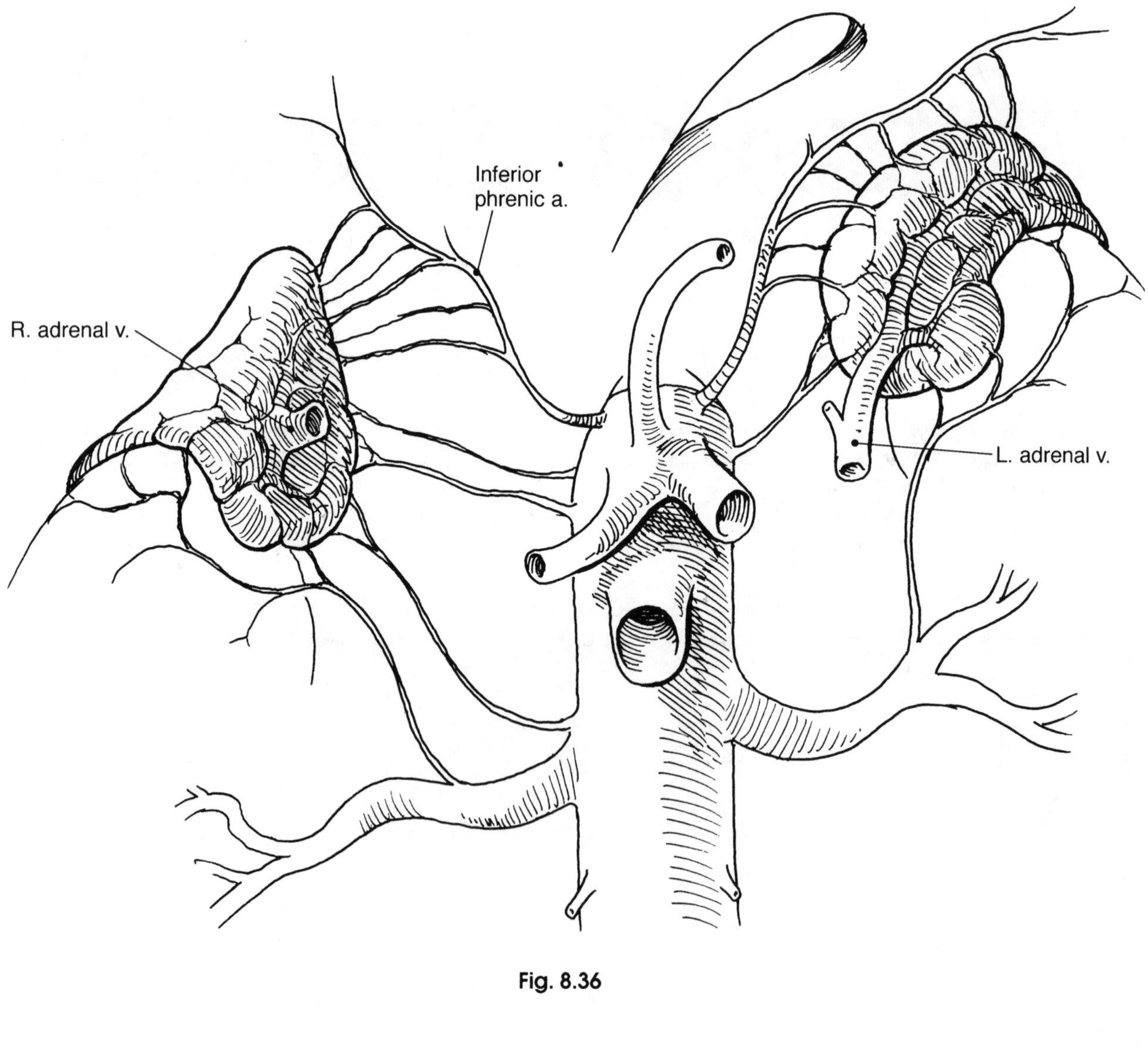

Fig. 8.36

The patient is given a bowel prep and perioperative antibiotics. Immediately prior to surgery a ureteral catheter is placed under fluoroscopy and its balloon tip inflated in the renal pelvis to aid in locating the ureter. The position of the balloon is marked on the skin to guide trochar placement. Foley catheter and nasogastric tubes are placed along with pneumatic compression stockings and the patient is positioned on the operating table.

The patient is initially placed supine on a deflatable beanbag with the arms extended and pneumoperitoneum is achieved. A large (11 or 12 mm) umbilical port is placed for the laparoscope followed by a large midclavicular subcostal and a small midclavicular port below the level of the umbilicus placed under direct vision. The patient is then secured in the lateral decubitus position with the beanbag, restraints and cushioning and two small upper and lower anterior axillary line ports are placed (Fig. 8.37). The surgeon stands in front of the patient with the assistant opposite and the camera operator below the surgeon. The surgeon works through the two midclavicular line ports and the assistant through the anterior axillary line ports.

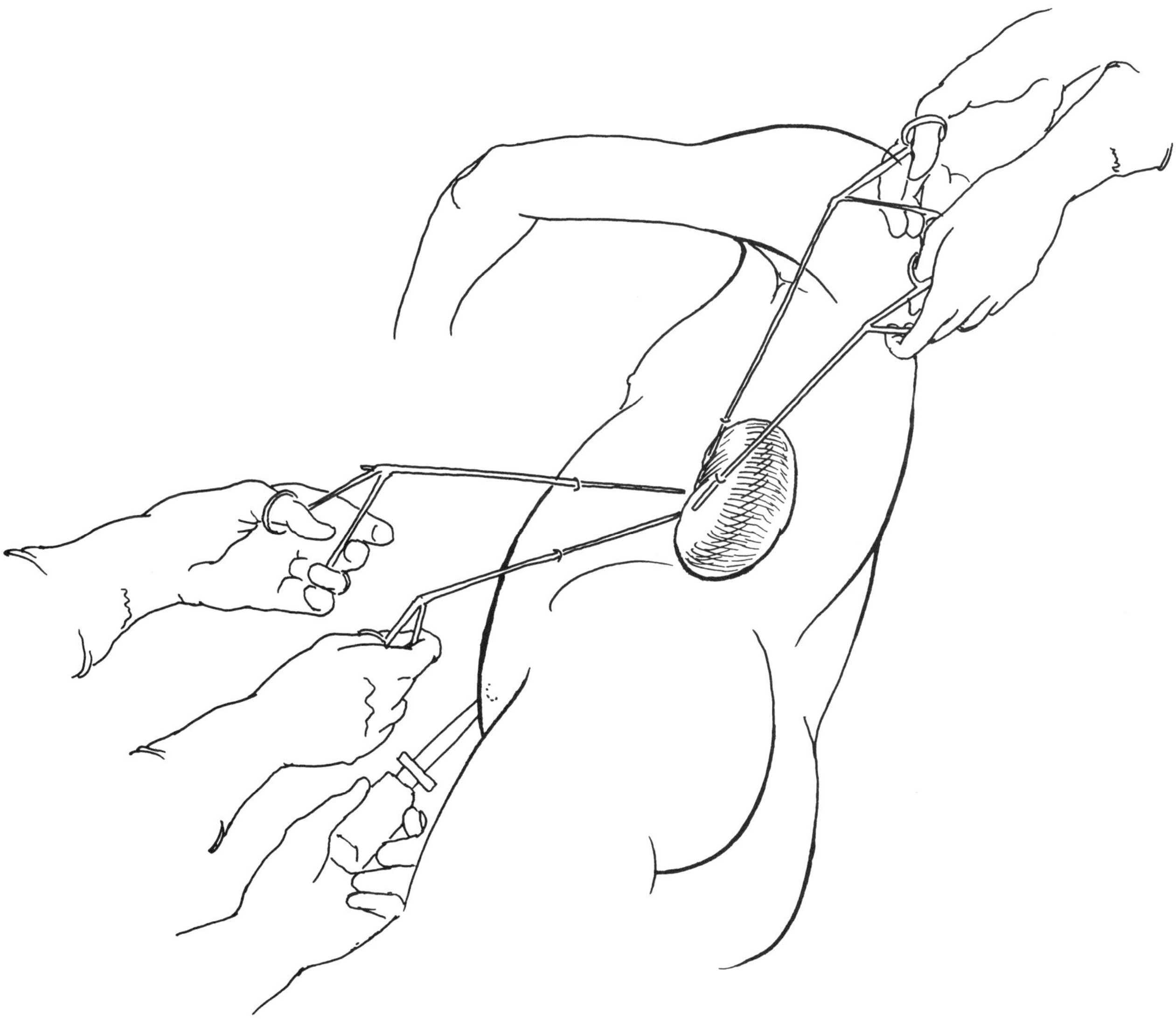

Fig. 8.37

The full length of the colonic peritoneal reflection is opened and the hepatic or splenic flexure is mobilized (Fig. 8.38A,B). The fusion fascia of the colon is opened as far medially as possible, exposing the renal fascia below it. On the right, the duodenum is elevated off the medial portion of the kidney. If the ureter is not evident below the kidney or at the level of the iliac bifurcation, it can be identified by manipulating the ureteral catheter.

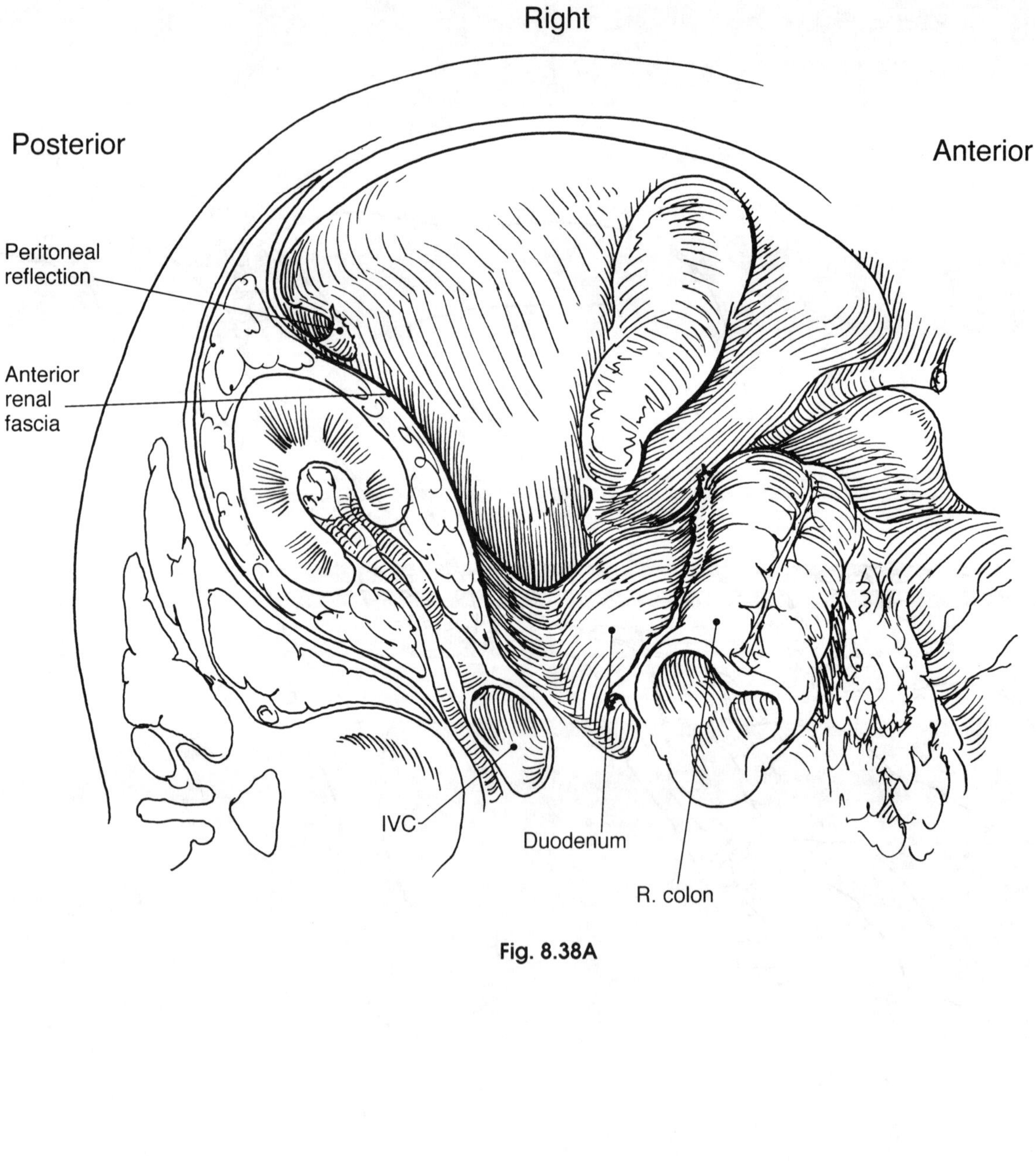

Fig. 8.38A

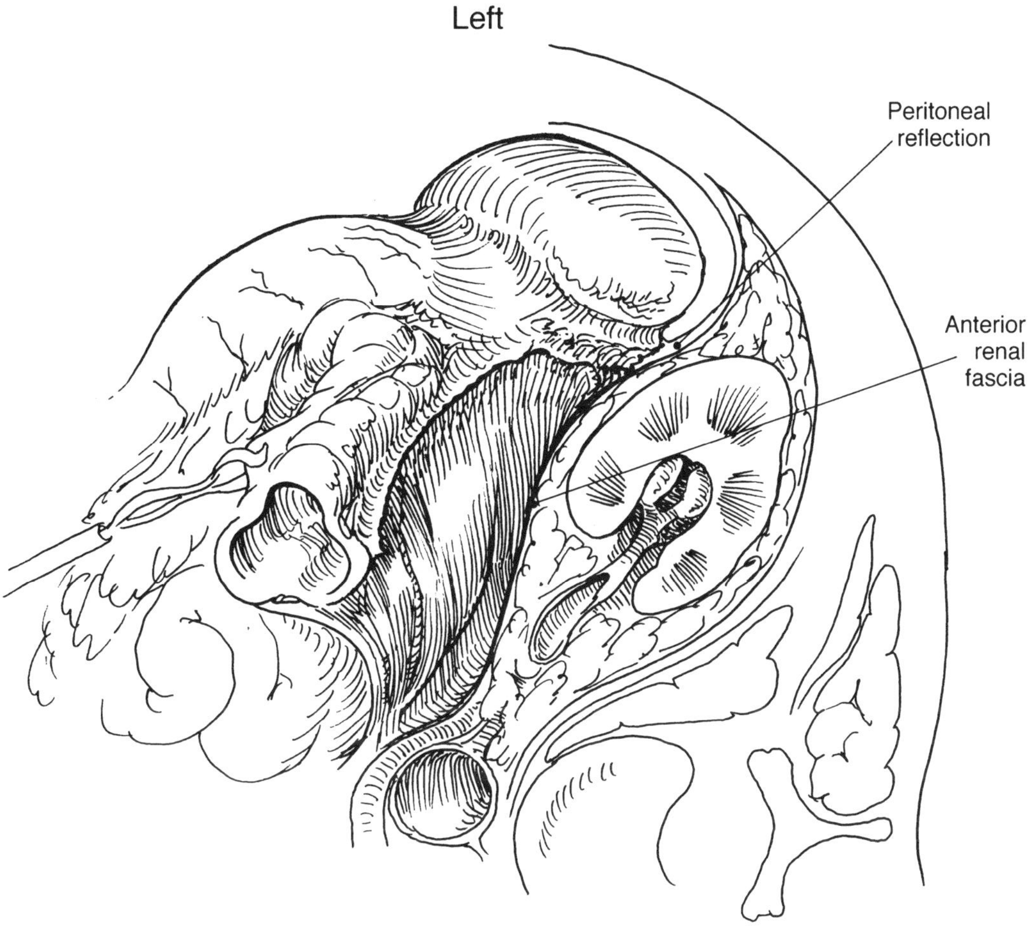

Fig. 8.38B

A segment of ureter is dissected free and retracted anterolaterally to guide dissection up to the renal pelvis (Fig. 8.39).

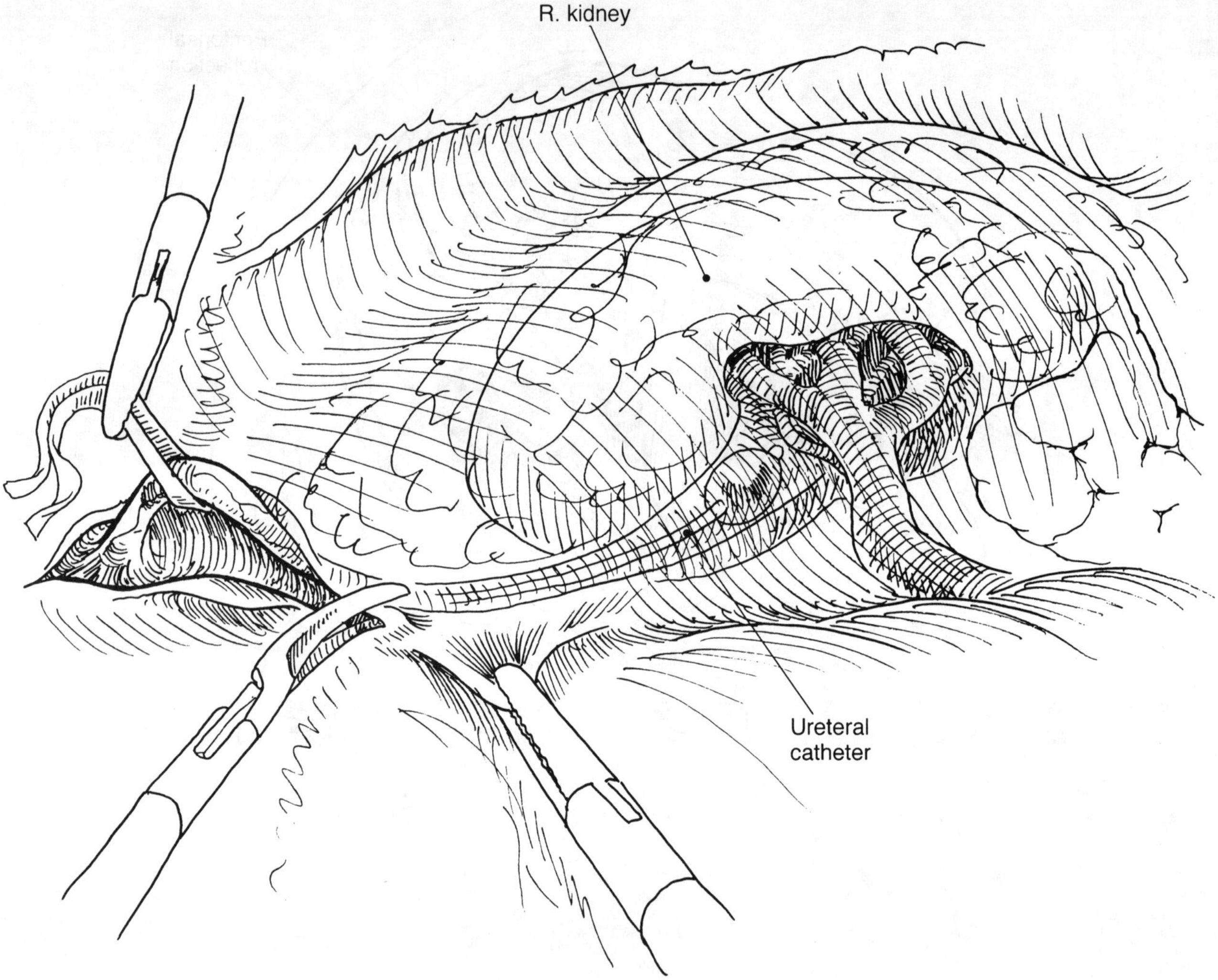

Fig. 8.39

The renal fascia over the lower pole of the kidney is opened, the lower pole is dissected free first, and dissection is continued around the margins of the kidney (Fig. 8.40). Once the kidney is mobilized, the assistant can

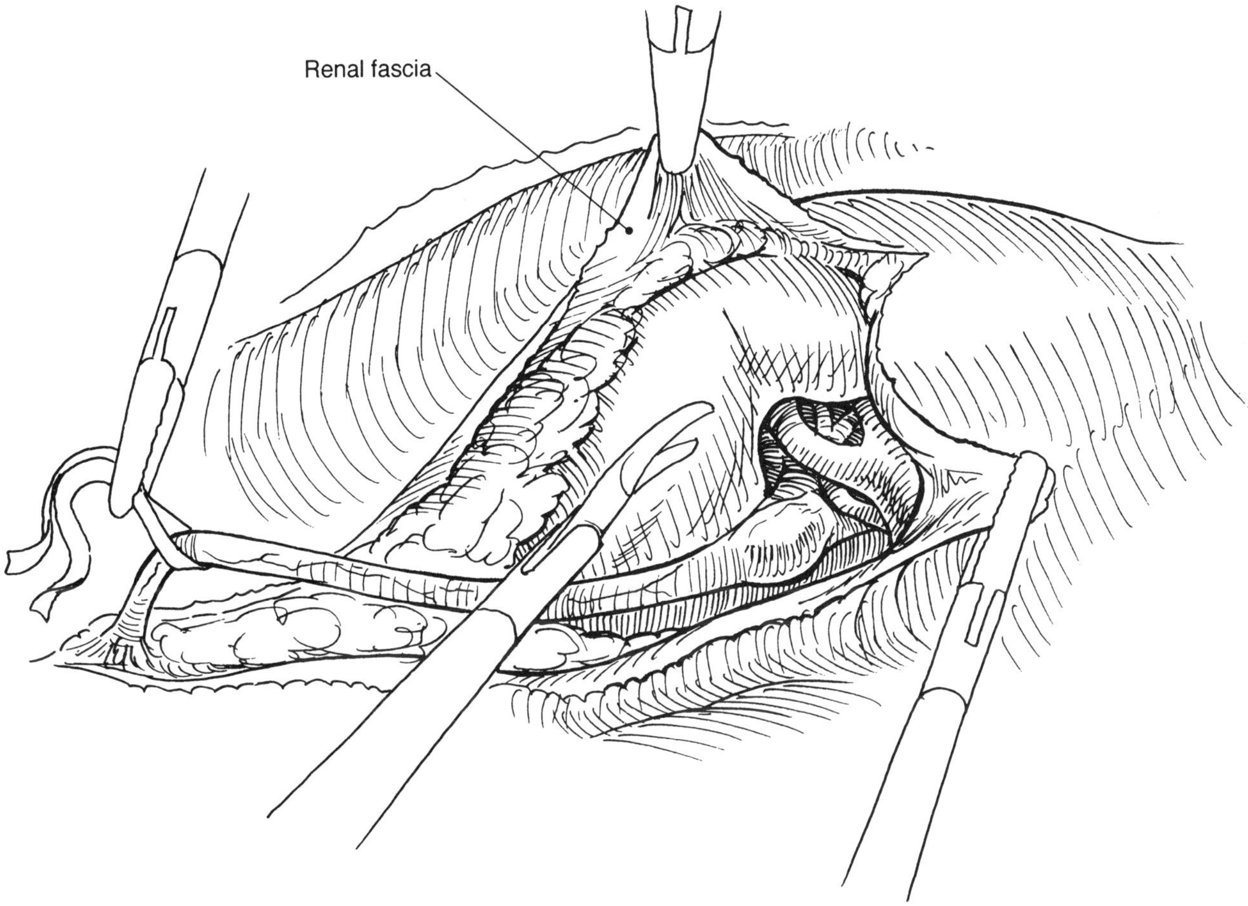

Fig. 8.40

apply lateral retraction to both poles, opening up the area of the hilar vessels (Fig. 8.41). Careful dissection of the perihilar fat exposes the renal vein and its branches. The main renal vein is mobilized to expose the renal artery.

On the right, the artery may already have bifurcated behind the inferior vena cava. On the left, the artery is most often found deep to the upper margin of the vein. The artery is secured first with two or three 9mm clips proximally and two distally and divided. An additional loop ligature is not an unreasonable precaution. Failure of the renal vein to deflate after arterial transection may indicate the presence of an additional artery that has not been exposed. A linear vascular stapler may also be used to individually secure and divide the renal vessels. Mass transection may result in a major arterio-venous fistula in the high flow renal vessels.

Once the arteries have been divided, clips are applied to the vein. On the left, the adrenal and gonadal veins and any lumbar venous branch are divided first followed by the main renal vein. A wide vein may be secured by alternating clips from opposite sides, by stapling or by clipping smaller distal branches individually. Dissection is carefully completed on the medial side of the kidney, watching for accessory vessels.

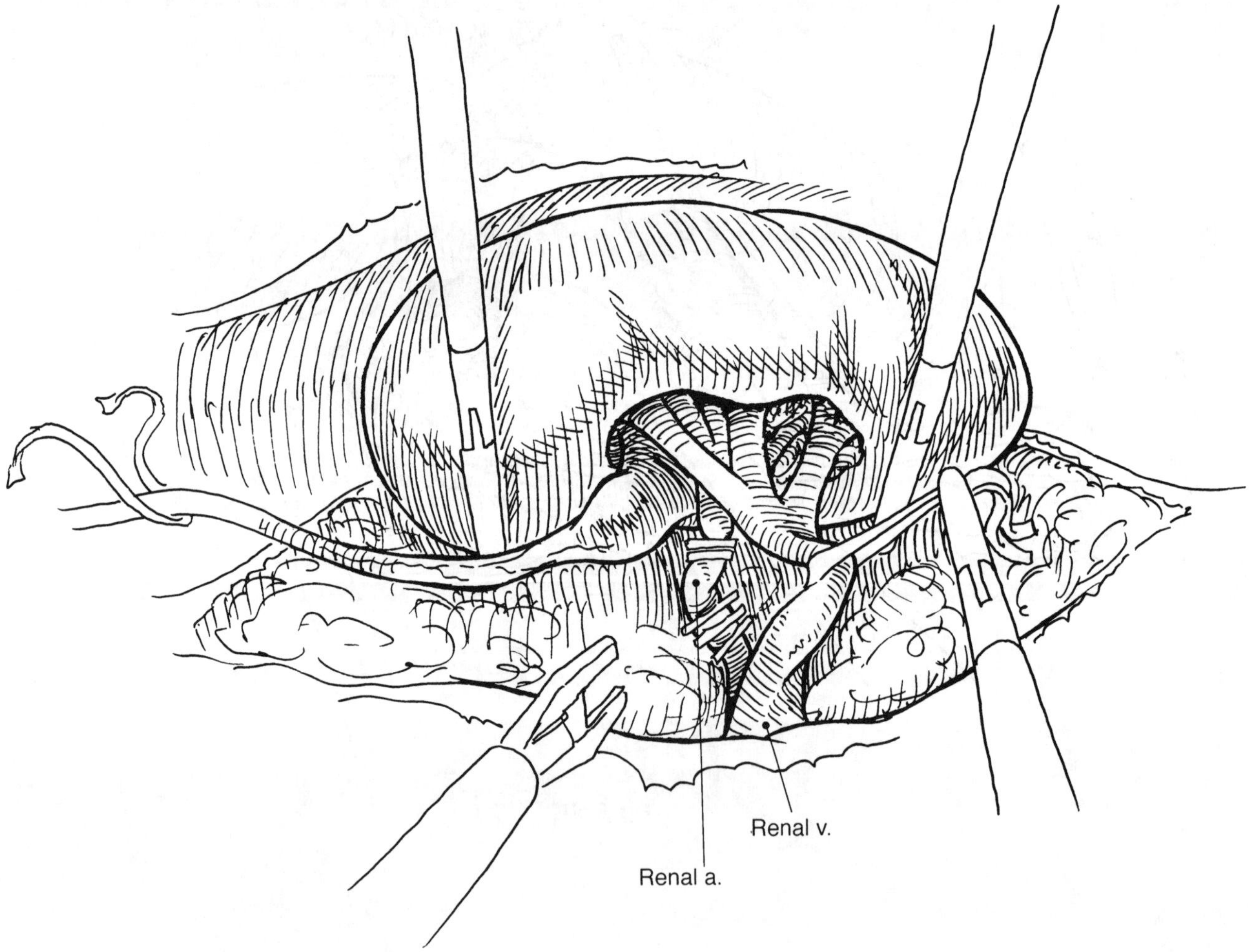

Fig. 8.41

After the kidney is completely free, the ureteral catheter is removed and the ureter is clipped and transected (Fig. 8.42). The ureter is used as a handle to place the kidney above the liver or spleen while a sturdy sac is inserted through the large upper midclavicular line port. The kidney is placed in the sac, and the drawstring is tightened. The laparoscope is changed to the large midclavicular line port, and the neck of the sac is pulled into the umbilical port. The patient is turned back to the supine position, and the umbilical trochar is removed exposing the sac at the abdominal wall. The sac is opened and held firmly up against the abdominal wall while the morcellator is introduced and pressed up against the kidney. The kidney is morcellated under direct observation until it is fully evacuated and the sac can be withdrawn through the port site.

The procedure is completed with the standard steps for exiting the abdomen.

Adrenalectomy

Small to medium (~10 cm or less) benign (incidental tumors, functioning or non-functioning cortical adenomas) adrenal tumors are the optimal candidates for laparoscopic adrenalectomy at the present time. Larger tumors have an increased probability of being malignant, and adrenal tumors, like the gland itself, are friable and prone to shed cells during manipulation. Small and moderate size pheochromocytomas can be done laparoscopically. With the availability of CT scanning, exploration of the abdomen for ectopic sites is no longer a necessary part of operation for pheochromocytoma and a contraindication to a laparoscopic approach. However, malignant and large pheochromocytomas should be done open both from an oncological point of view and because these lesions are highly vascular and can stimulate a dense pericapsular desmoplastic reaction

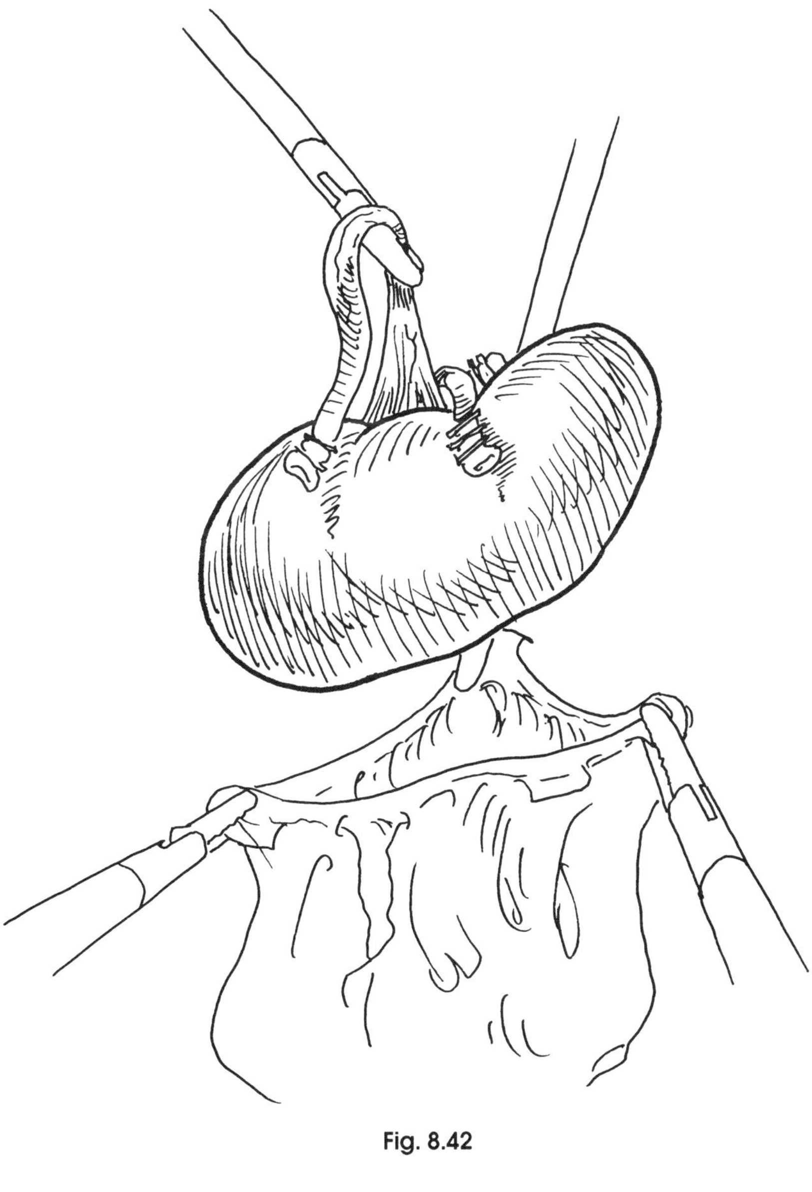

Fig. 8.42

(Pertsemlidis). Similarly, the 10% of pheochromocytomas that are extra-adrenal should be done open because they can be difficult to locate along the aorta and sometimes lie between the aorta and vena cava. They are also more likely to be malignant (constituting 50% of malignant pheos). Only those who are well versed in open adrenalectomy should perform the laparoscopic operation.

When operating for pheochromocytoma, whether the adrenal vein is divided first or last is not an issue of norepinephrine release for two reasons. Modern pharmacological control minimizes and compensates for hormone output during manipulation, and venous collaterals to renal capsular veins allow continued hormone release even if the adrenal vein is divided. However, initial experience in laparoscopic adrenalectomy in which the vein was left for last raised concerns about injury to the vein during manipulation, and those few surgeons with experience in this procedure are now dividing the vein first (Gagner, personal communication).

The following examples of left and right adrenalectomy (as performed by Gagner) use a lateral approach. The adrenal glands are shown in their normal shape without tumors for clarity. Basic patient preparation including bowel prep is the same as described for nephrectomy above. Specific endocrine concerns are addressed as appropriate for each patient.

For left adrenalectomy, the patient is placed in the left lateral decubitus position with slight reverse Trendelenburg (Fig. 8.43). Insufflation is accomplished in the subcostal midclavicular line, and the first 11-mm trochar is placed. Using all large trochars allow for shifts in the camera position as necessary. A 30-degree laparoscope is used. Under direct vision, additional trochars are placed in the anterior and posterior axillary lines between the ribs and the iliac crest. The surgeon stands in front of the patient and operates through the two lateral trochars. The crescentic distribution of trochars around the costal margin outlines the line of incision if the patient needs to be opened.

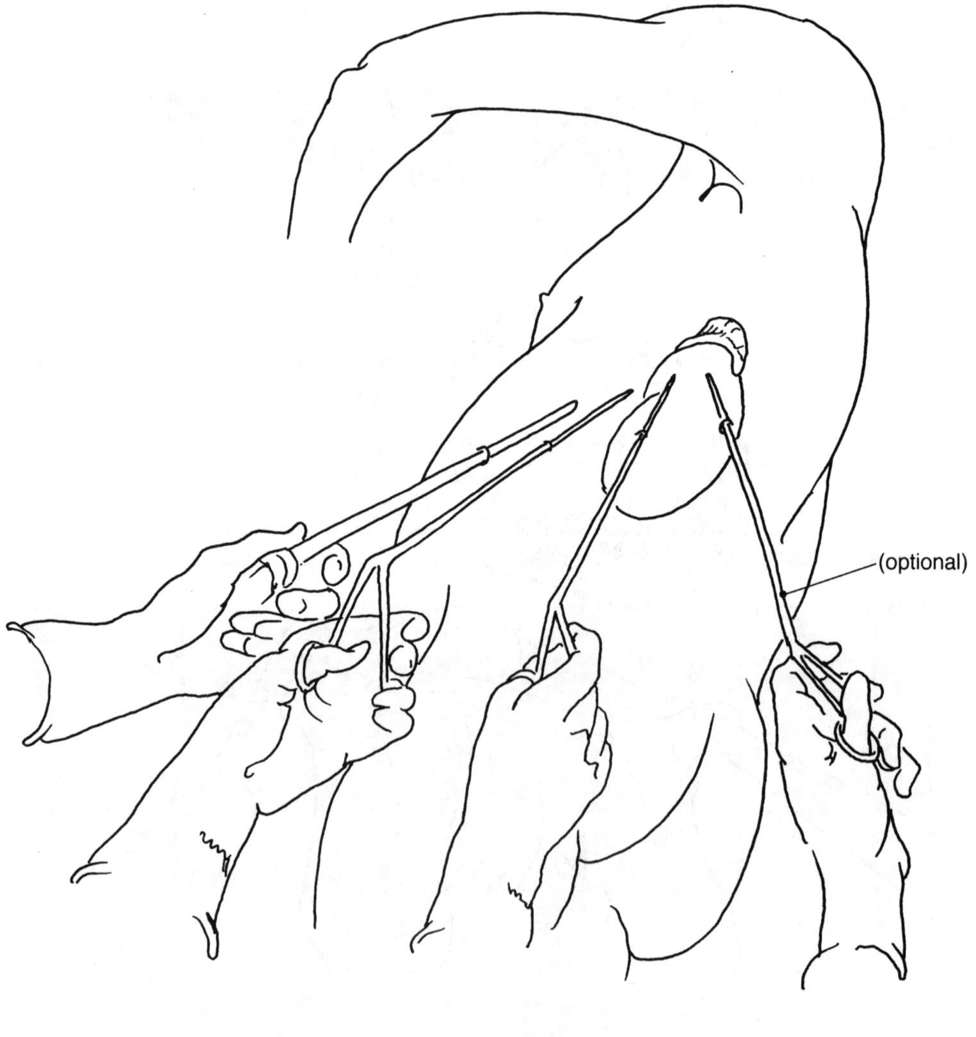

Fig. 8.43

The splenic flexure of the colon is dissected down by opening the peritoneal reflection (Line of Toldt) and proceeding up across the phrenocolic ligament (Fig. 8.44). The splenic flexure drops away, revealing the renal fascia and the bulge of the kidney below. A fourth trochar may be placed more posterolaterally over the kidney to retract the spleen but gravity usually provides sufficient exposure.

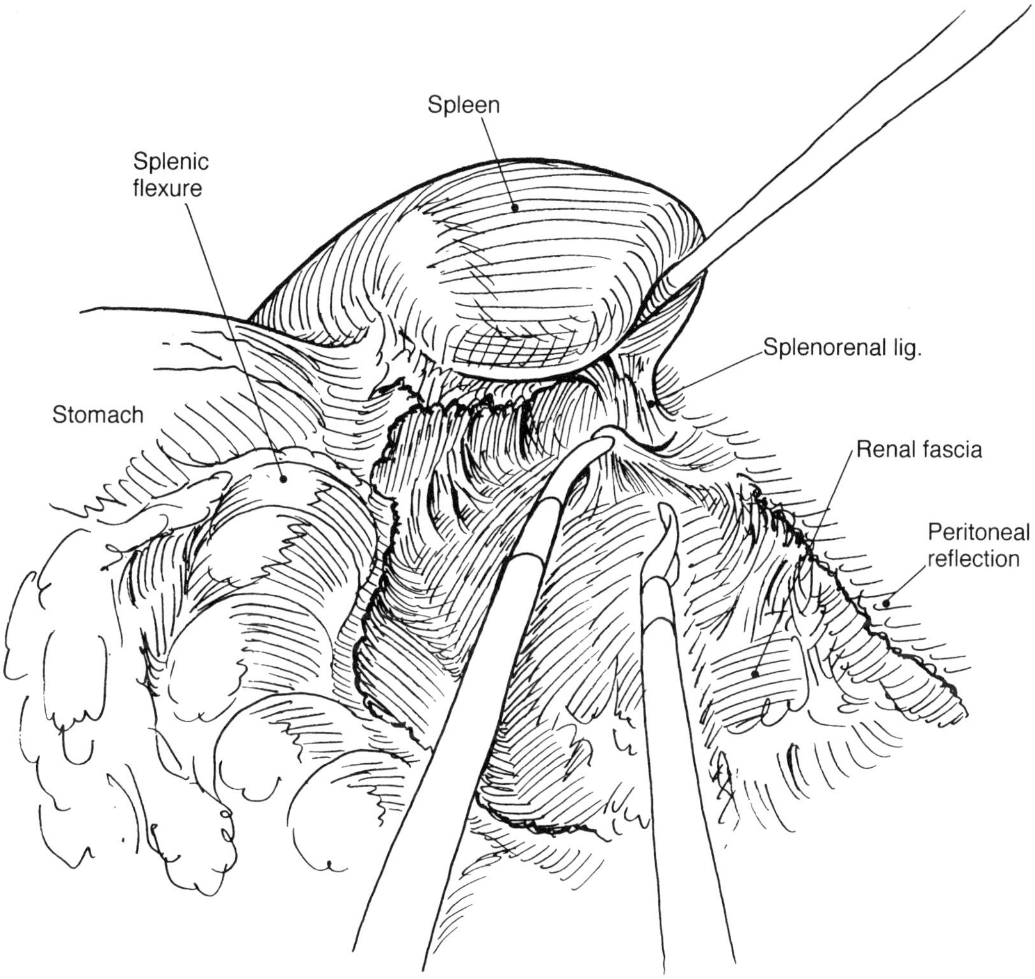

Fig. 8.44

The splenorenal ligament is opened upward along the outer margin of the kidney and the underlying renal fascia is opened, exposing the lateral border of the adrenal gland within the perinephric fat (Fig. 8.45). The adrenal gland is difficult to differentiate from periadrenal fat by color and is best identified by the firm feel of the edge of the gland. Because of the delicate nature of the gland, the technique of dissection is to tease the surrounding tissue away from the gland.

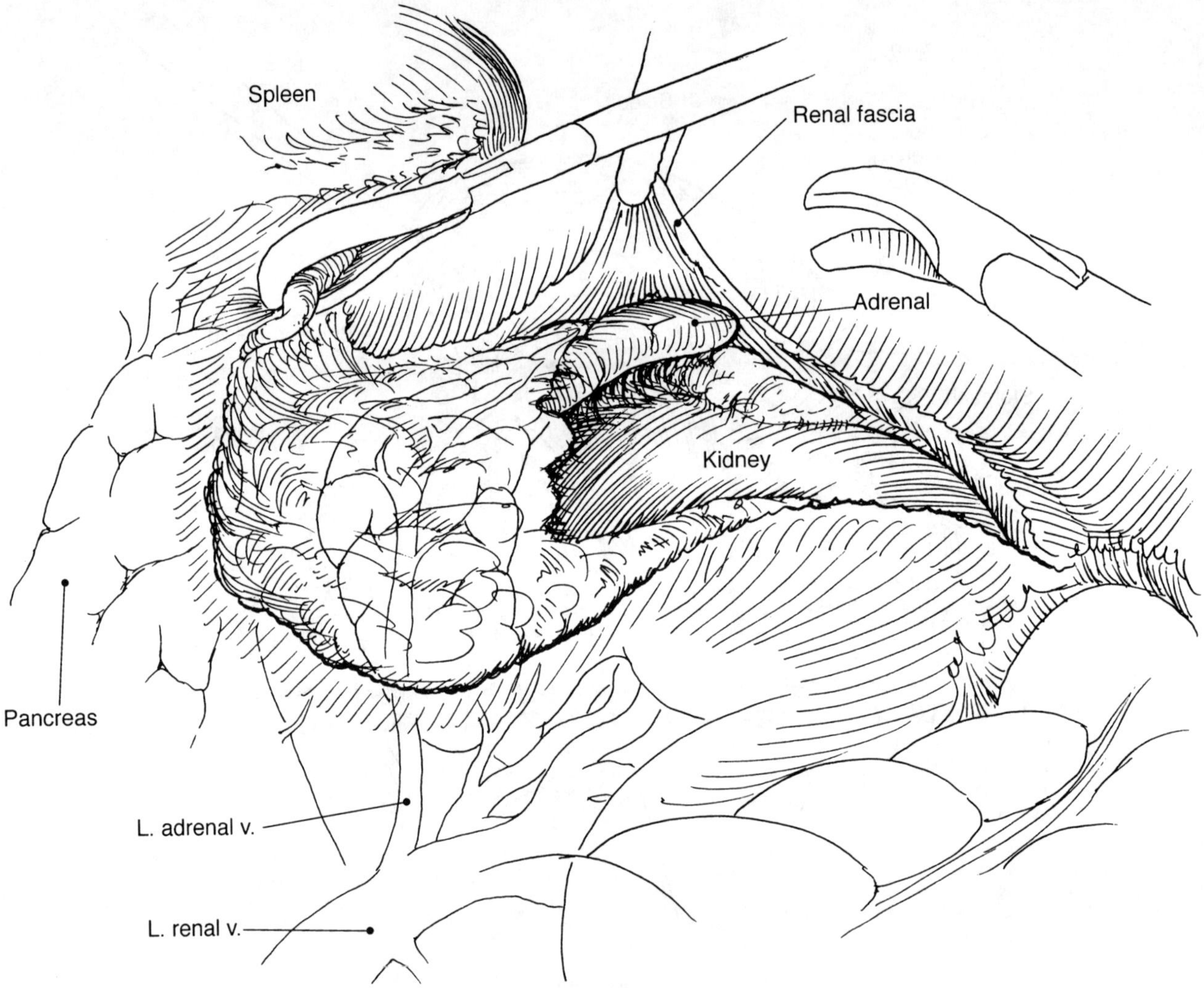

Fig. 8.45

The tissue over the anterior and inferior portion of the gland is dissected from lateral to medial to expose the adrenal vein draining into the left renal vein (Fig. 8.46). the vein is isolated, watching for the branch of the left inferior phrenic vein that often joins it. The vein is doubly clipped with large clips proximally and singly clipped distally and divided. There is occasionally an accessory inferior vein draining into the renal vein. Dissection is then begun at the medial border of the adrenal gland and proceeds around the remaining margins of the gland from medially to laterally, moving away from the clipped adrenal vein. Dissection is kept close to the areolar adrenal capsule. On the undersurface of the gland the layer of fat separating the adrenal from the

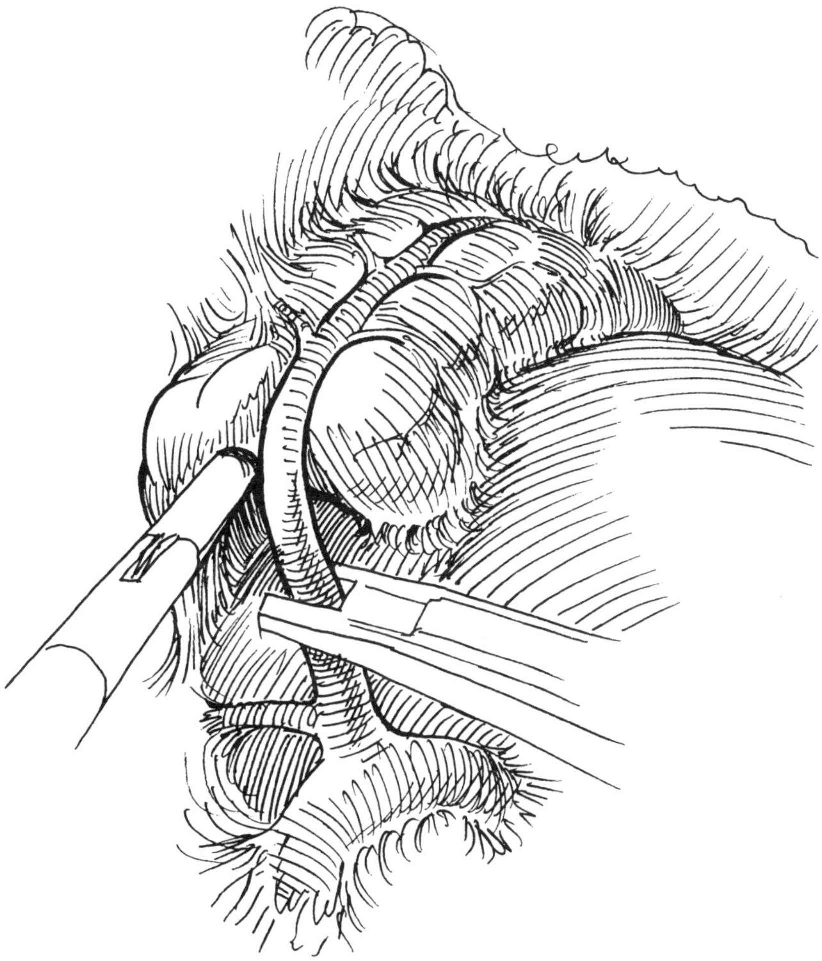

Fig. 8.46

kidney is left on the kidney side. As it is mobilized, the gland is gently grasped and manipulated with atraumatic forceps. Small vessels are cauterized or clipped until the gland is attached only at its posterolateral extremity (Fig. 8.47). The remaining attachment is divided, the area checked for hemostasis and the gland is removed in a sac. The incision is widened slightly if necessary. If there is concern about hemostasis, a closed system drain may be placed (Chapter 2). Standard desufflation and closure protocol are then followed.

To do a right adrenalectomy, which can be done under the same anesthesia (except for bilateral pheochromocytomas which should be staged), the patient is turned to the right lateral decubitus position. The surgeon initially stands in front of the patient and ports are placed in a mirror image of the left sided ports.

The surgeon, operating through the anterior and posterior axillary line ports, opens the peritoneum at the lateral margin of the right kidney bulge. The fourth trochar is placed posterolaterally. The additional port is

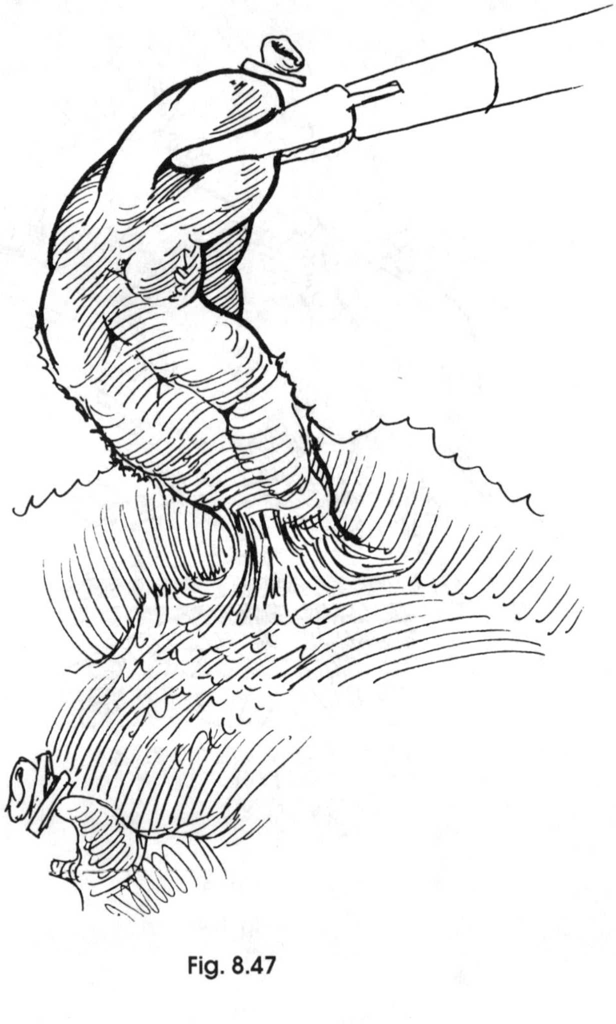

Fig. 8.47

used for liver retraction. Near the upper pole of the kidney, the right triangular ligament of the liver is opened and the dissection continued medially along the inferior leaf of the coronary ligament up to the inferior vena cava (Fig. 8.48). The renal fascia is opened, and the liver is gently elevated and carefully dissected off the retrohepatic portion of the adrenal gland, exposing its anterolateral surface. There may be some adherence between the surface of the gland and the liver. The camera is shifted according to the area being dissected. The subcostal position is best for visualizing the inferior pole of the adrenal, and the dorsal position is best for visualizing the superior pole of the gland. The surgeon stands on the side of the patient opposite the camera postion to work.

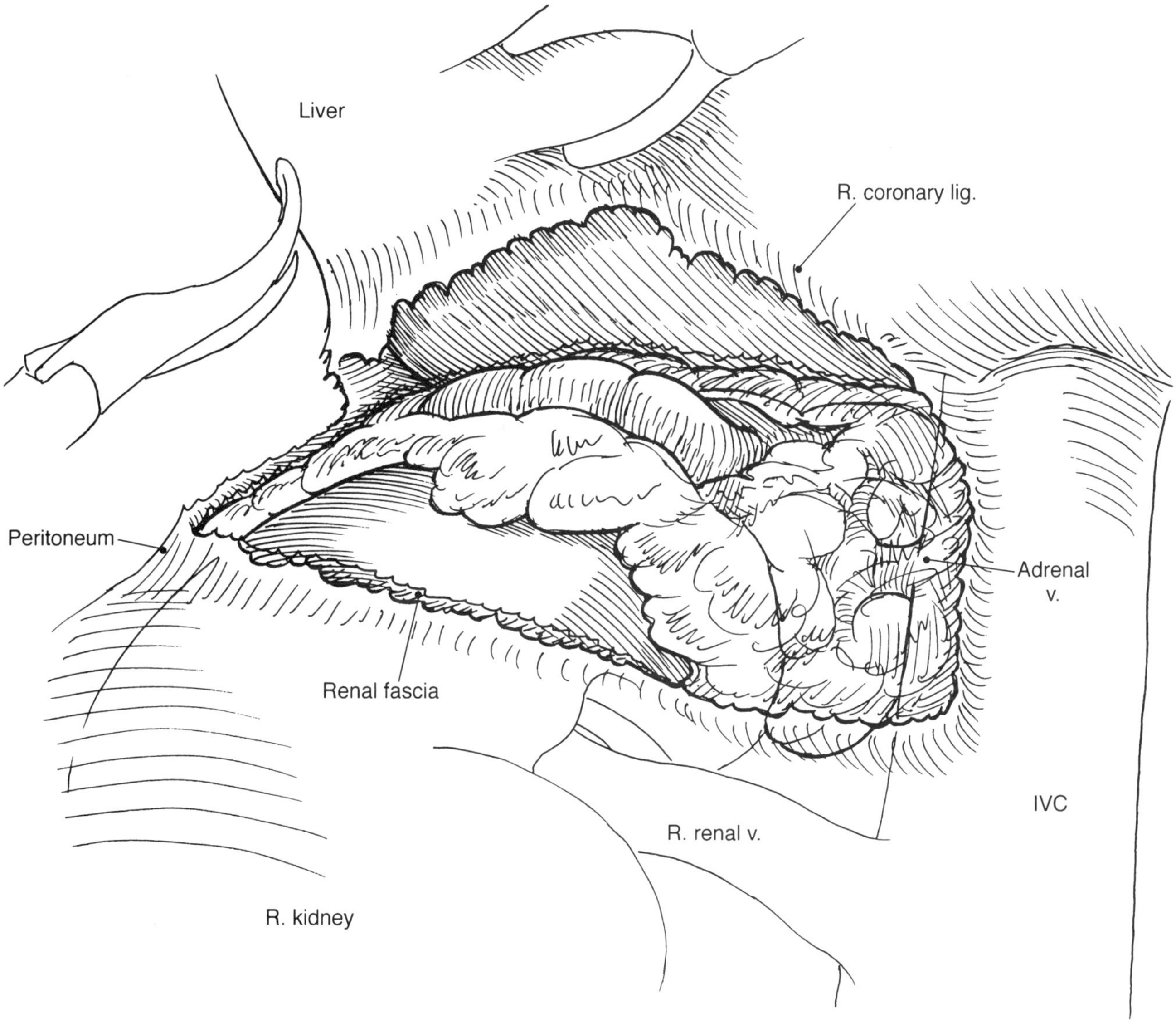

Fig. 8.48

With the surgeon in the posterior position and the camera subcostal, the medial surface of the gland is partially separated from the inferior vena cava to expose the short right adrenal vein (Fig. 8.49). The adrenal vein is doubly clipped with large clips medially and singly clipped laterally and divided. A large or short right adrenal vein might require division by the linear stapler with a vascular load. The surgeon shifts to the anterior

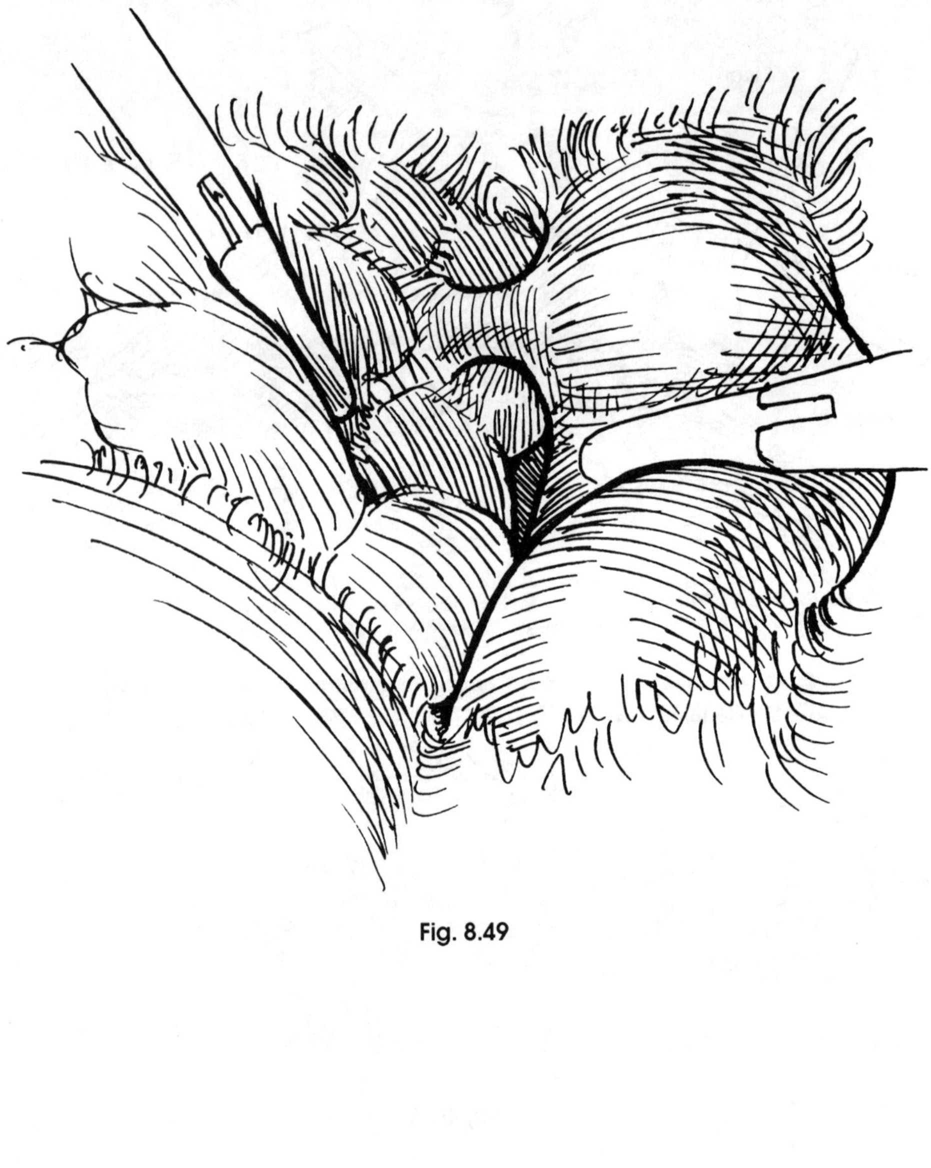

Fig. 8.49

position as dissection proceeds from inferior and medial to superior and lateral until the last attachments are divided laterally (Fig. 8.50). After hemostasis is checked, the gland is placed in a sac and extracted.

Varicocele

Introduction

Varicocele, a dilatation of the pampiniform plexus of veins in the spermatic cord, is found in 15% of the general male population. An association of varicocele with infertility is inferred from the much higher incidence in infertile men and the observation that about 40% of men with persistent varicoceles will develop infertility. Even though the great majority of clinically apparent varicoceles occur on the left, the defects in spermatogenesis are bilateral. Whether this is due to generalized scrotal warming, crossing vessels, or a subclinical right varicocele is not clear. A substance produced by the affected testis may act on the other in both undescended testis and varicocele. The size of the varicocele does not seem to be directly proportional to infertility, with small varicoceles being equally implicated.

The pathophysiology of varicocele related infertility is not completely understood. Idiopathic varicocele dilatation usually begins at puberty (late left varicocele formation is sometimes a sign of a left renal tumor occluding the left spermatic vein at its junction with the left renal vein) and is mainly found on the left. The left spermatic vein normally drains into the left renal vein, and the increased pressure in this system may rarely be explained

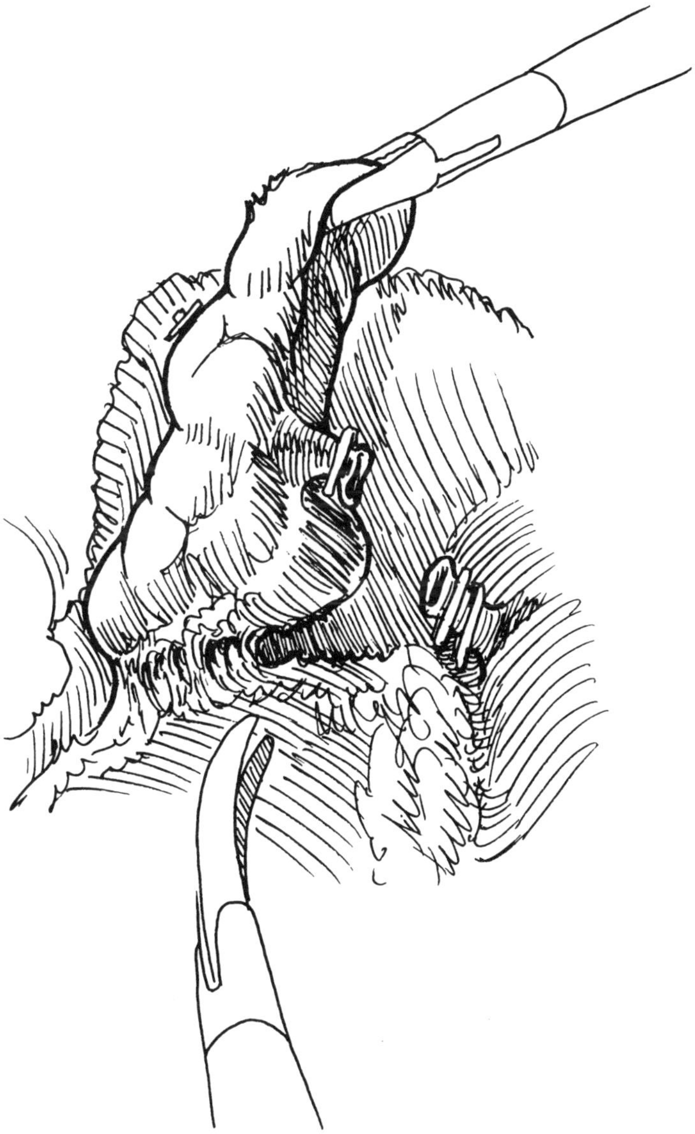

Fig. 8.50

by a congenital venous anomaly like a renal aortic venous collar. In the absence of such an anomaly, compression of the left renal vein by the superior mesenteric artery and/or compression of the left common iliac vein by the right common iliac artery have been proposed as mechanisms. In addition, protective venous valves, which when present are usually found near the renal vein, are present in only half of individuals. Collateral pelvic venous connections may also provide increased spermatic venous volume. Reflux spermatic venous blood flow appears to be the final common event leading to increased scrotal temperature and spermatic impairment. The defect appears to be progressive with time.

The apparent association between varicocele and male infertility is strengthened by the fact that ablation of the dilated veins results in significant improvement in sperm parameters and increase in impregnation. Established methods of ablation include transvenous embolization or sclerosis, and surgical ligation. Ligation has been done high, in the pelvic retroperitoneal space or low in the inguinal canal. Total interruption of the internal spermatic vessels compared to preservation of the internal spermatic artery has been shown in both open and laparoscopic approaches to have no detrimental effect on the testis and to have a lower recurrence rate. The higher recurrence rate with the selective approach is probably due to missing a vein. High ligation of only the internal spermatic veins is associated with a 10 to 20% perisistence or recurrence compared with a 1 to 3% recurrence (Dudai) with combined ligation of internal and external spermatic veins. Scrotal ligation, another option, is not commonly used. The surgical approaches have been more successful than the transvenous route. The more recent advent of the laparoscopic approach has added the advantages of superior exposure and lower morbidity but has the disadvantage of general anesthesia and the associated higher cost (although the procedure can be done under epidural at low pressure). To successfully and safely apply any of the approaches, the anatomy involved should be fully understood.

Anatomy

The venous drainage of the scrotum and its contents is a rich network with multiple interconnections. Retrograde perfusion of the spermatic vein radiographically demonstrates flow through collaterals to the vessels of the vas deferens, deep circumflex iliac, superficial epigastric, obturator, saphenous and pelvic veins (Fig. 8.51). Multiple veins draining the testicle and epididymis form the pampiniform plexus of the spermatic cord.

The veins, vas deferens, spermatic artery, lymphatics and autonomic nerves of the cord are wrapped in the thin sheath of internal spermatic fascia derived from the transversalis fascia layer of the abdominal wall. The vas deferens is surrounded by its own fine venous plexus which interconnects with the testicular veins. Surrounding the spermatic cord is the layer of cremaster muscle and fascia derived from the internal oblique muscle. This layer too contains veins that accompany the cremasteric/external spermatic artery and genital branch of the genitofemoral nerve. The external spermatic fascia, derived from the external oblique aponeurosis at the superficial inguinal ring, encircles the inner two layers. The scrotum itself drains to the internal pudendal system medially and to the external pudendal veins laterally.

The fine veins of the vas drain into the pelvic plexus of veins around the bladder and prostate. The cremasteric or external spermatic veins drain into the inferior epigastric vein and collaterally into the proximal branches of the greater saphenous vein (superficial external pudendal, superficial epigastric and superficial circumflex iliac veins). Reflux from the external spermatic veins has been demonstrated in 30% of individuals with varicoceles. The inferior epigastric vein drainage route affords communication with a pubic branch (connecting to the obturator vein) and, through the external iliac, to the deep circumflex iliac vein. The scrotal veins drain to the external and internal pudendal veins. Acute venous occlusion results in the same degree of testicular ischemia as arterial occlusion. Thus the critical element in reducing testicular venous blood flow is achieving the

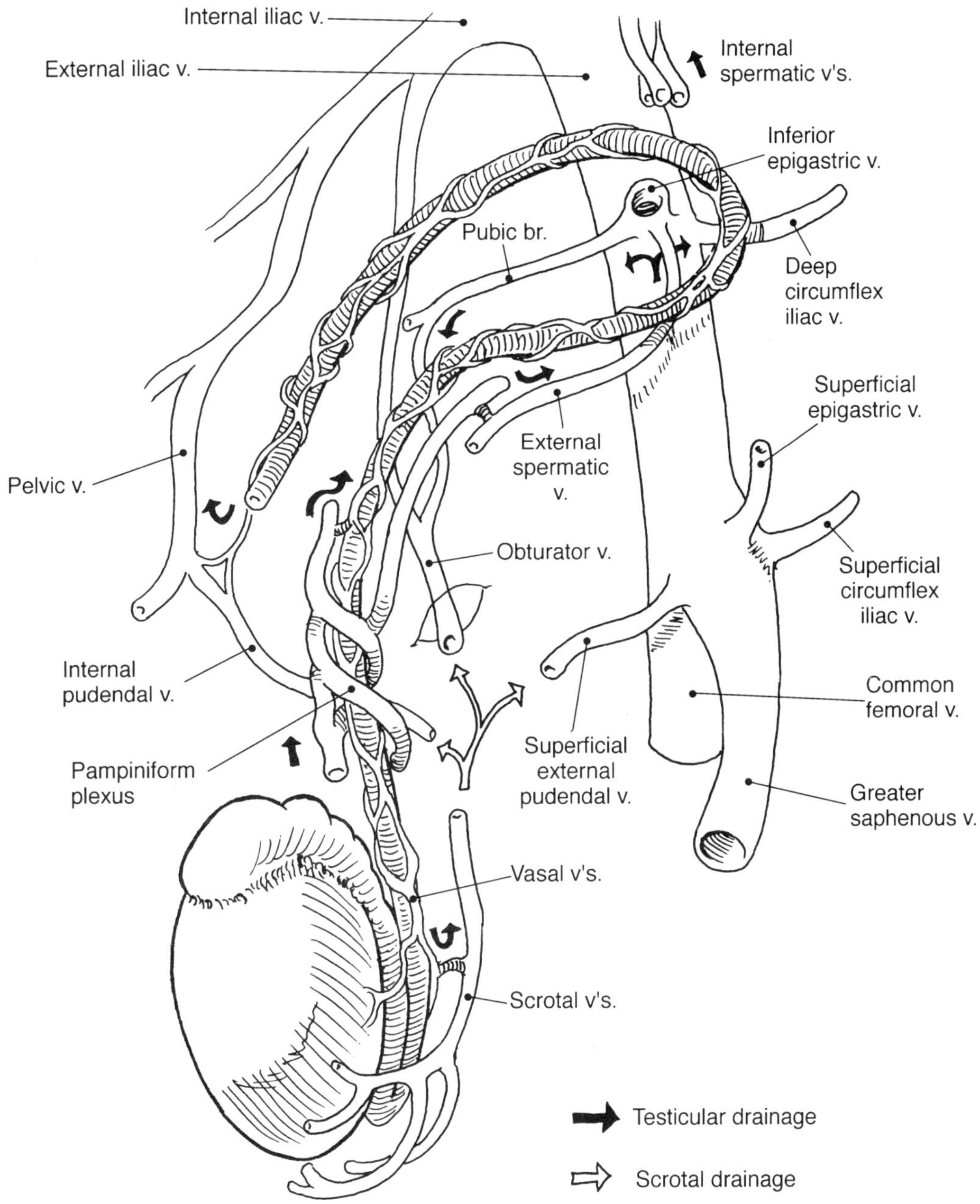
Internal iliac v.
External iliac v.
Internal spermatic v's.
Inferior epigastric v.
Pubic br.
Deep circumflex iliac v.
Superficial epigastric v.
External spermatic v.
Pelvic v.
Obturator v.
Superficial circumflex iliac v.
Internal pudendal v.
Common femoral v.
Superficial external pudendal v.
Pampiniform plexus
Greater saphenous v.
Vasal v's.
Scrotal v's.
Testicular drainage
Scrotal drainage

Fig. 8.51

correct degree of venous interruption. Failure to appreciate the extent of collateral venous pathways often leads to an inadequate surgical interruption.

As the veins of the pampiniform plexus ascend and enter the inguinal canal, they decrease in number to three or four. They cross through the deep inguinal ring (the neck of the evaginated transversalis fascia around the spermatic cord) and cross the distal external iliac artery to reach the psoas muscle in the plane between transversalis fascia and peritoneum (Fig. 8.52). The spermatic vein on the right drains into the inferior vena cava below the right renal vein. On the left, the spermatic vein crosses beneath the root of the sigmoid mesocolon and ascends to drain into the left renal vein.

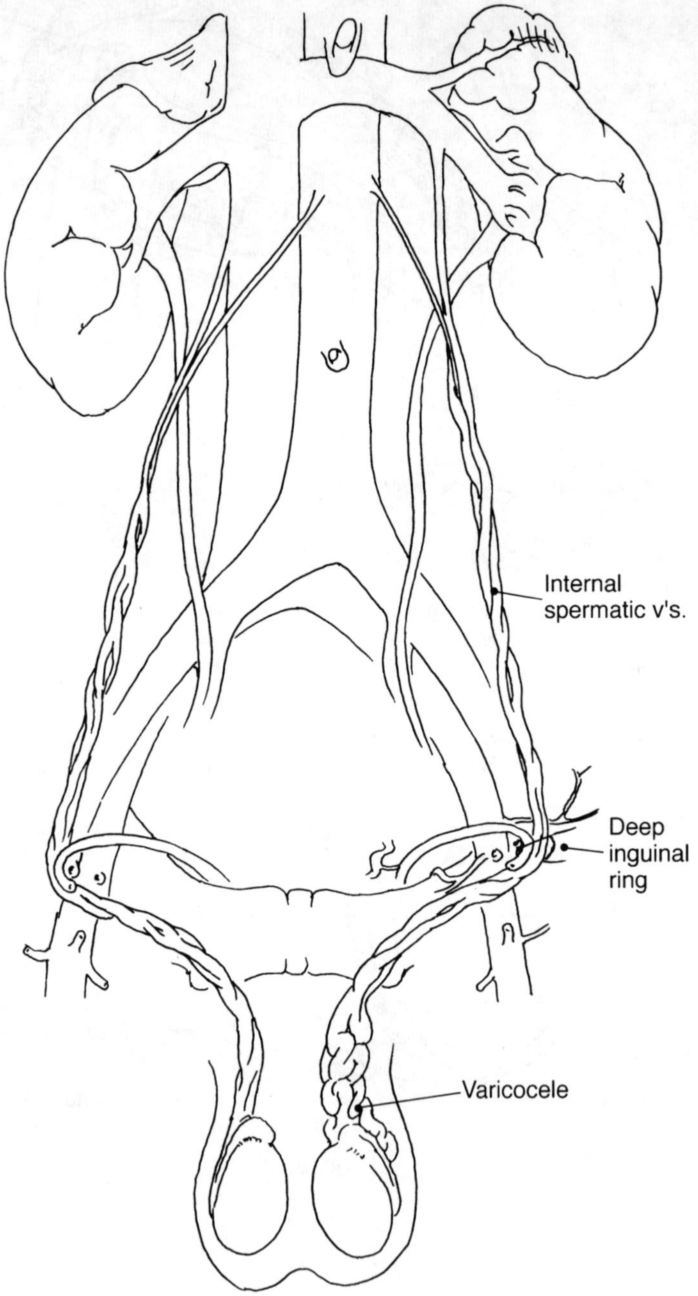

Fig. 8.52

The arterial supply to the spermatic cord and testicle comes from the internal spermatic and external spermatic arteries and the artery of the vas (Fig. 8.53). Arterial supply to the scrotum comes from the internal and external pudendal arteries. The spermatic arteries arise from the anterolateral walls of the aorta below the renal arteries (Fig. 8.52). They join the spermatic veins, descend on the psoas muscles, cross on top of the terminal external iliac arteries and enter the deep inguinal rings. In its lower abdominal course, the spermatic artery lies with two to three branches of the spermatic vein. It may be difficult to distinguish visually from the veins and is difficult to separate and preserve.

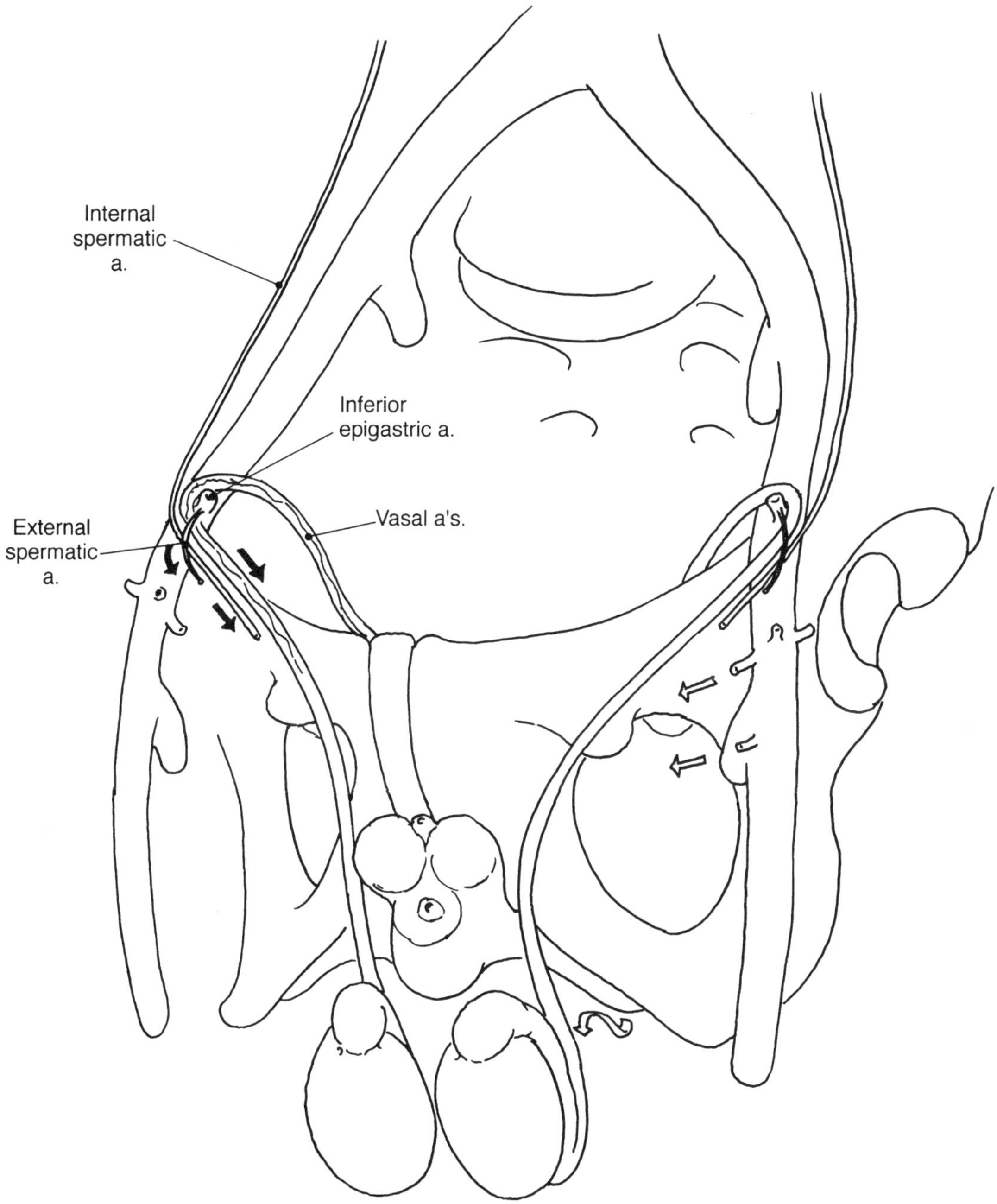

Fig. 8.53

In the spermatic cord (beginning at the deep inguinal ring where the vas and vessels converge) the spermatic artery lies among the veins of the pampiniform plexus (Fig. 8.54). Distally the artery branches and becomes more tortuous before reaching the epididymis and testis. It anastomosis with the artery of the vas, primarily at the tail of the epididymis. This connection is tenuous in some individuals. The artery of the vas usually arises from the superior vesicle artery in the pelvis and lies on the surface of the vas through its course. It anastomosis in two thirds of individuals with the external spermatic artery running just inside the cremaster layer.

The external spermatic artery arises from the proximal inferior epigastric artery and penetrates the transversalis fascia near the deep inguinal ring. There it is joined by the genital branch of the genitofemoral nerve. In the inguinal canal, the two structures lie between the cremaster and the internal spermatic fascia on the caudal side of the cord. They are sacrificed when this strip of cremaster is resected during hernia repair. Collateral flow from the scrotal arterial supply does not provide significant collateral support for the viability of the testis. Sacrifice of the internal spermatic artery by mass ligation of the internal spermatic vessels on the distal psoas dur-

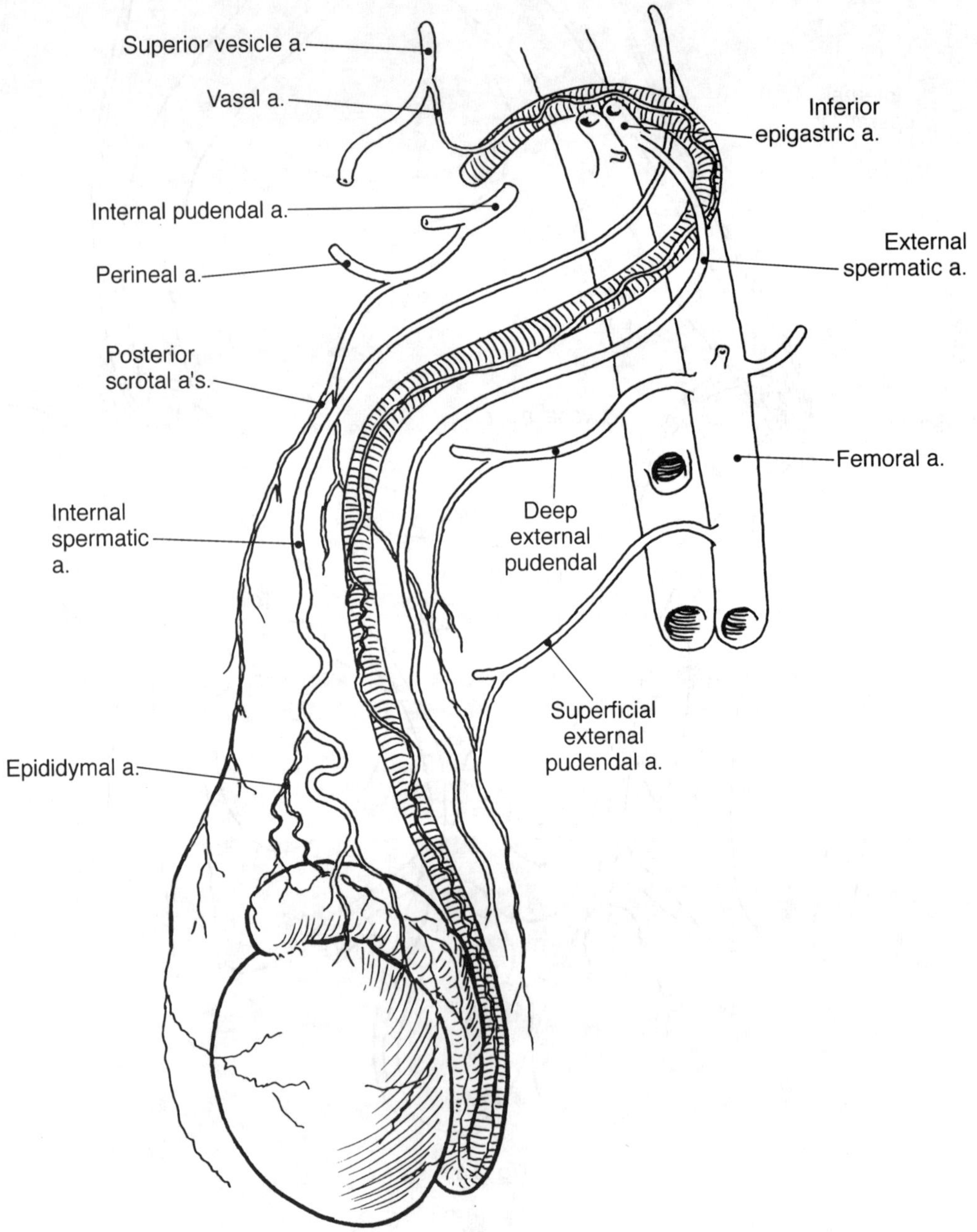

Fig. 8.54

ing varicocele ligation has not caused compromise of testicular viability in clinical practice. The vasal and external spermatic collaterals are primarily responsible for sustaining the testicle after division of the internal spermatic artery.

Varicocele Ligation

An umbilical camera port and two para-rectus ports are positioned as for hernia repair (see Fig. 3.36) to provide the proper working range for one or both suprainguinal areas (Fig. 8.55).One or both of the lateral ports must be large enough to accommodate the clip applier. The surgeon stands on the side opposite the site of ligation and operates through the two ports closest to him or her after the camera is shifted to the side of the pathology. The objective is to interrupt the accessible internal spermatic veins and collaterals.

Adhesions between the sigmoid colon and the lower abdominal wall often need to be divided to gain expo-

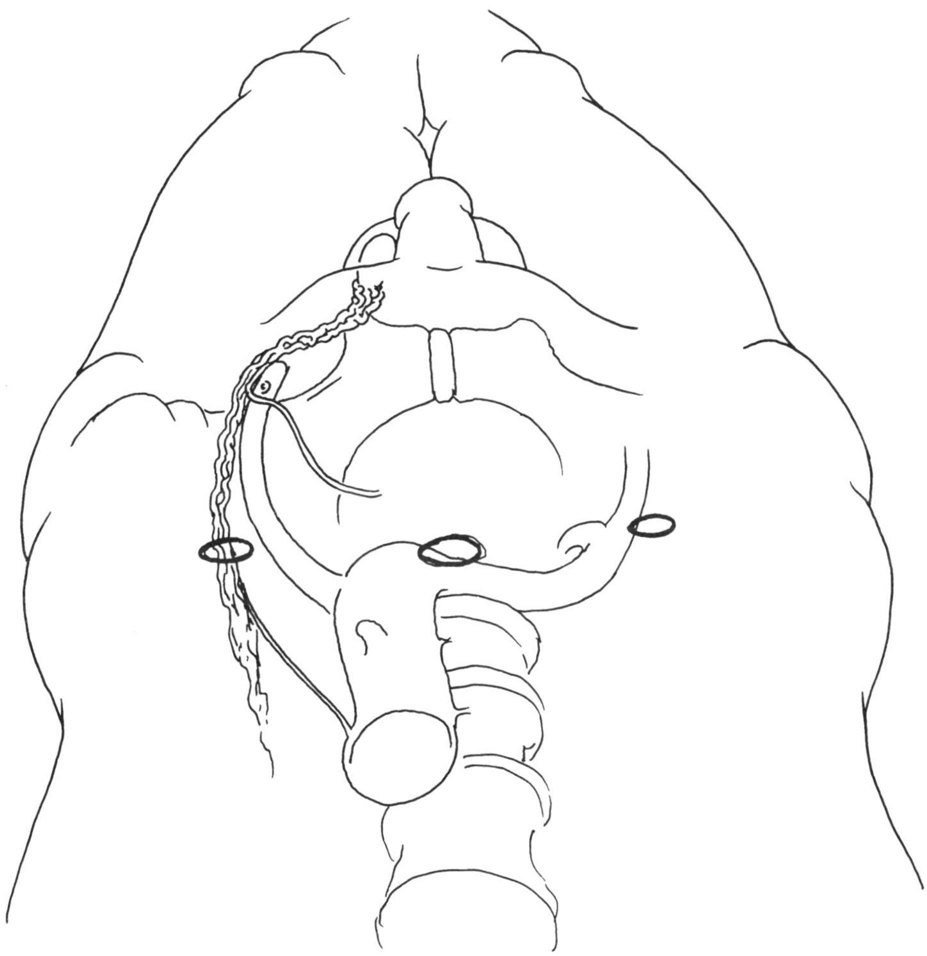

Fig. 8.55

sure of the distal psoas muscle, external iliac vessels and groin area on the left. An incision is made in the peritoneum just medial to the internal spermatic vascular bundle and is extended distally across the trifurcation point and up between the inferior epigastric vessels and the medial margin of the deep inguinal ring (Fig. 8.56). Exposure must be adequate to identify venous collaterals. Care must be taken to avoid injury to the vas and to the aberrant obturator artery found in 20% of individuals.

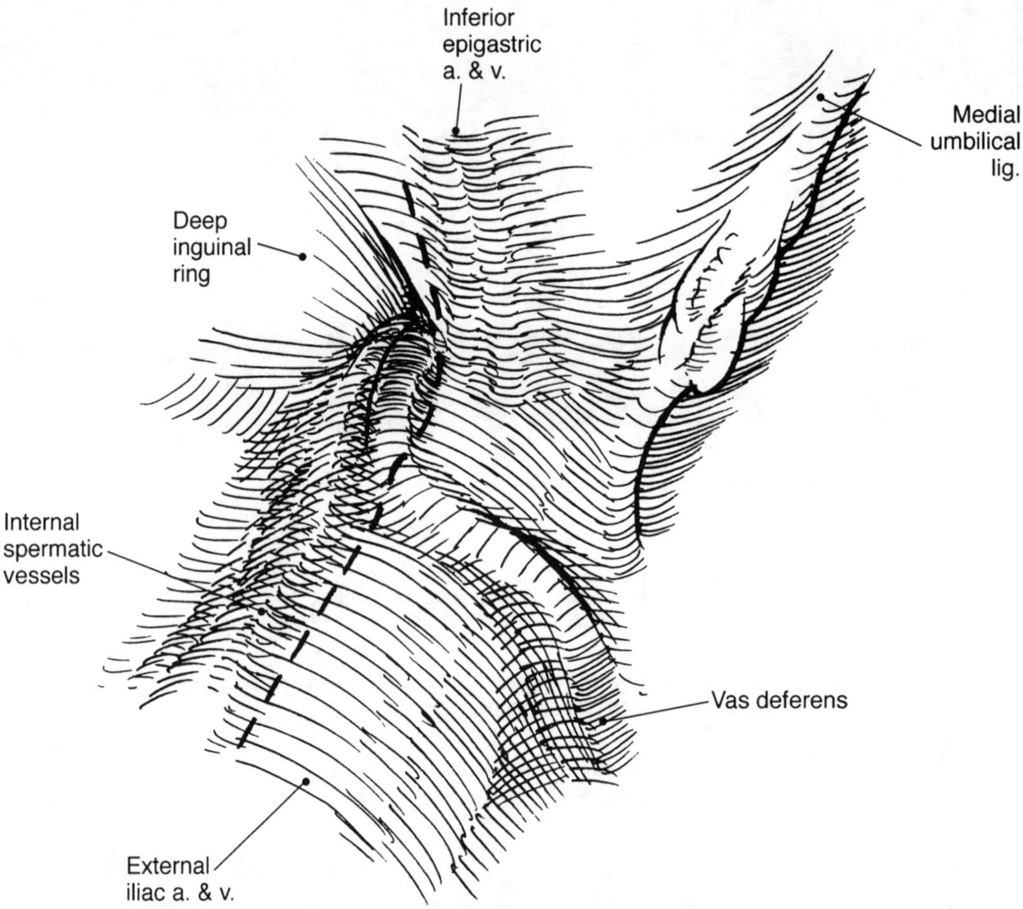

Fig. 8.56

The internal spermatic vascular bundle is isolated by blunt dissection taking care to avoid the genitofemoral nerve (Fig. 8.57). The artery may either be spared or included with mass ligation of the bundle. Mass ligation of internal and external spermatic vessels has proven safe to date (Dudai). Mass ligation allows completion of

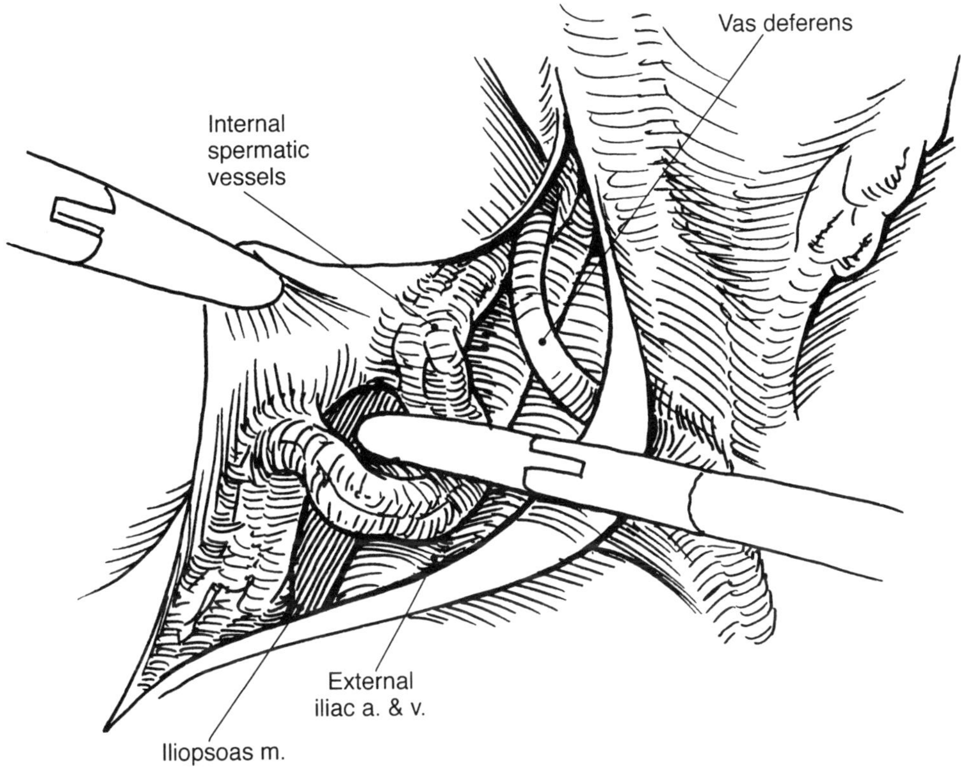

Fig. 8.57

one side in about 15 minutes. Separating the artery from the veins is the most delicate and time consuming part of the procedure (Fig. 8.58). If the artery cannot easily be identified by inspection, the Doppler probe may be helpful.

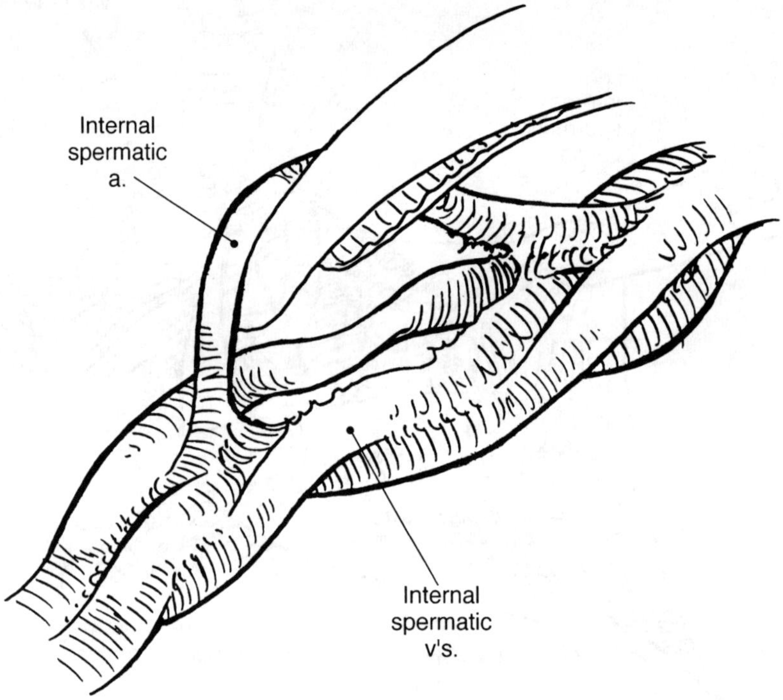

Fig. 8.58

The spermatic veins or the entire bundle are clipped or bipolar coagulated and divided along with pelvic collateral channels (Fig. 8.59A).

The external spermatic vein may be obliterated by applying bipolar cautery to the inferior epigastric vessels medial to the deep inguinal ring close to their origin (Fig. 8.59B). Dividing the external spermatic veins avoids the 10 to 20% recurrence or persistence seen with internal spermatic vein interruption alone. Unless it is possible to identify and clip the vein alone, the artery is also compromised by this technique. These steps leave the fine vasal veins, cremasteric collaterals to

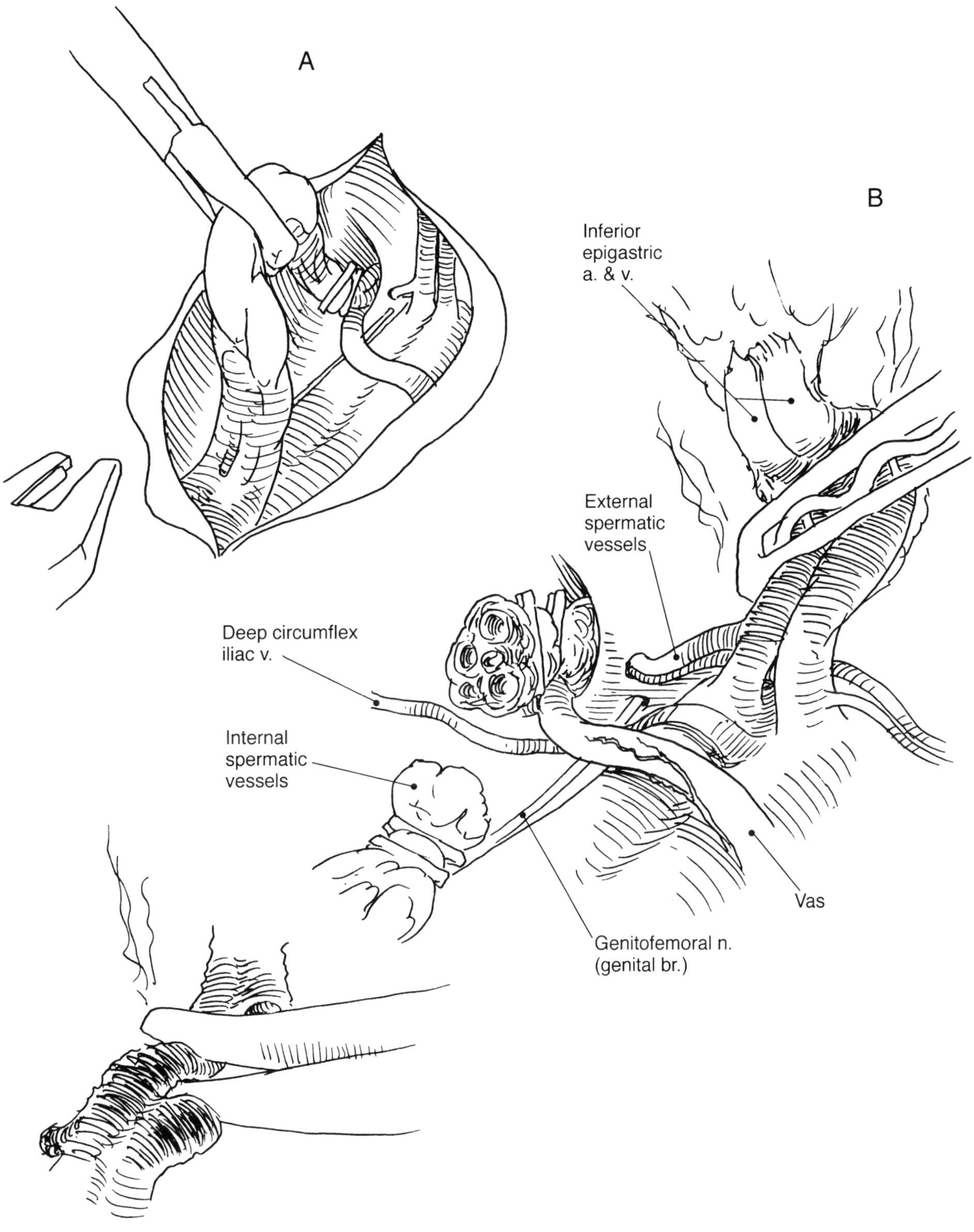

Fig. 8.59

the proximal saphenous branches and scrotal collateral veins intact.

The laparoscopic approach provides clear and easy access to the retroperitoneal internal spermatic vessels and collaterals with decreased surgical morbidity. A further advantage is access to both sides at no additional cost. The procedure can be done under epidural anesthesia, and all 5 mm ports can be used (with a 5mm camera and clip applier). If mass ligation continues to prove safe, the time and cost disadvantages may be eliminated.

Chapter 8: The Urologic System

EMBRYOLOGY

O'Rahilly R, Muller F. Human Embryology and Teratology. New York: Wiley-Liss, 1992:193-224.

Skandalakis JE, Gray SW. Embryology for Surgeons. Baltimore: Williams & Wilkins, 1984:594-847.

ANATOMY

Bergman RA, et. al. Compendium of Human Anatomic Variation. Baltimore: Urban & Schwawrzenberg , 1988: 81-83,91,92,408-416.

Clemente C. Gray's Anatomy, 13th American Ed. Philadelphia: Lea & Febiger, 1985:792,832,834,1515-1581.

Hinman Jr. F. Atlas of Urosurgical Anatomy. Philadelphia: WB Saunders Co., 1993:4-28,233-344,390-407.

Kadir S. Diagnostic Angiography 1986:387-411,429-433.

Lee QF, et al. Fascial planes and compartments of the posterior abdomen. Clin Anat 1990;3:1-15.

McMinn RMH, Hutchings RT. Color Atlas of Human Anatomy. Chicago: Yearbook Medical Publishers, 1977: 236-252.

LAPAROSCOPIC NEPHRECTOMY

Das S, et al. Laparoscopic nephroureterectomy for end-stage reflux nephropathy in a child. Surg Laparosc Endosc 1993;3:462-469.

Kavoussi LR, Clayman R. Laparoscopic renal surgery: nephrectomy, nephroureterectomy, and ureterolysis. In Gomella, LG, ed., et. al. Laparoscopic Urologic Surgery. New York: Raven Press Ltd., 1994:151-160.

McDougall EM, Clayman RV: Laparoscopic nephrectomy, nephroureterectomy, and partial nephrectomy. In: Das, S, Crawford, ed. Urologic Laparoscopy. Philadelphia: WB Saunders Co., 1994:127-140.

Scott-Conner C, Dawson DL. Operative Anatomy. Philadelphia: JB Lippincott Co., 1993:497-515.

Winfield HN, et al. Urological laparoscopic surgery. The Journal of Urology, 1991;146:941-948.

LAPAROSCOPIC ADRENALECTOMY

deCanniere L, et al. From laparoscopic training on an animal model to retroperitoneoscopic or coelioscopic adrenal and renal surgery in human. Surg Endosc 1995;9: 387-391.

Gagner M, et al. Laparoscopic Adrenalectomy. Surg Endosc 1993;7:122.

Gagner M, et al. Laparoscopic adrenalectomy: The importance of a flank approach in the lateral decubitus position. Surg Endosc 1994;8:135-138.

Pertsemlidis D. Minimal access versus open adrenalectomy. (editorial). Surg Endosc 1995;9:384-386.

Stoker ME, et al. Laparoscopic adrenal surgery. Surg Endosc 1995;9:387-391.

Suzuki K, et al. Laparoscopic surgery for adrenal tumors, in Das, S, Crawford, Editor. Urologic Laparoscopy. Philadelphia: WB Saunders Co., 1994:211-221.

LAPAROSCOPIC VARICOCELE LIGATION

Dudai M, et al. Laparoscopic simultaneous ligation of internal and external spermatic veins for varicocele. J Urol 1995;153:704-705.

Donovan Jr JF, Winfield HN. Laparoscopic varix ligation, in Gomella, LG, ed., et. al. Laparoscopic Urologic Surgery. New York: Raven Press Ltd., 1994:137-149.

Hagood PG, Parra RO. Laparoscopic varicocelectomy, in Das, S, Crawford, ed. Urologic Laparoscopy. Philadelphia: WB Saunders Co., 1994:119-126.

Hinman Jr. F. Atlas of Urosurgical Anatomy. Phila.: WB Saunders Co., 1993:489-490,501-502.

Kuypers P, et al. Valveless testicular veins: a possible etiological factor in varicocele. Clin Anat 1992;5:113-118.

Index